NEURODEVELOPMENTAL MECHANISMS IN PSYCHOPATHOLOGY

This volume represents a burgeoning perspective on the origins of psychopathology, one that focuses on the development of the human central nervous system. The contemporary neurodevelopmental perspective assumes that mental disorders result from etiologic factors that alter the normal course of brain development. Defined here in its broadest sense, neurodevelopment is a process that begins at conception and extends throughout the lifespan. We now know that it is a complex process and that its course can be altered by a host of factors, ranging from inherited genetic liabilities to psychosocial stressors.

This book features the very best, cutting-edge thinking in the converging fields of developmental neuroscience and developmental psychopathology. The developmental window represented is broad, extending from the prenatal period through adulthood, and the authors cover a broad range of etiologic factors and a spectrum of clinical disorders. Moreover, the contributors do not hesitate to use the opportunity to hypothesize about underlying mechanisms and to speculate on future research directions.

Dante Cicchetti is the Shirley Cox Kearns Professor of Psychology, Psychiatry, and Pediatrics and Director of Mt. Hope Family Center at the University of Rochester in New York. He is founding editor of the journal *Development and Psychopathology*, editor of the *Rochester Symposium on Developmental Psychopathology*, Vols. I–IX (with S. L. Toth), and editor of *Developmental Psychopathology*, Vols. I and II (with D. Cohen).

Elaine F. Walker is the Samuel Candler Dobbs Professor of Psychology and Neuroscience at Emory University in Atlanta, Georgia. She is also the editor of *Schizophrenia: A Life-Span Perspective* and co-editor of *Progress in Experimental Personality and Psychopathology Research* (with R. Dworkin and B. Cornblatt).

Neurodevelopmental Mechanisms in Psychopathology

Edited by

Dante Cicchetti
University of Rochester

Elaine F. Walker
Emory University

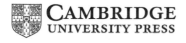
CAMBRIDGE
UNIVERSITY PRESS

PUBLISHED BY THE PRESS SYNDICATE OF THE UNIVERSITY OF CAMBRIDGE
The Pitt Building, Trumpington Street, Cambridge, United Kingdom

CAMBRIDGE UNIVERSITY PRESS
The Edinburgh Building, Cambridge CB2 2RU, UK
40 West 20th Street, New York, NY 10011-4211, USA
477 Williamstown Road, Port Melbourne, VIC 3207, Australia
Ruiz de Alarcón 13, 28014 Madrid, Spain
Dock House, The Waterfront, Cape Town 8001, South Africa

http://www.cambridge.org

First published 2003

Printed in the United States of America

Typefaces Stone Serif 9/12 pt. *and* Avenir   *System* LaTeX 2_ε [TB]

A catalog record for this book is available from the British Library.

Library of Congress Cataloging in Publication data

Neurodevelopmental mechanisms in psychopathology / editors,
Dante Cicchetti, Elaine F. Walker.
    p. cm.
Includes bibliographical references and index.
ISBN 0-521-80225-3 – ISBN 0-521-00262-1 (pb.)
1. Mental illness – Etiology.   2. Schizophrenia – Pathophysiology.
3. Schizophrenia – Etiology.   4. Developmental neurobiology.
5. Psychology, Pathological.   I. Cicchetti, Dante.   II. Walker, Elaine F.
RC454.4 .N486   2003
616.89′071–dc21   2002031209

ISBN 0 521 80225 3 hardback
ISBN 0 521 00262 1 paperback

Contents

Contributors

Jocelyne Bachevalier, Ph.D.
Department of Neurobiology and Anatomy
University of Texas Health Science Center

Francine M. Benes, M.D., Ph.D.
Department of Psychiatry
Harvard Medical School

Alan S. Brown, M.D.
Department of Psychiatry
Columbia University

Tyrone D. Cannon, Ph.D.
Department of Psychology
University of California, Los Angeles

Dennis Charney, M.D.
Mood and Anxiety Disorders Research
    Program
National Institute of Mental Health

Dante Cicchetti, Ph.D.
Mt. Hope Family Center
University of Rochester

John N. Constantino, M.D.
Department of Psychiatry
Washington University School of Medicine

Nancy A. Dreschel, D.V.M.
Department of Biobehavioral Health
Pennsylvania State University

Sherryl H. Goodman, Ph.D.
Department of Psychology
Emory University

Douglas A. Granger, Ph.D.
Department of Biobehavioral Health
Pennsylvania State University

Matti Huttunen, M.D.
Social Science Research Institute
University of Southern California

Joan Kaufman, Ph.D.
Department of Psychiatry
Yale University School of Medicine

Matcheri S. Keshavan, M.D.
Western Psychiatric Institute and Clinic
University of Pittsburgh School of Medicine

Jean King, Ph.D.
Department of Psychiatry
University of Massachusetts

Harold W. Koenigsberg, M.D.
Department of Psychiatry
Mount Sinai School of Medicine

Gary W. Kraemer, Ph.D.
Department of Kinesiology
University of Wisconsin-Madison

Gabriele S. Leverich, Ph.D.
Biological Psychiatry Branch
National Institute of Mental Health

Seymour Levine, Ph.D.
Department of Psychology
University of California – Davis

He Li, Ph.D.
Biological Psychiatry Branch
National Institute of Mental Health

Katherine A. Loveland, Ph.D.
Department of Psychiatry and Behavioral
    Sciences
University of Texas Health Science Center

Ricardo Machón, Ph.D.
Social Science Research Institute
University of Southern California

Dario Maestripieri, Ph.D.
Committee on Human Development
University of Chicago

Linda C. Mayes, M.D.
Yale Child Study Center
Yale University

Keith McBurnett, Ph.D.
Department of Psychiatry
University of Chicago

Sarnoff A. Mednick, Ph.D.
Social Science Research Institute
University of Southern California

Colleen F. Moore, Ph.D.
Department of Psychology
University of Wisconsin – Madison

Robin M. Murray, Ph.D.
Institute of Psychiatry
Kings College London

Chiara Nosarti, Ph.D.
Institute of Psychiatry
Kings College London

Robert M. Post, M.D.
Biological Psychiatry Branch
National Institute of Mental Health

Deidre Reynolds, M.D.
Mount Sinai School of Medicine
Department of Psychiatry

Larry Rifkin, Ph.D.
Institute of Psychiatry
Kings College London

Isabelle M. Rosso, Ph.D.
Department of Psychiatry
Harvard Medical School

Angela Scarpa, Ph.D.
Department of Psychology
Virginia Polytechnic Institute

Jason Schiffman, M.A.
Social Science Research Institute
University of Southern California

Mary L. Schneider, Ph.D.
Department of Kinesiology and Psychology
University of Wisconsin – Madison

Elizabeth A. Shirtcliff, C.Phil.
Department of Biobehavioral Health
Pennsylvania State University

Larry J. Siever, M.D.
Department of Psychiatry
Mount Sinai School of Medicine

Mark Smith, Ph.D.
Experimental Station, DuPont
    Pharmaceutical
National Institute of Mental Health

Linda Patia Spear, Ph.D
Center for Developmental Psychobiology
Binghamton University

Ezra S. Susser, M.D., Dr.P.H.
Department of Psychiatry
Columbia University

Kay Thomas, Ph.D.
Social Science Research Institute
University of Southern California

Richard D. Todd, Ph.D., M.D.
Division of Child Psychiatry
Washington University School of Medicine

Deborah Walder, M.A.
Department of Psychology
Emory University

Irwin D. Waldman, Ph.D.
Department of Psychology
Emory University

Elaine F. Walker, Ph.D.
Department of Psychology
Emory University

Kim Wallen, Ph.D.
Department of Psychology
Emory University

Anna Ward, M.A.
Yale Child Study Center
Yale University

Susan R. B. Weiss, Ph.D.
Biological Psychiatry Branch
National Institute of Mental Health

Guoqiang Xing, Ph.D.
Department of Psychiatry Uniformed
    Services
National Institute of Mental Health

Li-Xin Zhang, Ph.D.
Biological Psychiatry Branch
National Institute of Mental Health

Preface

This volume represents a burgeoning perspective on the origins of psychopathology, one that focuses on the development of the human central nervous system (CNS). The contemporary *neurodevelopmental* perspective assumes that mental disorders result from etiologic factors that alter the normal course of brain development. Defined here in its broadest sense, neurodevelopment is a process that begins at conception and extends throughout the lifespan. We now know that it is a complex process and that its course can be altered by a host of factors, ranging from inherited genetic liabilities to psychosocial stressors. This knowledge has challenged clinical researchers to devise novel methodologies aimed at identifying links in this chain of events that can lead to psychopathology.

Neurodevelopmental perspectives on psychopathology have become increasingly dominant as a consequence of major advances in both basic animal research and clinical investigations of human populations. Basic research efforts have succeeded in elucidating amazing facets of brain development that extend from the molecular to the behavioral levels of analysis. For example, using animal models, basic scientists have documented the long-term effects of prenatal and postnatal events on brain structure and function and have shown how these effects vary as a function of hereditary factors. They also have demonstrated that there are significant behavioral sequela of aberrant neurodevelopment. At the same time, clinical research has yielded extensive evidence that prenatal and early childhood factors are associated with subsequent risk for psychopathology. For example, within the past two decades, there have been numerous reports of correlations between prenatal complications and psychological functioning in adulthood. There are obvious points of convergence between the findings yielded by these basic and clinical research endeavors, and the result has been an increasing focus on the neurodevelopmental origins of psychopathology.

Inspired by this plethora of new theories and empirical findings, the editors of this volume organized a conference on neurodevelopmental aspects of psychopathology. The plan was to assemble a group of investigators who shared a primary interest in the field, including *basic* researchers who employ animal models to shed light on neurodevelopment and *clinical* researchers who study developmental factors in human psychopathology. The chief goals were to examine cutting-edge findings and to chart the directions for future research efforts. The meeting took place at Emory University in

1999. Generous financial support was provided by the Essel Foundation, the William T. Grant Foundation, the Janssen Research Foundation, and the Spunk Fund. In addition, invaluable guidance was provided by Constance and Stephen Lieber, two philanthropic leaders in the field of mental health research.

What began as a relatively modest plan to assemble a small group of investigators quickly blossomed into a conference that was attended by more than eighty scientists. More than twenty distinguished investigators, representing those at the forefront of their fields, presented their most recent work. They were encouraged to stretch their imaginations and to share their speculations on the evolution of the field. They did so, and in the process we believe they set the stage for the next decade of research on neurodevelopmental aspects of psychopathology.

This volume presents a collection of chapters that evolved from presentations at the conference. The chapters feature the very best thinking in the converging fields of developmental neuroscience and developmental psychopathology. The developmental window represented in the chapters is broad, extending from the prenatal period through adulthood, and the authors cover a broad range of etiologic factors and a spectrum of clinical disorders. Moreover, it is obvious that the contributors did not hesitate to use the opportunity to hypothesize about underlying mechanisms and to speculate on future research directions.

The first chapters, written by Mayes and Ward and by Nosarti, Rifkin, and Murray, address basic mechanisms in the prenatal and neonatal development of the human nervous system and the implications for subsequent behavioral development across the lifespan. The authors of these chapters have heightened our understanding of the intricate processes involved in fetal and neonatal brain development. Further, their work sheds light on the myriad factors that can perturb the early development of brain structures that are known to play a role in human emotion and cognition. The chapter by Spear takes us into a later period associated with significant neuromaturational change – adolescence. It is clear that the postpubertal brain is undergoing pervasive changes that result in a new pattern of cortical circuitry. Although advances in cognitive function emanate from these changes, they may also set the stage for heightened vulnerability for certain forms of mental disorder.

Chapters by Brown and Susser, Rosso and Cannon, and Shiffman, Mednick, Machón, Huttunen, Thomas, and Levine, present recent empirical findings on the associations of prenatal and perinatal events with adult psychiatric disorders. Through careful longitudinal research, these investigators have demonstrated relations between early insults to the developing CNS and mental health in adulthood. They show us how latent congenital vulnerabilities can lay dormant until later developmental events trigger their expression.

In the next section, the focus shifts to animal models. In chapters authored by Schneider, Moore, and Kraemer and by Maestripieri and Wallen the investigators describe the results of experimental research programs that are helping to clarify the mechanisms involved in the genesis of psychopathology. By manipulating exposure to nonoptimal environmental influences, the authors are able to provide strong support for the importance of early experience for later psychological functioning. In the final chapter in this section, Bachevalier and Loveland present experimental evidence derived from brain-lesioned monkeys and propose a developmental model of autism based on this animal work.

The next group of chapters focus on general models of the nature of genetic and environmental influences on the developmental course of psychopathology. Todd and Constantino suggest new approaches to conceptualizing genetic influences on development and psychopathology. In his chapter, Waldman explicates a number of behavioral and molecular genetic research strategies that may aid in our understanding of the neurodevelopmental contributors to psychopathology. Granger, Dreschel, and Shirtcliff explore the immune system and its impact on brain function, and they describe the myriad of ways in which viral and bacterial agents might give rise to aberrations in neurodevelopment that could lead to behavioral disorders. In his chapter, Keshavan draws our attention to adolescence as a sensitive neurodevelopmental period. He offers a convincing argument for the pivotal nature of adolescence in the genesis of major mental illnesses. In her chapter, Benes discusses the interaction of several neurotransmitter systems during childhood and adolescence and describes how stress can influence an individual's vulnerability for the development of psychopathology. In their chapter, McBurnett, King, and Scarpa describe research on neuroendocrine functioning and the emergence of conduct disorder and substance abuse disorders. Relatedly, Cicchetti illustrates how child maltreatment, a chronic social stressor, affects neuroendocrine functioning and the emergence of psychopathology.

In the final section of chapters, the authors address the developmental course of some specific mental disorders: personality disorders, schizophrenia, depression, bipolar illness, and posttraumatic stress disorder. The neural underpinnings of diverse personality disorders, which are often the developmental prelude to Axis I mental disorders, are discussed by Siever, Koenigsberg, and Reynolds. In chapters by Goodman, by Kaufman and Charney, by Post, Leverich, Weiss, Zhang, Xing, Li, and Smith, and by Walker and Walder we see how different syndromes of psychopathology can arise from interactions between specific constitutional liabilities and environmental factors that impinge on the individual.

The nature of the theoretical shift this volume represents is brought into clearer focus when we examine key theoretical papers published prior to 1980. These landmark theoretical models foreshadowed contemporary developments in the field. In 1973, Hagop Akiskal and William McKinney published a seminal paper in *Science* entitled, "Depressive disorders: Toward a unified hypothesis." In this paper, the authors began by briefly reviewing the major theoretical perspectives of the time: psychoanalytic, interpersonal, object relations, learning, and "biogenic amine" theories. They proceeded to argue that each of these theories deals with a different level of analysis and that there are important interactions among the various levels. They criticized the notion of a single initial cause for depression, and emphasized the importance of bidirectional interrelations among brain, behavior, and experience. Along the same lines, in 1977, Joseph Zubin and Bonnie Spring published a paper entitled, "Vulnerability: A new view of schizophrenia." They argued that schizophrenia is best understood as a disorder that arises from the dynamic interaction between constitutional vulnerabilities and stressful experiences. In support of this, they presented evidence that both biological and environmental factors contribute to schizophrenia, apparently interacting at multiple levels. Both of these papers were widely cited, stimulating a great deal of discussion in the field. The arguments were intuitively appealing. Yet, in the 1970s, there was very little empirical evidence for neural mechanisms that might subserve interactional influences. It had been demonstrated that biological factors (genetics and

Basic Mechanisms in Prenatal, Perinatal, and Postnatal Neurodevelopmental Processes and Their Associations with High-Risk Conditions and Adult Mental Disorders broader interpretation, teratology is the study of perinatal developmental injury or abnormal development and of the factors including birth accidents and genetic mutations that increase the risk of developmental injury (Wilson, 1977). In this broader interpretation, the field covers a vast range encompassing the impact of exposures to exogenous agents or events during specific developmental phases on physical and functional outcomes. The outcomes may range from death, physical malformation, growth abnormalities, and disruption in function in all organ systems including the central nervous system. Among the agents or events of interest are both prescribed and illicit drugs, industrial chemicals, environmental pollutants, irradiation, viral infections, traumas such as preterm birth, and psychological conditions such as increased perinatal stress or maternal depression/deprivation.

An even more recent research specialty is neurobehavioral teratology, which investigates the developmental impact of exposure to similar exogenous agents or events during different critical periods on the developing brain, and hence, on the offspring's psychological development (Vorhees, 1986). Neurobehavioral teratology examines agents (or events) capable of producing deficits in cognitive functioning or other measures of neurobehavioral performance in the absence of gross malformations of the central nervous system. The impact of individual exposures is assessed at varying distances in time from the original fetal exposure. The field became a distinctive branch of teratology when behavioral effects were suggested as the subtler outcome in a continuum of prenatal insults (Spyker, 1975). For example, studies of the impact on infant neurodevelopmental functioning of human exposure to radiation or methyl mercury or preclinical animal models on the effects of early experiential differences in handling on behavior were early examples of neurobehavioral teratologic studies as methodological approaches distinct from general teratology (Butcher, 1985; Vorhees, 1986). Up until that point, teratology had focused on fetal death and malformations, but neurobehavioral teratology emphasized functional disruption at exposures far below those capable of causing structural, physical malformations. Neurobehavioral teratology also emerged with the increasing need to regulate new drugs, and environmental and industrial exposures after the identification of thalidomide as a teratogen in the early 1960s (Adams, 1999). With the recognition of thalidomide as a drug with no toxicity in the adult but severe teratogenic effects for the fetus, the USDA began to require the evaluation of new drugs in pregnant experimental animals. Necessarily then, standards for determining teratogenicity were required; and debate ensued as to whether the labeling of an agent as a teratogen would be restricted to lethal effects, morphological abnormalities, growth retardation, and observable functional impairments, or would more subtle and sometimes later-appearing neurobehavioral functional disruptions at lower doses also be considered in the standards for defining an agent as a teratogen, an issue still largely unsettled in the regulatory arena (Adams, 1999; Vorhees, 1986c).

Given this emphasis on effects at lower exposure doses, much of the methodology of the discipline is focused on understanding the probability for a given outcome or the assessment of risk, and studies are directed toward establishing dose-response relations or the level at which there are no discernable effects for a given agent. The phrase "no discernable" is key, for this of course varies with the outcome selected for study. As a field, neurobehavioral teratology adds developmental psychology and developmental neuroscience to the multidisciplinary mixture of fields studying birth defects and developmental injuries in general; and despite the title "neurobehavioral teratology," the field has grown far beyond a strictly neurobehavioral or cognitive emphasis with a focus primarily on mental retardation to include functional neuroimaging, neuro-physiology, neurochemistry, and neuropsychology and an emphasis on a continuum of deficits in a number of developmental and behavioral domains. Indeed, interest in developmental injury from a psychological/behavioral point of view has provided a significant incentive to understanding the normal or expectable features of early per-ceptual, social-emotional, and cognitive processes and how to measure more accurately and specifically these developmental domains.

Not surprisingly, with such a diverse range of exposures from discrete pharamaco-logic treatments to psychosocial events such as overwhelming stress and an equally broad range of possible neurobehavioral outcomes, there is no one consensual focus or methodological standard in the field. Neurobehavioral teratologic questions about de-velopmental injury are approached from two broad perspectives (Adams, 1999; Vorhees & Mollnow, 1987). One perspective examines a question by its presumed causes, that is, by grouping subjects into those with and without the presumed cause of injury or exposure. In this perspective, studies may examine the prevalence of neurobehavioral deficits in the exposed individuals and attempt to establish relationships between the amount and timing of exposure and the severity of the deficit.

Another perspective studies questions of development injury not through the pu-tative cause but rather through the target organ, system, or function of injury. Hence, subjects of study are grouped by their functional impairment, and the programmatic study is to understand the various mechanisms and routes to that particular functional impairment. Investigations focused on this perspective may also use exposure models to understand the relationships between, for example, disruption in specific brain re-gions and impairments in related functional systems – again a focus on mechanism, but in this case mechanisms of normal ontogeny studied through exposure models. These two broad orientations may lead to different research questions, findings, and interpre-tations inasmuch as one focuses on outcome while the other emphasizes mechanism. The most productive approach to any investigation of developmental injury brings a combination of these two perspectives and a plurality of methods to the research questions.

The fundamental logic of questions from neurobehavioral teratology specifically and teratology in general is does exposure to A during a specific phase of development cause B, C, and/or D immediately or later in development. (Or in the language of mechanism, does disruption in process A during a specific phase of development lead to disruptions in functions B, C, and/or D later in development.) Importantly, one agent, A, may produce several different outcomes (e.g., outcomes B, C, and/or D) depending on dose or amount of exposure, and there may be different dose-response curves for the different outcomes. Functional behavioral or psychological changes may occur at lower doses than abnormal growth or major disruptions in organogenesis and the shape of the dose-response curves may also be different depending on the outcome (Vorhees & Mollnow, 1987; also see section below). There are several examples of these kinds of direct causative models for both functional and physical outcomes. These include prenatal rubella exposure and its association with deafness and mental retardation, or the classic example of prenatal thalidomide exposure and severe malformations of limb development. In these models, there is a clear association between a specific exposure to a discrete toxin and a clearly defined and easily identified endpoint or outcome.

However, many, if not all, of the more contemporary questions capturing much of the interest in neurobehavioral teratology are those that involve far more complex models of exposure, timing, and outcome assessment. These are not always clearly direct causality models and hence are not easily approached with standard research designs. The exposures are neither specific nor discrete, the outcomes are not uniformly present even with documented exposure, and the severity or extent of the deformation or developmental abnormality is variable. In these more complex models, interactions between the exposure agent or event and the environment are central. That is, does the environment in one way or another moderate the fetus's or child's risk of exposure as well as vulnerability to the potentially toxic effects of exposure and at the same time, determine other risk factors that may also mediate the severity of any exposure-related outcome.

For example, even the question of malnutrition and its effect on fetal outcome is not a straightforward question of exposure and effect. Malnutrition more often occurs among very poor or displaced populations who are usually considerably stressed and isolated from adequate medical and prenatal care. These conditions may further compound the impact of malnutrition on fetal development in a way that would not occur theoretically if malnutrition occurred in isolation or in the absence of social displacement and chronic stress. Similarly, a more contemporary question regarding the effects of maternal antidepressants on infant neurodevelopmental integrity is also made more complex by the possible relations between maternal depression, heightened perinatal stress, and altered maternal-infant care. Even in questions of exposure to industrial chemicals or environmental pollutants, there may be a number of mediating and moderating factors that diminish or increase the likelihood of exposure and the severity of the outcome. And there is perhaps no better (and no more confounded) illustration of interactive neurobehavioral teratology models in humans than those involving the putative teratogenic effects of drug abuse during pregnancy.

In this chapter, we shall discuss ten basic principles central to any neurobehavioral teratology investigation. In a classic paper, Wilson outlined the basic principles of teratological investigations and Vorhees later adapted these to neurobehavioral teratology studies in preclinical models (Vorhees & Mollnow, 1987; Wilson, 1973; Wilson, 1977). In this review, we will further adapt or expand upon these principles to underscore the particular application to human studies. These principles, also outlined in Table 1.1, include:

1. Delineating the possible mechanisms of teratogenic effect.
2. Defining the specific teratogenic agent.
3. Specifying the timing of the exposure.
4. Defining the nature of the exposure.
5. Delineating the range of susceptibility and response relationships.
6. Selecting those groups at greater or lesser risk for exposure.
7. Considering the environmental context and conditions most related to the exposure.
8. Defining the outcomes most likely related to the mechanism of action of the exposure agent or event.
9. Considering when exposure-related outcomes are most likely to be apparent.
10. Taking into account those conditions that ameliorate or exacerbate any exposure-related functional outcomes.

Table 1.1. Principles of Behavioral Teratology

1. **Delineating the Possible Mechanisms of Teratogenic Effect:** Agents that are behaviorally teratogenic should act on the developing CNS by specific mechanisms.
2. **Defining the Specific Teratogenic Agent:** Not all agents that produce malformations are necessarily behavioral teratogens. Only those agents that produce either teratogenic or psychoactive CNS effects are capable of producing behavioral teratogenic effects.
3. **Specifying the Timing of the Exposure:** Based on the principle of critical periods, the type and magnitude of the behavioral teratogenic effect will depend on the stage of CNS development when exposure occurs.
4. **Defining the Nature of the Exposure:** The type and magnitude of the behavioral teratogenic effect depends on the type of agent, frequency and amount of use, and route of administration.
5. **Delineating Dose-Response Relationships and the Range of Susceptibility:** The type and severity of the behavioral effects depends on the dose of the agent reaching the developing central nervous system. Behavioral teratogenic effects are usually demonstrable at levels of exposure below that causing other malformations if the exposure agent is capable of causing behavioral changes.
6. **Selecting Those Groups at Greater or Lesser Risk for Exposure and Susceptibility to Effects:** How exposed groups are identified influences the likelihood of finding greater or lesser behavioral teratogenic effects. Individual genetic differences in the exposed individual or organism also influence the type and magnitude of behavioral teratogenic effect.
7. **Considering the Environmental Context and Conditions Most Related to the Exposure:** The magnitude and type of a behavioral teratogenic effect (and the likelihood of finding such an effect) depends on environmental factors.
8. **Selecting Outcomes Most Likely Related to the Mechanism of Action of the Exposure Agent or Event:** Behavioral teratogenic effects are expressed as impaired cognitive, perceptual, or social-emotional function or delayed maturation of capacities in these domains and the chosen outcomes for study should be linked to the proposed mechanism of CNS teratogenesis rather than selecting "broad band" measures of CNS function.
9. **Considering When Exposure Related Outcomes Are Most Likely to Be Apparent:** Not all behavioral teratogenic effects are apparent in the perinatal period. Some are evident later in development when environmental demands on specific functional domains are higher or when periods of developmentally time CNS reorganization are occurring.
10. **Taking Into Account Those Conditions that Ameliorate or Exacerbate Any Exposure Related Functional Outcomes:** Some behavioral teratogenic effects may be exacerbated or ameliorated by other exposures or environmental conditions such as how the organism is handled or parented or other unexpected events such as illnesses that occur after the exposure period.

These principles do cut across animal and human models (Vorhees & Mollnow, 1987), although the methodological challenges are different and sometimes more complex in the human model. Throughout the discussion of these principles, we shall draw in particular on studies of the problem of prenatal cocaine exposure, which especially illustrates the principles of defining the independent variable (Table 1.1, principle 4), delineating dose-response relations (principle 5), defining cohorts based on risk of exposure (principle 6), and specifying the environmental context and conditions most related to the exposure (principle 7). Studies of prenatal cocaine exposure in human models that are informed by preclinical investigations are paradigmatic of contemporary neurobehavioral teratology perspectives. In our concluding section, we will suggest future directions for these kinds of models of behavioral teratogenicity in humans.

CENTRAL PRINCIPLES IN NEUROBEHAVIORAL TERATOLOGY STUDIES

One of the important legacies of the early stages of the field of neurobehavioral teratology is its initial "applied" nature as in, for example, the issues regarding the establishment of regulatory standards for drugs and chemicals. Because of this applied, practical beginning, in many of the early toxicological studies in both animal and human models, little attention was given to some critical methodological issues that presented potential prenatal and postnatal confounding variables (Nelson, 1990). The thalidomide tragedy notwithstanding, in most instances, establishing in humans clear links between prenatal exposures and immediate physical, neurological, or later developmental and psychological outcomes is fraught with significant methodological problems. Animal models of exposure offer some solutions to a number of these methodological issues while at the same time preclinical models may not adequately model the complexity of the human exposure situation. Thus, that only a few human environmental neurobehavioral teratogens have been identified (e.g., methyl mercury, PCBs, lead, alcohol) is not necessarily evidence for human invulnerability to teratogenic effects but rather that very few agents have actually been rigorously evaluated with appropriate methodological standards. For example, of at least 70,000 chemicals in regular commercial use, perhaps only 10 percent (excluding pharmaceutical agents) have been studied for their neurotoxic or neurobehavioral teratogenic potential (Dietrich, 1999; Rees, Francis, & Kimmel, 1990). Similarly, despite the number of psychoactive drugs that may be used during pregnancy and despite concerns regarding their potential teratogenic effects, for most, data are inconclusive (Levy & Koren, 1990, 1992) at least in part because of significant methodological issues. The following principles play a role in essentially every question regarding potential neurobehavioral teratogens.

Delineating Possible Mechanisms of Effect. While it perhaps seems obvious that it is important to consider the possible mechanisms of teratogenic effects of any given agent, it is not always the case particularly in studies of the human model that mechanisms of effect are either specified or hypothesized beyond the general expectation or assumption that, for example, psychoactive drugs administered during active CNS neurogenesis should be potentially teratogenic (see also below). This assumption not only ignores consideration of specificity of effect on particular CNS regions and functions, but also does not permit a more hypothesis-driven consideration of the possible domains of outcome to study. The notion that specifying mechanisms of effect on CNS that will be manifest in behavioral/psychological function does make that presumption that there are neurochemical and/or neuroanatomical, structural changes in the brain as a result of exposure to a particular agent which are in turn manifest in postnatal behavior and psychological functions. Often these possible mechanisms of action are defined not through investigations of the specific teratogen but rather through studies of other agents with similar mechanisms of action in the brain. For example, the potential effects of cocaine on developing monoaminergic systems in the fetal brain have been delineated more through in vitro and in vivo studies of monoaminergic regulation of neurogenesis, neuronal migration, and synaptogenesis rather than through direct study of disruptions in fetal brain structure-function relations with cocaine exposure (Mayes, 1999).

Parenthetically, because studies defining the mechanisms of action of a drug or of aspects of CNS ontogeny often are accomplished by investigators not strictly studying teratologic questions, it is paramount that any behavioral teratologic study be framed as an interdisciplinary endeavor and incorporate findings from investigations of basic mechanisms of action into the study's conceptual basis. It is on this point that the fault line between the two perspectives cited earlier is the most evident, that is, between teratologic studies focused on outcome and those focused on mechanisms of disruption leading to developmental injuries. Once mechanisms of effect become the focus, it is possible to think of groups of teratogens rather than considering each teratogen as unique. For instance, there may be a group of teratogens that affect primarily cortical layering or neuronal migration, others in which the mechanism of action is primarily at the level of second messenger systems in dopaminergic pathways. It is of course also possible that one teratogenic agent may share several different mechanisms, and the relevant outcomes vary according to the mechanism most active at a particular time in development. For example, despite our emphasis on monoaminergic systems in the prenatal cocaine exposure model, cocaine acts on several other systems in the adult and developing brain. These include glutamate receptors, neuropeptides including the opioids dynorphin and enkephalin and nonopioids such as substance-P, and at the level of ion-channel transmission (Kreek, 1996; Reith, 1988; Shippenberg & Rea, 1997; White, Hu, Zhang, & Wolf, 1995; Ye, Liu, Wu, & McArdle, 1997). Very little work has been done on these systems in the fetal animal model, but based on these other mechanisms of action in the CNS, it is possible that these may also be involved in mechanisms of teratogenesis for cocaine and other pharmacologically similar stimulants.

Another salient and related point regarding teratologic mechanisms is the notion that all types of embryopathy are expressed through a set of final common pathways (Wilson, 1973, 1977). For example, it has long been observed that there is a definable and finite, albeit long, set of birth defects because of disruptions in basic processes of embryogenesis. Some disruptions in embryonic processes are not compatible with fetal survival and result in spontaneous abortion (Warkany, 1978). Other disruptions in embryonic ontogenesis are compatible with survival, albeit with physical and functional malformations evident at delivery or shortly afterward. Embryonic events necessary for normal development include closure of the neural plates, rotation and fusion of the palate, or rotation of the heart tube, and there are many ways these processes may be disrupted. But for these and other examples, the final common pathway is disruption of the morphogenetic process that results in these closure or rotation processes. Failure of closure or rotation may produce neural tube defects, congenital heart malformations, or cleft palate. While there may be hundreds, if not thousands, of drugs or other exposures that may alter these morphogenetic processes and result in a neural tube or heart defect, these malformations are not unique to the particular drug or agent.

This same argument may well apply to behavioral teratogenic questions (Vorhees & Mollnow, 1987). There may also be a finite number of disruptions in neural ontogeny and hence a finite number of final common behavioral disruptions that occur in the infant and young child. Thus, agents that are chemically very different may produce behavioral profiles that are quite similar based on similar mechanisms of effect on neural ontogenetic processes. For example, cocaine and commonly prescribed psychoactive drugs for anxiety and depression, the selective serotonin reuptake inhibitors, share in part a common mechanism of effect on monoaminergic systems described above and hence may show a similar effect on some aspects of fetal neural development. Of course, early neurobehavioral functional abnormalities may interact with environmental conditions to modify the behavioral profile which does make the range of behavioral outcomes broader and more complex; and better methods of assessment also improves the fidelity of behavioral profiles as the same teratogenic agent is studied over time. Nonetheless, it is still an important and parsimonious principle to think about the outcomes of exposures to different teratogens in terms of final common behavioral profiles that may be the same across different exposure agents.

One other mechanism of effect, preconceptional or transgenerational effects, deserves mention though it is not well studied in any behavioral teratologic investigations. First, there are effects on offspring behavior from paternal rather than maternal exposure (Adams, Fabricant, & Legator, 1981). These are transmitted through exposure effects on male sperm and hence exposure effects through mutagenesis. Such mechanisms have been suggested for prenatal alcohol effects (Abel, 1992). Others have also suggested that transgenerational effects on behavior, that is, effects transmitted across more than one generation, may be mediated again by mutagenesis (Vorhees & Mollnow, 1987), though it may also be that a vulnerability to, for example, addiction is transmitted across generations not because of mutagenesis but rather through a genetically conveyed vulnerability that also conveys a vulnerability to other behavioral outcomes or phenotypes also associated with the specific genetic polymorphisms (see below).

Defining the Specific Teratogenic Agent. Not all agents that produce teratogenic effects in organ systems other than the brain are necessarily behavioral teratogens, though with increasingly refined methods of study, behavioral effects may be apparent. Thalidomide may be a notable example of the latter (McBride, 1977). Despite the dramatic limb reduction deformity, evidence is less clear regarding psychological developmental effects, although a reduction in IQ appears present after allowing for the impact of physical disabilities (McFie & Robertson, 1973). Conversely, only those agents that produce either teratogenic or psychoactive CNS effects are capable of producing behavioral teratogenic effects. While this may seem obvious, it is worth considering for a moment. All evidence to date suggests that all agents that result in CNS structural malformations at higher doses are also behavioral teratogens at lower doses.

Whether or not all psychoactive drugs are also potential structural and behavioral teratogens in the developing fetus is less clear. There are certainly instances of psychoactive drugs that apparently produce behavioral teratogenic effects, even effects on growth, but not apparent structural malformations. Examples include diazepam (Kellogg, Tervo, Ison, Parisi, & Miller, 1980), phenobarbital (Middahugh, 1986), neuroleptics (Vorhees, Brunner, & Butcher, 1979), and some pesticides (Mactutus & Tilson, 1986). Cocaine may also be an example, though at high doses cocaine may contribute to cerebral vascular accidents in the fetus because of vasoconstriction (Moore, Sorg, Miller, Key, & Resnik, 1986; Woods, Plessinger, & Clark, 1987) and cause structural malformations based on a mechanism that is different from the one associated with behavioral teratogenic effects. Hence, the absence of any data suggesting structural malformations for a given psychoactive drug cannot be taken as evidence against behavioral teratogenesis. Furthermore, since behavioral effects typically occur at doses lower than those effecting growth or morphogenesis (see below), safety studies need to consider the possibility of functional disruption even at low, and presumably safe, doses.

At the same time, it is an error to assume that every psychoactive agent necessarily produces behavioral teratogenic (or for that matter teratogenic) effects in the developing central nervous system. There are a number of examples of psychoactive drugs that do not appear to be behaviorally teratogenic, albeit with the accumulated evidence to date. Acetazolamide, an anticonvulsant, appears to be one such example (Butcher, Hawver, Burbacher, & Scott, 1975); acetazolamide is associated with limb deformities but apparently not behavioral teratogenic effects.

Specifying the Timing of Exposures. Defining the timing of exposure is critical because of differing windows of vulnerability in the developing fetus. These "windows" are based on differing phases of central nervous system development. CNS ontogeny reflects a complex interaction among genetic factors, neurochemical substrates, and environmental conditions (Kosofsky, 1991). At least eight stages describe the processes that occur in each part of the developing brain: neural plate induction, neuronal and glial cell proliferation, cell migration, cell aggregation, neuronal maturation, neuronal connectivity including synaptogenesis, cell death, and process elimination (pruning). Within each of these phases, there are parallel processes of metabolic differentiation and maturation, and genes taking their regulatory cues from the immediate neurochemical (and experiential) environment regulate the onset/offset of each phase. As a more general map in humans, cell proliferation occurs between two and four months gestation for neurons and five months gestation to one year postnatally for glia; neuronal migration takes place primarily between three and five months gestation. Between six months gestation to several years postnatally, the brain is in a protracted organizational phase establishing neuronal connectivity and pruning less utilized connections or synapses to enhance other patterns of connectivity (Volpe, 1987). The timing (gestational and/or postnatal) of potentially toxic exposures determines the possible developmental consequences. Exposures occurring during the first half of gestation affect cytogenesis and histogenesis, while those exposures occurring in the latter half of pregnancy and postnatally influence growth and structural/functional differentiation. Exposures throughout both periods have "interactive" effects inasmuch as altering early events during the cytogenesis phase will also alter events downstream that are regulated by the completion of earlier phases. Brain development in the second half of gestation and the early postnatal period is characterized by both *progressive* (e.g., synaptogenesis and neuronal maturation) and *regressive* (e.g., cell death and pruning) processes. Blocking, delaying, extending, or shortening either progressive or regressive events will have probable (and different) effects on immediate structure/function relations, on related genetic regulatory processes, and on neuromaturational events downstream that are dependent on earlier events.

Behavioral teratologic studies are implicitly based on the concept of critical periods or on defining periods of maximum or specific vulnerability to a specific insult. Ontogenetic processes (at the biochemical, cellular, structural, or functional level) are most vulnerable to disruption during their earliest and most active phases. And the window of maximal vulnerability also depends on the mechanism of action of the potential teratogen. That is, if the primary mechanism of action of a given drug is disruption of thymidine and uridine incorporation as, for example, is suggested for cocaine (Garg, Turndorf, & Bansinath, 1993), then the period of maximum vulnerability for the human fetus will be during neurogenesis and neuronal proliferation in the first trimester. Some windows of vulnerability are relatively short, others longer. For instance, there is a relatively narrow window during fetal development during which some agents can sufficiently alter neural plate closure so that brain and spinal cord malformations such as spina bifida occur (Warkany, Lemire, & Cohen, 1981). Behavioral teratologic questions are typically focused on more subtle types of structural and functional deficits that may not be visible on gross or even general microscopic inspection. There may also be several critical windows of vulnerability for any one potential teratogen, for many drugs disrupt neural ontogeny at several different stages and thus, depending on the timing of the exposure, the developmental process that is primary at that time will be most disrupted. Cocaine, for example, may have direct effects on neurogenesis, on neuronal migration, and on synaptogenesis – processes that cut across several critical windows of neural ontogeny. As with understanding mechanisms of teratogenesis, understanding critical periods or windows of vulnerability is based as much in the basic developmental neuroscience as in studies of toxicology. Indeed, toxicological studies may inform basic models of neural ontogeny and provide data that can be used to refine and narrow windows of vulnerability. Broadly defined neurogenesis phases may at times be too inclusive to allow more accurate definition of period-specific vulnerabilities. For example, within the broad phase of neuronal migration, there are many smaller windows and phase-specific processes such as the generation of radial glial cells, that may define mechanism-specific critical periods. Of equal importance, early disruptions in certain ontogenetic processes may have functional effects long after the exposure has stopped inasmuch as the interactions among systems and functional organization of processes continues to be affected by the early disruption. Continued histogenesis, functional organization, and brain (as well as other organ) growth through synaptogenesis and synaptic pruning continue long after birth including well into puberty. Thus, early ontogenetic alterations may have long-lasting effects without continued exposure to the teratogen.

For behavioral teratologic studies, a distinction between experience-expectant and experience-dependent or -sensitive is also important (Greenough, 1991; Greenough, Black, Klintsova, Bates, & Weiler, 1999; Greenough, Black, & Wallace, 1987). Experience-expectant processes are those that require certain experiences or events at one or more critical windows during ontogeny to develop fully. The classic postnatal example is the failure of the visual apparatus to develop without proper light exposure. Experience-dependent processes are those developmental events or phases that respond to experience and activity with enhanced development such as experience-sensitive synaptogenesis that occurs with enriched stimulating environments. Experience-dependent refers to incorporation of learned environmental information that is unique to the individual. The neural basis of this process appears to involve active formation of new synaptic connections in response to the events providing the information to be stored. Given that a considerable amount of neural development occurs in the human infant postnatally and in the first years of life, the concept of experience-dependent periods is particularly relevant for teratogenic studies of human exposures. Additionally, for humans, many exposures are not limited to the prenatal period, and exposure during the postnatal period may also occur during a phase-specific period of vulnerability. Postnatal teratogenic exposures include to some licit and illicit drugs such as nicotine, crack, or marijuana through passive inhalation, to prescribed psychoactive drugs through breast milk, or to parental stress or depression through caregiving interactions.

Defining the Nature of the Exposure. All questions regarding the effects of prenatal exposure to agents or events have the dilemma of defining the route, amount, and duration of exposure. For nonillicit, prescribed drugs, these definitions may be relatively straightforward. The dosage, frequency, and route of administration are prescribed and known and the patient's compliance with the prescribed regimen and individual pharmacokinetic variation in the metabolism of the drug are the sources of variance in the amount of exposure. However, for events such as exposure to maternal stress, the exposure issues are complex: when can the "exposure" be said to begin and end, what defines a potentially teratogenic level of maternal stress, and by what metric. Similarly, defining amount and duration of exposure for environmental toxins such as PCBs can be equally difficult and problematic.

For human models of prenatal illicit drug exposure, defining the independent exposure variable may be the single most problematic issue in neurobehavioral teratologic studies (Mayes & Fahy, 2001). Substance abusers typically do not report consistently or reliably the frequency or amount of their drug use (Babor, Brown, & delBoca, 1990; Chasnoff, Landress, & Barrett, 1990; Grissom, 1997; Weiss, et al., 1998). Various strategies have been devised to improve the reliability of self-reports of substance use including use of time-lines, careful training of interviewers, narrow windows for retrospective recall (Callahan, et al., 1992; Carey, 1997; Richardson & Day, 1994; Rogers & Kelly, 1997). Even with these more sophisticated interviewing strategies, self-reports of single or polydrug use typically though not uniformly (Richardson, Day, & McGauhey, 1993) underestimate the amount of exposure, particularly of illicit drugs.

Frequency of exposure obtained through self-report histories is usually expressed as a number of days per unit time (e.g., per month, use in last thirty days, use per week). Self-reports are typically though not universally augmented with toxicologic sampling of urine for drugs such as cocaine, marijuana, or opiates. Repeated toxicology screening through a pregnancy may provide some confirmation and/or identification of users and not uncommonly toxicologic screens are obtained from both infant and mother at the time of delivery. Urine toxicology provides a relatively narrow window on use. For example, for cocaine users, urine toxicology is typically positive no longer than thirty-six hours after use and that window varies for other drugs. For cocaine, infants' meconium and/or hair (infant's or mother's) have gained some support as particularly good samples to ascertain or confirm infant exposure because they provide a longer window for ascertaining exposure. Some data suggest that meconium or hair from the newborn may be a reliable measure of exposure as far back as mid-first trimester (Callahan, et al., 1992; Graham, Koren, Klein, Schneiderman, & Greenwald, 1989; Kline, Ng, Schittini, Levin, & Susser, 1997; Ostrea, 1995). However, despite early enthusiasm for these kinds of longer window measures and despite their obvious utility, they do not provide a reliable quantitative estimate of exposure.

Indeed, quantity or amount of exposure is particularly difficult to estimate reliably in studies of illicit drug exposure – or for that matter in industrial or environmental toxin exposures. Estimates of amount of drug per time of use are as problematic as frequency of use when obtained by self-report. Toxicologic assays typically do not provide sufficiently accurate quantitative assays to permit the definition of a more quantitative exposure variable. But it is an important variable since between individuals and for any one person, "dose" or amount per use varies enormously. There are obviously no standards for how illicit drugs are sold – how pure or how diluted with other ingredients that may be active or inert. Thus, even if an addict presents a more or less accurate account of frequency and amount of use, there are few to no reliable indices of how concentrated the drug was and what the carrier or substance for cutting the pure drug might have been.

With these various problems in obtaining accurate estimates of frequency and amount of exposure, the majority of studies of prenatal exposure to date have defined the independent exposure variable as a dichotomous one – exposed or not exposed. Grouping all exposed infants and children together obscures potential dose-related effects inasmuch as including those only minimally may reduce the likelihood of detecting exposure effects in the exposed group. Thus, a growing number of studies are attempting to create some metric of heavy, moderate, and light use to examine dose-related effects that follow either linear or nonlinear models (for example, see Frank, Augustyn, & Zuckerman, 1998; King, et al., 1995; Tronick, Frank, Cabral, Mirochnick, & Zuckerman, 1996).

A third problem in the definition of exposure variables in substance abuse models is maternal polydrug use. Rarely do addicts use one drug only. While they may consider one drug of abuse their primary drug, polydrug use and exposure is the rule rather than the exception. For example, for cocaine users, a very typical combination is alcohol and tobacco in combination with cocaine. The same issues of defining frequency and amount of use for each drug pertain, but also there are questions of interactive effects among drugs such as alcohol with cocaine and the resulting metabolite cocethylene. And a related problem specific to studies of prenatal exposure is obtaining reliable estimates of frequency and amount of exposure by trimester. Different drugs have different effects during the three trimesters of pregnancy. For example, in the first trimester, prenatal cocaine exposure may have a direct effect on neuronal migration and brain structure formation, whereas in the third trimester the central nervous system effect may be on synaptogenesis in specific brain regions (Dow-Edwards, Freed, & Milhorat, 1988; Frank, et al., 1998; Mayes & Bornstein, 1995). Related to breaking down exposure by trimester is continued exposure postnatally. Particularly among agents that may be inhaled passively (e.g., crack, tobacco, marijuana), postnatal exposure is relatively common (for example, see Bender, et al., 1995; Kjarasch, Glotzer, Vinci, Wietzman, & Sargent, 1991; Lustbader, Mayes, McGee, Jatlow, & Roberts, 1998).

Route of use presents another consideration in defining the exposure. While total amount is always an important metric in defining severity of exposure, amount of time above a certain peak blood level may also be important in some models of teratogenicity. Stated another way, the teratogenic effect may not be carried by cumulative amount of exposure time but only by those times when the level of exposure is above a certain threshold. Certain aspects of fetal alcohol effects may follow this threshold rather than the linear dose-related model. Blood levels peak at different points following use, depending on the preferred route of use. In animal models, intraperitoneal administration results in a very different blood level compared to subcutaneous, and both are different from gastric lavage. Furthermore, regardless of route of administration, fetal cocaine levels are different from the maternal one – lower for subcutaneous administration (Spear, Kirstein, & Frambes, 1989) but higher for intraperitoneal (DeVane, Simpkins, Miller, & Braun, 1989). In humans, intravenous use as with heroin or smoking crack with rapid absorption through the pulmonary vascular bed provides rapid and large peak blood levels to both mother and fetus. Few to no studies, particularly of cocaine where the routes of use may be quite varied, have examined differences in outcome depending on preferred method of use.

That route of use may influence the peak blood level to which the developing brain is exposed raises another issue regarding definitions of the independent variable, the pharmacokinetics of how the agent is handled in the body. Even knowing how much drug is administered or used over a given period of time and by what route does not fully define how much active drug reaches the fetal brain and over what period of time. Pharmacokinetic factors including absorption, metabolism, tissue uptake, protein binding, and excretion are each critical in determining the neural toxicity for any given agent. For example, some drugs do not readily or fully cross the placenta to the fetal circulation and thus, maternal blood levels, even if available, will not accurately reflect fetal blood levels. Some drugs are differentially metabolized by adults so that for one mother, a given dose results in a lower blood level than for another individual. Typically, in human studies, these individual pharmacokinetic factors are very difficult to take into account, particularly in the case of illicit drugs. A few studies examining the teratogenic effects of, for example, selective serotonin reuptake inhibitors during the immediate perinatal and postnatal period have examined maternal and infant cord blood, and breast milk drug levels (Kristensen, et al., 1999; Schmidt, Olesen, & Jensen, 2000), but far more consideration needs to be given to incorporating pharmacokinetic principles into human studies.

Delineating and Dose-Response Relationships and the Range of Susceptibility. Implicit in these considerations regarding dose, frequency, route of administration, and pharmacokinetics is establishing dose-response relations for the effects of the teratogen on the developing brain. What is the relationship between the appearance of teratogenic effects and the amount and duration of exposure? While only a few studies report clear dose-response relationships, there are a few teratogens for which these reports are consistent, including alcohol, vitamin A, and phenytoin (Abel, 1992; Vorhees, 1974; Vorhees, 1986d). Dose-response relationships are not always evident for behavior, though failure to detect such may be a reflection of study methods rather than the absence of a relationship (Nelson, 1981; Vorhees, 1986b). For many drugs such as dilantin (phenytoin; Vorhees, 1986a), the behavioral dose-response window is narrow and the curve steep. That is, the window of effect is so narrow that the model may seem one of an all-or-none effect – any exposure results in a teratogenic effect – and there is only a small difference between a dose at which only behavioral effects are evident and the dose at which structural malformations appear. Careful studies within this narrow window may nonetheless produce a graded model of severity of effect depending on dose. Other drugs that seem to act as behavioral teratogens such as diazepam produce behavioral effects far below the doses that are structurally toxic (Driscoll, Ferre, Fernandez-Terucl, & Levi de Stein, 1995; Kellogg, et al., 1980; Wee & Zimmerman, 1983).

For human models, establishing dose-response curves is problematic for all the reasons cited earlier. It is difficult to establish dosage and timing with any reliability, and the fetus may be concomitantly exposed to other agents, both pharmacologic and experiential (e.g., maternal malnutrition, depression, acute stress), that surely alter the dose-response relation for the target drug. Limits in behavioral assessment may also be a factor in the difficulties in establishing dose-response curves for both humans and preclinical models. Behavioral assessment techniques detect functional changes within the context of the experimental situation and the limits of the task. For example, tests of response inhibition usually reflect the child's performance in a quiet, structured, supportive laboratory setting and do not reflect how these capacities function in a real world setting such as a classroom. The converse is also true. An individual's performance on a certain task may be so poor because of impairments in related and necessary capacities that it is difficult to detect any effect on the function in question. For instance, tasks of short-term verbal memory, another executive function that may be impaired with prenatal cocaine exposure, may place demands on children's receptive and expressive language capacities that are in turn often markedly impaired in part because of severe environmental deprivation. The child's poor performance on verbal working memory tasks does not necessarily reflect a severe behavioral teratogenic effect of the drug.

Also, related to the issue of dose-response for behavioral effects is a point touched on earlier – the relation between dose-response curves for behavioral effects and those for other structural teratogenic effects from the same drug. It is important to note that this is not the same point as the common and probably erroneous assumption that behavioral teratogenic effects occur at lower doses than all other dose-response relationships for teratogenesis or embryotoxicity (Vorhees & Mollnow, 1987). It appears only the case that if a drug is a behavioral teratogen, the behavioral effects occur at lower doses than any structural effects, though for effects on growth, the two dose-response curves may be quite close, even superimposed. The latter appears to be true for example for cocaine, for which effects on growth and on behavior appear in preclinical models at essentially the same dose.

The dose-response relations for behavioral teratogenesis, growth retardation, and structural malformations have several other implications (Vorhees, 1986c; Wilson, 1973). Figure 1.1 (adapted from Vorhees, 1986c) shows a family of hypothetical dose-response curves for different outcomes A, B, & C at different doses. The X-axis shows dose of drug and the Y-axis the percentage of individuals with the outcome. For any single curve, the percentage increases with increasing dose. (An important caveat is that this figure shows essentially linear relations for the three outcomes. Different outcomes may have different curves both in slope and in shape.) For the family of curves taken together, as the dose increases, more individuals begin to show not only outcome A but also B and then C. At very high doses, 100 percent of exposed individuals may theoretically show outcome A, nearly 100 percent will show B, and 50 percent C. Of course, it may also be that outcome C is so devastating, that is, the structural malformations are so profound, that more subtle psychological functional disruptions are obscured. At lower doses in which only outcome A, the behavioral outcome, is evident, there will also be a proportion of unaffected individuals whether these studies are done in preclinical models using members of a litter or in human models using children matched on relevant characteristics. Thus, at sufficiently low doses to produce relatively "pure" behavioral

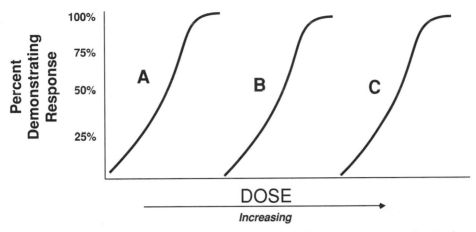

Figure 1.1. Hypothetical Dose-Response Curves for Different Outcomes (Behavioral to Structural)

teratogenic effects, there will be a dilution factor contributing to an underestimation of the true magnitude of the potential behavioral teratogenicity.

There are also individual differences in susceptibility to the effects of a behavioral teratogen, that is, even at lower doses where a dose-response curve might predict 40 percent of individuals would be affected, some individuals show greater or lesser magnitude of effect. These individual differences in susceptibility reflect both genetically and experientially determined individual differences in the fetus and in the maternal-fetal unit (see also below). For humans, better prenatal care and prenatal nutrition may be one experiential factor that modifies fetal susceptibility to, for example, the behavioral teratogenic effects of cocaine or other illicit drugs. Thus, even for the single behavioral teratogen dose-response curve, there is really a family of curves defined by these individual differences in susceptibility. Also, for any one behavioral teratogen, there is a family of curves for individual behavioral effects – one curve for effects on information processing, another for changes in emotional regulation, and yet another for alterations in attentional control.

Selecting Those Groups at Greater or Lesser Risk of Exposure and Susceptibility to Effects. How samples are identified, recruited, and maintained are crucial questions for any study of potentially teratologic agents. For example, if the question pertains to exposure to a particular environmental toxin, defining the area of possible exposure and the possible routes of exposure determine the sample selection strategies. Is it more appropriate to recruit among factory workers who were assigned to the area where the potential toxin was most concentrated and compare those to workers in other areas of the factory who presumably were not exposed? Or is it more appropriate to compare all factory workers to other members in the community and create a graded index of exposure? Is there something about selection to work in the potentially toxic area that interacts with the potential behavioral outcomes? For example, are workers in that area lower paid, perhaps less educated, at greater risk for substance use and depression? Do workers who were more likely to have been exposed tend to participate in the study more than those whose exposure was less clear?

These kinds of questions are relevant to every study attempting to relate exposures to later outcomes. They are also relevant to preclinical models in which the particular genetic strain or previous environmental experience of a group of animals may influence their behavioral response and function before and after the exposure. Sample selection issues have a special valence in studies of substance abuse and prenatal exposure. The valence relates to severity of exposure, compliance with the study and/or treatment, and overall psychosocial burden. Samples recruited from substance abuse clinics, while practical and convenient, present several potential detection biases. For one, patients attending substance abuse clinics or seeking help for their addiction may represent a group of more motivated or more distressed addicts. There is no readily available way to compare those recruited to substance users from the same population not recruited. More general screening strategies such as through a prenatal care or pediatric clinic afford a broader based sampling approach that may include mild to moderate as well as heavy users. On the other hand, including mild to moderate users without attempting to classify their amount of use may likely dilute the percentage of children who may show behavioral effects if the groups are contrasted only as "exposed" or "not exposed." There are no clear solutions to selection biases. These are always more or less present particularly in human teratogenic studies and may or may not limit the generalizability of findings.

A related issue is the link between genetic factors and either the fetus's susceptibility to teratogenic effects of exposure or the adult's susceptibility to exposure, or what Vorhees paraphrasing Wilson's classic principles has labeled the principle of genetic and environmental determinism (Vorhees, 1986b). In animal models, some inbred strains of mice have a greater incidence of birth defects in response to specific exposures, while others show none or a very low response to exposures (Kapron & Trasler, 1997). Selection of these highly susceptible or resistant strains influences the judgments regarding the teratogenicity of a particular agent and very few studies have been conducted that compare in a single experiment the response of different strains to a single teratogen (Vorhees, 1986b). Similar differences in susceptibility seem to pertain for behavioral effects as well and have been reported for alcohol (Gilliam, Kotch, Dudek, & Riley, 1988; Ginsburg, Yanai, & Sze, 1975) and also possibly for diazepam (Driscoll, et al., 1995). Although not well researched, it is also clear that in humans, susceptibility to teratogens such as alcohol or the retinoids varies across individuals and the manifestations of the purported effects may vary in severity and extent (Adams, 1999). These differences are probably due to differences in adult as well as fetal genotype that, for example, may regulate metabolism of the agent in question. Genotypic differences may also regulate the activation of compensatory mechanisms in response to the severity of the insult – the more compensation, the less severe the eventual insult.

Genetic differences in an adult's susceptibility to exposure are possible in several situations. For example, there may well be genetic differences in susceptibility to substance abuse and addiction. Several polymorphisms of dopamine receptors and transporter genes have been associated with addictive behaviors, substance abuse generally, and cocaine and/or alcohol abuse specifically. The A1 allele of the D_2 receptor has been associated more frequently with alcoholism, addictive behaviors, cocaine dependence specifically, and the severity of addiction (Berrettini & Persico, 1996; Comings, et al., 1991; Compton, Anglin, Khalsa-Denison, & Paredes, 1996; Goldman, Urbanek, Guenther, Robin, & Long, 1997; Noble, 1993; Noble, et al., 1993; Smith, et al., 1992; Uhl,

Persisco, & Smith, 1992). Alleles of the D_4 receptor (belonging to the D_2 like group) have also been reported more frequently among substance abusers (George, Cheng, Nguyen, Israel, & O'Dowd, 1993; Muramatsu, Higuchi, Murayama, Matsushita, & Hayashida, 1996). Polymorphisms of the dopamine transporter gene have been associated with cocaine abuse and cocaine-induced paranoia (Gelernter, Kranzler, Satel, & Rao, 1994) as well as attentional and anxiety disorders (Gill, Daly, Heron, Hawi, & Fitzgerald, 1997; Rowe, et al., 1998). Increased susceptibility to the effects of chronic stress as manifest by the symptom cluster of posttraumatic stress disorder may also be conveyed by the same allele of the D_2 receptor (Comings, Muhleman, & Gysin, 1996). The functional significance of this particular dopamine receptor allele is not entirely clear, though carriers of the A1 allele may show reduced receptor density (Noble, Blum, Ritchie, Montgomery, & Sheridan, 1991).

To be sure, substance abuse is not likely to be a monogenic disorder. Rather, it is more likely that these particular alleles working in concert with other genes and environmental contexts convey increased risk for substance abuse in a *certain proportion* of substance users. However, this increased genetic risk is particularly relevant to the offspring of those affected and addicted individuals, for they may convey the same genetic risk (and susceptibility to addiction) to their children. Moreover, the association of this constellation of alleles with susceptibility to the pathogenic effects of stress and to disordered attention and anxiety regulation suggests that this profile of behaviors seen more often among prenatally cocaine-exposed children may for some reflect a genetically based functional alteration in the dopamine system apart from or in addition to the effects of cocaine on monoaminergic ontogeny. Similar attentional/arousal profiles might occur in non–drug-exposed children in the comparison groups who carry these dopamine receptor/transporter alleles. Also, recruiting subjects among heavily addicted populations may oversample for carriers of these different alleles and hence oversample for children who may either be more vulnerable to the behavioral teratogenic properties of cocaine and/or show arousal/attentional regulatory difficulties at least in part on a genetic basis. And of course, in this example, a genetic vulnerability to substance abuse changes the postnatal as well as prenatal environment for the fetus so that there is a potential interaction between the conveyed genetic and environmental alteration that increases the impact of the teratogenic exposure.

The Environmental Context and Conditions Most Related to the Exposure. Sample selection issues and considering the environmental context related to the exposure are closely related issues and particularly important in the human model. In animal models, cross-fostering designs are available to sort through a direct effect of the teratogen on infant behavior versus an indirect effect through alterations in maternal behavior (Vorhees, 1986b; Vorhees & Butcher, 1982). But these models are not available experimentally in studies of humans where often the teratogenic agent may be a marker for particularly compromised environmental conditions that impact how adults are able to care for the infant postnatally. For example, substance abuse of one or multiple drugs rarely occurs isolated from other developmentally salient environmental factors. Parental health during pregnancy is usually compromised and more often than not, substance-using mothers receive little to no prenatal care. Nearly all drugs of abuse during pregnancy may at the very least influence fetal growth and contribute to intrauterine growth retardation and perhaps prematurity (see below for detailed discussions

under individual drugs). Postnatally, important covariates include those broadly describing parental/caregiving function. Indeed, variables such as ongoing parental substance use, neglect and abuse, parental depression, exposure to violence as witness or
victim, homelessness, parental separation and loss are common events for children
growing up in substance-using homes. It is naïve conceptually and statistically to discuss all of these events simply as covariates of prenatal substance exposure. While
they usually co-occur with substance use, they may or may not be related to the outcome of interest. On the other hand, many of these variables probably serve as either
mediators or moderators of the relation between prenatal exposure and later neurocognitive outcome (Baron & Kenny, 1986; Frank, Bresnahan, & Zuckerman, 1993). For
example, infants exposed prenatally to cocaine (see section below as well) appear more
likely to have disorders of arousal or emotional regulation (Mayes, Grillon, Granger, &
Schottenfeld, 1998). The strength of the relationship between prenatal cocaine exposure and the expression of this particular vulnerability may be mediated by the quality
of postnatal care the infant and young child receives.

Considering mediating and moderating variables also brings up the issue of interactive as well as main effect models. Traditionally, neurobehavioral teratology studies
have relied on main effect conceptualizations: How much of the variance of a given
neurodevelopmental outcome is explained by the prenatal exposure status? While important and a first step, most developmental questions relating to prenatal exposure
are probably better addressed as interactions. For example, as already cited, interactions
between caregiving and prenatal exposure may explain more of the variance in neurodevelopmental outcome than main effects alone. Interactions among a given genetic
predisposition (e.g., for attentional disorders), exposure to drugs in utero, and postnatal
neglect define another cluster of effects that are both more generalizable than single
effect, exposure models, and more biologically plausible.

Similarly, the concepts of equifinality and multifinality are particularly important in
considering the relation of environmental conditions (Cicchetti & Rogosch, 1999). Derived from general systems theory, these concepts capture the diversity of developmental pathways possible from a single event or associated with a particular presentation.
In terms of equifinality, a number of different pathways or events may lead to a similar
presentation. So for example, while a particular neurobehavioral teratogen may have
effects on attentional systems with a resulting behavioral profile of impulsivity and
distractability, a similar profile may also result from the impact of a chaotic, neglectful
environment postnatally or the interaction between a level of biological vulnerability
conveyed by the exposure and the environmental conditions into which the infant is
born. Conversely, in terms of multifinality, it is possible to have a given vulnerability
conveyed by a biological event or exposure that is not as severe because of a more
supportive, caring environment for the child. Once again, in cross-fostering animal
models, the impact of these different contexts can be somewhat controlled experimentally but in the human model, these different conditions are crucial variables.

**Selecting Outcomes Most Likely Related to the Mechanism of Action of the Expo-
sure Agent.** This principle has been implicit in several earlier points and in some ways
is obvious. However, outcome variables and timing of outcome measurement have varied widely in traditional neurobehavioral teratology studies in both human and animal
models. Especially in human studies, scientific investigations often reflect cultural or

public biases regarding the harmful nature of the exposure. For example, in studies of substance abuse, longstanding fears regarding the presumed harmful effects of drugs such as alcohol or opium and deep-seated biases that fetuses would pay the price of their mothers' ill ways and misfortunes are often reflected in the initial reports of serious damage in prenatally exposed infants (Mayes, Granger, Bornstein, & Zuckerman, 1992). Indeed, in many instances, hypotheses take shape first in the emotional climate of public fear and conviction about how a given drug affects the adult addict and, thus, how it must by downward extension affect the fetus, infant, and young child.

Because of the effects of public opinion and social standards on the shape and emphasis of scientific studies, the first reports about the consequences of prenatal exposure to a given drug or related environmental toxin often describe far more deleterious and severe outcomes than are true once larger and more carefully defined samples are examined. Later hypotheses are also usually revised based on neurobiologic models for the mechanism of action of the drug or toxin, and the pendulum often swings toward more cautious appraisals of the effects, if any, of a particular prenatal exposure. Thus, the first probands of any epidemic or new illness are often the most severe, most obvious, and least representative of the natural history of a condition. This observation is not limited to neurobehavioral teratology, but nonetheless is particularly relevant to considerations of the effects of drugs such as alcohol, opiates, or cocaine (Day & Richardson, 1993). Studies of the teratologic effects of nearly every drug of abuse have shown this swing in emphasis with the most recent, and perhaps most dramatic example being cocaine (Day & Richardson, 1993; Hutchings, 1993; Mayes, et al., 1992).

Just as profiles of first cohorts may present a picture of more severe impairment, so are the initial outcome variables of study often more globally defined and less linked to hypotheses about pharmacologic action of the drug. The most common neurobehavioral measures are those focusing on cognitive or sensorimotor impairments but less often are specific cognitive functions such as aspects of executive function or affective or social domains chosen for study. For example, besides physical or morphologic impairment, neurobehavioral studies of prenatal drug exposure have most often focused on global measures of intelligence and general developmental functions such as memory, school performance, and incidence of maladaptive behavior. More recently, studies of in utero drug exposure have begun to utilize more functional measures such as reaction time and to focus on individual components of more general functions (e.g., visual versus auditory attention). Outcome measures such as these may be more reflective of hypotheses that are directly linked to understanding the site of action of the drug in the central nervous system.

Finally, it is important to make explicit again that potential behavioral teratogens may exert their effects through different mechanisms acting simultaneously, even interactively. Most often assumed is a direct effects model in which the teratogen directly impairs a specific area of function in the CNS or otherwise. (And parenthetically, even stating a "direct" effect on CNS is far too global a statement that does not allow for the remarkable complexity of any effect on developing neural tissue. As already outlined, the levels of effect in the central nervous system span direct toxicity to developing cells, impaired synapse or connectivity, to facilitated or impaired induction of genes that in turn regulate neural development.)

A second, less often explicitly discussed model is one in which the potential teratogen contributes to a domain of vulnerability that is expressed or not depending on the degree of stress in the environment (a version of multifinality). In this instance, selection of outcome measures needs to assess function both at baseline and under novel challenges. A third model particularly relevant to conditions in which the potential teratogen is also a drug of abuse is that the drug itself may not be teratogenic for the developing fetus. Rather, in this third model, it may be that the context of drug abuse so alters the child's caregiving environment that any presumed teratogenicity is actually expressed through the effects of environmental chaos and deprivation. Outcome assessment needs then to include measures of environmental function such as child-caregiver interaction and/or interviews with parents regarding their perception and understanding of the child's behavior. Assessing environmental function is one of the most difficult challenges in studies of substance-abusing families and at the same time one of the most critical for our efforts to understand how the postnatal environment potentially compounds the potential biological vulnerabilities conveyed by the child's prenatal exposure (Mayes, 1995; Mayes & Bornstein, 1995).

Considering When Exposure-Related Outcomes Are Most Likely to Be Apparent.
Not all behavioral teratogenic effects are apparent in the perinatal period. Some are evident later in development when environmental demands on specific functional domains are higher or when periods of developmentally timed CNS reorganization are occurring. Some neurobehavioral changes are apparent in prepubertal animals and apparently disappear by adulthood, others persist, and a few appear later in development. For example, in the case of fetal diazepam exposure, some effects are not apparent until young adulthood or late adolescence (Kellogg, 1991). In this context, it is important to highlight two general principles. First, the central nervous system continues to develop after the cessation of exposure. Acute differences in neurobiological function and behavior may endure or attenuate with ongoing neural development. Second, compensatory processes are pervasive in central nervous system development. Without these continual microadjustments and compensations that occur during normal neural ontogeny, more functional impairments and developmental failures might occur than is indeed the case. With early drug exposures, these same compensatory mechanisms may promote substantial realignment or correction within other neural systems to allow for the return of some functions. These compensations may not be without costs and may not restore the organism to an average or fully functional state. Indeed, it may be that such neural compensations stabilize functioning under basal conditions, but with stress or challenge, continued deficits may be most apparent (Spear, 1997; Spear, Campbell, Snyder, Silveri, & Katovic, 1998).

Some effects on the CNS may also only be manifest at later stages of development. These are often referred to as latent or "sleeper" effects and examples of these are found both in studies of prenatal alcohol and marijuana exposure (Day, et al., 1994). Certain developmental stages mark periods of neurological reorganization (e.g., puberty, early school age, later half of the first year) and often prove to be important times to look for either latent or exacerbated effects of prenatal exposure. Within latent effects are those functional impairments that are apparent only under stressful, challenging, or novel conditions and are not apparent at baseline. In the work on cocaine in animal models, a considerable body of evidence has accumulated that this pattern may be particularly relevant to the neurotoxicity of cocaine (Spear, et al., 1998).

That subjects may not show possible exposure effects until later and also that early effects may disappear with subsequent development are both strong arguments for longitudinal designs as opposed to cross-sectional samples. Of course, especially in human models, longitudinal designs are more expensive both in terms of actual financial resources and personnel time. Investigative investment is considerable and the time it takes to attain definitive findings or useable results is often long. Maintaining compliance with a cohort is paramount, but challenging especially when the groups studied are populations with considerable comorbid psychopathology and sociodemographic risks such as substance-abusing populations. Especially for studies of neurodevelopmental outcome, it is a challenge to create designs with measures that sample similar behavioral phenomena across developmental phases yet have sufficient fidelity to capture the sometimes subtle changes in function that are potential effects of the teratogen. But cross-sectional designs run the risk of not highlighting important "growth" trends within individuals and of falsely attributing absence or presence of effects. Additionally, while a necessity of scientific study, reporting cross-sectional findings from partial samples in a longitudinal cohort also runs the risk of a bias in the selection of those individuals for the one-time comparison. Again, these cross-sectional snapshots of the data are warranted and important to hypothesis-generating and communication within the scientific community, but these do not adequately describe developmental trajectories within individuals who may have had a discrete perinatal exposure that nonetheless may alter many developmental events downstream years later.

Taking Into Account Those Conditions That Ameliorate or Exacerbate Any Exposure-Related Functional Outcomes. Nearly all behavioral teratogenic effects may be exacerbated or ameliorated by other exposures or environmental conditions such as how the organism is handled or parented or other unexpected events such as illnesses that occur after the exposure period. These issues are particularly important for studies of prenatal drug exposure, for they not only complicate any attempts to relate delays or impairments in postnatal development directly to the prenatal exposure, but more importantly these various postnatal factors are an essential part of the larger context of the substance abusing and hence exposure variable. After children are born, substance abuse has the potential to disrupt parenting behavior, as many abused drugs impede awareness of and sensitivity to environmental cues, interfere with emotion regulation, judgment, aspects of executive functioning, and impair motor skills (Lief, 1985; Miller, Smyth, & Mudar, 1999; Seagull, et al., 1996; Tucker, 1979). All of these capacities are central to providing timely, responsive, and stable parenting for a child. In addition to the direct effects of substance-abuse on parenting behaviors, many parenting problems among substance-abusing adults are also a function of specific psychological and environmental factors that co-occur with the substance abuse (Bernstein & Hans, 1994; Hans, Bernstein, & Henson, 1999; Lester, Boukydis, & Twomey, 2000).

Within the last fifteen years it has become apparent that many substance-abusing individuals suffer from a variety of comorbid psychiatric impairments, such as depression, anxiety, and personality disorders (Kessler, et al., 1997; Rounsaville, et al., 1991; Verheul, et al., 2000), many of which go unidentified and untreated (Kessler, et al., 1996); some have argued that the use of substances such as cocaine and alcohol represents an attempt to treat the symptoms of these disorders. Moreover, for the majority of addicted women, the onset of their psychopathology typically predates their first pregnancy (Beckwith, Howard, Espinosa, & Tyler, 1999; Howard, Beckwith, Espinosa, & Tyler, 1995; Luthar, Cushing, Merikangas, & Rounsaville, 1998) and the onset of substance abuse (Hans, et al., 1999). The nature and type of the psychiatric impairments comorbid with substance abuse may have profound effects both on the individual's choice of drug and on their ability to stop the substance abuse and to lead a more adaptive life (Glantz, 1992; Ziedonis, 1992). Recognizing the underlying psychiatric/psychological contributions to substance abuse may also clarify potential genetic factors that will be influential for the substance-abusing adult's children. For example, a certain proportion of adults using cocaine may do so because stimulant effects ameliorate their problems with attention that are characteristic of attention deficit disorder (Clure, et al., 1999; Khantzian, 1983; Khantzian, Gawin, Kleber, & Riordan, 1984). Similar problems with attention in their children may be due to a potential genetic loading for attention deficit disorder, and may not be related either to the effects of a cocaine-using parenting environment or to the teratogenic effects of cocaine on the child's brain.

Comorbid maternal psychopathology may contribute to greater impairments in parenting interactions among substance-abusing adults compared to non–substance abusers and to those substance abusers with no co-existing psychiatric disturbance. For example, a study of cocaine- and opiate-using mothers and their children found that many of the women had comorbid psychiatric disturbance, and these impairments were significantly related to their children's lower levels of social function and higher levels of disruptive behavior (Luthar, et al., 1998). In another study using a sample of inner-city opioid-addicted mothers, over half of the women met criteria for a personality disorder, and over a third of the sample met criteria for either current or past history of major depression. These diagnoses were linked to insensitive, unresponsive, and punitive parenting styles. Perhaps most important, the children of mothers with comorbid psychopathology (and particularly antisocial personality disorder) rated their mothers as being highly rejecting of them (Hans, et al., 1999). Findings such as these point to the importance of not considering drug use alone as the single determining variable for observed differences in maternal interactive behaviors, but rather as a marker for several predictor variables that are more often associated with substance abuse.

Additional factors comprising adult and parenting function among substance-using adults are the confluence of conditions relating to extreme poverty, homelessness, prostitution, and violence. Multiple studies from substance abuse treatment programs document the high incidence of unemployment and less than a high school education among participating substance-abusing women (Hawley & Disney, 1992). In this population, the rate of unemployment has been shown as high as 96 percent (Suffet & Brotman, 1976). Many report few to no friendships or contacts with supportive persons who are not also substance abusers, and substance-abusing adults often describe long-standing social detachment (Tucker, 1979). The level of violence in substance-abusing families, particularly between women and their spouses or male friends, is markedly high and exposes children to a considerable amount of witnessed violence (Brookoff, O'Brien, Cook, Thompson, & Williams, 1997; Regan, Leifer, & Finnegan, 1982). Notably, there are few data about how often children in substance-abusing families are being reared by a single mother, although the quoted percentages usually exceed 70 percent (Boyd & Mieczkowski, 1990), or how often and in what ways fathers are involved. The reluctance of many substance-abusing adults to reveal details about their households contributes in part to this lack of knowledge, but it also reflects in part the broader lack of adequate data about the family structure in substance-abusing households – how many adults usually care for a child, how many households may a child move among, how often are substance-abusing mothers and their children virtually homeless (Mayes, 1995).

FUTURE DIRECTIONS

The field of neurobehavioral teratology has grown steadily in the last decade, and studies of human models are becoming far more sophisticated in their appreciation of basic developmental neuroscience and the need to consider developmental mechanisms of neural ontogeny as well as simple toxicology. Advances in developmental neuroscience are supporting the development of behavioral and neuropsychological techniques that also permit a more sophisticated approach to behavioral assessment post-exposure. More sophisticated neuroimaging as well as behavioral assessment techniques are making it feasible to examine structural CNS changes in the live subject and to target outcome measures based on the presumed mechanisms of effect. A third area of advance in the field has been the gradual appreciation that for many if not all perinatal exposures, there are critical interactions between the exposure condition and the environment caring for the child. Thus, particularly in humans, rarely are teratogenic exposures simple, discrete, and easily classified. Those investigators embarking on questions about potential behavioral teratogenicity would be well served to reach for the following goals:

1. *Multidisciplinary investigative teams.* The understanding of processes of neural ontogeny has expanded exponentially in the last decade. More information regarding phases of fetal and postnatal brain development has led to refined understanding of vulnerable and critical phases. Developmental neuroscientists can provide the expertise for informed and mechanism-driven hypotheses. Similarly, with the explosion in developmental neuroscience has come a rapid growth in increasingly specific and refined methods for assessing neurocognitive, social, and emotional functions in children. Developmental psychologists and neuropsychologists are essential members of this multidisciplinary team. Other important members of this team are developmental geneticists who can begin to address questions of genetic sources of individual variation in susceptibility to exposures.

2. *Look to preclinical models.* Many have commented on the great divide that usually exists between scientists developing animal models and scientists studying humans. Surely there are marked differences in methods and interpretation of findings and caution always needs to be exerted when translating from preclinical to human models. Nonetheless, many of the methodological issues that are important considerations in the preclinical model also raise the consciousness (if not the frustration) of those studying humans. Examples include thoughts about route of exposure, about the effects of handling, and strain (or genetic) differences. Preclinical models may provide ground for hypotheses in the human model and suggest the most salient mechanisms of effect (Spear, 1993). Although it may not be possible to have those using animal models as active members of the research team, it is important

that the research team be informed and seek consultation from those working with and developing animal models.

3. *Ask mechanism as well as outcome questions.* As we have implied throughout this chapter, studies of potential teratogens may also inform studies of normative developmental processes. This is particularly true if the investigator considers mechanisms of effect and looks for common mechanisms among groups of teratogens. For example, instead of asking how does cocaine influence arousal regulation in exposed children, the mechanism question is does early disruption of the balance between dopaminergic and noradrenergic systems compromise the regulation of prefrontal cortical function in times of stress or challenge (Mayes, 1999). In this way, the question shifts to consideration of how early changes in the ontogeny of dopaminergic and noradrenergic systems compromises later functions and cocaine exposure becomes only one model for how such systems might be disrupted. In other words, this emphasis shifts the investigative team away from solely looking for effects of one agent or another to understanding how disruptions in developmental processes at one or more phases are expressed later in behavior and psychology. Investigators then begin to think about the many ways such disruptions may occur and then look beyond finding specific, discrete teratogens. An emphasis on mechanism moves the field beyond categorizing agents or events as to their "unique" toxicity, an endeavor that potentially does not inform developmental science beyond an increasingly detailed but unintegrated catalogue of sources of developmental injury.

4. *Place exposures in a context.* As we have stated repeatedly, most prenatal exposures are part of a broader context. Adults come to their addictions, their stressful lives, their depression, exposure to environmental toxins as part of a complex, interactive series of events and circumstances. It is a useful, if not overwhelming, scholarly exercise to think through the many preconditions and susceptibility factors for exposures. It is also a crucial challenge for the field to develop strategies and methods for adequately assessing the experiential contexts of different exposures and, even more important, including those environmental variables in statistical models relating exposure to outcome. In human studies, we should be past simple questions of "does X cause Y" but rather should be addressing problems such as "under what conditions is Y more likely to be associated with X versus Z." Here again the concepts of equifinality and multifinality are crucial (Cicchetti & Rogosch, 1999). It is very possible for a given behavioral profile such as arousal regulatory difficulties with impairments in attention to be the result of several different events, including interactions between a prenatal exposure to a given agent and the environmental conditions into which the child was born. Conversely, in terms of multifinality, it is also possible for a child to have a particular vulnerability conveyed by exposure to a teratogenic agent or event during pregnancy (e.g., fetal hypoxia or premature delivery) but that vulnerability is less severely expressed because of the supportive and nurturing environment in which the child lives.

5. *Think dose-response.* Once again, this is a concept more readily studied in the preclinical model, but at least considering it in the human model will force investigators to refine their definition and assessment of their exposure variable. It is crucial for human studies to move beyond a simple metric of exposed–nonexposed to a more sophisticated measurement of amount, timing, and fluctuations in exposures. Seek to study subjects with a range of exposures from the most severe to mild. Also,

where possible consider biological assays of exposure including blood and urine (and breast milk) toxicologies or drug levels.

6. *Look to more sophisticated, mechanism-informed outcome measures.* While in recent years, human studies of potential behavioral teratogens have moved somewhat beyond standard measures of global cognitive abilities or early developmental competencies, there is much work still to be done. This is a latent goal of the interdisciplinary teams that brings to the discussion individuals studying basic developmental processes such as prefrontal cortical functions, affect regulation, social attribution, or specific attachment and parenting behaviors. Also, incorporating challenge techniques such as evoked potentials or startle, functional imaging, biopsychological measures such as heart rate variability, or neurochemistry such as cortisol response allows investigators to study a given domain such as arousal regulation from multiple perspectives. Our ability to characterize functionally important and relevant polymorphisms in families will soon make it imperative to study behavioral genetics profiles – linking phenotype to genotype – as a part of behavioral teratogenic questions.

7. *Move beyond demographic characterizations of environment to examining process.* As we have suggested throughout this review, studies of substance abuse are particularly good examples of how a child's parenting environment exacerbates or ameliorates the teratogenically conveyed vulnerability. But the field is quite far from being able to characterize parenting environments adequately by, for example, proximal measures of parenting behaviors and/or of parents' ability to take their child's perspective. Assessing the child's caregiving environment is a very large undertaking and often is more complex and arduous than the assessment of specific neuropsychological functions. Nonetheless, it is crucial to be able to build models of mediating and moderating effects of early exposures.

8. *Link basic studies with clinical interventions.* This final recommendation or goal is not foreshadowed in what has been said thus far, but represents a shared and implied goal of all teratogenic investigations – to either minimize exposure risk or ameliorate the deleterious effects of the exposure on subsequent development. It is not necessarily the case that investigators studying the effects of a given exposure will also be studying the interventions – indeed, this may not be possible. But just as investigators studying children and their mothers need to collaborate with basic scientists in the definition of basic mechanisms of effects, so should they collaborate with clinicians helping these children and families. Information from behavioral teratologic studies can inform the design and implementation of psychiatric, pediatric, and educational interventions for these children and their families. And clinicians can further add to hypothesis refinement by providing observations from their individual experience with a child and family over time.

Neurobehavioral teratology is a field still in its own developmental transitions, particularly as new methods emerge for studying the elements of complex behaviors and developmental neuroscience continues to elucidate structure-function relations in early brain ontogeny. The field promises fertile intellectual and investigative ground for developmentalists seeking models to study the impact of early developmental disruptions or shifts in expected ontogenetic patterns as well as models for studying up close the process of biology-environment interaction.

REFERENCES

Abel, E. L. (1992). Paternal exposure to alcohol. In *Perinatal substance abuse: Research findings and clinical implications* (ed. Sonderegger, T. B.), pp. 132–160. Baltimore: Johns Hopkins University Press.

Adams, J. (1999). On neurodevelopmental disorders: Perspectives from neurobehavioral teratology. In *Neurodevelopmental disorders* (ed. Tager-Flusberg, H.), pp. 452–468. Cambridge, Mass.: MIT Press.

Adams, P. M., Fabricant, J. D., & Legator, M. S. (1981). Cyclophosphamid-induced speratogenic effects detected in the F1 generation by behavioral testing. *Science* 211, 80–82.

Babor, T. F., Brown, J., & delBoca, F. K. (1990). Validity of self-reports in applied research on addictive behaviors: Fact or fiction? *Behavioral Assessment* 12, 5–31.

Baron, R. & Kenny, D. (1986). The moderator-mediator variable distinction in social psychological research: Conceptual, strategic, and statistical considerations. *Journal of Personality and Social Psychology* 51, 1173–1182.

Bauer, W. (1957, 1979). *A Greek-English lexicon of the New Testament and early christian literature.* Chicago: University of Chicago Press.

Beckwith, L., Howard, J., Espinosa, M., & Tyler, R. (1999). Psychopathology, mother-child interaction, and infant development: Substance-abusing mothers and their offspring. *Development and Psychopathology* 11, 715–725.

Bender, S. L., Word, C. O., DiClemente, R. J., Crittenden, M. R., Persaud, N. A., & Ponton, L. E. (1995). The developmental implications of prenatal and/or postnatal crack cocaine exposure in preschool children: A preliminary report. *Journal of Developmental and Behavioral Pediatrics* 16, 418–424.

Bernstein, V. & Hans, S. (1994). Predicting the developmental outcome of two-year-old children born exposed to methadone: Impact of social-environmental risk factors. *Journal of Clinical Child Psychology* 23, 349–359.

Berrettini, W. & Persico, A. (1996). Dopamine D2 receptor gene polymorphisms and vulnerability to substance abuse. *Biological Psychiatry* 40, 144–147.

Boyd, C. & Mieczkowski, T. (1990). Drug use, health, family, and social support in "crack" cocaine users. *Addictive Behavior* 15, 481–415.

Brookoff, D., O'Brien, K., Cook, C. S., Thompson, T. D., & Williams, C. (1997). Characteristics of participants in domestic violence. *Journal of the American Medical Association* 277, 1369–1373.

Butcher, R. E. (1985). A historical perspective on behavioral teratology. *Neurobehavior, Teratology, & Toxicology* 7, 537–540.

Butcher, R. E., Hawver, K., Burbacher, T., & Scott, W. (1975). Behavioral effects from antenatal exposure to teratogens. In *Aberrant development in infancy: Human and infant studies* (ed. Ellis, N. R.). Hillsdale, N.J.: Erlbaum.

Callahan, C. M., Grant, T. M., Phipps, P., Clark, G., Novack, A. H., Streissguth, A. P., & Raisys, V. A. (1992). Measurement of gestational cocaine exposure: Sensitivity of infants' hair, meconium, and urine. *Journal of Pediatrics* 120, 763–768.

Carey, K. (1997). Clinical rating scales for substance abuse. *Psychiatric Services* 48, 106–107.

Chasnoff, I., Landress, H., & Barrett, M. (1990). The prevalence of illicit drug or alcohol use during pregnancy and discrepancies in mandatory reporting in Pinellas County, Florida. *New England Journal of Medicine* 322, 1202–1206.

Cicchetti, D. & Rogosch, F. A. (1999). Psychopathology as risk for adolescent substance use disorders: A developmental psychopathology perspective. *Journal of Clinical Child Psychology* 28, 355–365.

Clure, C., Brady, K. T., Saladin, M. E., Johnson, D., Waid, R., & Rittenbury, M. (1999). Attention deficit/hyperactivity disorder and substance use: Symptoms pattern and drug choice. *American Journal of Drug and Alcohol Abuse* 25, 441–448.

Comings, D. E., Comings, B. G., Muhleman, D., Dietz, G., Shahbahrami, B., Tast, D., Knell, E., Kocsis, P., Baumgarten, R., Kovacs, B. W., Levy, D. L., Smith, M., Borison, R. K., Evans, D., Klein, D. N., MacMurray, J., Tosk, J. M., Sverd, J., Gysin, R., & Flanagan, S. D. (1991). The Dopamine D2 receptor locus as a modifying gene in neuropsychiatric disorders. *Journal of the American Medical Association* 266, 1793–1800.

Comings, D. E., Muhleman, D., & Gysin, R. (1996). Dopamine receptor (DRD2) gene and suscepti-bility to postraumatic stress disorder: A study and replication. *Biological Psychiatry* 40, 368–372.

Compton, P. A., Anglin, M. D., Khalsa-Denison, E., & Paredes, A. (1996). The D2 dopamine receptor gene, addiction, and personality: Clinical correlates in cocaine abusers. *Biological Psychiatry* 39, 302–304.

Day, N. & Richardson, G. (1993). Cocaine use and crack babies: Science, the media, and miscom-munication. *Neurotoxicology and Teratology* 15, 293–294.

Day, N., Richardson, G., Goldschmidt, L., Robles, N., Taylor, P., Stoffer, D., Cornelius, M., & Geva, D. (1994). The effect of prenatal marijuana exposure on the cognitive development of offspring at age three. *Neurotoxicology and Teratology* 16, 169–175.

DeVane, C. L., Simpkins, J. W., Miller, R. L., & Braun, S. B. (1989). Tissue distribution of cocaine in the pregnant rat. *Life Sciences* 45, 1271–1276.

Dietrich, K. N. (1999). Environmental toxins and child development. In *Neurodevelopmental dis-orders* (ed. Tager-Flusberg, H.), pp. 469–490. Cambridge, Mass.: MIT Press.

Dow-Edwards, D. L., Freed, L. A., & Milhorat, T. H. (1988). Stimulation of brain metabolism by perinatal cocaine exposure. *Devopmental Brain Research* 42, 137–141.

Driscoll, P., Ferre, P., Fernandez-Teruel, A., & Levi de Stein, M. (1995). Effects of prenatal diazepam on two-way avoidance behavior, swimming navigation and brain levels of benzodiazepine-like molecules in male Roman high- and low-avoidance rats. *Psychopharmacology* 122, 51–57.

Frank, D. A., Augustyn, M., & Zuckerman, B. (1998). Neonatal neurobehavioral and neuroanatomic correlates of prenatal cocaine exposure. Problems of dose and confounding. *Annals of the New York Academy of Science* 846, 40–50.

Frank, D. A., Bresnahan, K., & Zuckerman, B. S. (1993). Maternal cocaine use: Impact on child health and development. *Advances in Pediatrics* 40, 65–99.

Garg, U. C., Turndorf, H., & Bansinath, M. (1993). Effect of cocaine on macromolecular syntheses and cell proliferation in cultured glial cells. *Neuroscience* 57, 467–472.

Gelernter, J., Kranzler, H. R., Satel, S. L., & Rao, P. A. (1994). Genetic association between dopamine transporter protein alleles and cocaine-induced paranoia. *Neuropsychopharmacology* 11, 195–200.

George, S., Cheng, R., Nguyen, T., Israel, Y., & O'Dowd, B. (1993). Polymorphisms of the D4 dopamine receptor alleles in chronic alcoholism. *Biochemical and Biophysical Research Commu-nications* 196, 107–1114.

Gill, M., Daly, G., Heron, S., Hawi, Z., & Fitzgerald, M. (1997). Confirmation of association between attention deficit hyperactivity disorder and a dopamine transporter polymorphism. *Molecular Psychiatry* 2, 311–313.

Gilliam, D. M., Kotch, L. E., Dudek, B. C., & Riley, E. P. (1988). Ethanol teratogenesis in mice selected for differences in alcohol sensitivity. *Alcohol* 5, 513–519.

Ginsburg, B. E., Yanai, J., & Sze, P. Y. (1975). A developmental genetic study of the effects of alcohol consumed by parent mice on the behavior and development of their offspring. In *Proceedings of the Fourth Annual Alcoholism Conference of the National Institute on Alcohol Abuse and Alcoholism*, pp. 183–204. Washington, D.C.: Department of Health, Education, and Welfare.

Glantz, M. D. (1992). A developmental psychopathology model of drug abuse vulnerability. In *Vulnerability to Drug Abuse* (ed. Glantz, M. D. and Pickens, R. W.), pp. 389–418. Washington, D.C.: American Psychological Association Press.

Goldman, D., Urbanek, M., Guenther, D., Robin, R., & Long, J. C. (1997). Linkage and association of a functional DRD2 variant and DRD2 markers to alcoholism, substance abuse, and schizophrenia in Southwestern American indians. *American Journal of Medical Genetics* 74, 386–394.

Graham, K., Koren, G., Klein, J., Schneiderman, J., & Greenwald, M. (1989). Determination of gestational cocaine exposure by hair analysis. *Journal of the American Medical Association* 262, 3328–3330.

Greenough, W. T. (1991). Experience as a component of normal development: Evolutionary con-siderations. *Developmental Psychology* 27, 14–17.

Greenough, W. T., Black, J. E., Klintsova, A., Bates, K. E., & Weiler, I. J. (1999). Experience and plasticity in brain structure: Possible implications of basic research findings for developmental disorders. In *The changing nervous system: Neurobehavioral consequences of early brain disorders* (ed. Broman, S. H. and Fletcher, J. M.), pp. 51–70. New York: Oxford University Press.

Greenough, W. T., Black, J. E., & Wallace, C. S. (1987). Experience and brain development. *Child Development* 58, 539–559.

Grissom, G. (1997). Treatment outcomes in inpatient and substance abuse programs. *Psychiatric Annals* 27, 113–118.

Hans, S. L., Bernstein, V. J., & Henson, L. G. (1999). The role of psychopathology in the parenting of drug-dependent women. *Development and Psychopathology* 11, 957–977.

Hawley, T. L. & Disney, E. R. (1992). Crack's children: The consequences of maternal cocaine abuse. *Social Policy Report of the Society for Research in Child Development* 6, 1–22.

Howard, J., Beckwith, L., Espinosa, M., & Tyler, R. (1995). Development of infants born to cocaine-abusing women: Biologic/maternal influences. *Neurotoxicology and Teratology* 17, 403–411.

Hutchings, D. E. (1993). The puzzle of cocaine's effects following maternal use during pregnancy: Are there reconcilable differences? [see comments]. *Neurotoxicology and Teratology* 15, 281–286.

Kapron, C. M. & Trasler, D. G. (1997). Genetic determinants of teratogen-induced abnormal development in mouse and rat embryos in vitro. *International Journal of Developmental Biology* 41, 337–344.

Kellogg, C. K. (1991). Postnatal effects of prenatal exposure to psychoactive drugs. *Pre- & Peri-Natal Psychology Journal* 5, 233–251.

Kellogg, C., Tervo, D., Ison, J., Parisi, T., & Miller, R. K. (1980). Prenatal exposure to diazepam alters behavioral development in rats. *Science* 207, 205–207.

Kessler, R. C., Crum, R. M., Warner, L. A., Nelson, C. B., Schulenberg, J., & Anthony, J. C. (1997). Lifetime co-occurrence of DSM-III-R alcohol abuse and dependence with other psychiatric disorders in the National Comorbidity Survey. *Archives of General Psychiatry* 54, 313–321.

Kessler, R. C., Nelson, C. B., McGonagle, K. A., Edlund, M. J., Frank, R. G., & Leaf, P. J. (1996). The epidemiology of co-occurring addictive and mental disorders: Implications for prevention and service utilization. *American Journal of Orthopsychiatry* 66, 17–31.

Khantzian, E. J. (1983). An extreme case of cocaine dependence and marked improvement with methylphenidate treatment. *American Journal of Psychiatry* 140, 784–785.

Khantzian, E. J., Gawin, F., Kleber, H. D., & Riordan, C. E. (1984). Methylphenidate treatment of cocaine dependence – a preliminary report. *Journal of Substance Abuse Treatment* 1, 107–112.

King, T. A., Perlman, J. R., Laptook, A. R., Rollins, N., Jackson, G., & Little, B. (1995). Neurologic manifestations of in utero cocaine exposure in near-term and term infants. *Pediatrics* 96, 259–264.

Kjarasch, S. J., Glotzer, D., Vinci, R., Wietzman, M., & Sargent, T. (1991). Unsuspected cocaine exposure in children. *American Journal of Diseases of Children* 145, 204–206.

Kline, J., Ng, S., Schittini, M., Levin, B., & Susser, M. (1997). Cocaine use during pregnancy: Sensitive detection by hair assay. *American Journal of Public Health* 87, 352–358.

Kosofsky, B. (1991). The effect of cocaine on developing human brain. *National Institute Drug Abuse Monograph Series* 114, 128–143.

Kreek, M. J. (1996). Cocaine, dopamine, and the endogenous opioid system. *Journal of Addictive Diseases* 15, 73–96.

Kristensen, J. H., Ilett, K. F., Hackett, L. P., Yapp, P., Paech, M., & Begg, E. J. (1999). Distribution and excretion of fluoxetine and norfluoxetine in human milk. *British Journal of Clinical Pharmacology* 48, 521–527.

Lester, B. M., Boukydis, C. Z., & Twomey, J. (2000). Maternal substance abuse and child outcome. In *Handbook of infant mental health* (ed. Zeanah, C. H.), pp. 161–175. New York: Guilford Press.

Levy, M. & Koren, G. (1990). Obstetric and neonatal effects of drugs of abuse. *Emergency Medicine Clinics of North America* 8, 633–652.

Levy, M. & Koren, G. (1992). Clinical toxicology of the neonate. *Seminars in Perinatology* 16, 63–75.

Lief, N. R. (1985). The drug user as parent. *International Journal of the Addictions* 20, 63–97.

Lustbader, A. S., Mayes, L. C., McGee, B. A., Jatlow, P., & Roberts, W. L. (1998). Incidence of passive exposure to crack/cocaine and clinical findings in infants seen in an outpatient service. *Pediatrics* 102, 1.

Luthar, S. S., Cushing, G., Merikangas, K. R., & Rounsaville, B. J. (1998). Multiple jeopardy: Risk and protective factors among addicted mothers' offspring. *Development and Psychopathology* 10, 117–136.

Mactutus, C. F. & Tilson, H. A. (1986). Psychogenic and neurogenic abnormalities after perinatal insecticide exposure: A critical review. In *Handbook of behavioral teratology* (ed. Riley, E. P. and Voorhees, C. V.), pp. 335–383. New York: Plenum.

Mayes, L. C. (1995). Substance abuse and parenting. In *The handbook of parenting* (ed. Bornstein, M.), pp. 101–125. Hillsdale, N.J.: Erlbaum.

Mayes, L. C. (1999). Developing brain and in-utero cocaine exposure: Effects on neural ontogeny. *Development and Psychopathology* 11, 685–714.

Mayes, L. C. & Bornstein, M. H. (1995). Developmental dilemmas for cocaine-abusing parents and their children. In *Mothers, babies, and cocaine: The role of toxins in development* (ed. Lewis, M. and Bendersky, M.), pp. 251–272. Hillsdale, N.J.: Erlbaum.

Mayes, L. C. & Fahy, T. (2001). Prenatal drug exposure and cognitive development. In *Environmental effects on cognitive abilities* (ed. Sternberg, R. J. and Grigorenko, E. L.), pp. 189–220. Mahwah, N.J.: Erlbaum.

Mayes, L. C., Granger, R. H., Bornstein, M. H., & Zuckerman, B. (1992). The problem of prenatal cocaine exposure. A rush to judgment. *Journal of the American Medical Association* 267, 406–408.

Mayes, L. C., Grillon, C., Granger, R., & Schottenfeld, R. (1998). Regulation of arousal and attention in preschool children exposed to cocaine prenatally. *Annals of the New York Academy of Science* 846, 126–143.

McBride, W. G. (1977). Thalidomide embryopathy. *Teratology* 16, 79–82.

McFie, J. & Robertson, J. (1973). Psychological test results of children with thalidomide deformities. *Developmental Medicine and Child Neurology* 15, 719–727.

Middahugh, L. D. (1986). Prenatal phenobarbital: Effects on pregnancy and offspring. In *Handbook of behavioral teratology* (ed. Riley, E. P. and Voorhees, C. V.), pp. 243–263. New York: Plenum.

Miller, B. A., Smyth, N. J., & Mudar, P. J. (1999). Mothers' alcohol and other drug problems and their punitiveness toward their children. *Journal of Studies on Alcohol* 60, 632–642.

Moore, T. R., Sorg, J., Miller, L., Key, T. C., & Resnik, R. (1986). Hemodynamic effects of intravenous cocaine on the pregnant ewe and fetus. *American Journal of Obstetrics and Gynecology* 155, 883–888.

Muramatsu, T., Higuchi, S., Murayama, M., Matsushita, S., & Hayashida, M. (1996). Association between alcoholism and the dopamine D4 receptor gene. *Journal of Medical Genetics* 33, 113–115.

Nelson, B. K. (1981). Dose/effect relationships in developmental neurotoxicology. *Neurobehavioral Toxicology and Teratology* 3, 255.

Nelson, B. K. (1990). Origins of behavioral teratology and distinctions between research on pharmaceutical agents and environmental/industrial chemicals. *Neurotoxicology and Teratology* 12, 301–305.

Noble, E. P. (1993). The D2 dopamine receptor gene: A review of association studies in alcoholism. *Behavioral Genetics* 23, 119–129.

Noble, E. P., Blum, K., Khalsa, M. E., Ritchie, T., Montgomery, A., Wood, R. C., Fitch, R. J., Ozkaragoz, T., Sheridan, P. J., Anglin, M. D., Paredes, A., Treiman, L. J., & Sparkes, R. S. (1993). Allelic association of the D2 dopamine receptor gene with cocaine dependence. *Drug and Alcohol Dependence* 33, 271–285.

Noble, E. P., Blum, K., Ritchie, T., Montgomery, A., & Sheridan, P. J. (1991). Allelic association of the D2 dopamine receptor gene with receptor binding characteristics in alcoholism. *Archives of General Psychiatry* 48, 648–654.

Ostrea, E. M. (1995). Meconium drug analysis. In *Mothers, babies and cocaine: The role of toxins in development* (ed. Lewis, M. and Bendersky, M.), pp. 179–202. Hillsdale, N.J.: Erlbaum.

Oxford English Dictionary, 2nd edition (ed. Simpson, J. A. and Weiner, E. S. C.). Oxford: Oxford University Press, 1989.

Rees, D. C., Francis, E. Z., & Kimmel, C. A. (1990). Scientific and regulatory issues relevant to assessing risk for developmental neurotoxicity: An overview. *Neurotoxicology and Teratology* 12, 175–181.

Regan, D., Leifer, B., & Finnegan, L. (1982). Generations at risk: Violence in the lives of pregnant drug abusing women. *Pediatric Research* 16, 91.

Reith, M. E. A. (1988). Cocaine receptors on monoamine transporters and sodium channels. *NIDA Research Monograph* 88, 23–41.

Richardson, G. & Day, N. (1994). Detrimental effects of prenatal cocaine exposure: Illusion or reality? *Journal of the American Academy of Child and Adolescent Psychiatry* 33, 28–34.

Richardson, G., Day, M., & McGauhey, P. (1993). The impact of prenatal marijuana and cocaine use on the infant and child. *Clinical Obstetrics and Gynecology* 36, 302–318.

Rogers, R. & Kelly, K. S. (1997). Denial and misreporting of substance abuse. In *Clinical assessment of malingering and deception* (ed. Rogers, R.), pp. 108–129. New York: Guilford Press.

Rounsaville, B. J., Anton, S. F., Carroll, K., Budde, D., Prusoff, B. A., & Gawin, F. (1991). Psychiatric disorders of treatment-seeking cocaine abusers. *Archives of General Psychiatry* 48, 43–51.

Rowe, D. C., Stever, C., Gard, J. M., Cleveland, H. H., Sanders, M. L., Abramowitz, A., Kozol, S. T., Mohr, J. H., Sherman, S. L., & Waldman, I. D. (1998). The relation of the dopamine transporter gene (DAT1) to symptoms of internalizing disorders in children. *Behavior Genetics* 28, 215–225.

Schmidt, K., Olesen, O. V., & Jensen, P. N. (2000). Citalopram and breast-feeding: Serum concentration and side effects in the infant. *Biological Psychiatry* 47, 164–165.

Seagull, F. N., Mowery, J. L., Simpson, P. M., Robinson, R. R., Martier, S. S., Sokol, R. J., & McGarver-May, D. G. (1996). Maternal assessment of infant development: Associations with alcohol and drug use in pregnancy. *Clinical Pediatrics* 35, 621–628.

Shippenberg, T. S. & Rea, W. (1997). Sensitization to the behavioral effects of cocaine: modulation by dynorphin and kappa-opioid receptor agonists. *Pharmacology, Biochemistry and Behavior* 57, 449–455.

Smith, S. S., OHara, B. F., Persico, A. M., Gorelick, D. A., Newlin, D. B., Vlahov, D., Solomon, L., Pickens, R., & Uhl, G. R. (1992). Genetic vulnerability to drug abuse: The D2 dopamine receptor Taq I B1 restriction length polymorphism appears more frequently in polysubstance abusers. *Archnives of General Psychiatry* 49, 723–727.

Spear, L. P. (1993). Missing pieces of the puzzle complicate conclusions about cocaine's neurobehavioral toxicity in clinical populations: Importance of animal models [comment]. *Neurotoxicology and Teratology* 15, 307–309; discussion 311–302.

Spear, L. P. (1997). Neurobehavioral abnormalities following exposure to drugs of abuse during development. In *Drug addiction and its treatment: Nexus of neuroscience and behavior* (ed. Johnson, B. A. and Roache, J. D.), pp. 233–255. Philadelphia: Lippincott-Raven.

Spear, L. P., Campbell, J., Snyder, K., Silveri, M., & Katovic, N. (1998). Animal behavior models. Increased sensitivity to stressors and other environmental experiences after prenatal cocaine exposure. *Annals of the New York Academy of Science* 846, 76–88.

Spear, L. P., Kirstein, C. L., & Frambes, N. A. (1989). Cocaine effects on the developing central nervous system: Behavioral, psychopharmacological, and neurochemical studies. *Annals of the New York Academy of Science* 562, 290–307.

Spyker, J. M. (1975). Behavioral teratology and toxicology. In *Behavioral toxicology* (ed. Weiss, B. and Laties, V. G.), pp. 311–344. New York: Plenum.

Suffet, F. & Brotman, R. (1976). Employment and social disability among opiate addicts. *American Journal of Drug and Alcohol Abuse* 3, 387–395.

Tronick, E. Z., Frank, D. A., Cabral, H., Mirochnick, M., & Zuckerman, B. (1996). Late dose-response effects of prenatal cocaine exposure on newborn neurobehavioral performance. *Pediatrics* 98, 76–83.

Tucker, M. B. (1979). A descriptive and comparative analysis of the social support structure of heroin addicted women. Addicted women: Family dynamics, self-perceptions, and support systems (ed. NIDA), pp. 37–76. Washington, D.C.: U.S. Government Printing Office.

Uhl, G. R., Persisco, A. M., & Smith, S. S. (1992). Current excitement with D2 dopamine receptor gene alleles in substance abuse. *Archives General Psychiatry* 49, 157–160.

Verheul, R., Kranzler, H. R., Poling, J., Tenne, H., Ball, S., & Rounsaville, B. J. (2000). Co-occurrence of Axis I and Axis II disorders in substance abusers. *Acta Psychiatrica Scandinavica* 101, 110–118.

Volpe, J. (1987). *Neurology of the newborn*. Phildelphia: WB Saunders.

Vorhees, C. V. (1974). Some behavioral effects of maternal hypervitaminosis A in rats. *Teratology* 10, 269–274.

Vorhees, C. V. (1986). Origins of behavioral teratology. In *Handbook of behavioral teratology* (ed. Riley, E. P. and Vorhees, C. V.), pp. 3–22. New York: Plenum.

Vorhees, C. V. (1986a). Behavioral teratology of anticonvulsant and antianxiety medications. In *Handbook of behavioral teratology* (ed. Riley, E. P. and Vorhees, C. V.). New York: Plenum.

Vorhees, C. V. (1986b). Principles of behavioral teratology. In *Handbook of behavioral teratology* (ed. Riley, E. P. and Vorhees, C. V.), pp. 23–48. New York: Plenum.

Vorhees, C. V. (1986c). Comparison and critique of government regulations for behavioral teratology. In *Handbook of behavioral teratology* (ed. Riley, E. P. and Vorhees, C. V.). New York: Plenum.

Vorhees, C. V. (1986d). Behavioral teratology of anticonvulsant and antianxiety medications. In *Handbook of behavioral teratology* (ed. Riley, E. P. and Vorhees, C. V.), pp. 211–242. New York: Plenum.

Vorhees, C. V., Brunner, R. L., & Butcher, R. E. (1979). Psychotropic drugs as behavioral teratogens. *Science* 205, 1220–1225.

Vorhees, C. V. & Butcher, R. E. (1982). Behavioral teratogenicity. In *Developmental toxicology* (ed. Snell, K.). New York: Praeger.

Vorhees, C. V. & Mollnow, E. (1987). Behavioral teratogenesis: Long-term influences on behavior from early exposure to environmental agents. In *Handbook of infant development* (ed. Osofsky, J.), pp. 913–971. New York: Wiley.

Warkany, J. (1977). History of teratology. In *General principles and etiology*, vol. 1 (ed. Wilson, J. G. and Fraser, F. C.), pp. 3–45. New York: Plenum.

Warkany, J. (1978). Terathanasia. *Teratology* 17, 187–192.

Warkany, J., Lemire, R. J., & Cohen, M. M. (1981). *Mental retardation and congenital malformations of the central nervous system*. Chicago: Year Book Medical Publishers.

Wee, E. L. & Zimmerman, E. F. (1983). Involvement of GABA in palate morphogenesis and its relation to diazepam teratogenesis in two mouse strains. *Teratology* 28, 15–22.

Weiss, R. D., Najavits, L. M., Greenfield, S. F., Soto, J. A., Shaw, S. R., & Wyner, D. (1998). Validity of substance use self-reports in dually diagnosed outpatients. *American Journal of Psychiatry* 155, 127–128.

White, F. J., Hu, X. T., Zhang, X. F., & Wolf, M. E. (1995). Repeated administration of cocaine or amphetamine alters neuronal responses to glutamate in the mesoaccumbens dopamine system. *Journal of Pharmacology & Experimental Therapeutics* 273, 445–454.

Wilson, J. G. (1973). *Environment and birth defects*. New York: Academic Press.

Wilson, J. G. (1977). Current status of teratology – General priniciples and mechanisms derived from animal studies. In *Handbook of teratology*, vol. 1 (ed. Wilson, J. G. and Fraser, F. C.), pp. 47–74. New York: Plenum.

Woods, J. R., Jr., Plessinger, M. A., & Clark, K. E. (1987). Effect of cocaine on uterine blood flow and fetal oxygenation. *Journal of the American Medical Association* 257, 957–961.

Ye, J. H., Liu, P. L., Wu, W. H., & McArdle, J. J. (1997). Cocaine depresses GABAA current of hippocampal neurons. *Brain Research* 770, 169–175.

Ziedonis, D. M. (1992). Comorbid psychopathology and cocaine addiction. In *Clinician's guide to cocaine addiction* (ed. Kosten, T. R. and Kleber, H. D.), pp. 335–358. New York: Guilford Press.

TWO

The Neurodevelopmental Consequences of Very Preterm Birth

Brain Plasticity and Its Limits

Chiara Nosarti, Larry Rifkin, and Robin M. Murray

In this chapter, we will discuss the long-term consequences of being born very early or very small. This issue is relevant to those interested in developmental psychopathology as this area of research emphasizes the understanding of the mechanisms underlying the development of pathology in high-risk individuals, as well as the pathways to competent adaptation despite exposure to conditions of adversity.

Studies in the United States and others have shown that rates of low birth weight increase with decreasing socioeconomic status (e.g., Paneth, 1995). At the individual level, women belonging to lower socioeconomic strata are at significantly higher risk of preterm delivery, even after controlling for other known risk factors such as weight, weight gain, alcohol and tobacco consumption, ethnicity, parity, and source of prenatal care. At the geographic level, for any defined area, the more socioeconomically disadvantaged the population, the higher the incidence of preterm delivery and low birth weight. Socio-demographic factors, such as maternal education and family income, may be related to a less favorable neuropsychological outcome in low birth weight and preterm children, as well as in normal birth weight children (Sameroff, Seifer, Barocas, Zax, & Greenspan, 1987). In addition, a considerable proportion of preterm children are treated by intensive care and sustain some brain injuries and subsequent neurological and neuropsychological impairment. However, even in the absence of major neurological deficits, preterm and low birth weight children seem to be at risk of developing a variety of cognitive and behavioral problems in childhood. The population that will be explored in this chapter is thus at increased biological risk; in other words, it is vulnerable to the development of neuropsychological deficits prior to their actual emergence.

Biological risk is an important concept in developmental neuropsychology, as before a psychopathological condition manifests, specific aspects of development may depart from their usual course and form the basis for subsequent pathology (Cicchetti & Rogosch, 1996; Sroufe, 1989). Preterm and low birth weight children, being at biological risk, may have difficulties in coping and successfully adapting to their environment in the course of development, and the relationship with their caregivers may be negatively affected (Bennet, 1987). Individuals at high biological risk are not always maladjusted, as in several instances they reach normal adaptation:

According to the principle of resilience (e.g., Cicchetti and Garmezy, 1993), such individuals may still be able to overcome severe stressors and develop successful functioning.

It is important to understand the contributing factors to adaptive or maladaptive outcomes in any individual, the various degrees in which these factors affect different individuals, such as heterogeneity in outcome (concept of multifinality), and the way several different pathways may lead to similar outcomes (concept of equifinality, e.g., Cicchetti & Cannon, 1999; Cicchetti & Rogosch, 1996). The understanding of both adaptation and maladaptation is central to developmental psychopathology, as this approach emphasizes the mutual interplay between normality and psychopathology. In order to elucidate psychopathology, it is necessary to have an understanding of the normal functioning used as a term of comparison. Therefore, not only can the study of normal biological, social, and psychological adaptation be useful in identifying, treating, and hopefully preventing the development of psychopathology, but also the departures from normal adaptation, which characterize psychopathology, can improve our understanding of normal development.

In this chapter we will particularly focus on a study in which we are investigating the neurological, neuroradiological, cognitive, and behavioral outcomes of large groups of very preterm individuals who have now reached adolescence.

EARLY EVENTS AND ADULT PSYCHOSIS

Over the last two decades, there has been a good deal of research into whether exposure to pre- and perinatal complications predisposes individuals to later psychiatric disorders, particularly schizophrenia (Lewis & Murray, 1987; McGrath & Murray, 1995; McNeil & Kaij, 1978). Most of the studies which have addressed this question have been small retrospective case-control studies in which series of schizophrenic patients have been compared with other psychiatric patients, siblings, or normal controls (see Geddes & Lawrie, 1995). The vast majority of such studies have reported a positive association between a range of pre- and perinatal complications (collectively termed obstetric complications or OCs) and schizophrenia; however, these studies have been much criticized (e.g., Sacker, Done, Crow, & Golding, 1995).

A recent large meta-analysis of individual data from eleven studies using similar methodology (Geddes et al., 1999) confirmed that adult schizophrenics are more likely than controls to have experienced OCs; unfortunately, the data on OCs was again obtained from mothers retrospectively. Two studies examined the birth records of population cohorts and compared those who became schizophrenic with those who did not, and initially reported no association between OCs and schizophrenia. However, the methodology and interpretation of the first, by Sacker et al. (1995), was contentious, whereas the second group of investigators (Buka, Tsuang, & Lipsitt, 1993) subsequently reversed their conclusions after more detailed and systematic enquiry (Buka & Fan, 1999).

Three recent large epidemiological studies have helped to clarify the issue and address the criticisms raised about previous research. The first, by Jones, Rantakallio, Hartikainen, Isohanni, and Sipila (1998), reviewed the psychiatric status of all children born in North Finland in 1966 and showed that those babies deemed to be of low birth weight (defined as $< 2,000$ g) were 6.2 times more likely to develop schizophrenia, after adjusting for possible confounders such as sex, socioeconomic status at birth, maternal depression, and maternal smoking. Perinatal brain damage carried a 6.9 times increased risk.

Subsequently, Hultman, Sparen, Takei, Murray, and Cnattingius (1999) examined potential risk factors for schizophrenia and affective and reactive psychosis. These included: (a) pregnancy and delivery factors; (b) child characteristics and season of birth; as well as (c) mother characteristics. This study had a large population based case-control design, which included all children born during 1973–1979 in Sweden. Data were extracted from the national birth register, which contains information on 99 percent of all births in Sweden. For each subject diagnosed with schizophrenia, affective and reactive psychosis, five controls were assessed. Being small for gestational age and maternal bleeding during pregnancy were associated with increased risk of schizophrenia in males; the case was not so strong for females. Affective and reactive forms of psychosis were only weakly associated with OCs.

In a second Swedish study, Dalman, Allebeck, Cullberg, Grunewald, and Koster (1999) carried out a large longitudinal study of individuals born during 1973–1977 who received a diagnosis of schizophrenia during 1987–1995 ($n = 238$). Risk factors were grouped according to three different etiologic mechanisms: malnutrition during foetal life, extreme prematurity, and hypoxia or ischemia. The results implicated all three etiologic mechanisms, although the effects were only modest. The most important risk factor for schizophrenia, after controlling for all potential confounders, was pre-eclampsia.

Numerous brain imaging studies have shown that patients with schizophrenia have an excess of cerebral structural abnormalities. Reductions in whole brain volume, cortical grey matter, temporal lobe, hippocampal/amygdala formation, and increases in lateral and third ventricle volumes are the most commonly reported findings (e.g., Lawrie & Abukmeil, 1998; Velakoulis et al., 1999; Wright et al., 2000). Some, but not all, studies have reported that those schizophrenic patients with obvious brain abnormalities are particularly likely to have experienced OCs (reviewed by McGrath & Murray, 1995). Perhaps the clearest evidence comes from a study in which Stefanis et al. (1999) compared volumetric magnetic resonance imaging (MRI) measurements of the hippocampi in two groups of schizophrenic patients and normal controls. The first group was comprised of patients with no family history of schizophrenia but who had experienced OCs. The second group was made up of patients with no history of OCs but who came from families multiply affected with schizophrenia. Thus, the study compared two groups of schizophrenic patients, respectively, at high obstetric and genetic risk. Reduction of the left hippocampal volume was associated with schizophrenia, but only in patients with a history of OCs. A graded relationship was observed between hippocampal volume and the onset of psychosis: the smaller the volume, the earlier the onset.

The above studies obviously raise the questions of (a) whether subjects exposed to obstetric hazards grow up to have an increased risk of psychotic illness in particular, and psychiatric illness in general; and (b) whether any associations between obstetric hazards and psychiatric illness are mediated by structural brain damage incurred in the pre- or perinatal period.

PRETERM AND LOW BIRTH WEIGHT BABIES

To our knowledge, no adequate study has taken a series of babies who are exposed to severe obstetric complications and prospectively followed them into adult life with brain imaging both at birth and at follow-up. This is mainly because high-quality neuroimaging techniques are a relatively recent invention. Nevertheless, it is unfortunate because the advent of neonatal care has meant that increasing numbers of babies exposed to severe obstetric hazards are now surviving.

Prevalence, Survival, and Mortality

The percentage of babies who are being born preterm and surviving in Western countries varies according to the center investigated, as well as to the criteria used for defining preterm birth. For instance, in Western Australia, Hagan, Benninger, Chiffings, Evans, and French (1996) reported that 1.4 percent of all births occurred at less than thirty-three weeks of gestation. In Scotland, a study by Magowan, Bain, Juszczak, and McInneny (1998), which defined preterm as all singleton deliveries from twenty-four to thirty-six weeks, reported a percentage of 5.4 percent.

Wide differences are also found in the percentages of infants born of low birth weight, partly because various definitions of low birth weight births have been used. The most frequently used categories are low birth weight (LBW, i.e., those infants weighing less than 2,500 g); very low birth weight (VLBW, i.e., those weighing less than 1,500 g); and extremely low birth weight (ELBW, i.e., those weighing less than 1,000 g). Guyer, MacDorman, Martin, Peters, and Strobino (1998) reported LBW births constituted 7.5 percent of all live births in 1997 in the United States. Infants weighing less than 2,000 g at birth represented 2.3 percent of all live births in Merseyside, United Kingdom in 1980–1981 (Hutton, Pharoah, Cooke, & Stevenson, 1997).

Infants born at a very early gestational age are much more likely to survive than they were a few decades ago (e.g., Allen, Donohue, & Dusman, 1993; Rennie, 1996). For example, Emsley, Wardle, Sims, Chiswick, and D'Souza (1998) reported that between 1984–1989 and 1990–1994, there was an increase from 27 percent to 42 percent in survival to discharge of infants born at twenty-three to twenty-five weeks of gestational age. Increased survival of infants weighing less than 800 g has also been reported: By 1987, 43 percent of such babies born in England and Wales survived to one year compared with 32 percent five years earlier (Alberman & Botting, 1991). Similarly, the mortality of VLBW neonates fell from 56.4 percent of live births in 1971 to 21.1 percent in 1991 (Alberman, 1974; Staples & Pharoah, 1994). Table 2.1 shows VLBW births in Alabama as a percentage of total births according to birth weight: 1,000–1,499 g, 500–999 g, and less than 500 g. As can be seen, over twenty years there was a 2.5-fold increase in the percentage of total births made up by infants weighing less than 500 g at birth, as well as a significant increase in the proportion of births that such infants comprised (0.04 percent to 0.23 percent). Such encouraging figures have been brought about by advances in neonatal care, which has focused its attention on very small and very premature babies.

However, as early as 1961, Drillien predicted that the increased survival of preterm and VLBW infants would be associated with an increase in the prevalence of physical impairment. This prediction has been proven correct; an increase in absolute numbers

Table 2.1. Very Low Birth Weight Births as a Percentage of Total Births, By Birth Weight, and Outcome: Adapted from Phelan, Goldenberg, Alexander, and Cliver (1998)

	Birth Weight					
	< 500 g		500–999 g		1,000–1,499 g	
Year	% Total Births	% Live Births	% Total Births	% Live Births	% Total Births	% Live Births
1974	.20	.04	.72	.41	.94	.77
1977	.21	.06	.72	.42	.80	.68
1980	.33	.09	.81	.55	.77	.63
1984	.37	.13	.85	.62	.76	.66
1988	.46	.17	.84	.61	.91	.81
1990	.46	.15	.82	.59	.96	.84
1991	.41	.16	.82	.62	.94	.84
1992	.45	.18	.98	.70	.88	.79
1993	.47	.20	.90	.64	.95	.86
1994	.51	.23	.90	.68	1.01	.92

of impaired infants has occurred, and the improved survival rate has not been found to modify the rate of physical disability (Hack et al., 1994). In a review of the outcome literature, Escobar, Littenburg, and Pettiti (1991) reported the prevalence of major handicap of VLBW and very preterm children in the 1960s and 1970s to be 6–8 percent, with studies from the United States reporting higher rates of disability than those from Europe; the median rate of cerebral palsy among all the cohorts studied was 7.7 percent. In the 1990s, the prevalence of disability was reported as being between 5 and 16 percent (Korkman, Liikanen, & Fellman, 1996). The smallest (i.e., weighing less than 750 g) and least mature (i.e., those born before 25 weeks of gestation) babies are at particularly high risk of permanent handicap, comprising up to 40 percent of the cases in one series (Hack & Fanaroff, 1999). These authors reported no improvement in the neurodevelopmental outcomes of such infants.

Brain Injury

With the introduction of new brain imaging technology, several patterns of brain injury were identified in the preterm and LBW brain. One of the first brain imaging studies of neonates in the United States was by Papile, Burstein, Burstein, and Koffler (1978), who carried out computed tomography (CT) brain scans of VLBW infants who had suffered brain hemorrhage. Pape et al. (1979) carried out the first UK study, using a linear-array real-time ultrasound (US) scanner; 23 percent of the preterm infants investigated had cerebral lesions, including germinal matrix (GM) and intraventricular hemorrhages (IVH), hydrocephalus, and infarction of the periventricular region and cerebral cortex.

Hemorrhages into the germinal matrix or ventricles, or both, are often grouped together as periventricular hemorrhage (PVH). This is seen typically in infants born at less than 32–33 weeks gestation; the more immature the infant, the higher the risk of PVH. Neonatal ultrasonography shows PVH to occur in around 46 percent of very preterm infants (Stewart, Thorburn, Lipscomb, & Amiel-Tison, 1983), whereas it is rare in mature infants. PVH normally involves the GM, a transient embryonic structure (it involutes at 34 weeks) of the telencephalon that proliferates the neuroblasts and glioblasts, which provides the basis for the organization of the cortex. At the end of the second trimester, the GM is among the most metabolically active regions of the brain. GM tissue is sited over the caudate nucleus of the thalamus and is separated from the cerebrospinal fluid of the lateral ventricles only by a single layer of ependyma. Hemorrhage may remain localized in the GM or may rupture through the overlying ependymal cell layer into the lateral ventricles. Depending on the extent of the bleeding, the hemorrhage may fill up and expand the ventricular system, follow the course of the cerebrospinal fluid (CSF) to emerge in the subarachnoid space (i.e., the layer of tissue situated or occurring between the arachnoid and the pia mater) overlying the brain stem and cerebellum, or may occasionally emerge in the white matter. Bleeding in the caudothalamic region is responsible for most of the intracerebral extensions of the hemorrhage. White matter hemorrhage does not appear to be a direct result of extension of blood from the adjacent ventricle, but rather damage in white matter seems to be a prerequisite for ependymal rupture and continuity between the ventricular cavity and adjacent white matter.

Anoxic-ischemic injury to the brain is the most dreaded consequence of perinatal asphyxia. Grey matter lesions are classically seen since these neurons are extremely sensitive to asphyxia (disruption of oxygen delivery to the fetus), and may occur in both the cerebral cortex and deep grey matter (thalamus, basal ganglia, and brain stem). Involvement of the deep grey matter is seen more often in infants, particularly preterm infants, than in adults suffering from anoxia and/or ischemia. This probably reflects the fact that in the infant, the neurons in the deep nuclei are more mature and metabolically active than those in the cortex and thus more susceptible to ischemia.

White matter is the site of significant damage in preterm and LBW infants, and such injury represents the main cause of neonatal mortality and long-term neurological impairment in them (Perlman, 1998). White matter is largely composed of axons grouped together into fibre bundles and is easily distinguishable from grey matter in the adult brain, as the presence of myelin gives it its color. In the infant, and the preterm infant specifically, myelination is incomplete and therefore the grey/white matter distinction is not as obvious.

The neonatal brain shows different reactions to physiological insult according to gestational age. The prominence of white matter injury may occur because the myelination process is more susceptible to injury than is already formed myelin. Not infrequently, premature infants suffering a hypotensive episode will also develop white matter infarcts, which are called periventricular leukomalacia (PVL); this is a frank necrosis in white matter and includes a variety of glial cell reactions (Banker & Larroche, 1962). PVL affects 15–20 percent of VLBW infants (Baud et al., 1999; Perlman, 1998), and can be recognized by fairly well demarcated yellow-white chalky lesions, which are typically located bilaterally in the white matter, characteristically at the corners of the lateral ventricles. Since loss of myelin leads to ventricular dilatation, there is considerable overlap between the effects of IVH and PVL. With increased gestational age, the risk of PVL decreases: by thirty-two weeks of gestation, the periventricular vascular supply has expanded substantially and PVL is more rare (Fanaroff & Hack, 1999).

However, hemorrhagic infarction of the white matter is not always periventricular in location. Merrill, Piccuch, Fell, Barkovich, and Goldstein (1998) reported that cerebellar hemorrhage is found in 10–25 percent of autopsy specimens from VLBW infants. Skullerud and Westre (1986) identified pontosubicular neuronal necrosis (PSN, affecting the subiculum of the hippocampus and the gray matter of the ventral pons) as a solitary lesion in about 35 percent of preterm infants coming to postmortem, whereas Paneth, Rudelli, Kazam, and Monte (1994) reported a lower figure of 16 percent. The same authors found basal ganglia necrosis in 17 percent of their sample. These abnormalities frequently overlap.

Recent magnetic resonance imaging (MRI) studies have reported brain abnormalities in over half of preterm and LBW samples. For instance, Maalouf et al. (1999) performed MRI scans in a group of preterm infants (gestational age < 30 weeks) during the first forty-eight hours of life and found that 76 percent of infants had ventricular enlargement, 83 percent had squaring of the anterior or posterior horns of the lateral ventricles, 38 percent had a widened interhemispheric fissure or extracerebral space, and 76 percent had diffuse and high signal intensity in the white matter, indicating cerebral atrophy.

Krageloh-Mann et al. (1999) examined a group of twenty-nine children aged 5.5 to 7 years and found abnormal MRI results in 65.5 percent of the sample. These abnormalities included periventricular lesions (65.5%), especially PVL (58.6%), and cerebellar atrophy (10.3%).

Cooke and Abernethy (1999) investigated brain structure in adolescence in a subgroup of VLBW infants with learning disorders. 87/137 (64%) subjects and 8/26 (30%) controls were examined. Differences were found between subjects and controls, with subjects having smaller brain volume and smaller size of their corpora callosa. There was no relationship with cognitive, behavioral, and motor measures. This study, however, did not allow for findings to be generalized across LBW populations as the subject sample was recruited on the basis of cognitive impairment and the control group was very small.

To summarize, very preterm birth is associated with an increased risk of brain injury, and recent MRI studies have demonstrated high rates of brain abnormalities in individuals born preterm compared to full-term controls (Cooke & Abernethy, 1999; Maalouf et al., 1999; Stewart et al., 1999). The abnormalities reported include ventricular dilatation, thinning of the corpus callosum with specific involvement of the posterior body (splenium), abnormal white matter signal, and decreased white matter volume. Hippocampal abnormalities have also been reported in postmortem studies (Fuller, Guthrie, & Alvord, 1983). These abnormalities may reflect neonatal hypoxic-ischemic damage, and the vulnerability of the developing cerebral gray and white matter in the last trimester of gestation to hypoxic-ischemic damage. In support of this hypothesis, Krageloh-Mann et al. (1999) observed low oxygen delivery to the brain in 63 percent of school-age children with abnormal MRI scans, compared to 12.5 percent with normal MRI.

OUTCOME IN CHILDHOOD

Neurological Impairments

Neurological abnormalities are clearly more common in preterm and LBW individuals than the child population as a whole. In general, the most severe abnormalities are found during the first months of life, but they later decrease with age (Gherpelli,

Ferreira, & Costa, 1993). An excess of specific deficits such as poor visual-motor integration and visuo-spatial deficits has been reported (Saigal, Szatmari, Rosenbaum, Campbell, & King, 1991; Teplin, Burchinal, Johnson-Martin, Humphry, & Kraybil, 1991). Of the LBW children in the Vancouver follow-up study, 42 percent had abnormal neurological signs at age $6^{1}/_{2}$ (Dunn, 1986): "Minimal brain dysfunction" was detected in 18.2 percent of the sample. This category included agnosias, apraxias, tone or reflex asymmetry, poor coordination of fine movements, and abnormal electroencephalogram (EEG).

Another follow-up study of LBW children, which excluded those with cerebral palsy, showed an excess of motor abnormalities, behavior problems, and "minor neurological signs" at six years. The signs included dystonia, dysdiadochokinesis, and mirror movements (Marlow, Roberts, & Cooke, 1989). Other studies (e.g., Calame, Fawer, Anderegg, & Perentes, 1985; Hadders-Algra, Touwen, & Huisjes, 1988; Hall, McLeod, Counsell, Thomson, & Mutch, 1995) found a similar range of impairments and disability, with most of the impairments being of the "minor" type.

Sommerfelt, Ellertsen, and Markestad (1996) studied a group of five-year-old children whose birth weight had been less than 2,000 g and found a sex-dependent frequency of neurological impairments. LBW boys showed more minor neurological signs than girls, and small head circumference at birth was associated with an increased frequency of minor neurological signs in LBW boys. A sex-dependent frequency has been found in a number of other studies (e.g., Ounsted, Moar, & Scott, 1988).

The prognostic significance of major impairments associated with spastic or athetoid cerebral palsy is obvious, in that those affected require lifelong support from health and social services. Rather less is known about the long-term prognosis for those with minor abnormalities, which do not cause obvious disability. As pointed out earlier, LBW and preterm children tend to have reduced educational attainment (e.g., Hadders-Algra et al., 1988; Hall et al., 1995) while LBW children without conventional disability use about twice the amount of medical services as controls in the first eight to nine years of life (Stevenson, McCabe, Pharoah, & Cooke, 1996). Such evidence suggests that so-called minor impairments may, in fact, have significant disruptive effects on development.

There seems to be an overrepresentation of left handers among VLBW school children (e.g., Fritsch, Winkler, Flanyek, & Muller, 1986; O'Callaghan, Burn, Mohay, Rogers, & Tudehope, 1993). At eight years, Saigal, Rosenbaum, Szatmari, and Hoult (1992) found non-right handedness (left and mixed) in 31 percent of ELBW children compared with 19 percent of full-term controls. In the ELBW children, non-right handedness was associated with neurological impairments but not with inferior school performance. Powls, Botting, Cooke, and Marlow (1996) observed that impaired manual dexterity was more common in VLBW non-right handers, but poor cognitive or educational outcomes were not associated with handedness. These results support the idea that in VLBW children, non-right handedness has a pathological origin, even though the exact relationship to perinatal events is yet to be specified.

To summarize, preterm and VLBW children are at risk of disruption of their normal processes of neurodevelopment because the immature brain is susceptible to injury in the neonatal period by factors including hypoxia, ischemia, sepsis, and undernutrition. Clinically, these infants are at risk of serious neurodevelopmental sequelae, and 6–8 percent go on to develop cerebral palsy or mental retardation (Stewart,

Reynolds, & Lipscomb, 1981) and 4 percent develop epilepsy (Amess et al., 1998). However, between 80 and 90 percent of survivors of neonatal intensive care are, in fact, free of conventional disability (Powls, Botting, Cooke, & Marlow, 1995). These children show an excess of neurological impairments, particularly on tests of motor performance, and are more likely to be considered "clumsy" than their term-born classmates (Goyen, Lui, & Woods, 1998; Luoma, Herrgard, & Martikainen, 1998): This finding has been termed *developmental coordination disorder* by some authors (Huh, Williams, & Burke 1998).

NEUROPSYCHOLOGICAL IMPAIRMENT

Studies looking at the neuropsychological outcome of VLBW and preterm children suggest that their performance as a whole is somewhat impaired on a variety of cognitive tests. The specificity of such cognitive defects is yet to be established and there remains controversy over whether these deficits are out of proportion to the generalized reduction in cognitive ability. These impairments, although not gross, imply considerable dysfunctioning across a range of variables relevant to adult adjustment (e.g., Hoy et al., 1992).

The majority of LBW children have intelligence quotients (IQs) within the normal range but nevertheless, as a group, such individuals score significantly lower than controls, even in studies which controlled for social class, and excluded children with severe neurological disabilities (e.g., Breslau, 1995; Breslau et al., 1994; Hack et al., 1992; Klein, Hack, & Breslau, 1989; Lloyd, Wheldall, & Perks, 1988; McCormick, 1989; Rickards et al., 1993; Skuse, 1999). Neuropsychological as well as neuromotor and behavioral functions can be differentially assessed according to the age group of the children investigated. It is important to take the children's age, as well as the criteria used to define group inclusion, into account when comparing studies.

Casiro et al. (1990) studied language development in a group of VLBW infants and matched full-term controls at one year of age. Thirty-nine percent of VLBW infants had significant language delays, as assessed by testing the infants' capability to understand simple questions, to recognize objects or body parts when named, to initiate speech-gesture games, to follow simple commands, and to imitate or use words consistently. VLBW infants also had attention problems and a variety of language-related impairments. In this study, language development was positively correlated with gestational age and five-minute Apgar scores (a rapid means of evaluating an infant's cardiopulmonary and neurologic function at set intervals after birth, routinely at one and five minutes), and negatively correlated with severity of intraventricular hemorrhage, bronchopulmonary dysplasia, and length of hospital stay. Furthermore, language delays were more often found in those individuals with mild to moderate neurological impairments.

An excess of specific deficits such as memory and language problems (Fritsch et al., 1986) and verbal deficits (Smith & Knight-Jones, 1990) has been identified in both VLBW and ELBW children attending primary school. Wolke and Meyer (1999), in a study with six-year-old preterm and full-term children, found that deficits in speech articulation and pre-reading skills were three to five times more frequent in the preterm group. However, other studies detected no differences. Aram, Hack, Hawkins, Weissman, and Borawski-Clark (1991) compared speech and language comprehension and production between VLBW and normal birth weight eight-year-old children. When children with major neurologic abnormalities were excluded, scores on the majority of speech and language measures did not significantly differ between subjects and controls. Selective cognitive or neuromotor deficits may partly explain the poor school performance in those whose full scale IQ is within the normal range (Hall et al., 1995; Klein, Hack, Gallacher, & Faneroff, 1985). In general, however, the percentage of preterm and LBW children receiving special education or being placed in special schools is increased (e.g., Schaap et al., 1999).

Selective memory deficits have been observed in LBW and preterm children. Luciana, Lindeke, Georgieff, Mills, and Nelson (1999) investigated nonverbal memory span, spatial working-memory abilities, planning, set-shifting, and recognition memory in preterm school-age children using the Cambridge Neuropsychological Testing Automated Battery. Relative to controls, preterm individuals showed lower scores on the spatial working-memory and planning tasks. They also demonstrated poorer pattern recognition as well as a shorter spatial memory span. The two groups did not differ in visual-discrimination learning or in spatial-recognition memory. A recent study by Isaacs et al. (2000) reported that VLBW adolescents had significantly lower scores on tests assessing episodic memory (i.e., memory for everyday events) than age-matched normal birth weight controls, independently of global cognitive functioning. Performance on verbal and nonverbal recall was similar between the two groups. Episodic memory deficits were associated with reductions in hippocampal size.

Children from progressively lower birth weight groups show increasing deficits in neuropsychological outcome. For instance, Breslau et al. (1994) found a gradient relationship with full-scale IQ in a LBW population at six years. The largest deficit was in those individuals born at 1,500 g or less, an intermediate deficit was found in those born between 1,501 and 2,000 g, and the least conspicuous deficit in those born between 2,001 and 2,500 g. Among the group at higher risk of adverse outcome, namely the ELBW group, poor school performance has been reported in up to 67 percent of cases (Ross, Lipper, & Auld, 1991; Stewart & Pezzani-Goldsmith, 1986; Stewart, Turcan, Rawlings, Hart, & Gregory, 1978). For preterm individuals, figures range between 16 percent (Kok, den Ouden, Verloove-Vanhorick, & Brand, 1998) and 38 percent (Stjernqvist & Svenningsen, 1999).

Weisglas-Kuperus, Baerts, Smrkovsky, and Sauer (1993) found that the results of neonatal neurological examination was the best predictor for cognitive development at one year of age in a cohort of VLBW infants regarded as being high risk according to cerebral neonatal ultrasound findings. From two years of age onward, LBW babies at high biological risk seemed able to compensate their cognitive problems if they had a favorable home environment. Children at low as well as high biological risk in a less stimulating home environment showed a decline in cognitive development.

The interaction between birth weight and social risk has also been investigated by Hack et al. (1992) in a sample of 249 VLBW school-age children (8 years) and 362 age-matched controls. The following areas were assessed: global intelligence, language, speech, reading, mathematics, spelling, visual and fine motor abilities, and behavior. VLBW had a statistically significant poorer performance on all tests, except speech and behavior. Even in VLBW children without major neurologic abnormality such differences persisted, with the exception of social competence, reading, and spelling. After controlling for global intelligence and neurological outcome, VLBW children had a poorer performance than did controls in expressive language, memory, visuo-motor, and fine motor function, and measures of hyperactivity. The results of a multiple regression analysis showed that social risk was the main predictor of neuropsychological outcome.

In order to provide a theoretical framework to their research, Lee and Barratt (1993) employed a "transactional model" of development, originally formulated by Sameroff and Chandler (1975). According to this model, preterm children with cognitive impairment exhibit a self-righting tendency during early childhood, and eventually environmental factors overshadow biological factors. Lee and Barratt found that the developmental problems in preschool preterm and LBW children diminish with age. They studied preterm and LBW children between five and eight years of age and matched full-term normal birth weight controls with respect to delays in cognitive functioning, including language and mathematical abilities. Preterm children seemed to have delays in cognitive functioning only until six years of age. Later in life, environmental factors seemed to account better for the degree of cognitive development than did perinatal variables. The transactional model of development will be discussed again toward the end of this chapter.

To summarize neuropsychological outcome, although the majority of VLBW and preterm children have IQ scores within the normal range, as a group, they are usually reported as having lower IQ than appropriately matched controls, even after controlling for possible confounds (e.g., Breslau, 1995; Breslau et al., 1994; Hack et al., 1992; Klein, Hack, & Breslau, 1989; Lloyd et al., 1988; McCormick, 1989; Rickards et al., 1993; Skuse, 1999). Regarding specific cognitive deficits, evaluation of neuropsychological outcomes of low birth weight and preterm children have found declines in language, fine motor, tactile, and attention skills (e.g., Breslau et al., 1996), and selective memory functioning (e.g., Briscoe, Gathercole, & Marlow, 1998; Luciana et al., 1999). These findings are not consistent. The employment of various neuropsychological batteries and study methodologies may account for different results. The hypothesis that the cognitive outcome of very preterm infants may be poorer than often reported has been put forward by Wolke, Ratschinski, Ohrt, and Riegel (1994). The authors evaluated the cognitive impairment of very preterm infants (< 32 weeks gestation or < 1,500 g birth weight) in a prospective population study (i.e., the Bavarian Longitudinal Study II). Cognitive outcome was assessed at 5, 20, and 56 months of age. Rates of cognitive impairment of 321 very preterm infants were obtained according to the published test norms, to scores of a full-term control group ($n = 321$), and to scores from a representative sample of children ($n = 431$) of the same birth cohort. IQ scores for these "concurrent" control groups were higher than those in the original standardization sample. Therefore, using the concurrent test norms, up to 2.4 times more very preterm children scored as being cognitively impaired than if the standardized norms had been used. In light of these findings, methodological issues of preterm and LBW outcome studies should always be taken into account when interpreting the results.

Behavioral Abnormalities

LBW and preterm infants are at increased risk of developing emotional, behavioral, and temperamental problems (Buka, Lipsitt, & Tsuang, 1992). The most consistent behavioral abnormalities found in LBW children are increased activity and poor attention.

Indeed, up to 30 percent (Pharoah, Stevenson, Cooke, & Stevenson, 1994; Stevenson, Blackburn, & Pharoah, 1999) have been reported to experience behavioral problems which meet the criteria for attention deficit hyperactivity disorder (ADHD). ADHD is a disorder characterized by deficits in sustained attention, overactivity, and impulsiveness (Taylor, 1998), together with impairment of higher order executive control functions (e.g., response inhibition) and motor timing (Barkley, 1997). Various studies have found an increased risk of ADHD in LBW populations (e.g., Breslau, 1995; Breslau et al., 1996; Szatmari, Saigal, Rosenbaum, Campbell, & King, 1990). Increased rates of emotional, conduct, and temperamental problems have also been reported (Breslau et al., 1996; Calame et al., 1986). LBW boys from socially disadvantaged backgrounds are at particular risk of developing ADHD (Breslau, 1995; Hall et al., 1995; Hutton et al., 1997).

Whitaker et al. (1997) studied the relation of neonatal cranial ultrasound abnormalities to psychiatric disorder at age six years in a group of children with birth weights of 501 to 2,000 g. Neonatal cranial ultrasound abnormalities were classified as 1 (no abnormality); 2 (isolated GM and/or IVH); and 3 (parenchymal lesions and/or ventricular enlargement with or without GM/IVH). Children with severe mental retardation were excluded. Analyses were conducted first in the entire sample and then in children with normal intelligence. Results indicated that 22 percent of the cohort had at least one psychiatric disorder, the most common being ADHD (15.6%). In the whole sample, white matter lesions and/or ventricular enlargement increased risk relative to no abnormality, independently of other biological and social predictors, for any disorder, ADHD, and tic disorders. Isolated GM/IVH was not related to psychiatric disorder at age six years. Non-US variables such as maternal smoking during pregnancy elevated risk for any psychiatric disorder. Male sex predicted any disorder and ADHD. In children of normal intelligence, white matter lesions/ventricular enlargement independently increased by four-fold the risk for any disorder, ADHD, and separation anxiety, independently of sex and socioeconomic status.

Weisglas-Kuperus et al. (1993) studied parent and medical professional reports of behavioral abnormalities among VLBW children aged 3½ years. Other variables controlled for included neonatal cerebral damage, cognition and social factors, that is, occupational status of the family, mother's education, family support, and ethnic background. VLBW children were more depressed and had increased affective problems according to parent report. The association between behavior and biological variables was indirect: Neonatal cerebral damage was related to cognitive development, which directly influenced behavioral problems. The authors suggested that depression in preschool VLBW children might have been associated with the reactions of the parents after their birth, and that attention problems might have been indirectly associated with brain damage via cognitive impairments. Thus, social as well as biological factors may mediate behavioral deficits found in LBW and preterm populations.

In 1995, Breslau published a review of eleven studies investigating psychiatric symptoms and disorders in LBW children. All studies were published after 1988 and included school-age LBW children born during and after the mid-1970s. Most studies excluded subjects with severe handicaps and those attending special schools (approximately 15% of the LBW population) as they aimed to identify the long-term sequelae of LBW children without obvious neurological impairment. Overall results showed that LBW children had greater hyperactivity and inattention problems than normal birth weight children, as measured by parents' and teachers' ratings. A positive association was also found between LBW and ADHD, as measured by the *Diagnostic and Statistical Manual of Mental Disorders* (*DSM-III-R*) (American Psychiatric Association, 1987). No association was found between LBW and other childhood disorders such as oppositional/defiant disorder, anxiety disorder, and conduct disorder, a condition characterized by a repetitive and persistent pattern of behavior in which the basic rights of others or major age-appropriate social norms are not respected. The evidence reviewed by Breslau (1995) suggested a possible gradient effect of LBW on ADHD, inattention and hyperactivity, in other words, the lower the birth weight, the more severe the behavioral problems.

To summarize, overall results from studies on the emotional and behavioral development of LBW and preterm children suggest that, as a group, such children are at increased risk of developing behavioral problems. The most frequent behavioral abnormalities include high activity levels and short attention spans, approximating the clinical diagnosis of ADHD. The recognition of behavioral problems in LBW and preterm sub-populations allows opportunity for the identification of high-risk groups and early intervention, which has been proven effective in randomized controlled studies. For instance, the Infant Health and Development Program (1990) successfully used a family-based educational curriculum and support program in order to reduce behavioral problems in LBW children. Targeted use of intervention programs may significantly improve the development of LBW and preterm populations.

THE UNIVERSITY COLLEGE HOSPITAL LONDON (UCHL) STUDY

It is clear from the above that we are still very ignorant of how preterm and LBW children fare when they reach adolescence and adulthood. Unfortunately, only a few studies have progressed beyond childhood. What is required is a long-term study, which combines detailed assessment of function from birth into adolescence, together with more definitive assessment of brain anatomy, and which is of sufficient size to allow an examination of the relationships between perinatal findings and adolescent deficits.

We have been carrying out such a study involving the examination at an average age of fifteen years, of a series of individuals who were born very preterm (before 33 weeks) and who entered the neonatal unit within one week of birth at University College London Hospital (UCLH) from 1979 onward ($n = 109$). Of this cohort, 4 died within 24 months; the remaining 105 were enrolled for long-term follow-up. At 15 years, 103 (98%) individuals were traced. Altogether, 76 (83%) agreed to attend for assessment. The cohort members who were unavailable for investigation did not differ from those studied in birth weight, gestational age at birth, sex ratio, mode of delivery, condition at birth, the need for mechanical ventilation, or neonatal cranial ultrasonographic findings. Forty-seven infants delivered in University College Hospital at term (38–42 weeks) in 1979–1980 were enrolled to act as controls for assessments made on the cohort at four years of age. They were matched for sex, parental social class (coded by the Registrar's General classification), ethnicity, deprivation of neighborhood, and age. None of these individuals had ultrasonographic imaging during the neonatal period. All individuals who were living in the United Kingdom ($n = 45$) were traced at fifteen years; twenty-two agreed to have MRI, although one refused on the day.

Our preterm subjects were the first series of infants to have neonatal ultrasound brain scanning performed and relatively crude linear-array apparatus was used. Forty-three percent were rated as having abnormal cranial ultrasound scans (Stewart, Thorburn, Hope, et al., 1983). After 1983, a mechanical sector scanner was used to give better resolution, especially of hypoxic-ischemic and white matter lesions. Extensive data were collected concerning pregnancy, labor, delivery, and the early neonatal period. Cognitive, behavioral, neurological, and social function was subsequently assessed in detail at one, four, and eight years of age.

Neurology

At one year of age, 79 percent of the cohort were judged to have no neurological abnormality, 10 percent had minor impairments not sufficient to cause disability, and 11 percent had major impairments with concomitant disability (Stewart et al., 1989). At four years, neurological abnormalities again classified as "major" or "minor" (Stewart et al., 1989). Major abnormalities, perhaps better termed "impairment with disability," included sensorineural hearing loss; amblyopia; and spastic tetraplegia, hemiplegia or paraplegia. Minor abnormalities were those considered not to cause disability, defined by the World Health Organization (1980) as "any restriction or lack (resulting from an impairment) of ability to perform an activity in the manner or within the range considered normal for a human being." The minor abnormalities, therefore, included disorders of muscle tone, tendon stretch reflexes, or cranial nerves.

The proportion of children in the cohort who showed major neurological impairments remained relatively constant at four years (15%) and eight years (12%) of age, as has been found in other studies (Tin, Wariyar, & Hey, 1997). Ultrasound evidence of areas of marked echodensity or echolucency (cysts) in brain parenchyma, usually adjacent to the ventricles (and thought to represent white matter damage), and ventricular dilatation or hydrocephalus were found to be potent predictors of major disability at one, four, and eight years (Costello et al., 1988; Roth et al., 1993; Stewart, Thorburn, Hope, et al., 1983).

In contrast to major abnormalities, minor abnormalities increased in prevalence from 10 percent at age one to 23 percent at the age of eight years (Roth et al., 1994). By the age of fourteen years, 66 percent of the cohort had an abnormal or equivocal neurological examination compared to 30 percent of the control group (Stewart et al., 1999). Once more the proportion of children with major neurological abnormality and disability stayed relatively constant, but the prevalence of minor neurological signs again increased in prevalence.

Two possible explanations for this increase have been suggested. First, the range of motor skills that normal individuals can perform (and which can therefore be tested for) increases with age; more abnormalities may therefore be revealed by the more comprehensive testing of older children. The second possibility is that lesions of the CNS acquired early in development may not have a significant effect until the neuronal systems that they involve reach developmental maturity. Some support for the latter comes, for example, from experiments involving newborn rats; when subjected to hippocampal lesions they appear relatively normal until they reach maturity, after which gross behavioral disturbance results (Sams-Dodd, Lipska, & Weinberger, 1997).

Neuropsychology

Although the mean full scale IQ of the very preterm subjects was well within the normal range at eight years, half the subjects showed neuropsychological evidence of poor interhemispheric interaction; indeed, this was the best predictor of poor school performance (Stewart, Thorburn, Hope, et al., 1983). These deficits were postulated to be due to damage to the posterior third of the corpus callosum, which lies adjacent to the periventricular region, the most common site for damage in the preterm infant. The application of a battery of neuro-motor tests designed to test interhemispheric transfer of cognitive information provided some support for this suggestion (Kirkbride, Baudin, Lorek, et al., 1994; Kirkbride, Baudin, Townsend, et al., 1994).

At age fifteen years, the very preterm subjects were significantly impaired relative to controls on only two measures of cognitive function: cognitive flexibility and phonemic verbal fluency (Rushe, Rifkin, Stewart, & Murray, 1998). IQ, naming, spelling, visuo-motor function, verbal, and visuospatial memory were not significantly impaired. Further group analyses were conducted on the preterm group data, in order to assess whether abnormal brain MRI at fifteen years had a significant effect on cognitive performance. The results showed that the cognitive performance of the preterm subjects was unrelated to the presence of gross brain abnormality, except that reading age was lower in those preterm individuals with abnormal scans (Stewart et al., 1999).

Psychiatric Outcome

Behavior was assessed at fifteen years, using the Rutter Behavioral Scale (Rutter, Tizard, & Whitmore, 1981) and the social adjustment scale of Cannon-Spoor, Potkin, and Wyatt (1982). Behavioral abnormalities were increased in a statistically significant way only in those preterm subjects with abnormal MRI scans. Premorbid adjustment problems were increased in subjects with equivocal and abnormal MRI, whereas preterm adolescents with normal MRI had adjustment scores similar to controls.

Neuroimaging

MRI scans were performed in all participating subjects at fifteen years. In a preliminary analysis, Stewart et al. (1999) reported on seventy-two cases and twenty-one full-term controls. MRI scans were "blindly" rated according to a structured format by two neuroradiologists. MRI scans were classified as normal (no detected abnormality), equivocal (negligible ventricular dilatation, or negligible thinning of the corpus callosum, or an isolated [single] white-matter signal) and abnormal (more than one parenchymal lesion, definite ventricular dilatation, or definite thinning or atrophy of the corpus callosum, reduced white matter or cortical volume, multiple areas of white matter signal changes, or intraparenchymal cysts).

Only 24 percent of very preterm adolescents were rated by the neuroradiologists as having normal MRI scans; 21 percent had equivocal and 56 percent had abnormal results; the percentages for controls were 71 percent, 24 percent, and 5 percent, respectively. In those preterm individuals with an MRI scan classified as abnormal, ventricular dilatation was observed in 80 percent of the cases, posterior trigonal dilatation in 73 percent, thinning of the corpus callosum with specific involvement of the posterior body (splenium) in 65 percent, abnormal white matter signal in 45 percent, and decreased white matter volume in 25 percent. Ventricular dilatation and thinning of the corpus callosum were correlated with each other and with other brain lesions, and may be regarded as markers of hypoxic-ischemic damage. Finding of white matter signal

Table 2.2. Regional Volumetric Measurements in cm^3 in the Preterm and Control Groups

Variable	Cases (N = 66)	Controls (N = 48)	Statistics
Mean (SD; 95% CI)			
Quantitative MRI Measures			
Whole brain volume	1297.59 (118.20; 1269.02–1326.16)	1384.72 (115.67; 1351.22–1418.22)	F = 13.76 p < 0.0001
White matter volume*	465.33 (72.02; 446.80–483.86)	470.61 (81.11; 448.89–492.34)	F = 3.73 p = 0.056
Cortical grey matter volume*	624.13 (84.98; 603.52–644.74)	707.63 (83.84; 683.46–731.80)	F = 11.51 p < 0.001
Lateral ventricles*	22.39 (20.87; 18.41–26.37)	9.46 (5.65; 4.79–14.12)	F = 29.86 p = 0.0001
Cortical grey/white matter ratio*	1.38 (0.32; 1.30–1.50)	1.55 (0.35; 1.46–1.65)	F = 7.82 p = 0.006
Left hippocampus*	2.33 (0.49; 2.21–2.45)	2.65 (0.67; 2.47–2.87)	F = 6.77 p = 0.020
Right hippocampus*	2.17 (0.57; 2.03–2.2)	2.57 (0.68; 2.38–2.78)	F = 11.29 p = 0.003

* After controlling for whole brain volume and gender.
Nosarti et al., 2002

abnormalities may reflect the scattered patchy gliosis secondary to ischemic damage (Hope et al., 1988).

The volume of cerebral structures was quantitatively measured in sixty-seven of the very preterm subjects and forty-eight full-term controls. The very preterm individuals had significantly decreased whole brain and cortical grey matter volumes; their mean lateral ventricular volumes were more than twice as large as those of the control subjects (Nosarti et al., 2002). Preterm adolescents also had bilaterally decreased hippocampal (Nosarti et al., 2002) and cerebellar volumes (Allin et al., 2001) when compared with full-term controls. Some of the regional brain measurements are shown in Table 2.2.

Preterm adolescents had decreased callosal volume, specifically the posterior quarter (Nosarti, 2001), compared with full-term controls, confirming the qualitative findings (Stewart et al., 1999). This could be the basis for the poor interhemispheric interaction previously noted (Roth et al., 1994), possibly due to hemorrhagic or hypoxic-ischaemic damage to the splenium of the corpus callosum.

All preterm individuals had neonatal ultrasound brain scanning, and adolescent MRI results were investigated in relation to ultrasound results. Of the thirteen cases with neonatal ultrasound showing lesions definitely or presumably caused by hypoxic-ischemic damage (i.e., ventricular dilatation, hydrocephalus, and cerebral atrophy), twelve had equivocal (two cases) or abnormal (ten cases) MRI scans in adolescence; a positive predictive value of 94 percent. However, the sensitivity of prediction of equivocal or abnormal MRI in adolescence for definite or presumed hypoxic/ischemic injury on neonatal ultrasound scans was only 22 percent. Fifty-five cases had abnormal adolescent MRI scans, of whom only twelve had been reported as having abnormal neonatal cranial ultrasounds. Neonatal characteristics (i.e., birth weight, gestational age, method of delivery, and Apgar scores) did not differentiate between the three MRI classifications.

Therefore, although abnormal neonatal ultrasound predicted abnormal adolescent brain MRI in this preterm sample, many subjects who had not had neonatal ultrasound anomalies were reported to have brain abnormalities in adolescence, and these subjects were not predicted by other neonatal parameters. To our knowledge, there are no other reports of predictors of abnormal MRI in adolescence of preterm individuals.

BRAIN PLASTICITY AND ITS LIMITS

The UCHL study shows that over half of the very preterm children who reach adolescence have brain scans which neuroradiologists regard as abnormal. They also show some neurological, cognitive, and psychiatric problems, but these are not as severe as might have been predicted from seeing their MRI scans. This is initially surprising, as is the fact that no clear association was found between the brain structural and neurological outcomes.

Perhaps these findings may be explained by neural plasticity (i.e., the process whereby compensatory neural events facilitate the re-organization of existing brain tissue). Healing responses include: establishment of new limiting membranes that function as boundaries and creation of conditions conducive to rapid sprouting of neurites that underlie circuit reorganization (Ide et al., 1996). Such circuit reorganization occurs in the perinatal lesion model in the rodent, as demonstrated by Coltman, Earley, Shahar, Dudek, and Ide (1995), who observed collateral sprouting in the molecular layer of the hippocampal dentate gyrus as early as six days after a lesion.

Studies on the visual system of the cat have demonstrated that remaining areas of the brain are able to take over functions which are lost following brain damage in both adults and neonates; however, neonates show better behavioral recovery than adults (Spear, 1996). The neonatal brain has exuberant pathways that normally disappear during development. Initial research in neurotrophic substances (i.e., involved in the nutrition or maintenance of neural tissue) suggests that at least part of the answer is that neurotrophin receptors are more present early in life and not in adulthood, and these receptors rescue cells following brain damage (Lindholm, 1994). As a result, it may be possible for neurotrophins to act preferentially on cells in young animals. This action may be at a distance, attracting new cells to grow and new projections to a target, or maintaining existing projections that would retract otherwise.

However, other authors have argued that early lesions or deprivation not only result in alteration of connections, but can produce more dramatic atrophy or cell loss (Himes & Tessler, 1989). How developmental stage influences plastic responses to brain injury is not clear. Cusick (1996) suggested that early peripheral lesions may deprive central neurons of essential trophic factors (i.e., pertaining to nutrition), accentuate naturally occurring central cell death, and result in smaller central representations. In addition, throughout all stages of development, the capacity for reorganization may be spatially limited and depend on the size or pattern of the peripheral injury.

In humans, research has attempted to clarify both the extent and limitations of functional and neural plasticity by assessing a variety of functional skills in children who sustained brain injury at a very early age. The majority of the research to date has focused on the development and/or recovery of language function. Mariotti, Iuvone, Torrioli, and Silveri (1998) studied language skills in a patient who had an early left hemispherectomy. Language was only marginally impaired in comparison to controls matched for IQ. Vargha-Khadem et al. (1997) studied the case of a boy with Sturge-Weber Syndrome affecting the left hemisphere. This condition is a congenital syndrome characterized by a facial birthmark and neurological abnormalities; it is often associated with intracranial calcification, cognitive deficits, hemiplegia, and epilepsy. In early childhood, the boy investigated by Vargha-Khadem and colleagues failed to develop speech, and his comprehension of single words and simple commands remained stationary at an age equivalent of three to four years. However, after left hemidecortication at age $8^{1}/_{2}$ years, the boy suddenly began to acquire speech and language skills. Presumably in the absence of the left, the right hemisphere mediates verbal language.

Overall, research suggests that when brain damage is sustained to the left hemisphere in infancy, there is good functional recovery of language function. If the injury is sustained in middle childhood, however, adult-like aphasic symptoms occur (e.g., Hecaen, 1983). This suggests that the ability of the brain to compensate for injury depends in part on the stage of maturation at which the injury is sustained. During normal brain development, neural systems responsible for certain cognitive behaviors progress from diffuse, undifferentiated systems to specialized systems. The bulk of this "fine tuning" process occurs during the last trimester of gestation and a few years postnatally (Aram & Eisele, 1992). However, the process of maturation of the brain continues up to the age of fifteen years, with evidence that the frontal and occipital cortices do not fully mature until twenty years of age (Neville, 1993). Myelin accumulation occurs late in gestation and after birth, and the speed of myelination differs between the various connecting systems of the brain (Girard, Raybaud, & du Lac, 1991). The child's brain is characterized by incomplete myelination and increased synaptic density, increased glucose metabolism and cerebral blood flow (CBF), which are about 50 percent above the adult level at ages eight to twelve (Chiron et al., 1992). The frontal lobe is the latest to mature; through synaptic pruning the adult pattern is reached at around age eighteen to twenty. The earlier the injury, therefore, the greater the availability of alternative neural substrates to take over the role of neural substrate for certain cognitive functions. Aram and Eisele (1992) suggested that a consequence of such reorganization/alteration of the structure-function relationship might be that complex cognitive functions, which are acquired later in development, suffer due to a lack of synaptic sites.

As noted earlier, the prevalence of disability appears to increase in preterm children as they grow older, possibly due to the greater range and complexity of normal skills expected and hence of deficits which may be revealed on testing (e.g., Palfrey, Singer, Walker, & Butler, 1987; Roth et al., 1994; Stewart & Kirkbride, 1996). Furthermore, an early brain lesion can have different functional consequences as the individual advances in age. Rankin, Aram, and Horwitz (1981) investigated three children with left hemisphere lesions, who showed initial delays in expressive language, and testing six to eight years later showed significant deficits in syntactic production and comprehension. Along similar lines, animal studies show that a lesion may remain relatively silent until the neuronal system affected reaches a degree of maturity, at which point abnormal behavior results. For example, in nonhuman primates, experimental damage to the dorsolateral prefrontal cortex has little measurable effect on delayed response learning until the animals reach adulthood (Goldman, 1971). Similarly, as mentioned earlier, newborn rats subjected to hippocampal lesions appear relatively normal until they reach maturity, after which gross behavioral disturbance results (Sams-Dodd et al.,

1997). Some researchers believe that in humans, certain early lesions may produce little impairment in childhood, but profound behavioral disturbance in adult life (Weinberger, 1987). Recent studies with humans have supported this hypothesis. For instance, Anderson, Bechara, Damasio, Tranel, and Damasio (1999) investigated the social and moral behavior of two young adults who received focal nonprogressive prefrontal damage before sixteen months of age. These individuals showed no behavioral abnormalities up to the age of three years, but had severely impaired social behavior despite normal basic cognitive abilities later on in life.

INTEGRATIVE SUMMARY AND FUTURE DIRECTIONS

We have used the UCHL study of the biological and cognitive outcomes of very preterm infants who survived after neonatal intensive care to illustrate research on risk conditions and neuropsychological and behavioral abnormalities observed in these individuals in childhood and adolescence. This study, and others like it, are beginning to elucidate the adolescent outcome of a population whose mortality is continuously decreasing thanks to advances in neonatal care. However, many questions are still unanswered. For example, the adult function of individuals born very preterm is largely unknown. Up to know, our research remains speculative with respect to specific mechanisms associating perinatal data with later neuropsychological and behavioral outcomes, as well as neurodevelopmental anomalies and later maladaptation or psychopathology.

Zigler and Glick (1986) argue that a central tenet of developmental psychopathology is the possibility for an individual to move between pathological and nonpathological forms of functioning. The determinants of such movement within a continuum of functioning are important for the understanding of ontogenetic processes. Therefore it will be interesting to prospectively follow cohorts such as that from UCHL through early adult life since, for instance, this is the period of maximum risk for disorders such as schizophrenia and bipolar affective disorder. A prospective study design such as ours could allow for the investigation of already identified risk factors. For instance, future work to provide insight into the very long-term consequences of preterm birth could include repeated MRI analyses (e.g., every decade), as well as comprehensive neuropsychological assessments. In this way several areas of functioning could be elucidated, such as the association between decreased brain volume and increased ventricular size, decreased cognitive reserve, and the possible risk of degenerative disorders such as Alzheimer's disease.

The study of neuronal activity in preterm populations using functional MRI (fMRI) techniques would provide the opportunity to ascertain differences in the degree, profile, and specificity of possible impairments in this group. In order to validate the neurodevelopmental model of schizophrenia, we are currently planning an fMRI investigation with three groups of subjects (preterm adolescents, age-matched individuals with first-onset schizophrenia, and normal controls) using cognitive tasks involving episodic memory, which has been reported to be impaired both in patients with schizophrenia (Rushe, Woodruff, Murray, & Morris, 1999) and individuals born preterm (Isaacs et al., 2000). We predict that preterm adolescents and those with schizophrenia will be particularly likely to show similarities in abnormal neuronal activity, compared with healthy full-term controls. Attenuated activation is expected in the hippocampus (Heckers,

Rauch, & Goff, 1988), prefrontal cortex (Lepage, Ghaffar, & Nyberg, 2000), and cerebellum (Fiez, 1996).

The UCHL study attempts to adequately assess multiple domains of development, both within and outside the individual. Cicchetti and Cannon (1999) and Cicchetti and Rogosch (1996) emphasize the importance of understanding the differentiation, integration, and organization of biological and cognitive and behavioral development in order to put the individual investigated in context and facilitate the identification of the etiology, course, outcomes, and therapeutic intervention for high-risk conditions and pathologies. However, a danger to any multidisciplinary research is that the team possesses more strength in some areas of expertise than others. For instance, our neuropsychological assessment tends to investigate broad areas of functioning rather than specific deficits. The extent of the demands of multiple assessments on participating subjects certainly, yet unavoidably, limits the areas investigated, as is often the case in research with human subjects. The longitudinal nature of the study is also a factor that needs to be taken into account.

Another important gap in our knowledge is the extent to which data collected in the neonatal period can predict adolescent and adult deficits in neurological, cognitive, and psychosocial function. To date, ultrasound results have successfully predicted MRI results in adolescence, but other neonatal variables have failed to do so. Neuropsychological variables at age one, four, and eight are being investigated in relation to quantitative MRI results (Nosarti et al., 2002). The identification of possible predictors of outcome would help neonatal pediatricians to develop preventative strategies as well as focus their efforts on those particular infants at greatest risk of adolescent and adult impairments. Subsequently, remedial educational and psychological help could be directed to such individuals throughout childhood. The efficacy of both prevention and intervention services should be regularly evaluated.

A guiding theory for preterm and LBW research could be found in the transactional model (Cicchetti & Schneider-Rosen, 1986; Sameroff & Chandler, 1975), which stresses the importance of transacting genetic, constitutional, biological, biochemical, psychological, and environmental factors in determining behavior. According to the transactional model, there exists a dynamic transaction between these various factors, which forms the basis of a developmental framework that shapes individual organization. A main tenet of this model is that multiple factors operate together through a hierarchy of dispositions. Individual and environmental characteristics are bi-directionally influenced, that is, the individual is influenced by the environment and adapts to it, but also the environment is influenced and modified by the characteristics of the individual. An example is given by the observation of infants' temperament, which is transformed into a range of attachment organizations determined by the caregiver's variation in responses (e.g., Goldsmith & Alansky, 1987). Later on in development, children's organizational systems may affect the way they respond to external stimuli, that is, positive or negative, and the long-term processes of adjustment or maladjustment.

Within a transactional model framework the heterogeneity in outcomes found in preterm individuals could be studied in association with vulnerability factors. External (e.g., familial and social) and internal (e.g., genetic, temperamental, psychological) factors can be regarded as sources of vulnerability if they serve to direct the individual toward maladaptation. Via the process of ontogenesis, these vulnerability factors may promote psychopathology.

REFERENCES

Alaghband-Rad, J., McKenna, K., Gordon, C., Albus, K., Hamburger, S., Rumsey, J., Lenane, M., & Rapaport, J. (1995). Childhood onset schizophrenia: the severity of premorbid course. *Archives of General Psychiatry, 43*, 1273–1283.

Alberman, E. (1974). Stillbirths and neonatal mortality in England and Wales by birthweight 1953–71. *Health Trends, 6*, 14–17.

Alberman, E., & Botting, B. (1991). Trends in prevalence and survival of very low birthweight infants, England and Wales: 1983–7. *Archives of Disease in Childhood, 66*, 1304–1308.

Allen, M.C., Donohue, P.K., & Dusman, A.E. (1993). The limit of viability – neonatal outcome of infants born at 22 to 25 weeks' gestation. *New England Journal of Medicine, 329*, 1597–1601.

Allin, M.P.G., Matsumoto, H., Santhouse, A.M., Nosarti, C., Al-Asady, M.H.S., Stewart, A.L., Rifkin, L., & Murray, R.M. (2001). Cognitive and motor function and the size of the cerebellum in adolescents born very preterm. *Brain, 124*, 60–66.

American Psychiatric Association. (1987). *Diagnostic and statistical manual of mental disorders: DSM-III-R. 3rd Ed.* Washington, D.C.: American Psychiatric Association.

Amess, P.N., Baudin, J., Townsend, J., Meek, J., Roth, S.C., Neville, B.G., Wyatt, J.S., & Stewart, A. (1998). Epilepsy in very preterm infants: neonatal cranial ultrasound reveals a high-risk subcategory. *Developmental Medicine and Child Neurology, 40*, 724–730.

Anderson, S.W., Bechara, A., Damasio, H., Tranel, D., & Damasio, A.R. (1999). Impairment of social and moral behavior related to early damage in human prefrontal cortex. *Nature Neuroscience, 11*, 1032–1037.

Aram, D.M., & Eisele, J.A. (1992). Plasticity and recovery of higher cognitive function following early brain damage. In F. Boller & J. Grafman (Eds.), *Handbook of neuropsychology, Vol. 6* (pp. 73–91). Amsterdam: Elsevier.

Aram, D.M., Hack, M., Hawkins, S., Weissman, B.M., & Borawski-Clark, E. (1991). Very-low-birthweight children and speech and language development. *Journal of Speech and Hearing Research, 34*, 1169–1179.

Banker, B.Q., & Larroche, J.C. (1962). Periventricular leukomalacia of infancy: a form of neonatal anoxic encephalopathy. *Archives of Neurology, 7*, 386–410.

Barkley, R.A. (1997). Behavioural inhibition, sustained attention, and executive functions: constructing a unifying theory of ADHD. *Psychological Bulletin, 121*, 65–94.

Baud, O., Foix-L'Helias, L., Kaminski, M., Audibert, F., Jarreau, P.H., Papiernik, E., Huon, C., Lepercq, J., Dehan, M., & Lacaze-Masmonteil, T. (1999). Antenatal glucocorticoid treatment and cystic periventricular leukomalacia in very premature infants. *New England Journal of Medicine, 341*, 1190–1196.

Bennet, F.C. (1987). The effectiveness of early intervention for infants at increased biological risk. In M.J. Guralnick, & F.C. Bennet (Eds.), *The effectiveness of early intervention for at risk and handicapped children* (pp. 79–109). New York: Academic Press.

Blackman, J.A. (1991). Neonatal intensive care: is it worth it? Developmental sequelae of very low birthweight. *Paediatric Clinics of North America, 38*, 1497–1511.

Breslau, N. (1995). Psychiatric sequelae of low birth weight. *Epidemiological Reviews, 17*, 96–106.

Breslau, N., Brown, G.G., Del Dotto, J.E., Kumar, S., Ezhuthachan, S., Andreski, P., & Hufnagle, K.G. (1996). Psychiatric sequelae of low birth weight at 6 years of age. *Journal of Abnormal Child Psychology, 24*, 385–400.

Breslau, N., Del Dotto, J.E., Brown, G.G., Kumar, S., Ezhuthachan, S., Hufnagle, K.G., & Peterson, E.L. (1994). A gradient relationship between low birth weight and IQ at age six years. *Archives of Pediatrics and Adolescent Medicine, 148*, 377–383.

Briscoe, J., Gathercole, S.E., & Marlow, N. (1998). Short-term memory and language outcomes after extreme prematurity at birth. *Journal of Speech, Language and Hearing Research, 41*, 654–666.

Buka, S.L., & Fan, A.P. (1999). Association of prenatal and perinatal complications with subsequent bipolar disorder and schizophrenia. *Schizophrenia Research, 39*, 113–119.

Buka, S.L., Lipsitt, L.P, & Tsuang, M.T. (1992). Emotional and behavioural development of low birth-weight infants. In S.L. Friedman & M.D. Sigman (Eds.), *Annual advances in applied developmental psychology, Volume 6* (pp. 187–214). Norwood, N.J.: Ablex Publishing.

Buka, S.L., Tsuang, M.T., & Lipsitt, L.P. (1993). Pregnancy/delivery complications and psychiatric diagnosis. A prospective study. *Archives of General Psychiatry, 50,* 151–156.

Calame, A., Fawer, C.L., Anderegg, A., & Perentes, E. (1985). Interaction between perinatal brain damage and processes of normal development. *Developmental Neuroscience, 7,* 1–11.

Calame, A., Fawer, C.L., Claeys, V., Arrazola, L., Ducret, S., & Jounin, L. (1986). Neurodevelopmental outcome and school performance of very low birthweight infants at eight years of age. *European Journal of Pediatrics, 145,* 461–466.

Cannon-Spoor, H.E., Potkin, S.G., & Wyatt, K.J. (1982). Measurement of premorbid adjustment in chronic schizophrenia. *Schizophrenia Bulletin, 8,* 470–484.

Casiro, O.G., Moddemann, D.M., Stanwick, R.S., Panikkar-Thiessen, V.K., Cowan, H., & Cheang, M.S. (1990). Language development of very low birth weight infants and fullterm controls at 12 months of age. *Early Human Development, 24,* 65–77.

Chiron, C., Raynaud, C., Maziere, B., Zilbovicius, M., Laflamme, L., Masure, M.C., Dulac, O., Bourguignon, M., & Syrota, A. (1992). Changes in regional cerebral blood flow during brain maturation in children and adolescents. *Journal of Nuclear Medicine, 33,* 696–703.

Cicchetti, D. (1984). The emergence of developmental psychopathology. *Child Development, 55,* 1–7.

Cicchetti, D., & Cannon, T.D. (1999). Neurodevelopmental processes in the ontogenesis and epigenesis of psychopathology. *Development and Psychopathology, 11,* 375–393.

Cicchetti, D., & Garmezy, N. (Eds.). (1993). Milestones in the development of resilience [Special issue]. *Development and Psychopathology, 5,* 497–774.

Cicchetti, D., & Rogosch, F. (Eds.). (1996). Developmental pathways [Special Issue]. *Development and Psychopathology, 8,* 597–896.

Cicchetti, D., & Schneider-Rosen, K. (1986). An organisational approach to childhood depression. In M. Rutter, C. Izard & P. Read (Eds.), *Depression in young people, clinical and developmental perspectives* (pp. 71–134). New York: Guilford Press.

Coltman, B.W., Earley, E.M., Shahar, A., Dudek, F.E., & Ide, C.F. (1995). Factors influencing mossy fibre collateral sprouting in organotypic slice cultures of neonatal mouse hippocampus. *Journal of Comparative Neurology, 362,* 209–222.

Cooke, R.W.I., & Abernethy, L.J. (1999). Cranial magnetic resonance imaging and school performance in very low birth weight infants in adolescence. *Archives of Disease in Childhood: Fetal and Neonatal Edition, 81,* F116–F121.

Costello, A.M. de L., Hamilton, P.A., Baudin, J., Townsend, J., Bradford, B.C., Stewart, A.L., & Reynolds, E.O.R. (1988). Prediction of neurodevelopmental impairment at four years from brain ultrasound appearance of very preterm infants. *Developmental Medicine and Child Neurology, 30,* 711–722.

Cusick, C.G. (1996). Extensive cortical reorganisation following sciatic nerve injury in adult rats versus restricted reorganisation after neonatal injury: implications for spatial and temporal limits on somatosensory plasticity. *Progress in Brain Research, 108,* 379–390.

Dalman, C., Allebeck, P., Cullberg, J., Grunewald, C., & Koster, M. (1999). Obstetric complications and the risk of schizophrenia: a longitudinal study of a national birth cohort. *Archives of General Psychiatry, 56,* 234–240.

Drillien, C.M. (1961). Incidence of physical and mental handicaps in school age children of very low birth weight. *Paediatrics, 27,* 452–464.

Dunn, H.G. (Eds.). (1986) *Sequelae of low birth weight, the Vancouver study.* London: MacKeith Press.

Elman, I., Sigler, M., Kronenberg, J., Lindenmayer, J.P., Doron, A., Mendlovic, S., & Gaoni, B. (1998). Characteristics of patients with schizophrenia successive to childhood attention deficit hyperactivity disorder. *Israel Journal of Psychiatry and Related Sciences, 35,* 280–286.

Emsley, H.C.A., Wardle, S.P., Sims, D.G., Chiswick, M.L., & D'Souza, S.W. (1998). Increased survival and deteriorating developmental outcome in 23 to 25 week old gestation infants, 1990–4 compared with 1984–9. *Archives of Disease in Childhood: Fetal and Neonatal Edition, 78,* F99–F104.

Escobar, G.J., Littenburg, B., & Pettiti, D.B. (1991). Outcome among surviving very low birth weight infants: a meta-analysis. *Archives of Disease in Childhood, 66,* 204–211.

Fanaroff, A.A., & Hack, M. (1999). Periventricular leukomalacia – prospects for prevention. *New England Journal of Medicine, 341,* 1229–1231.

Fiez, J.A. (1996). Cerebellar contributions to cognition. *Neuron, 16,* 13–15.

Fritsch, G., Winkler, E., Flanyek, A., & Muller, W.D. (1986). [Neurologic, psychologic and logopedic follow-up of 6- to 8-year-old former premature infants with a birth weight below 1,501 g]. *Monatsschrift Kinderheilkunde, 134,* 687–691.

Fuller, P.W., Guthrie, D., & Alvord, E.C. (1983). A proposed neuropathological basis for learning disabilities in children born prematurely. *Developmental Medicine and Child Neurology, 25,* 214–231.

Geddes, J.R., & Lawrie, S.M. (1995). Obstetric complications and schizophrenia: a meta-analysis. *British Journal of Psychiatry, 167,* 786–793.

Geddes, J.R., Verdoux, H., Takei, N., Lawrie, S.M., Bovet, P., Eagles, J.M., Heun, R., McCreadie, R.G., McNeil, T.F., O'Callaghan, E., Stober, G., Willinger, U., & Murray, R.M. (1999). Schizophrenia and complications of pregnancy and labour: an individual patient data meta-analysis. *Schizophrenia Bulletin, 25,* 413–423.

Gherpelli, J.L., Ferreira, H., & Costa, H.P. (1993). [Neurological follow-up of small-for-gestational age newborn infants. A study of risk factors related to prognosis at one year of age]. *Arquivos de Neuro-Psiquiatria, 51,* 50–58.

Girard, N., Raybaud, C., & du Lac, P. (1991). MRI study of brain myelination. *Journal of Neuroradiology, 18,* 291–307.

Goldman, P.S. (1971). Functional development of the prefrontal cortex in early life and the problem of plasticity. *Experimental Neurology, 32,* 366–387.

Goldsmith, H.H., & Alansky, J.A. (1987). Maternal and infant predictors of attachment: a meta-analytic review. *Journal of Consulting and Clinical Psychology, 55,* 805–816.

Goyen, T.A., Lui, K., & Woods, R. (1998). Visual-motor, visual-perceptual, and fine motor outcomes in very-low-birthweight children at 5 years. *Developmental Medicine and Child Neurology, 40,* 76–81.

Guyer, B., MacDorman, M.F., Martin, J.A., Peters, K.D., & Strobino, D.M. (1998). Annual summary of vital statistics – 1997. *Pediatrics, 102,* 1333–1349.

Hack, M., Breslau, N., Aram, D., Weissman, B., Klein, N., & Borawski-Clark, E. (1992). The effect of very low birth weight and social risk on neurocognitive abilities at school age. *Journal of Developmental and Behavioral Pediatrics, 13,* 412–420.

Hack, M., & Fanaroff, A.A. (1999). Outcomes of children of extremely low birthweight and gestational age in the 1990s. *Early Human Development, 53,* 193–218.

Hack, M., Taylor, G., Klein, N., Eiben, R., Schatschneider, C., & Mercuri-Minich, N. (1994). School-age outcomes in children with birth weights under 750 g. *The New England Journal of Medicine, 331,* 753–759.

Hadders-Algra, M., Touwen, B.C.L., & Huisjes, H.J. (1988). Perinatal risk factors and minor neurological dysfunction: significance for behavioural and school achievement at nine years. *Developmental Medicine and Child Neurology, 30,* 482–491.

Hagan, R., Benninger, H., Chiffings, D., Evans, S., & French, N. (1996). Very preterm birth – a regional study. Part 2: The very preterm infant. *British Journal Obstetrics and Gynaecology, 103,* 239–245.

Hall, A., McLeod, A., Counsell, C., Thomson, L., & Mutch, L. (1995). School attainment, cognitive ability and motor function in a total Scottish very-low-birthweight population at 8 years: a controlled study. *Developmental Medicine and Child Neurology, 37,* 1037–1050.

Hecaen, H. (1983). Acquired aphasia in childhood: revisited. *Neuropsychologia, 21,* 581–587.

Heckers, S., Rauch, S.L., & Goff, D. (1988). Impaired recruitment of the hippocampus during conscious recollection in schizophrenia. *Nature Neuroscience, 1,* 318–323.

Himes, B.T., & Tessler, A. (1989). Death of some dorsal root ganglion neurons and plasticity of others following sciatic nerve section in adult and neonatal rats. *Journal of Comparative Neurology, 284,* 215–230.

Hope, P.L., Gould, S.J., Howard, S., Hamilton, P.A., Costello, A.M. de L., & Reynolds, E.O.R. (1988). Precision of ultrasound diagnosis of pathologically verified lesions in the brain of very preterm infants. *Developmental Medicine and Child Neurology, 30,* 457–471.

Hoy, E.A., Sykes, D.H., Bill, J.M., Halliday, H.L., McClure, B.G., & Reid, M.M. (1992). The social competence of very-low-birthweight children: teacher, peer, and self-perceptions. *Journal of Abnormal Child Psychology, 20,* 123–150.

Huh, J., Williams, H.G., & Burke, J.R. (1998). Development of bilateral motor control in children with developmental coordination disorders. *Developmental Medicine and Child Neurology, 40,* 474–484.

Hultman, C.H., Sparen, P., Takei, N., Murray, R.M., & Cnattingius, S. (1999). Prenatal and perinatal risk factors for schizophrenia, affective psychosis, and reactive psychosis of early onset: case-control study. *British Medical Journal, 318,* 421–425.

Hutton, J.L., Pharoah, P.O., Cooke, R.W., & Stevenson, R.C. (1997). Differential effects of preterm birth and small gestational age on cognitive and motor development. *Archives of Disease in Childhood: Fetal and Neonatal Edition, 76,* F75–81.

Ide, C.F., Scripter, J.L., Coltman, B.W., Dotson, R.S., Snyder, D.C., & Jelaso, A. (1996). Cellular and molecular correlates to plasticity during recovery from injury in the developing mammalian brain. *Progress in Brain Research, 108,* 365–377.

Infant Health and Development Program. (1990). Enhancing the outcomes of low birth weight premature infants: a multisite randomized trial. *Journal of the American Medical Association, 263,* 3035–3042.

Isaacs, E.B., Lucas, A., Chong, W.K., Wood, S.J., Johnson, C.L., Marshall, C., Vargha-Khadem, F., & Gadian, D.G. (2000). Hippocampal volume and everyday memory in children of very low birth weight. *Pediatric Research, 47,* 713–720.

Jones, P., Rantakallio, P., Hartikainen, A.L., Isohanni, M., & Sipila, P. (1998). Schizophrenia as a long-term outcome of pregnancy, delivery, and perinatal complications: a 28-year follow-up of the 1966 north Finland general population birth cohort. *American Journal of Psychiatry, 155,* 355–364.

Kirkbride, V., Baudin, J., Lorek, A., Meek, J., Penrice, J., Townsend, J., Roth, S., Edwards, D., McCormick, D., Reynolds, O., & Stewart, A. (1994). Motor tests of interhemispheric control and cognitive function in very preterm infants at eight years. *Pediatric Research, 36,* 20A.

Kirkbride, V., Baudin, J., Townsend, J., Roth, S.C., McCormick, D.C., Edwards, A.D., Reynolds, O., & Stewart, A. (1994). Abnormalities of corpus callosal function in very preterm infants at eight years (Abstract). *Early Human Development, 38,* 234–235.

Klein, N.K., Hack, M., & Breslau, N. (1989). Children who were very low birth weight: development and academic achievement at nine years of age. *Journal of Developmental and Behavioral Pediatrics, 10,* 32–37.

Klein, N., Hack, M., Gallacher, J., & Faneroff, A. (1985). Pre-school performance of children with normal intelligence who were very low birth weight infants. *Pediatrics, 75,* 531–537.

Kok, J.H., den Ouden, A.L., Verloove-Vanhorick, S.P., & Brand, R. (1998). Outcome of very preterm small for gestational age infants: the first nine years of life. *British Journal of Obstetrics and Gynaecology, 105,* 162–168.

Korkman, M., Liikanen, A., & Fellman, V. (1996). Neuropsychological consequences of very low birth weight and asphyxia at term: follow-up until school-age. *Journal of Clinical and Experimental Neuropsychology, 18,* 220–233.

Krageloh-Mann, I., Toft, P., Lunding, J., Andresen, J., Pryds, O., & Lou, H.C. (1999). Brain lesions in preterms: origin, consequences and compensation. *Acta Paediatrica, 88,* 897–908.

Lawrie, S.M., & Abukmeil, S.S. (1998). Brain abnormality in schizophrenia. A systematic and quantitative review of volumetric magnetic resonance imaging studies. *British Journal of Psychiatry, 172,* 110–120.

Lee, H., & Barratt, M.S. (1993). Cognitive development of preterm low birth weight children at 5 to 8 years old. *Journal of Developmental and Behavioral Pediatrics, 14,* 242–249.

Lepage, M., Ghaffar, O., & Nyberg, L. (2000). Prefrontal cortex and episodic memory retrieval mode. *Proceedings of the National Academy of Science USA, 97,* 506–511.

Lewis, S.W., & Murray, R.M. (1987). Obstetric complications, neurodevelopmental deviance, and risk of schizophrenia. *Journal of Psychiatric Research, 21,* 413–421.

Lindholm, D. (1994). Role of neurotrophins in preventing glutamate induced neuronal cell death. *Journal of Neurology, 242,* S16–18.

Lloyd, B.W., Wheldall, K., & Perks, D. (1988): Controlled study of intelligence and school performance of very low birth weight children from a defined geographical area. *Developmental Medicine and Child Neurology, 30,* 36–42.

Luciana, M., Lindeke, L., Georgieff, M., Mills, M., & Nelson, C.A. (1999). Neurobehavioral evidence for working-memory deficits in school-aged children with histories of prematurity. *Developmental Medicine and Child Neurology, 41,* 521–533.

Luoma, L., Herrgard, E., & Martikainen, A. (1998). Neuropsychological analysis of the visuomotor problems in children born preterm at < or = 32 weeks of gestation: a 5-year prospective follow-up. *Developmental Medicine and Child Neurology, 40,* 21–30.

Maalouf, E.F., Duggan, P.J., Rutherford, M.A., Counsell, S.J., Fletcher, A.M., Battin, M., Cowan, F., & Edwards, A.D. (1999). Magnetic resonance imaging of the brain in a cohort of extremely preterm infants. *Journal of Pediatrics, 135,* 351–357.

Magowan, B.A., Bain, M., Juszczak, E., & McInneny, K. (1998). Neonatal mortality amongst Scottish preterm singleton births (1985–1994). *British Journal Obstetrics and Gynaecology, 105,* 1005–1010.

Mariotti, P., Iuvone, L., Torrioli, M.G., & Silveri, M.C. (1998). Linguistic and non-linguistic abilities in a patient with early left hemispherectomy. *Neuropsychologia, 36,* 1303–1312.

Marlow, N., Roberts, B.L., & Cooke, R.W. (1989). Motor skills in extremely low birth weight children at the age of 6 years. *Archives of Disease in Childhood, 64,* 839–847.

McCarley, R.W., Wible, C.G., Frumin, M., Hirayasu, Y., Levitt, J.J., Fischer, I.A., & Shenton, M.E. (1999). MRI anatomy of schizophrenia. *Biological Psychiatry, 45,* 1099–1119.

McCormick, M.C. (1989). Long term follow-up of infants discharged from neonatal intensive care units. *Journal of the American Medical Association, 261,* 1767–1772.

McGrath, J., & Murray, R.M. (1995). Risk factors for schizophrenia from conception to birth. In S.R. Hirsch & D.R. Weinberger (Eds.), *Schizophrenia* (pp. 187–205). Oxford: Blackwell.

McNeil, T.F., & Kaij, L. (1978). Obstetric factors in the development of schizophrenia. In C. Wynne, R.L. Cromwell & S. Matthyss (Eds.), *The nature of schizophrenia* (pp. 38–51). New York: Wiley.

Merrill, J.D., Piecuch, R.E., Fell, S.C., Barkovich, A.J., & Goldstein, R.B. (1998). A new pattern of cerebellar hemorrhages in preterm infants. *Pediatrics, 102,* E62.

Murray, R.M. (1994). Neurodevelopmental schizophrenia: the rediscovery of dementia praecox. *British Journal of Psychiatry, 165,* 6–12.

Neville, H.J. (1993). Neurobiology of cognitive and language processing: Effects of early experience. In M.H. Johnson (Eds.), *Brain development and cognition: a reader* (pp. 424–448). Oxford: Blackwell.

Nosarti, C., Al-Asady, M.H.S., Frangou, S., Stewart, A.L., Murray, R.M., & Rifkin, L. (1999, September). Hippocampal volumetric measurements in very preterm adolescents compared to age-matched full term controls. ESMRMB '99. 16th annual meeting of the European Society for Magnetic Resonance in Medicine and Biology. Seville.

Nosarti, C., Al-Asady, M.H.S., Frangou, S., Stewart, A.L., Rifkin, L., & Murray, R.M. (2002). Adolescents who were born very preterm have decreased brain volumes. *Brain, 125,* 1616–1623.

Nosarti, C., Rifkin, L., Rushe, T.M., Woodruff, P.W.R., Stewart, A.L., & Murray, R.M. (2001). Corpus callosum size in adolescents who were born very preterm. *Pediatric Research, Special Supplement*: *First World Congress Fetal Origins of Adult Disease*, July 2001, 50(1).

O'Callaghan, M.J., Burn, Y.R., Mohay, H.A., Rogers, Y., & Tudehope, D.I. (1993). Handedness in extremely low birth weight infants: aetiology and relationship to intellectual abilities, motor performance and behaviour at four and six years. *Cortex, 29,* 629–637.

Ounsted, M., Moar, V.A., & Scott, A. (1988). Neurological development of small-for-gestational age babies during the first year of life. *Early Human Development, 16,* 163–172.

Palfrey, J.S., Singer, J.D., Walker, D.A., & Butler, J.A. (1987). Early identification of children's special needs: a study in five metropolitan communities. *Journal of Pediatrics, 111,* 651–659.

Paneth, N. (1995). The problem of low birth weight. In *The future of children, Vol. 5.* Los Altos, Calif.: David and Lucile Packard Foundation.

Paneth, N., Rudelli, R., Kazam, E., & Monte, W. (1994). *Brain damage in the preterm infant.* Cambridge, UK: MacKeith Press/Cambridge University Press.

Pape, K.E., Blackwell, R.J., Cusick, G., Sherwood, A., Houang, M.T., Thorburn, R.J., & Reynolds, E.O. (1979). Ultrasound detection of brain damage in preterm infants. *Lancet, 1,* 1261–1264.

Papile, L.A., Burstein, J., Burstein, R., & Koffler, H. (1978). Incidence and evolution of subependymal and intraventricular hemorrhage: a study of infants with birthweights less than 1,500 g. *Journal of Pediatrics, 92,* 529–534.

Perlman, J.M. (1998). White matter injury in the preterm infant: an important determination of abnormal neurodevelopment outcome. *Early Human Development, 53*, 99–120.

Pharoah, P.O., Stevenson, C.J., Cooke, R.W., & Stevenson, R.C. (1994). Prevalence of behaviour disorders in low birth-weight infants. *Archives of Disease in Childhood, 70*, 271–274.

Phelan, S.T., Goldenberg, R., Alexander, G., & Cliver, S.P. (1998). Perinatal mortality and its relationship to the reporting of low-birthweight infants. *American Journal of Public Health, 88*, 1236–1239.

Powls, A., Botting, N., Cooke, R.W., & Marlow, N. (1995). Motor impairment in children 12 to 13 years old with a birthweight of less than 1250 g. *Archives of Disease in Childhood: Fetal and Neonatal Edition, 73*, F62–F66.

Powls, A., Botting, N., Cooke, R.W., & Marlow, N. (1996). Handedness in very-low-birthweight (VLBW) children at 12 years of age: relation to perinatal and outcome variables. *Developmental Medicine and Child Neurology, 38*, 594–602.

Rankin, J.M., Aram, D.M., & Horwitz, S.J. (1981). Language ability in right and left hemiplegia children. *Brain and Language, 14*, 292–306.

Rennie, J.M. (1996). Perinatal management at the lower margin of viability. *Archives of Disease in Childhood, 74*, F214–F218.

Rickards, A.L., Kitchen, W.H., Doyle, L.W., Ford, G.W., Kelly, E.A., & Callanan C. (1993). Cognitive school performance, and behaviour in very low birth weight and normal weight children at eight years of age: a longitudinal study. *Journal of Developmental Behavioral Pediatrics, 14*, 363–368.

Rifkin, L., Lewis, S.W., Jones, P.B., Toone, B., & Murray, R.M. (1994). Low birth weight and schizophrenia. *British Journal of Psychiatry, 165*, 357–362.

Ross, G., Lipper, E., & Auld, P. (1991). Educational status and school related abilities of very low birth weight premature children. *Pediatrics, 88*, 1125–1134.

Roth, S.C., Baudin, J., McCormick, D.C., Edwards, A.D., Townsend, J., Stewart, A.L., & Reynolds, E.O.R. (1993). Relation between ultrasound appearance of the brain in very preterm infants and neurodevelopmental impairment at eight years. *Developmental Medicine and Child Neurology, 35*, 755–768.

Roth, S.C., Baudin, J., Pezzani-Goldsmith, M., Townsend, J., Reynolds, E.O., & Stewart, A.L. (1994). Relation between neurodevelopmental status of very preterm infants at one and eight years. *Developmental Medicine and Child Neurology, 36*, 1049–1062.

Rushe, T., Rifkin, L., Stewart, A., & Murray, R.M. (1998, August). Cognitive outcome for adolescents born very preterm: relationship to MRI at 14–15 and ultrasound status at birth. Paper presented at the Annual Congress of Paediatrics. Amsterdam, Naederlands.

Rushe, T.M., Woodruff, P.W., Murray, R.M., & Morris, R.G. (1999). Episodic memory and learning in patients with chronic schizophrenia. *Schizophrenia Research, 35*, 85–96.

Rutter, M., Tizard, J., & Whitmore, K. (1981). *Education, health and behaviour.* Melbourne: Kreiger.

Sacker, A., Done, D.J., Crow, T.J., & Golding, J. (1995). Antecedents of schizophrenia and affective illness. Obstetric complications. *British Journal of Psychiatry, 166*, 734–741.

Saigal, S., Rosenbaum, P., Szatmari, P., & Hoult, L. (1992). Non-right handedness among ELBW and term children at eight years in relation to cognitive function and school performance. *Developmental Medicine and Child Neurology, 34*, 425–433.

Saigal, S., Szatmari, P., Rosenbaum, P., Campbell, D., & King, S. (1991). Cognitive abilities and school performance of extremely low birth weight children and matched control children at age eight years: a regional study. *Journal of Pediatrics, 118*, 751–760.

Sameroff, A.J., & Chandler, M.J. (1975). Reproductive risk and the continuum of caretaking casualty. In F.D. Horowitz (Eds.), *Review of child development research, Vol. 4* (pp. 187–244). Chicago: University of Chicago Press.

Sameroff A.J., Seifer, R., Barocas, R., Zax, M., & Greenspan, S. (1987). Intelligence quotient scores of 4-year-old children: social environmental risk factors. *Pediatrics, 79*, 343–350.

Sams-Dodd, F., Lipska, B.K., & Weinberger, D.R. (1997). Neonatal lesions of the rat ventral hippocampus result in hyperlocomotion and deficits in social behaviour in adulthood. *Psychopharmacology, 132*, 303–310.

Schaap, A.H., Wolf, H., Bruinse, H.W., Smolders-de Haas, H., van Ertbruggen, I., & Treffers, P.E. (1999). School performance and behaviour in extremely preterm growth-retarded infants. *European Journal of Obstetrics, Gynecology and Reproductive Biology, 86*, 43–49.

Skullerud, K., & Westre, B. (1986). Frequency and prognostic significance of germinal matrix hemorrhage, periventricular leukomalacia, and pontosubicular necrosis in preterm neonates. *Acta Neuropathologica, 70,* 257–261.

Skuse, D. (1999). Survival after being born too soon, but at what cost? *Lancet, 354,* 1999–2000.

Smith, A.E.A., & Knight-Jones, E.B. (1990). The abilities of very low birth weight children and their classroom controls. *Developmental Medicine and Child Neurology, 32,* 590–561.

Sommerfelt, K., Ellertsen, B., & Markestad, T. (1996). Low birthweight and neuromotor development: a population based, controlled study. *Acta Paediatrica, 85,* 604–610.

Spear, P.D. (1996). Neural plasticity after brain damage. *Progress in Brain Research, 108,* 391–408.

Sroufe, L.A. (1989). Pathways to adaptation and maladaptation: Psychopathology as developmental deviation. In D. Cicchetti (Ed.), *Rochester Symposium of Developmental Psychopathology, Vol. 1. The emergence of a discipline* (pp. 13–40). Hillsdale, N.J.: Erlbaum.

Staples, B., & Pharoah, P.O. (1994). Child health statistical review. *Archives of Disease in Childhood, 71,* 548–554.

Stefanis, N., Frangou, S., Yakeley, J., Sharma, T., O'Connell, P., Morgan, K., Sigmudsson, T., Taylor, M., & Murray, R. (1999). Hippocampal volume reduction in schizophrenia: effects of genetic risk and pregnancy and birth complications. *Biological Psychiatry, 46,* 697–702.

Stevenson, C.J., Blackburn, P., & Pharoah, P.O. (1999). Longitudinal study of behaviour disorders in low birthweight infants. *Archives of disease in childhood: Fetal and Neonatal Edition, 81,* F5–F9.

Stevenson, R.C., McCabe, C.J., Pharoah, P.O., & Cooke, R.W. (1996). Cost of care for a geographically determined population of low birthweight infants to age 8–9 years. I. Children without disability. *Archives of Disease in Childhood, 74,* F114–F117.

Stewart, A.L., Costello, A.M., Hamilton, P.A., Baudin, J., Townsend, J., Bradford, B.C., & Reynolds, E.O. (1989). Relationship between neurodevelopmental status of very preterm infants at 1 and 4 years. *Developmental Medicine and Child Neurology, 31,* 756–765.

Stewart, A., & Kirkbride, V. (1996). Very preterm infants at fourteen years: relationship with neonatal ultrasound brain scans and neurodevelopmental status at age one year. *Acta Paediatrica. Supplement, 416,* 44–47.

Stewart, A., & Pezzani-Goldsmith, M. (1986). Long term outcome of extremely low birth weight infants. In C. Amiel-Tison & A. Grenier (Eds.), *Neurologic assessment within the first year of life* (pp. 151–166). New York: Oxford University Press.

Stewart, A.L., Reynolds, E.O.R., & Lipscomb, A.P. (1981). Outcome for infants of very low birth weight: survey of world literature. *Lancet, i,* 1038–1041.

Stewart, A.L., Rifkin, L., Amess, P.N., Kirkbride, V., Townsend, J.P., Miller, D.H., Lewis, S.W., Kingsley, D.P.E., Moseley, I.F., Foster, O., & Murray, R.M. (1999). Brain structure and neurocognitive and behavioral function in adolescents who were born very preterm. *Lancet, 353,* 1653–1657.

Stewart, A.L., Thorburn, R.J., Hope, P.L., Goldsmith, M., Lipscomb, A.P., & Reynolds, E.O.R. (1983). Ultrasound appearance of the brain in very preterm infants and neurodevelopmental outcome at 18 months of age. *Archives of Disease in Childhood, 58,* 598–604.

Stewart, A.L., Thorburn, R.J., Lipscomb, A.P., & Amiel-Tison, C. (1983). Neonatal neurologic examinations of very preterm infants: comparison of results with ultrasound diagnosis of periventricular hemorrhage. *American Journal of Perinatology, 1,* 6–11.

Stewart, A., Turcan, D., Rawlings, G., Hart, S., & Gregory S. (1978). Outcome for infants at high risk of major handicap. In K. Elliot & M. O'Connor (Eds.), *Major mental handicap: Methods and costs of prevention. Ciba Foundation Symposium No: 59 (new series)* (pp. 151–171). North Holland: Elsevier.

Stjernqvist, K., & Svenningsen, N.W. (1999). Ten-year follow-up of children born before 29 gestational weeks: health, cognitive development, behaviour and school achievement. *Acta Paediatrica, 88,* 557–562.

Szatmari, P., Saigal, S., Rosenbaum, P., Campbell, D., & King, S. (1990). Psychiatric disorders at five years among children with birth weights less than 1,000 g: a regional perspective. *Developmental Medicine and Child Neurology, 32,* 954–962.

Taylor, E. (1998). Clinical foundations of hyperactivity research. *Behavioural Brain Research, 94,* 11–24.

Teplin, S.W., Burchinal, M., Johnson-Martin, N., Humphry, R.A., & Kraybil, E.N. (1991). Neurodevelopmental, health and growth status at age six years of children with birth weights less than 1001 g. *Journal of Pediatrics, 118,* 768–777.

Tin, W., Wariyar, U., & Hey, E. (1997). Changing prognosis for babies of less than 28 weeks' gestation in the north of England between 1983 and 1994. *British Medical Journal, 314,* 107–111.

Vargha-Khadem, F., Carr, L.J., Isaacs, E., Brett, E., Adams, C., & Mishkin, M. (1997). Onset of speech after left hemispherectomy in a nine-year-old boy. *Brain, 120,* 159–182.

Velakoulis, D., Pantelis, C., McGorry, P.D., Dudgeon, P., Brewer, W., Cook, M., Desmond, P., Bridle, N., Tierney, P., Murrie, V., Singh, B., & Copolov, D. (1999). Hippocampal volume in first-episode psychoses and chronic schizophrenia: a high-resolution magnetic resonance imaging study. *Archives of General Psychiatry, 56,* 133–141.

Weinberger, D.R. (1987). Implications of normal brain development for the pathogenesis of schizophrenia. *Archives of General Psychiatry, 44,* 660–669.

Weisglas-Kuperus, N., Baerts, W., Smrkovsky, M., & Sauer, P.J. (1993). Effects of biological and social factors on the cognitive development of very low birth weight children. *Pediatrics, 92,* 658–665.

Weisglas-Kuperus, N., Koot, H.M., Baerts, W., Fetter, W.P., & Sauer, P.J. (1993). Behaviour problems of very low-birthweight children. *Developmental Medicine and Child Neurology, 35,* 406–416.

Whitaker, A.H., Van-Rossem, R., Feldman, J.F., Schonfeld, I.S., Pinto-Martin, J.A., Tore, C., Shaffer, D., & Paneth, N. (1997). Psychiatric outcomes in low-birth-weight children at age 6 years: relation to neonatal cranial ultrasound abnormalities. *Archives of General Psychiatry, 54,* 847–856.

Wolke, D., & Meyer, R. (1999). Cognitive status, language attainment, and prereading skills of 6-year-old very preterm children and their peers: the Bavarian Longitudinal Study. *Developmental Medicine and Child Neurology, 41,* 94–109.

Wolke, D., Ratschinski, G., Ohrt, B., & Riegel, K. (1994). The cognitive outcome of very preterm infants may be poorer than often reported: an empirical investigation of how methodological issues make a big difference. *European Journal of Pediatrics, 153,* 906–915.

World Health Organization. (1980). *International classification of impairments, disabilities and handicaps.* Geneva: WHO.

Wright, I. C., Rabe-Hesketh, S., Woodruff, P.W.R., David, A.S., Murray, R.M., & Bullmore, E.T. (2000). Meta-analysis of regional brain volumes in schizophrenia. *American Journal of Psychiatry, 157,* 16–25.

Zigler, E., & Glick, M. (1986). *A developmental approach to adult psychopathology.* New York: Wiley.

THREE

Neurodevelopment During Adolescence

Linda Patia Spear

Adolescence is a time of considerable change. Adolescents undergo periods of rapid growth and emergence of secondary sexual characteristics, along with sometimes sudden changes in behavior and mood. These obvious visible signs of adolescence are mirrored by at least as dramatic internal alterations that include substantial increases in hormone release as well as notable changes in the brain. Indeed, adolescents rival newborns in the sheer magnitude of the developmental transformations occurring in their brains.

It is interesting to note that, to the extent relevant data are available, many of these neural changes – as well as certain related behavioral ramifications – are seen across adolescents of a variety of species. Thus, although we often think of adolescence as being a characteristic phase of human development, similarities across species in the neurobehavioral features of this developmental transition have led to the suggestion that certain adolescent-typical behaviors (and their neural underpinnings) may have been evolutionarily conserved. The transformations occurring in the adolescent brain may not only facilitate characteristic adolescent behaviors, but may also alter the expression of psychopathology as at-risk individuals traverse this developmental period.

DEFINITION AND TIMING OF ADOLESCENCE

Adolescence can be defined as the gradual transformation from youth/dependency to adulthood/independency. Adolescence is not synonymous with puberty. The physiological processes associated with the attainment of sexual maturation – puberty – occur during a relatively restricted interval within the broader adolescent period, with a timing that varies considerably among individuals. Because no single event signals the onset or termination of adolescence, precise boundaries of this period are difficult to determine. The age range from 12–18 years is commonly considered prototypic adolescence in humans, with less agreement in the margins outside this age range. The entire second decade has been defined as adolescence according to some investigators (Petersen, Silbereisen, & Sörensen, 1996), with ages up to twenty-five years being considered late adolescence by others (e.g., Baumrind, 1987).

Time periods termed as adolescence have likewise been identified in other mammalian species such as rats (approximate postnatal days [P] 28–42) and monkeys

(2–4 years), although again the absolute boundaries of this gradual transition are difficult to determine precisely (see Spear, 2000a, for discussion). Although ontogenetic periods corresponding to the developmental transition commonly called adolescence can be identified in nonhuman animals, none of these other species of course demonstrates the full complexity of human brain, behavior, or psychopathology evident during adolescence (or at any other time in life, for that matter). Yet, as we shall see, there are considerable similarities between human adolescents and adolescents of other mammalian species in terms of developmental history and genetic constraints, as well as behavioral, neural, and hormonal characteristics – similarities driven perhaps in part by common evolutionary pressures.

ADOLESCENT BEHAVIOR, HORMONES, AND EVOLUTION

Adolescents behave differently from individuals at other ages. A change in the focus of social interactions is a characteristic hallmark of adolescence, with adolescents of a variety of species showing increased social interactions with peers, sometimes associated with increases in conflicts with parents (e.g., Csikszentmihalyi, Larson, & Prescott, 1977; Primus & Kellogg, 1989; Steinberg, 1989). Adolescents from a broad range of species including humans also exhibit increases in behaviors classified as risk taking or sensation/novelty seeking (Adriani, Chiarotti, & Laviola, 1998; Trimpop, Kerr, & Kirkcaldy, 1999).

Adolescent-typical behavioral features that are seen across species may have evolved in part to facilitate the adolescent transition to maturity. For example, peer-directed interactions serve to develop new skills and social support (e.g., Galef, 1977; Harris, 1995), whereas risk taking has been suggested to increase the probability of reproductive success among males of a variety of species, including humans (Wilson & Daly, 1985). Risk taking (and shifts in social affiliation) may also provide the impetus to explore new and broader areas away from the home. Emigrating from the home area to territory far from genetically related individuals is one successful strategy to avoid inbreeding depression – that is, the lower viability associated with expression of recessive genes in offspring derived from the mating of closely related individuals (Bixler, 1992; Moore, 1992). Indeed, in most species of birds and mammals, members of at least one gender leave the natal area prior to reproducing (Keane, 1990). Behaviors serving to facilitate emigration by sexually emergent adolescents may have been retained during evolution to avoid inbreeding and enhance species survival and viability. Yet, this considerable species benefit seemingly may be at considerable cost to individual adolescents, given the increased mortality rates associated with risk taking and emigration into new regions with uncertain resources and unknown dangers (e.g., Crockett & Pope, 1993; Irwin & Millstein, 1992).

It has long been assumed that adolescent behaviors are driven largely by "raging hormones." And indeed, the chemistry of the body undergoes considerable modification during the adolescent period. Pubertal-associated hormonal changes include dramatic gender-specific rises in gonadal steroids (estrogen and testosterone). These pubertal increases in gonadal hormones are stimulated by a reinstatement of pituitary release of luteinizing hormone (LH) and follicle stimulating hormone (FSH), release that was pronounced during the early postnatal period but suppressed throughout childhood (see Brooks-Gunn & Reiter, 1990, for review). Other adolescent hormonal changes include increases in growth hormone (GH) release (e.g., Brook & Hindmarsh, 1992; Gabriel, Roncancio, & Ruiz, 1992) as well as an early prepubertal rise in adrenal androgens (including hormones such as androstenedione and dehydroepiandrosterone, often called "neurosteroids" for their potent actions on the nervous system; Parker, 1991). There is also emerging evidence for a postpubertal increase in release of the stress-associated hormone, cortisol (e.g., see Cicchetti & Walker, 2001; Walker & Walder, *this volume*) that may in part reflect an adolescent-associated increase in stressor responsiveness (see Spear, 2000a).

Common folklore has long assumed that the dramatic pubertal-associated increases in sex-related hormones largely drive adolescent behavior. The data, however, do not support a simple "raging hormones" explanation. Based on an extensive review of the literature comparing adolescent behavior with levels of a variety of gonadal steroids and adrenal androgens, Susman and colleagues concluded: "At the folk-wisdom level, hormonal changes are associated with behavioral change in adolescents. The empirical evidence confirming this link is almost nonexistent" (1987, p. 1,114). This conclusion still largely holds today, with evidence for at best only small direct effects of androgens and estrogens on adolescent behavior (e.g., Graber & Brooks-Gunn, 1996), including a linkage of adrenal androgens with certain adjustment problems in adolescence (see Susman & Ponirakis, 1997).

With the realization that sex-related hormones are responsible for only a limited amount of behavioral change during adolescence, attention has turned to other potential contributors. As discussed later in this chapter (see also Cicchetti & Walker, 2001; Walker & Walder, *this volume*), adolescence-associated increases in stress hormones or sensitivity to stressors may support the emergence of adolescent-typical behaviors (as well as symptom expression in adolescents at risk for mental disorders). Dramatic adolescent-associated alterations in brain, including numerous stress-sensitive brain regions, are also likely contributors to unique adolescent-typical behaviors. Indeed, given the pronounced transformations occurring in the brain during adolescence, it would be surprising if the behaviors of adolescents did not differ from those of other aged individuals. Some of these dramatic adolescent-associated alterations in brain are reviewed in the next sections.

NEURAL CHARACTERISTICS OF ADOLESCENCE

From its very beginnings early in embryogenesis until old age, the nervous system is in a dynamic state of change. Although small numbers of neurons continue to be formed throughout life (Eriksson et al., 1998; Kempermann & Gage, 2000), the vast majority of neurons date their birth to the prenatal period. Migration of these neurons to their final location and their differentiation through the elaboration of dendritic and axonal processes continues well into the postnatal period (see Nowakowski & Hayes, 1999, for review). Although much initial neural differentiation, formation of glial support cells and their myelination of neural axons, and related growth in brain size occurs during the first 3–4 years postnatally, brain maturation is by no means complete at that time. Myelination continues until at least the third decade, along with a progressive decline in the proportion of cerebral gray matter to white matter (Jernigan & Sowell, 1997). Other measures reveal changes in brain until at least 70–80 years of age (Blinkov & Glezer, 1968, cited by Nowakowski & Hayes, 1999).

Although the brain undergoes dynamic change throughout life, these alterations are by no means linear, with periods of rapid neural transformation amidst intervals of more modest change. Moreover, not all of this neural development is progressive: Some earlier formed connections are transient and some neurons are ultimately destined for elimination as development proceeds. During the early postnatal period, such overproduction and pruning may allow the developing nervous system to maximize appropriate connections and eliminate those projections or neurons that have been unsuccessful in establishing suitable associations (see Nowakowski & Hayes, 1999, for review). Following on the heels of a period of more modulated change during childhood, the brain again undergoes a metamorphosis during adolescence, a transformation characterized by both progressive and regressive alterations.

Adolescence, Synapse Elimination, and Metabolic Decline. Adolescence is associated with the loss of a considerable number of synapses. The magnitude of this decline is difficult to fathom. Rakic and colleagues (1994) have estimated that as many as 30,000 synapses may be lost per second over the entire cortical region during portions of the pubertal/adolescent period in primate brain, eventually resulting in a decline by nearly half of the average number of synapses present per cortical neuron prior to the adolescent period. Such synaptic downsizing has been reported not only in nonhuman primates (Bourgeois, Goldman-Rakic, & Rakic, 1994; Rakic, Bourgeois, & Goldman-Rakic, 1994) but also in humans, with substantial synaptic declines in human neocortex occurring between seven and sixteen years (e.g., Huttenlocher, 1979). The scarcity of postmortem tissue from developing humans has not permitted a more precise detailing of the timeline for this decline.

Although the functional implications of a massive pruning of synapses during adolescence remain speculative, it has been suggested that these relatively late developmental changes reflect ongoing brain plasticity, allowing the developing brain to be sculpted to meet the particular environmental demands to which it is exposed (Rakic, et al., 1994). One should be cautious, however, about assuming that this phase is analogous to the period of "overproduction followed by pruning" (see Rakic et al., 1994) seen during the prenatal and early postnatal periods. Synaptic complements maintained for years prior to being pruned during adolescence would seemingly have played some functional role in juvenile brain prior to their adolescent demise. The pruning during adolescence thus may not so much reflect the culling of nonproductive synapses, but rather an active restructuring that may serve to promote a more mature pattern of brain effort. More synapses and connections are not necessarily better, some forms of mental retardation being associated with an unusually high number of synapses (Goldman-Rakic, Isseroff, Schwartz, & Bugbee, 1983).

Cortical pruning may be one of a number of developmental changes in adolescent brain that serve to refine brain effort during adolescence. Associated with this apparent refinement of effort is a reduction in overall brain activation as more specific regions respond to stimuli typically activating broader brain regions in younger individuals. For instance, ontogenetic decreases in synaptic density in prefrontal regions have been suggested to be associated with developmental declines in the amount of prefrontal brain tissue activated during task performance through childhood and into adolescence (e.g., Casey, Giedd, & Thomas, 2000). Other ontogenetic changes occurring during adolescence include increases in the degree to which the two cerebral hemispheres can process information independently (Merola & Liederman, 1985) and in the extent of asymmetries in electroencephalograph (EEG) activity between the hemispheres (Anokhin, Lutzenberger, Nikolaev, & Birbaumer, 2000).

An increase in specificity of cortical responses may help minimize energy use and increase efficiency. A majority of synapses undergoing developmental elimination in neocortex are thought to be excitatory because of their asymmetrical appearance (Rakic et al., 1994). Along with this loss of excitatory input to cortex is a reduction in overall brain energy utilization. Measures that reflect the energy needed for brain activity, such as rates of glucose metabolism, blood flow, or oxygen utilization, are greatest in early childhood and decline gradually during adolescence to reach lower, adult-typical levels in humans (see Chugani, 1996, Feinberg, 1987 for review and references) and other species including rats (Tyler & van Harreveld, 1942) and cats (Chugani, 1994).

The relative size of the cellular (gray matter) component of some brain regions declines during adolescence as well. Structural MRI has revealed that ontogenetic declines in cerebral gray matter volume between childhood and adolescence are particularly pronounced in frontal brain regions (dorsal frontal and parietal areas of cortex (Rapoport et al., 1999; Sowell, Thompson, Holmes, Batth et al., 1999a). These changes have been suggested to reflect ontogenetic increases in regions segmenting as white matter rather than gray matter in the adolescents (Sowell et al., 1999a), a suggestion reminiscent of the evidence for developmental increases through adolescence in white matter density in numerous cortical fiber tracks, including the corpus callosum (e.g., Paus et al., 1999; Giedd, Blumenthal, Jeffries, Rajapakse et al., 1999a). In contrast to the developmental decline in gray matter volume of frontal brain regions, volumes in the amygdala and hippocampus increase during childhood and adolescence, with volume changes in the amygdala more prominent in males whereas increases in the hippocampus are more pronounced in females (Giedd, Castellanos, Rajapakse, Vaituzis, & Rapoport, 1997). The adolescent brain is a brain in the process of becoming leaner, more efficient, and less energy consuming.

Developmental Changes in Prefrontal Cortex (PFC). Among the areas of brain undergoing considerable remodeling during adolescence is the prefrontal region of the neocortex. Recent functional (fMRI) MRI work has provided evidence for a functional frontalization with age during the course of normal maturation from adolescence to adulthood (Rubia et al., 2000), with a greater power of functional activation of prefrontal and frontal regions in adults than adolescents during performance of tasks normally activating these regions (e.g., delay task). Differences in the brain regions activated during a stop task were also noted between adolescents and adults, despite comparable performance across age.

Luna and colleagues (2001) used fMRI to examine age differences in brain activation during an oculomotor response-suppression task. Along with gradual ontogenetic increases in the ability to inhibit responding during performance of the task from childhood through adolescence and into adulthood, brain activation in frontal, parietal, striatal, and lateral cerebellar regions was found to be greater in adults than younger subjects. In contrast, prefrontal activation during performance of the task was more pronounced in adolescents than in children or adults. Luna and colleagues (2001) interpret these fMRI results to suggest that age-related improvements in task performance may be related to "maturation of integrated function among the neocortex, striatum, thalamus, and cerebellum."

Anatomical data provide evidence of structural changes in PFC during adolescence in a variety of species. The volume of PFC declines around adolescence in humans (Giedd, Blumenthal, Jeffries, Castellanos et al., 1999b; Jernigan, Trauner, Hesselink, & Tallal, 1991; Sowell, Thompson, Holmes, Jernigan, & Toga, 1999b) and rats (van Eden, Kros, & Uylings, 1990), while density of spines on pyramidal cells in human PFC have been found to decline between adolescence and adulthood (Mrzljak, Uylings, van Eden, & Judáš, 1990). As in other cortical regions, there is substantial pruning of synapses in PFC during adolescence, including the loss of many presumed glutaminergic excitatory synapses in humans (Huttenlocher, 1984) and nonhuman primates (Zecevic, Bourgeois, & Rakic, 1989). In rats as well, receptors for the NMDA form of the glutamate receptor in PFC show a considerable decline during adolescence, with a loss of about one-third of these receptors between the beginnings of adolescence to its end (Insel, Miller, & Gelhard, 1990).

In contrast to the decline in excitatory drive to PFC, input to PFC from dopaminergic (DA) neurons increases during adolescence in nonhuman primates to peak at levels considerably higher than seen earlier in life or in adulthood (Rosenberg & Lewis, 1994, 1995); comparable developmental increases in DA input to PFC through adolescence have also been reported in rats (Kalsbeek, Voorn, Buijs, Pool, & Uylings, 1988; Leslie, Robertson, Cutler, & Bennett, 1991). An adolescent-associated increase in input to PFC from this inhibitory neurotransmitter, DA, may further enhance the impact of a loss in PFC excitatory drive at this time.

Adolescent DA Systems. Alterations are not only evident in DA projections to PFC (often referred to as the mesocortical DA system), but also in projections of this neurotransmitter to other regions as well. These DA terminal regions include the striatum (with its substantial input from DA cell bodies in the substantia nigra), as well as mesolimbic areas that, like the mesocortical DA system, receive projections from DA cell bodies located largely in the ventral tegmental area. Adolescent-related changes in mesolimbic and mesocortical DA projection systems are receiving substantial attention because of the importance of these systems in modulating social behaviors, risk taking, and the rewarding effects of drugs, novelty, and other reinforcing stimuli (Koob, 1992; Koob, Robledo, Markou, & Caine, 1993; Le Moal & Simon, 1991), phenomena of particular relevance during adolescence. As discussed later, maturational changes in these regions during adolescence are also of interest because they have been suggested to contribute to the emergence of overt symptoms of schizophrenia and other disorders (e.g., Lipska & Weinberger, 1993a).

One indicator of adolescent-related transformations occurring in these DA terminal regions is a pronounced decline in numbers of certain DA receptor subtypes. These changes are particularly notable in the striatum, with developmental declines of one-third to one-half or more of the D1-like and D2-like receptors in human striatum from childhood until mature levels are reached in adulthood (Seeman et al., 1987). Although some work has failed to confirm a D2 receptor decline, ontogenetic decreases in D1 receptors from infancy to adulthood in humans have been reported by others (Montague, Lawler, Mailman, & Gilmore, 1999; Palacios, Camps, Cortés, & Probst, 1988). In rats as well, there is a reliable and well-characterized peak in D1 and D2 receptor binding in striatum during adolescence followed subsequently by a 30–75 percent decline to reach adult levels (Teicher, Andersen, & Hostetter, 1995; Tarazi, Tomasini, & Baldessarini, 1998, 1999; Tarazi & Baldessarini, 2000). Striatal binding to DA D4 receptors (Tarazi et al., 1998; Tarazi & Baldessarini, 2000), but not D3 receptors (Demotes-Mainard, Henry, Jeantet, Arsaut, & Arnauld, 1996), similarly appears to peak during adolescence and decline subsequently.

The evidence is mixed as to whether similar developmental declines in DA receptors are seen in mesolimbic (e.g., nucleus accumbens) and mesocortical brain regions. For instance, work reporting no clear evidence for DA receptor "overproduction" and pruning in rat accumbens (Teicher et al., 1995) contrasts with other data in the same species showing a peak in both D1 and D2 receptor binding during early adolescence at levels about one-third higher than in adulthood (Tarazi et al., 1998; Tarazi et al., 1999; Tarazi & Baldessarini, 2000). In the PFC of rat, findings showing a peak in DA D1 and D2 receptor binding from P40–60 followed by a protracted but considerable ontogenetic decline thereafter (Andersen, Thompson, Rutstein, Hostetter, & Teicher, 2000) differ from others reporting only a gradual ontogenetic increase in DA receptors (Tarazi et al., 1998, 1999; Tarazi & Baldessarini, 2000). Part of these discrepancies may be related to the ages examined, with for instance ontogenetic declines in D1 and D2 binding in PFC reported not to occur until after P60 by Andersen and colleagues (2000), whereas animals P60 and younger were the focus of the work by Tarazi & Baldessarini (2000). Taken together, these data support the tentative notion that binding to D1 and D2 DA receptors peaks early in adolescence and subsequently declines in striatum and perhaps the accumbens, whereas binding of these receptor subtypes remains elevated in PFC throughout adolescence, with later declines into adulthood.

Taken together, these data suggest that adolescence is associated with considerable change in binding capacity for DA in a variety of forebrain DA terminal regions. Although less explored, the functional coupling of these receptors to second messenger systems may also vary from that seen in the mature organism (Andersen & Teicher, 1999; Bolanos, Glatt, & Jackson, 1998). For instance, with some exceptions, D1 stimulatory and D2 inhibitory effects on adenylate cyclase activity were found to be less evident in adolescents than adults (Andersen & Teicher, 1999), although basal levels of cAMP were generally elevated in the adolescents. In addition to these changes in DA receptor binding and its functional consequences, developmental alterations in rates of DA synthesis and utilization also are evident, transformations that perhaps reflect an age-related shift in the balance between subcortical versus cortical DA projection systems, as discussed in the next section.

Developmental Shifts in the Balance Between Mesocortical and Mesolimbic DA Projection Systems. One consequence of the developmental increase in DA input to PFC during adolescence (Kalsbeek et al., 1988; Leslie et al., 1991; Rosenberg & Lewis, 1994, 1995) may be a compensatory decline in DA utilization in this brain region late in adolescence. For instance, rates of synthesis and turnover of DA are greater in the PFC of early adolescent than late adolescent rats (Andersen, Dumont, & Teicher, 1997; Boyce, 1996; although see also Leslie et al., 1991). It is interesting that an inverse ontogenetic pattern is seen in accumbens, where DA synthesis and turnover rates are lower early than late in adolescence (Andersen et al., 1997; Boyce, 1996). Such a developmental shift in the balance of DA activity between mesocortical (PFC) and mesolimbic (e.g., accumbens) forebrain regions during adolescence is reminiscent of the often reciprocal relationship between these forebrain DA terminal regions (Deutch, 1992; Lipska & Weinberger, 1993a; Wilkinson, 1997), with "expressed behavior (being) the result of the summed outcome of competing systems" (Whishaw, Fiorino, Mittleman, & Castaneda, 1992, p. 9). A developmental shift of this nature may be of particular significance for the adolescent, given the involvement of these stress-sensitive regions in the attribution of incentive value and reward-directed behaviors (e.g., Berridge & Robinson, 1998; Ikemoto & Panksepp, 1999; Koob et al., 1993). The accumbens, in particular, has been suggested to play a critical role in the processing of reinforcing stimuli and their behavioral implications (e.g., Berridge & Robinson, 1998; Schultz, 1998; Kalivas, Churchill, & Klitenick, 1993).

A shift in the balance of DA activity from mesolimbic to mesocortical regions early in adolescence would seemingly result in a transient lowering of DA function in mesolimbic brain regions during early adolescence. Functional insufficiencies in mesolimbic DA reward pathways have been linked to a reward deficiency syndrome (Gardner, 1999). According to Gardner (1999), abstinent drug users and other at-risk individuals with this syndrome "actively seek out not only addicting drugs but also environmental novelty and sensation as a type of behavioral remediation of reward deficiency" (p. 82). To the extent that adolescents demonstrate an age-related net decline in DA function in mesolimbic regions during early adolescence, they likewise may exhibit a qualitatively similar "reward deficiency syndrome," albeit transient and normally of notably lesser intensity (Spear, 2000a). Indeed, reports of feeling "very happy" drop by 50 percent between childhood and early adolescence (fifth to seventh grade), with adolescents also experiencing positive situations as less pleasurable than adults (Larson & Richards, 1994).

Such reward deficiencies would be expected to be particularly prominent in stressed adolescents. Mesocortical DA projections are more sensitive to activation by stressors than DA terminals in subcortical (mesolimbic and striatal) brain regions (e.g., Dunn, 1988). Hence, by selectively activating the mesocortical DA system, stressors would be expected to further tilt the balance toward relative DA predominance in mesocortical over mesolimbic brain regions during adolescence (e.g., Cabib & Puglisi-Allegra, 1996).

These speculations should be tempered by some caveats. First, both reductions and elevations in mesolimbic DA activity have been related to increases in drug-taking behavior. According to the reward deficiency syndrome, drug-seeking behavior is associated with deficits in mesolimbic DA systems (Gardner, 1999), whereas the traditional DA hypothesis of reward conversely predicts that drug seeking would be positively related to activity in mesolimbic DA systems (see Spanagel & Weiss, 1999, for review). It is possible that both associations may be evident, with both atypically low as well as unusually high DA levels leading to increased drug-taking behavior, a nonmonotonic relationship for which there is substantial precedent, given the high prevalence of inverted U-shaped relationships in psychopharmacology. Also, although there is considerable evidence for developmental alterations in mesocorticolimbic DA terminal regions and other related brain regions during adolescence, further work is needed to determine whether these changes indeed reflect a shift in balance between mesocortical and mesolimbic regions. Moreover, much of the work to date implicating a developmental shift in balance among mesocorticolimbic DA terminal regions has been derived from work with rodents, and it remains to be determined how well these findings represent developmental events occurring in human adolescents. Finally, developmental adjustments within these forebrain systems do not occur in a vacuum, but should be considered within a context of adolescent-associated adjustments in a variety of other neural systems, a few examples of which are given in the following section.

Alterations in Other Neural Systems. Although neural data in this age range are sparse for some systems, it nevertheless is clear that adolescent-associated transformations of brain are not restricted to alterations in forebrain DA projections and the pruning of excitatory (glutaminergic) input to neocortex as discussed in previous sections. Alterations in other neurotransmitter and neuromodulatory systems are also seen. For instance, adolescent (P30) rats have substantially (four-fold) lower turnover rates of serotonin (5-hydroxytryptamine, 5-HT) in the nucleus accumbens than younger (P10–15) or adult rats, an age effect not apparent in striatum (Teicher & Andersen, 1999). These findings are intriguing, given that certain characteristics associated with low 5-HT activity, such as stressor hyperresponsiveness, increased negative affect, hyperdipsia, increased alcohol drinking, and anxiety (see Depue & Spoont, 1986) are reminiscent of those attributes often ascribed to adolescents.

Receptors for cannabinoids, a class of psychoactive compounds that includes the active ingredients in marijuana, mature slowly during the postnatal period (Belue, Howlett, Westlake, & Hutchings, 1995; Rodríguez de Fonseca, Ramos, Bonnin, & Fernández-Ruiz, 1993). Cannabinoid receptor systems seem to undergo considerable functional maturation during the adolescent age range, with cannabinoid agonists inducing clear-cut behavioral effects in late adolescent (P45) and adult, but not pre-adolescent (P23) rats (Fride & Mechoulam, 1996a,b). Emergence of cannabinoid responsiveness during adolescence could potentially facilitate a developmental shift in balance between mesolimbic/striatal versus mesocortical DA systems, given evidence (at least in adult animals) for cannabinoid activation of mesocortical DA systems (Diana, Melis, & Gessa, 1998) contrasting with findings of a cannabinoid inhibition of DA-induced activation in striatum (Giuffrida et al., 1999).

The adolescent amygdala is also of considerable interest. Portions of the amygdala intimately connect with accumbens and other limbic and mesolimbic regions to form the "extended amygdala complex," circuitry thought to play important roles in reward and drug-related behaviors (Koob et al., 1993). There is an old and complex literature implicating developmental changes in the amygdala in the timing of puberty (see Moltz, 1975, for review). Research has also revealed substantial alterations in amygdala activity and its processing of stressful and emotional stimuli in adolescence. Work in laboratory animals has shown that adolescents (P26–40 rats) are much more likely to develop seizures following electrical stimulation of the amygdala than either younger or older animals (Terasawa & Timiras, 1968). Using increases in the expression of the immediate early gene c-fos as an index of neural activation, young adolescent (P28) rats were found to exhibit less stress-induced activation in certain regions of the amygdala than young adult (P60) rats (Kellogg, Awatramani, & Piekut, 1998).

In humans, studies using fMRI have shown that levels of negative affect and anxiety are correlated with activity in the amygdala (Davidson, Abercrombie, Nitschke, & Putnam, 1999). Such amygdalar activation in response to emotional stimuli, such as faces displaying fear, is seen in children, adolescents, and adults (e.g., see Baird et al., 1999), although there may be a change during adolescence in the extent of this activation. Killgore, Oki, and Yurgelun-Todd (2001) observed that when subjects looked at faces with emotional content, the amount of left amygdala activation declined during adolescence, an effect that reached significance only in females, although a similar trend was evident in males (Killgore et al., 2001). On the other hand, Thomas and colleagues (2001) reported that it was the adults who exhibited more left amygdala activation to emotional (fearful) than neutral faces, whereas children exhibited more activation of this region in response to neutral than fearful faces, data suggesting a presumptive increase during adolescence in left amygdala activation. In other research (Pine et al., 2001), adolescents were found to be similar to adults in the extent of amygdala activation by fearful faces. Clearly the picture is more confusing than illuminating at present, but research in this area seems to be progressing rapidly. Given that metabolic activity in the amygdala of humans is often inversely related to activity in cortical regions such as the PFC (Davidson et al., 1999), an intriguing area for further study is the notion of a potential adolescence-associated alteration in the pattern of PFC versus amygdala activation in the processing of stressful and emotional stimuli. Indeed, there are reports of different patterns of cortical activation during emotional processing when comparing younger and older adolescents (Killgore et al., 2001) as well as adolescents and adults (Pine et al., 2001).

This section will close by considering a neuromodulator that has received considerable recent attention: leptin. Leptin is a protein released by fat cells and is thought to serve as a satiety signal to the brain. Leptin levels often increase considerably during the growth spurt of adolescence (Lahlou, Landais, De Boissieu, & Bougnères, 1997; Mantzoros, Flier, & Rogol, 1997; but see also Ahima, Dushay, Flier, Prabakaran, & Flier, 1997; Cheung, Thornton, Nurani, Clifton & Steiner, 2001). Although not sufficient to trigger puberty alone, increasing levels of leptin are thought to "act in a permissive fashion" to indicate to the brain that metabolic reserves are sufficient to support pubertal maturation (Cheung et al., 1997). Increasing levels of leptin during adolescence may have broad impact on brain function. Leptin inhibits hypothalamo-pituitary-adrenal axis activity (Heiman, Chen, & Caro, 1998) while stimulating the hypothalamo-pituitary-gonadal axis (Blum, 1997). This protein also modulates activity of peptides, such as neuropeptide Y and corticotropin-releasing hormone, thought to regulate energy homeostasis (see Buchanan, Mahesh, Zamorano, & Brann, 1998, for review) and to play critical roles in modulating stress/emotional responding and in influencing drug responsivity (Koob, 1999; Koob & Heinrichs, 1999).

Developmental Alterations in Psychopharmacological Sensitivity. To the extent that adolescence is associated with developmental changes in the neural systems underlying the effects of some psychoactive drugs, it might be expected that adolescence would be associated with developmental changes in drug sensitivity. Indeed, this is the case for a number of psychoactive drugs, a few examples of which will be given here. The NMDA glutamate receptor antagonists phencyclidine (PCP) and ketamine do not produce hallucinations in prepubertal children, but do so in adults (Hirsch, Das, Garey, & de Belleroche, 1997). Adolescent humans and rats are more sensitive to neuroleptics than their adult counterparts (Spear, Shalaby, & Brick, 1980; Keepers, Clappison & Casey, 1983; Campbell, Baldessarini, & Teicher, 1988; Greenhill & Setterberg, 1993). At least in studies in laboratory animals, adolescents also appear to differ from adults in sensitivity to stimulant drugs (see Spear & Brake, 1983; Spear, 2000a, for review) and ethanol (see Spear, 2000b). Interestingly, the nature of the age-related alterations in responsiveness to ethanol varies with the response measure examined, and may reflect

differential development of the neural systems underlying these differing ethanol consequences. For instance, adolescents are more sensitive than adults to ethanol-related
disruptions of hippocampal plasticity and spatial memory (Swartzwelder, Wilson, &
Tayyeb, 1995a; Markwiese, Acheson, Levin, Wilson, & Swartzwelder, 1998), findings
linked to developmental "overexpression" of hippocampal glutamate/NMDA systems
(Swartzwelder, Wilson, & Tayyeb, 1995b). In contrast, the attenuated sensitivity of
adolescents to ethanol-induced sedation relative to adults (Little, Kuhn, Wilson &
Swartzwelder, 1996; Silveri & Spear, 1998) may be related in part to immaturity of
gamma-aminobutyric acid (GABA) inhibitory systems (Silveri & Spear, submitted).

As these few examples have illustrated, the dramatic transformations occurring in
adolescent brain may not only facilitate characteristic adolescent behaviors, but may
also alter the substrate for expression of the effects of a number of psychoactive drugs.

IMPLICATIONS OF ADOLESCENT-RELATED NEURAL ALTERATIONS ON EXPRESSION OF SYMPTOMATOLOGY

Adolescent-associated neural transformations may also alter the expression of psychopathology by a vulnerable brain. Indeed, as discussed in more detail elsewhere
in this volume, the expression of a variety of neuropsychological disorders and psychopathology changes during adolescence.

In some cases, symptomatology may at least partially abate during adolescence. For
instance, Tourette's syndrome tends to improve or resolve during adolescence (Kurlan,
1992). Only about 10 percent of cases of childhood epilepsy continue into adolescence
(see Saugstad, 1994). In work conducted in Rhesus monkeys, an adolescent-associated
improvement in outcome following early orbital frontal lesions was seen, with the
notable lesion-related deficits evident early in life resolving considerably as animals
reached maturity (Goldman, 1971).

More common than an improvement in outcome during adolescence is the converse, with overt symptomatology of some types of psychological disorders and early
brain damage only emerging during adolescence.

Schizophrenia. One well-known example is schizophrenia. Despite growing evidence
that schizophrenia is a disorder of largely fetal origin (see Bunney & Bunney, 1999,
for review), typical features of this disorder do not emerge fully until at least adolescence. The abnormal location of cortical neurons in the innermost layers of cortex
in the brains of schizophrenics is consistent with a disruption in neuronal migration
to neocortex during the second trimester (Akbarian et al., 1993; Jakob & Beckmann,
1986); similar evidence for disrupted migration in schizophrenia brain is evident in
other brain regions, including hippocampus (Conrad & Scheibel, 1987; Kovelman &
Scheibel, 1984). Among the chromosomal loci with linkage to schizophrenia are regions coding for genes regulating retinoids and retinoic acids, substances that modulate transcription of numerous genes critical for neural development and migration
(see Goodman, 1998). Such genetic factors may perhaps predispose the developing nervous system to be adversely affected by various environmental factors (such as prenatal
nutritional deficiencies, exposure to viruses, drug/toxin exposure), setting the stage for
the later emergence of overt symptomatology as the PFC and other forebrain regions
are sculpted during adolescence (see Lipska & Weinberger, 1993a, for review).

Cerebellar Cognitive Affective Syndrome. Cerebellar lesions in adults have been shown to impair executive functioning and affective regulation (e.g., Schmahmann & Sherman, 1998), presumably due to disruptions of neural circuits that include prefrontal cortex, thalamus, and cerebellum (Middleton & Strick, 2000, 2001). Although limited study populations have restricted the detail to which age effects could be explored, expression of this syndrome may intensify around adolescence. Deficits characteristic of this syndrome were more apparent in older than younger individuals within a group of 3–16-year-olds with cerebellar damage (Levisohn, Cronin-Golomb, & Schmahmann, 2000).

Other Disorders. A variety of other disorders are also associated with a largely adolescent onset, a few examples of which are given here. Eating disorders show a substantial increased incidence during adolescence, particularly among adolescent females (Brooks-Gunn & Attie, 1996). Adolescence is likewise associated with a considerable increase in the rates of depressive disorders and the emergence of a gender difference in these prevalence rates. Incidence of clinical depression in children is approximately 1 percent, and reaches adult levels of 8 percent by nineteen years of age (see Kutcher & Sokolov, 1995). Rates of depression are slightly greater during childhood in boys than girls, whereas greater prevalence rates in females emerge in adolescence and continue into adulthood (see Ge, Lorenz, Conger, Elder, & Simons, 1994, for discussion and references). Adolescents may also vary from other aged individuals in the physiological correlates of this depression. Depressed adolescents (and children) are less likely to hypersecrete cortisol than adult depressives (e.g., Puig-Antich, 1987; see Brooks-Gunn, Petersen, & Compas, 1995, for review and discussion). Depressive disorders in adolescence also appear to be more associated with serotonergic dysfunction, whereas disturbances in norepinephrine have been more closely linked with this disorder in adulthood (Kutcher & Sokolov, 1995).

Adolescent-Associated Emergence of Effects of Early Brain Damage in Laboratory Animals. Reminiscent of the emergence of overt signs of schizophrenia and the increased incidence of affective disorders in adolescent humans, laboratory animals have also been reported to "grow into their deficits" during the adolescent period following a variety of types of early brain damage. For instance, sparing of function early in life is evident after early dorsolateral lesions of the PFC in Rhesus monkeys, with consequences of the lesions becoming progressively more evident as the animal reaches maturity (Goldman, 1971). Analogous findings were observed following excitotoxic lesions of the medial PFC in neonatal (P7) rats; such lesions have little impact on behavior when animals are tested in mid-adolescence (P35), with lesion effects emerging by late adolescence/early adulthood (P56) (Flores, Wood, Liang, Quirion, & Srivastava, 1996). Similarly, emergence of stress hyperresponsiveness and DA-related abnormal behaviors is delayed until adolescence following neonatal excitotoxic lesions of the ventral hippocampus in rats, effects that have been speculated to result from lesion-induced disruptions in the development of stress sensitivity circuitry including the medial PFC (see Lipska & Weinberger, 1993b). Delayed emergence of consequences is also apparent following other types of early insults. For example, characteristic disruptions in stress responsiveness, arousal, and attention in rats exposed prenatally to diazepam often do not become apparent until the late adolescent period (Kellogg, 1991).

Although more tangential to the focus here, not only age at the time of examination, but also age at the time of brain damage is critical in influencing outcome. For instance, aphagia and adipsia resulting from lesions of the PFC in rats typically do not emerge unless animals are lesioned after adolescence (Kolb & Nonneman, 1976). Damage to DA systems induced by the neurotoxin 6-hydroxydopamine had only minor effects if the damage occurred prior to adolescence (P27 or younger), whereas comparable DA depletion in more mature rats caused profound behavioral impairment (aphagia, adipsia, akinesia, sensory neglect; Joyce, Frohna, & Neal-Beliveau, 1996). The hyper-responsiveness to stress and altered response to amphetamine challenge emerging in late adolescence following neonatal excitotoxic lesions of the hippocampus were not apparent after comparable lesions in adult rats (Lipska, Jaskiw, & Weinberger, 1993).

COMPENSATIONS AND STRESSORS: WHAT IS SPECIAL ABOUT ADOLESCENCE?

Why should the adolescent period be associated with developmental declines or emergences in the expression of certain types of psychopathology and lesion effects? There are a number of possibilities. It is possible that in some instances, impaired neural regions may not become functionally mature until adolescence, and hence consequences of damage to that region may not surface until adolescence. For instance, development in the prefrontal cortex continues through adolescence (Rubia et al., 2000), and hence it is possible that subtle perturbations there or in functionally associated brain regions might have few functional consequences until the region is sufficiently developed to express these deficits. Conversely, manifestation of some early appearing deficits may decline developmentally as brain activity during adolescence is restructured and refined to permit compensations for these deficits to emerge.

The restructuring of adolescent brain may also unveil early developmental compromises. The brain during early development shows considerable plasticity and may be able to adjust for some types of suboptimal developmental events triggered via a variety of genetic and environmental conditions. Such neural compensations may in some cases result in substantial masking of the functional consequences of the neural perturbation. But, as Goldman-Rakic and colleagues (1983) said: "there must be a 'price' to the behavioral sparing following early damage" (p. 331). One potential price is a delayed emergence of symptomatology. Some of these early ontogenetic compromises may be exposed decades later by the developmental shifts in patterns of neural activity among brain regions associated with the normal sculpting of brain during adolescence.

Another potential cost associated with compensatory neural reorganization early in life is a decrease in the organism's later ability to adapt to environmental challenges and stressors (e.g., Spear, Campbell, Snyder, Silveri, & Katovic, 1998). Increased sensitivity to stressors and environmental demands has been reported following a variety of developmental perturbations including perinatal stress (Cabib, Puglisi-Allegra, & D'Amato, 1993; Takahashi, Turner, & Kalin, 1992; Weinstock, 1997); as well as prenatal exposure to drugs including cocaine, ethanol, or diazepam (Kellogg, 1991; Mayes, Grillon, Granger, & Schottenfeld, 1998; Riley, 1990; Spear et al., in press). Such stressor vulnerability may be particularly pronounced during adolescence. Adolescence appears to be an unusually stressful life stage (see Spear, 2000a, for review) that may be associated with an increase in levels of activity of the hypothalamo-pituitary-adrenal axis, resulting in postpubertal rises in normative cortisol levels (e.g., see Walker & Walder, *this volume*, for reviews and references). Many of the neural regions undergoing developmental alterations during adolescence are highly sensitive to activation by stressors, including the PFC and other mesocorticolimbic DA terminal regions (Dunn, 1988). As discussed above, any adolescence-associated shift to greater mesocortical than subcortical DA transmission would be expected to be further exacerbated by stressors (see Spear, 2000a), given the greater stress sensitivity of the DA projections to PFC (Dunn, 1988). Early brain dysfunction may predispose certain individuals for the later development of schizophrenia and potentially other disorders by increasing their sensitivity to stressors during the vulnerable stage of adolescence (Bogerts, 1989; Lipska & Weinberger, 1993a; Walker & Diforio, 1997).

DIRECTIONS FOR FUTURE RESEARCH

Although there are tantalizing hints as to the magnitude and significance of the metamorphosis in brain during adolescence, areas yet to be investigated far exceed what is known. Even in those brain regions shown to undergo alterations during adolescence, the significance of these modifications and their relationship to development in other brain regions often remains to be explored. The hypothesis of a postulated shift in balance between mesocortical and mesolimbic brain regions during adolescence and the functional implications of such a developmental transition needs further detailed testing in laboratory animals and confirmation and extension to human adolescents (Spear, 2000). Particularly intriguing is recent fMRI work suggesting potential adolescent transitions in levels of activity in the amygdala and PFC during the processing of emotional or stressful stimuli (Killgore et al., 2001; Pine et al., 2001). Indeed, these two brain regions – the PFC and amygdala – are highly sensitive to stressful and emotional stimuli (e.g., Davidson et al., 1999; Dunn, 1988) and may be particularly important "players" in the adolescent-associated tranformation of brain. Yet, the fMRI data thus far examining amygdalar and frontal activation in response to emotional stimuli have yielded a mosaic of inconsistent ontogenetic findings (Killgore et al., 2001; Pine et al., 2001; Thomas et al., 2001). Clearly, more work is needed in this rapidly evolving research area.

In these studies, it is likely to become increasingly important to dissect the time course of specific adolescent-associated neurobehavioral changes within the broader adolescent period. The adolescent brain may not represent a static developmental state, but rather an unfolding series of neural alterations that differentially become expressed as adolescent development proceeds. For example, as discussed previously, developmental peaks and subsequent declines in DA D1 and D2 receptors may occur relatively early in adolescence in rat striatum and perhaps in accumbens (Tarazi et al., 1998, 1999; Tarazi & Baldessarini, 2000), whereas declines in these receptors in PFC may occur later, during the transition between late adolescence and adulthood (Andersen et al., 2000). Early adolescent rats likewise differ from older adolescents in regional rates of DA synthesis and turnover, with higher rates in PFC and lower rates in accumbens evident earlier than later in adolescence (Andersen et al., 1997; Boyce, 1996). As suggested by these data, it may be overly simplistic to view even the abbreviated adolescent period of rats, let alone human adolescence, as a single ontogenetic transition rather than a series of developmental alterations.

Much remains to be understood about stress responsivity during adolescence in terms of its behavioral, hormonal, and neural substrates. Is adolescence an unusually stressful life stage and/or are adolescents more reactive to environmental stressors? Do stressors during adolescence exacerbate or attenuate adolescent-associated alterations in neural activity in specific stress-sensitive brain regions, and what impact do these neural alterations have on expression of normative and atypical adolescent behaviors?

As findings in these areas are elaborated, it will be critical to consider their implications for the emergence during or shortly following adolescence of certain symptoms of brain damage and psychopathology. How might alterations in stressor responsivity and activity of the hypothalamo-pituitary-adrenal axis promote the expression of psychopathology? Can specific maturational events in the PFC, mesolimbic or other regions of the adolescent brain be linked with the appearance of specific lesion effects or symptoms of psychopathology during or following adolescence, or the precipitation by stressors of these effects? It will become possible to address these and other questions as more is learned about the brain of the adolescent and the way it responds to environmental demands. What is clear at this point is that the brain undergoes considerable sculpting and remodeling during adolescence. What remains a challenge is to detail the extent of this restructuring and its functional ramifications.

REFERENCES

Adriani, W., Chiarotti, F., & Laviola, G. (1998). Elevated novelty seeking and peculiar d-amphetamine sensitization in periadolescent mice compared with adult mice. *Behavioral Neuroscience, 112*, 1152–1166.

Ahima, R. S., Dushay, J., Flier, S. N., Prabakaran, D., & Flier, J. S. (1997). Leptin accelerates the onset of puberty in normal female mice. *Journal of Clinical Investigation, 99*, 391–395.

Akbarian, S., Bunney, W. E., Jr., Potkin, S. G., Wigal, S. B., Hagman, J. O., Sandman, C. A., & Jones, E. G. (1993). Altered distribution of nicotinamide-adenine dinucleotide phosphate-diaphorase cells in frontal lobe of schizophrenics implies disturbances of cortical development. *Archives of General Psychiatry, 50*, 169–177.

Andersen, S. L., Dumont, N. L., & Teicher, M. H. (1997). Developmental differences in dopamine synthesis inhibition by (±)-7-OH-DPAT. *Naunyn-Schmiedeberg's Archives of Pharmacology, 356*, 173–181.

Andersen, S. L., & Teicher, M. H. (1999, October). *Cyclic adenosine monophosphate (cAMP) changes dramatically across periadolescence and region.* Poster session presented at the annual meeting of the Society for Neuroscience, Miami Beach, Fla.

Andersen, S. L., Thompson, A. T., Rutstein, M., Hostetter, J. C., & Teicher, M. H. (2000). Dopamine receptor pruning in prefrontal cortex during the periadolescent period in rats. *Synapse, 37*, 167–169.

Anokhin, A. P., Lutzenberger, W., Nikolaev, A., & Birbaumer, N. (2000). Complexity of electrocortical dynamics in children: developmental aspects. *Developmental Psychobiology, 36*, 9–22.

Baird, A. A., Gruber, S. A., Fein, D. A., Maas, L. C., Steingard, R. J., Renshaw, P. F., Cohen, B. M., & Yurgelun-Todd, D. A. (1999). Functional magnetic resonance imaging of facial affect recognition in children and adolescents. *Journal of the American Academy of Child and Adolescent Psychiatry, 38*, 195–199.

Baumrind, D. (1987). A developmental perspective on adolescent risk taking in contemporary America. In C. E. Irwin, Jr. (Ed.), *Adolescent social behavior and health* (pp. 93–125). San Francisco: Jossey-Bass.

Belue, R. C., Howlett, A. C., Westlake, T. M. & Hutchings, D. E. (1995). The ontogeny of cannabinoid receptors in the brain of postnatal and aging rats. *Neurotoxicology and Teratology, 17*, 25–30.

Berridge, K. C., & Robinson, T. E. (1998). What is the role of dopamine in reward: Hedonic impact, reward learning, or incentive salience? *Brain Research Reviews, 28*, 309–369.

Bixler, R. H. (1992). Why littermates don't: The avoidance of inbreeding depression. *Annual Review of Sex Research*, *3*, 291–328.

Blinkov, S. M., & Glezer, I. I. (1968). *The human brain in figures and tables: A quantitative handbook*. New York: Plenum.

Blum, W. F. (1997). Leptin: The voice of the adipose tissue. *Hormone Research*, *48*, 2–8.

Bogerts, B. (1989). Limbic and paralimbic pathology in schizophrenia: Interaction with age- and stress-related factors. In S. C. Schulz & C. A. Tamminga (Eds.), *Schizophrenia: Scientific progress* (pp. 216–226). Oxford: Oxford University Press.

Bolanos, C. A., Glatt, S. J., & Jackson, D. (1998). Subsensitivity to dopaminergic drugs in peri-adolescent rats: A behavioral and neurochemical analysis. *Developmental Brain Research*, *111*, 25–33.

Bourgeois, J.-P., Goldman-Rakic, P. S., & Rakic, P. (1994). Synaptogenesis in the prefrontal cortex of rhesus monkeys. *Cerebral Cortex*, *4*, 78–96.

Boyce, W. T. (1996). Biobehavioral reactivity and injuries in children and adolescents. In M. H. Bornstein & J. L. Genevro (Eds.), *Child development and behavioral pediatrics* (pp. 35–58). Mahwah, N.J.: Erlbaum.

Brook, C. G., & Hindmarsh, P. C. (1992). The somatotropic axis in puberty. *Endocrinology and Metabolism Clinics of North America*, *21*, 767–782.

Brooks-Gunn, J., & Attie, I. (1996). Developmental psychopathology in the context of adolescence. In M. F. Lenzenweger & J. J. Haugaard (Eds.), *Frontiers of developmental psychopathology* (pp. 148–189). New York: Oxford University Press.

Brooks-Gunn, J., Petersen, A. C., & Compas, B. E. (1995). Physiological processes and the development of childhood and adolescent depression. In I. M. Goodyer (Ed.), *The depressed child and adolescent: Developmental and clinical perspectives* (pp. 81–109). Cambridge: Cambridge University Press.

Brooks-Gunn, J., & Reiter, E. O. (1990). The role of pubertal processes. In S. S. Feldman & G. R. Elliott (Eds.), *At the threshold: The developing adolescent* (pp. 16–53). Cambridge, Mass.: Harvard University Press.

Buchanan, C., Mahesh, V., Zamorano, P., & Brann, D. (1998). Central nervous system effects of leptin. *Trends in Endocrinology and Metabolism*, *9*, 146–150.

Bunney, W. E., Jr., & Bunney, B. G. (1999). Neurodevelopmental hypothesis of schizophrenia. In D. S. Charney, E. J. Nestler, & B. S. Bunney (Eds.), *Neurobiology of mental illness* (pp. 225–235). New York: Oxford University Press.

Cabib, S., & Puglisi-Allegra, S. (1996). Stress, depression and the mesolimbic dopamine system. *Psychopharmacology*, *128*, 331–342.

Cabib, S., Puglisi-Allegra, S., & D'Amato, F. R. (1993). Effects of postnatal stress on dopamine mesolimbic system responses to aversive experiences in adult life. *Brain Research*, *604*, 232–239.

Campbell, A., Baldessarini, R. J., & Teicher, M. H. (1988). Decreasing sensitivity to neuroleptic agents in developing rats: Evidence for a pharmacodynamic factor. *Psychopharmacology*, *94*, 46–51.

Casey, B. J., Giedd, J. N., & Thomas, K. M. (2000). Structural and functional brain development and its relation to cognitive development. *Biological Psychology*, *54*, 241–257.

Cheung, C. C., Thornton, J. E., Kuijper, J. L., Weigle, D. S., Clifton, D. K., & Steiner, R. A. (1997). Leptin is a metabolic gate for the onset of puberty in the female rat. *Endocrinology*, *138*, 855–858.

Cheung, C. C., Thornton, J. E., Nurani, S. D., Clifton, D. K., & Steiner, R. A. (2001). A reassessment of leptin's role in triggering the onset of puberty in the rat and mouse. *Neuroendocrinology*, *74*, 12–21.

Chugani, H. T. (1994). Development of regional brain glucose metabolism in relation to behavior and plasticity. In G. Dawson & K. W. Fischer (Eds.), *Human behavior and the developing brain* (pp. 153–175). New York: Guilford Press.

Chugani, H. T. (1996). Neuroimaging of developmental nonlinearity and developmental pathologies. In R. W. Thatcher, G. R. Lyon, J. Rumsey, & N. Krasnegor (Eds.), *Developmental neuroimaging: Mapping the development of brain and behavior* (pp. 187–195). San Diego: Academic Press.

Cicchetti, D., & Walker, E. F. (2001). Stress and development: Biological and psychological. *Development and Psychopathology*, *13*, 413–418.

Conrad, A. J., & Scheibel, A. B. (1987). Schizophrenia and the hippocampus: The embryological hypothesis extended. *Schizophrenia Bulletin, 13*, 577–587.

Crockett, C. M., & Pope, T. R. (1993). Consequences of sex differences in dispersal for juvenile red howler monkeys. In M. E. Pereira & L. A. Fairbanks (Eds.), *Juvenile primates* (pp. 104–118, 367–415). New York: Oxford University Press.

Csikszentmihalyi, M., Larson, R., & Prescott, S. (1977). The ecology of adolescent activity and experience. *Journal of Youth and Adolescence, 6*, 281–294.

Davidson, R. J., Abercrombie, H., Nitschke, J. B., & Putnam, K. (1999). Regional brain function, emotion and disorders of emotion. *Current Opinion in Neurobiology, 9*, 228–234.

Demotes-Mainard, J., Henry, C., Jeantet, Y., Arsaut, J., & Arnauld, E. (1996). Postnatal ontogeny of dopamine D3 receptors in the mouse brain: Autoradiographic evidence for a transient cortical expression. *Developmental Brain Research, 94*, 166–174.

Depue, R. A., & Spoont, M. R. (1986). Conceptualizing a serotonin trait: A behavioral dimension of constraint. *Annals of the New York Academy of Sciences, 487*, 47–62.

Deutch, A. Y. (1992). The regulation of subcortical dopamine systems by the prefrontal cortex: Interactions of central dopamine systems and the pathogenesis of schizophrenia. *Journal of Neural Transmission, 36*, 61–89.

Diana, M., Melis, M., & Gessa, G. L. (1998). Increase in meso-prefrontal dopaminergic activity after stimulation of CBI receptors by cannabinoids. *European Journal of Neuroscience, 10*, 2825–2830.

Dunn, A. J. (1988). Stress-related activation of cerebral dopaminergic systems. *Annals of the New York Academy of Sciences, 537*, 188–205.

Eriksson, P. S., Perfilieva, E., Björk-Eriksson, T., Alborn, A.-M., Nordborg, C., Peterson, D. A., & Gage, F. H. (1998). Neurogenesis in the adult human hippocampus. *Nature Medicine, 4*, 1313–1317.

Feinberg, I. (1987). Adolescence and mental illness. *Science, 236*, 507.

Flores, G., Wood, G. K., Liang, J.-J., Quirion, R., & Srivastava, L. K. (1996). Enhanced amphetamine sensitivity and increased expression of dopamine D2 receptors in postpubertal rats after neonatal excitotoxic lesions of the medial prefrontal cortex. *Journal of Neuroscience, 16*, 7366–7375.

Fride, E., & Mechoulam, R. (1996a). Developmental aspects of anandamide: Ontogeny of response and prenatal exposure. *Psychoneuroendocrinology, 21*, 157–172.

Fride, E., & Mechoulam, R. (1996b). Ontogenetic development of the response to anandamide and Δ-(9)-tetrahydrocannabinol in mice. *Developmental Brain Research, 95*, 131–134.

Gabriel, S. M., Roncancio, J. R., & Ruiz, N. S. (1992). Growth hormone pulsatility and the endocrine milieu during sexual maturation in male and female rats. *Neuroendocrinology, 56*, 619–628.

Galef, B. G., Jr. (1977). Mechanisms for the social transmission of food preferences from adult to weanling rats. In L. M. Barker, M. Best, & M. Domjan (Eds.), *Learning mechanisms in food selection* (pp. 123–148). Waco, Tex.: Baylor University Press.

Gardner, E. L. (1999). The neurobiology and genetics of addiction: Implications of the reward deficiency syndrome for therapeutic strategies in chemical dependency. In J. Elster (Ed.), *Addiction: Entries and exits* (pp. 57–119). New York: Russell Sage Foundation.

Ge, X., Lorenz, F. O., Conger, R. D., Elder, G. H., Jr., & Simons, R. L. (1994). Trajectories of stressful life events and depressive symptoms during adolescence. *Developmental Psychology, 30*, 467–483.

Giedd, J. N., Blumenthal, J., Jeffries, N. O., Castellanos, F. X., Liu, H., Zijdenbos, A., Paus, T., Evans, A. C., & Rapoport, J. L. (1999b). Brain development during childhood and adolescence: A longitudinal MRI study. *Nature Neuroscience, 2*, 861–863.

Giedd, J. N., Blumenthal, J., Jeffries, N. O., Rajapakse, J. C., Vaituzis, A. C., Liu, H., Berry, Y. C., Tobin, M., Nelson, J., & Castellanos, F. X. (1999a). Development of the human corpus callosum during childhood and adolescence: A longitudinal MRI study. *Progress in Neuro-Psychopharmacology & Biological Psychiatry, 23*, 571–588.

Giedd, J. N., Castellanos, F. X., Rajapakse, J. C., Vaituzis, A. C., & Rapoport, J. L. (1997). Sexual dimorphism of the developing human brain. *Progress in Neuro-Psychopharmacology & Biological Psychiatry, 21*, 1185–1201.

Giuffrida, A., Parsons, L. H., Kerr, T. M., Rodríguez de Fonseca, F., Navarro, M., & Piomelli, D. (1999). Dopamine activation of endogenous cannabinoid signaling in dorsal striatum. *Nature Neuroscience, 2*, 358–363.

Goldman, P. S. (1971). Functional development of the prefrontal cortex in early life and the problem of neuronal plasticity. *Experimental Neurology, 32*, 366–387.

Goldman-Rakic, P. S., Isseroff, A., Schwartz, M. L., & Bugbee, N. M. (1983). The neurobiology of cognitive development. In P. H. Mussen (Vol. Ed.), *Handbook of child psychology, Vol. II. Infancy and developmental psychobiology* (pp. 281–344). New York: Wiley.

Goodman, A. B. (1998). Three independent lines of evidence suggest retinoids as causal to schizophrenia. *Proceedings of the National Academy of Sciences of the United States of America, 95*, 7240–7244.

Graber, J. A., & Brooks-Gunn, J. (1996). Transitions and turning points: Navigating the passage from childhood through adolescence. *Developmental Psychology, 32*, 768–776.

Greenhill, L. L., & Setterberg, S. (1993). Pharmacotherapy of disorders of adolescents. *Psychiatric Clinics of North America, 16*, 793–814.

Harris, J. R. (1995). Where is the child's environment? A group socialization theory of development. *Psychological Review, 102*, 458–489.

Heiman, M. L., Chen, Y., & Caro, J. (1998). Leptin participates in the regulation of glucocorticoid and growth hormone axes. *Journal of Nutritional Biochemistry, 9*, 553–559.

Hirsch, S. R., Das, I., Garey, L. J., & de Belleroche, J. (1997). A pivotal role for glutamate in the pathogenesis of schizophrenia, and its cognitive dysfunction. *Pharmacology, Biochemistry and Behavior, 56*, 797–802.

Huttenlocher, P. R. (1979). Synaptic density of human frontal cortex – developmental changes and effects of aging. *Brain Research, 163*, 195–205.

Huttenlocher, P. R. (1984). Synapse elimination and plasticity in developing human cerebral cortex. *American Journal of Mental Deficiency, 88*, 488–496.

Ikemoto, S., & Panksepp, J. (1999). The role of nucleus accumbens dopamine in motivated behavior: A unifying interpretation with special reference to reward-seeking. *Brain Research Reviews, 31*, 6–41.

Insel, T. R., Miller, L. P., & Gelhard, R. E. (1990). The ontogeny of excitatory amino acid receptors in rat forebrain: I. N-methyl-d-aspartate and quisqualate receptors. *Neuroscience, 35*, 31–43.

Irwin, C. E., Jr., & Millstein, S. G. (1992). Correlates and predictors of risk-taking behavior during adolescence. In L. P. Lipsitt & L. L. Mitnick (Eds.), *Self-regulatory behavior and risk taking: Causes and consequences* (pp. 3–21). Norwood, N.J.: Ablex Publishing.

Jakob, H., & Beckmann, H. (1986). Prenatal developmental disturbances in the limbic allocortex in schizophrenics. *Journal of Neural Transmission, 65*, 303–326.

Jernigan, T. L., & Sowell, E. R. (1997). Magnetic resonance imaging studies of the developing brain. In M. S. Keshavan & R. M. Murray (Eds.), *Neurodevelopment & adult psychopathology* (pp. 63–70). Cambridge: Cambridge University Press.

Jernigan, T. L., Trauner, D. A., Hesselink, J. R., & Tallal, P. A. (1991). Maturation of human cerebrum observed in vivo during adolescence. *Brain, 114*, 2037–2049.

Joyce, J. N., Frohna, P. A., & Neal-Beliveau, B. S. (1996). Functional and molecular differentiation of the dopamine system induced by neonatal denervation. *Neuroscience and Biobehavioral Reviews, 20*, 453–486.

Kalivas, P. W., Churchill, L., & Klitenick, M. A. (1993). The circuitry mediating the translation of motivational stimuli into adaptive motor responses. In P. W. Kalivas & C. D. Barnes (Eds.), *Limbic motor circuits and neuropsychiatry* (pp. 237–287). Boca Raton, Fla.: CRC Press.

Kalsbeek, A., Voorn, P., Buijs, R. M., Pool, C. W., & Uylings, H. B. M. (1988). Development of the dopaminergic innervation in the prefrontal cortex of the rat. *Journal of Comparative Neurology, 269*, 58–72.

Keane, B. (1990). Dispersal and inbreeding avoidance in the white-footed mouse, *Peromyscus leucopus*. *Animal Behaviour, 40*, 143–152.

Keepers, G., Clappison, V., & Casey, D. (1983). Initial anticholinergic prophylaxis for acute neuroleptic induced extrapyramidal syndromes. *Archives of General Psychiatry, 40*, 1113–1117.

Kellogg, C. K. (1991). Postnatal effects of prenatal exposure to psychoactive drugs. *Pre- and Peri-Natal Psychology, 5*, 233–251.

Kellogg, C. K., Awatramani, G. B., & Piekut, D. T. (1998). Adolescent development alters stressor-induced Fos immunoreactivity in rat brain. *Neuroscience, 83*, 681–689.

Kempermann, G., & Gage, F. H. (2000). Neurogenesis in the adult hippocampus. In *Novartis Foundation Symposium 231: Neural Transplantation in Neurodegenerative Disease: Current Status and New Directions* (pp. 220–235). Chichester: John Wiley.

Killgore, W. D. S., Oki, M., & Yurgelun-Todd, D. A. (2001). Sex-specific developmental changes in amygdala responses to affective faces. *Neuroreport, 12*, 427–433.

Kolb, B., & Nonneman, A. J. (1976). Functional development of prefrontal cortex in rats continues into adolescence. *Science, 193*, 335–336.

Koob, G. F. (1992). Neural mechanisms of drug reinforcement. *Annals of the New York Academy of Sciences, 654*, 171–191.

Koob, G. F. (1999). Stress, corticotropin-releasing factor, and drug addiction. *Annals of the New York Academy of Sciences, 897*, 27–45.

Koob, G. F., & Heinrichs, S. C. (1999). A role for corticotropin releasing factor and urocortin in behavioral responses to stressors. *Brain Research, 848*, 141–152.

Koob, G. F., Robledo, P., Markou, A., & Caine, S. B. (1993). The mesocorticolimbic circuit in drug dependence and reward – a role for the extended amygdala? In P. W. Kalivas & C. D. Barnes (Eds.), *Limbic motor circuits and neuropsychiatry* (pp. 289–309). Boca Raton, Fla.: CRC Press.

Kovelman, J. A., & Scheibel, A. B. (1984). A neurohistological correlate of schizophrenia. *Biological Psychiatry, 19*, 1601–1621.

Kurlan, R. (1992). The pathogenesis of Tourette's syndrome: A possible role for hormonal and excitatory neurotransmitter influences in brain development. *Archives of Neurology, 49*, 874–876.

Kutcher, S., & Sokolov, S. (1995). Adolescent depression: Neuroendocrine aspects. In I. M. Goodyer (Ed.), *The depressed child and adolescent: Developmental and clinical perspectives* (pp. 195–224). Cambridge: Cambridge University Press.

Lahlou, N., Landais, P., De Boissieu, D., & Bougnères, P.-F. (1997). Circulating leptin in normal children and during the dynamic phase of juvenile obesity: Relation to body fatness, energy metabolism, caloric intake, and sexual dimorphism. *Diabetes, 46*, 989–993.

Larson, R., & Richards, M. H. (1994). *Divergent realities: The emotional lives of mothers, fathers, and adolescents*. New York: Basic Books.

Le Moal, M., & Simon, H. (1991). Mesocorticolimbic dopaminergic network: Functional and regulatory roles. *Physiological Reviews, 71*, 155–234.

Leslie, C. A., Robertson, M. W., Cutler, A. J., & Bennett, J. P., Jr. (1991). Postnatal development of D1 dopamine receptors in the medial prefrontal cortex, striatum and nucleus accumbens of normal and neonatal 6-hydroxydopamine treated rats: A quantitative autoradiographic analysis. *Developmental Brain Research, 62*, 109–114.

Levisohn, L., Cronin-Golomb, A., & Schmahmann, J. D. (2000). Neuropsychological consequences of cerebellar tumour resection in children: Cerebellar cognitive affective syndrome in a paediatric population. *Brain, 123*, 1041–1050.

Lipska, B. K., Jaskiw, G. E., & Weinberger, D. R. (1993). Postpubertal emergence of hyperresponsivenss to stress and to amphetamine after neonatal excitotoxic hippocampal damage: A potential animal model of schizophrenia. *Neuropsychopharmacology, 9*, 67–75.

Lipska, B. K., & Weinberger, D. R. (1993a). Cortical regulation of the mesolimbic dopamine system: Implications for schizophrenia. In P. W. Kalivas & C. D. Barnes (Eds.), *Limbic motor circuits and neuropsychiatry* (pp. 329–349). Boca Raton, Fla.: CRC Press.

Lipska, B. K., & Weinberger, D. R. (1993b). Delayed effects of neonatal hippocampal damage on haloperidol-induced catalepsy and apomorphine-induced stereotypic behaviors in the rat. *Developmental Brain Research, 75*, 213–222.

Little, P. J., Kuhn, C. M., Wilson, W. A., & Swartzwelder, H. S. (1996). Differential effects of ethanol in adolescent and adult rats. *Alcoholism: Clinical and Experimental Research, 20*, 1346–1351.

Luna, B., Thulborn, K. R., Munoz, D. P., Merriam, E. P., Garver, K. E., Minshew, N. J., Keshavan, M. S., Genovese, C. R., Eddy, W. F., & Sweeney, J. A. (2001). Maturation of widely distributed brain function subserves cognitive development. *Neuroimage, 13*, 786–793.

Mantzoros, C. S., Flier, J. S., & Rogol, A. D. (1997). A longitudinal assessment of hormonal and physical alterations during normal puberty in boys. V. Rising leptin levels may signal the onset of puberty. *Journal of Clinical Endocrinology and Metabolism, 82*, 1066–1070.

Markwiese, B. J., Acheson, S. K., Levin, E. D., Wilson, W. A., & Swartzwelder, H. S. (1998). Differential effects of ethanol on memory in adolescent and adult rats. *Alcoholism: Clinical and Experimental Research, 22*, 416–421.

Mayes, L. C., Grillon, C., Granger, R. & Schottenfeld, R. (1998). Regulation of arousal and attention in preschool children exposed to cocaine prenatally. *Annals of the New York Academy of Sciences, 846,* 126–143.

Merola, J. L., & Liederman, J. (1985). Developmental changes in hemispheric independence. *Child Development, 56,* 1184–1194.

Middleton, F. A., & Strick, P. L. (2000). Basal ganglia and cerebellar loops: Motor and cognitive circuits. *Brain Research Reviews, 31,* 236–250.

Middleton, F. A., & Strick, P. L. (2001). Cerebellar projections to the prefrontal cortex of the primate. *Journal of Neuroscience, 21,* 700–712.

Moltz, H. (1975). The search for the determinants of puberty in the rat. In B. E. Eleftheriou & R. L. Sprott (Eds.), *Hormonal correlates of behavior: A lifespan view* (pp. 35–154). New York: Plenum.

Montague, D. M., Lawler, C. P., Mailman, R. B., & Gilmore, J. H. (1999). Developmental regulation of the dopamine D1 receptor in human caudate and putamen. *Neuropsychopharmacology, 21,* 641–649.

Moore, J. (1992). Dispersal, nepotism, and primate social behavior. *International Journal of Primatology, 13,* 361–378.

Mrzljak, L., Uylings, H. B. M., van Eden, C. G., & Judáš, M. (1990). Neuronal development in human prefrontal cortex in prenatal and postnatal stages. In H. B. M. Uylings, C. G. van Eden, J. P. C. De Bruin, M. A. Corner, & M. G. P. Feenstra (Vol. Eds.), *Progress in brain research: Vol. 85. The prefrontal cortex: Its structure, function and pathology* (pp. 185–222). Amsterdam: Elsevier.

Nowakowski, R. S., & Hayes, N. L. (1999). CNS development: An overview. *Development and Psychopathology, 11,* 395–417.

Palacios, J. M., Camps, M., Cortés, R., & Probst, A. (1988). Mapping dopamine receptors in the human brain. *Neural Transmissions, 27,* 227–235.

Parker, L. N. (1991). Adrenarche. *Endocrinology and Metabolism Clinics of North America, 20,* 71–83.

Paus, T., Zijdenbos, A., Worsley, K., Collins, D. L., Blumenthal, J., Giedd, J. N., Rapoport, J. L., & Evans, A. C. (1999). Structural maturation of neural pathways in children and adolescents: In vivo study. *Science, 283,* 1908–1911.

Petersen, A. C., Silbereisen, R. K., & Sörensen, S. (1996). Adolescent development: A global perspective. In K. Hurrelmann & S. F. Hamilton (Eds.), *Social problems and social contexts in adolescence* (pp. 3–37). New York: Aldine de Gruyter.

Pine, D. S., Grun, J., Zarahn, E., Fyer, A., Koda, V., Li, W., Szeszko, P. R., Ardekani, B., & Bilder, R. M. (2001). Cortical brain regions engaged by masked emotional faces in adolescents and adults: An fMRI study. *Emotion, 1,* 137–147.

Primus, R. J., & Kellogg, C. K. (1989). Pubertal-related changes influence the development of environment-related social interaction in the male rat. *Developmental Psychobiology, 22,* 633–643.

Puig-Antich, J. (1987). Sleep and neuroendocrine correlates of affective illness in childhood and adolescence. *Journal of Adolescent Health Care, 8,* 505–529.

Rakic, P., Bourgeois, J.-P., & Goldman-Rakic, P. S. (1994). Synaptic development of the cerebral cortex: Implications for learning, memory, and mental illness. In J. van Pelt, M. A. Corner, H. B. M. Uylings, & F. H. Lopes da Silva (Vol. Eds.), *Progress in brain research: Vol. 102. The self-organizing brain: From growth cones to functional networks* (pp. 227–243). Amsterdam: Elsevier.

Rapoport, J. L., Giedd, J. N., Blumenthal, J., Hamburger, S., Jeffries, N., Fernandez, T., Nicolson, R., Bedwell, J., Lenane, M., Zijdenbos, A., Paus, T., & Evans, A. (1999). Progressive cortical change during adolescence in childhood-onset schizophrenia. *Archives of General Psychiatry, 56,* 649–654.

Riley, E. P. (1990). The long-term behavioral effects of prenatal alcohol exposure in rats. *Alcoholism: Clinical and Experimental Research, 14,* 670–673.

Rodríguez de Fonseca, F., Ramos, J. A., Bonnin, A., & Fernández-Ruiz, J. J. (1993). Presence of cannabinoid binding sites in the brain from early postnatal ages. *Neuroreport, 4,* 135–138.

Rosenberg, D. R., & Lewis, D. A. (1994). Changes in the dopaminergic innervation of monkey prefrontal cortex during late postnatal development: A tyrosine hydroxylase immunohistochemical study. *Biological Psychiatry, 36,* 272–277.

Rosenberg, D. R., & Lewis, D. A. (1995). Postnatal maturation of the dopaminergic innervation of monkey prefrontal and motor cortices: A tyrosine hydroxylase immunohistochemical analysis. *Journal of Comparative Neurology, 358*, 383–400.

Rubia, K., Overmeyer, S., Taylor, E., Brammer, M., Williams, S. C. R., Simmons, A., Andrew, C., & Bullmore, E. T. (2000). Functional frontalisation with age: Mapping neurodevelopmental trajectories with fMRI. *Neuroscience and Biobehavioral Reviews, 24*, 13–19.

Saugstad, L. F. (1994). The maturational theory of brain development and cerebral excitability in the multifactorially inherited manic-depressive psychosis and schizophrenia. *International Journal of Psychophysiology, 18*, 189–203.

Schmahmann, J. D., & Sherman, J. C. (1998). The cerebellar cognitive affective syndrome. *Brain, 121*, 561–579.

Schultz, W. (1998). Predictive reward signal of dopamine neurons. *Journal of Neurophysiology, 80*, 1–27.

Seeman, P., Bzowej, N. H., Guan, H.-C., Bergeron, C., Becker, L. E., Reynolds, G. P., Bird, E. D., Riederer, P., Jellinger, K., Watanabe, S., & Tourtellotte, W. W. (1987). Human brain dopamine receptors in children and aging adults. *Synapse, 1*, 399–404.

Silveri, M. M., & Spear, L. P. (1998). Decreased sensitivity to the hypnotic effects of ethanol early in ontogeny. *Alcoholism: Clinical and Experimental Research, 22*, 670–676.

Silveri, M. M., & Spear, L. P. (2001). *The effects of NMDA and GABA$_A$ pharmacological manipulations on ethanol sensitivity in immature and mature animals.* Manuscript submitted for publication.

Sowell, E. R., Thompson, P. M., Holmes, C. J., Batth, R., Jernigan, T. L., & Toga, A. W. (1999a). Localizing age-related changes in brain structure between childhood and adolescence using statistical parametric mapping. *Neuroimage, 9*, 587–597.

Sowell, E. R., Thompson, P. M., Holmes, C. J., Jernigan, T. L., & Toga, A. W. (1999b). In vivo evidence for post-adolescent brain maturation in frontal and striatal regions. *Nature Neuroscience, 2*, 859–861.

Spanagel, R., & Weiss, F. (1999). The dopamine hypothesis of reward: Past and current status. *Trends in Neuroscience, 22*, 521–527.

Spear, L. P. (2000a). The adolescent brain and age-related behavioral manifestations. *Neuroscience and Biobehavioral Reviews, 24*, 417–463.

Spear, L. P. (2000b). Adolescent period: Biological basis of vulnerability to develop alcoholism and other ethanol-mediated behaviors. In A. Noronha, M. Eckardt, & K. Warren (Eds.), *NIAAA Research Monograph 34: Review of NIAAA's Neuroscience and Behavioral Research Portfolio* (NIH Publication No. 00-4520, pp. 315–333). Washington, D.C.: U.S. Department of Health and Human Services.

Spear, L. P., & Brake, S. C. (1983). Periadolescence: Age-dependent behavior and psychopharmacological responsivity in rats. *Developmental Psychobiology, 16*, 83–109.

Spear, L. P., Campbell, J., Snyder, K., Silveri, M., & Katovic, N. (1998). Animal behavior models: Increased sensitivity to stressors and other environmental experiences after prenatal cocaine exposure. *Annals of the New York Academy of Sciences, 846*, 76–88.

Spear, L. P., Shalaby, I. A., & Brick, J. (1980). Chronic administration of haloperidol during development: Behavioral and psychopharmacological effects. *Psychopharmacology, 70*, 47–58.

Spear, L. P., Silveri, M. M., Casale, M., Katovic, N. M., Campbell, J. O., & Douglas, L. A. (in press). Cocaine and development: A retrospective perspective. *Neurotoxicology and Teratology.*

Steinberg, L. (1989). Pubertal maturation and parent-adolescent distance: An evolutionary perspective. In G. R. Adams, R. Montemayor, & T. P. Gullotta (Eds.), *Advances in adolescent behavior and development* (pp. 71–97). Newbury Park, Calif.: Sage Publications.

Susman, E. J., Inoff-Germain, G., & Nottelmann, E. D. (1987). Hormones, emotional dispositions, and aggressive attributes in young adolescents. *Child Development, 58*, 1114–1134.

Susman, E. J., & Ponirakis, A. (1997). Hormones – context interactions and anti-social behavior in youth. In A. Raine, P. A. Brennan, D. P. Farrington, & S. A. Mednick (Eds.), *Biosocial bases of violence* (pp. 251–269). New York: Plenum.

Swartzwelder, H. S., Wilson, W. A., & Tayyeb, M. I. (1995a). Age-dependent inhibition of long-term potentiation by ethanol in immature versus mature hippocampus. *Alcoholism: Clinical and Experimental Research, 19*, 1480–1485.

Swartzwelder, H. S., Wilson, W. A., & Tayyeb, M. I. (1995b). Differential sensitivity of NMDA receptor-mediated synaptic potentials to ethanol in immature versus mature hippocampus. *Alcoholism: Clinical and Experimental Research, 19*, 320–323.

Takahashi, L. K., Turner, J. G., & Kalin, N. H. (1992). Prenatal stress alters brain catecholaminergic activity and potentiates stress-induced behavior in adult rats. *Brain Research, 574*, 131–137.

Tarazi, F. I., & Baldessarini, R. J. (2000). Comparative postnatal development of dopamine D(1), D(2) and D(4) receptors in rat forebrain. *International Journal of Developmental Neuroscience, 18*, 29–37.

Tarazi, F. I., Tomasini, E. C., & Baldessarini, R. J. (1998). Postnatal development of dopamine and serotonin transporters in rat caudate-putamen and nucleus accumbens septi. *Neuroscience Letters, 254*, 21–24.

Tarazi, F. I., Tomasini, E. C., & Baldessarini, R. J. (1999). Postnatal development of dopamine D1-like receptors in rat cortical and striatolimbic brain regions: An autoradiographic study. *Developmental Neuroscience, 21*, 43–49.

Teicher, M. H., & Andersen, S. L. (1999, October). *Limbic serotonin turnover plunges during puberty.* Poster session presented at the annual meeting of the Society for Neuroscience, Miami Beach, Fla.

Teicher, M. H., Andersen, S. L., & Hostetter, J. C., Jr. (1995). Evidence for dopamine receptor pruning between adolescence and adulthood in striatum but not nucleus accumbens. *Developmental Brain Research, 89*, 167–172.

Terasawa, E., & Timiras, P. S. (1968). Electrophysiological study of the limbic system in the rat at onset of puberty. *American Journal of Physiology, 215*, 1462–1467.

Thomas, K. M., Drevets, W. C., Whalen, P. J., Eccard, C. H., Dahl, R. E., Ryan, N. D., & Casey, B. J. (2001). Amygdala response to facial expressions in children and adults. *Biological Psychiatry, 49*, 309–316.

Trimpop, R. M., Kerr, J. H., & Kirkcaldy, B. (1999). Comparing personality constructs of risk-taking behavior. *Personality and Individual Differences, 26*, 237–254.

Tyler, D. B., & van Harreveld, A. (1942). The respiration of the developing brain. *American Journal of Physiology, 136*, 600–603.

van Eden, C. G., Kros, J. M., & Uylings, H. B. M. (1990). The development of the rat prefrontal cortex: Its size and development of connections with thalamus, spinal cord and other cortical areas. In H. B. M. Uylings, C. G. van Eden, J. P. C. De Bruin, M. A. Corner, & M. G. P. Feenstra (Vol. Eds.), *Progress in brain research: Vol. 85. The prefrontal cortex: Its structure, function and pathology* (pp. 169–183). Amsterdam: Elsevier.

Walker, E. F., & Diforio, D. (1997). Schizophrenia: A neural diathesis-stress model. *Psychological Review, 104*, 667–685.

Walker, E. F., & Walder, D. (this volume). *Neurohormonal aspects of the development of psychotic disorders.*

Weinstock, M. (1997). Does prenatal stress impair coping and regulation of hypothalamic-pituitary-adrenal axis? *Neuroscience & Biobehavioral Reviews, 21*, 1–10.

Whishaw, I. Q., Fiorino, D., Mittleman, G., & Castaneda, E. (1992). Do forebrain structures compete for behavioral expression? Evidence from amphetamine-induced behavior, microdialysis, and caudate-accumbens lesions in medial frontal cortex damaged rats. *Brain Research, 576*, 1–11.

Wilkinson, L. S. (1997). The nature of interactions involving prefrontal and striatal dopamine systems. *Journal of Psychopharmacology, 11*, 143–150.

Wilson, M., & Daly, M. (1985). Competitiveness, risk taking, and violence: The young male syndrome. *Ethology and Sociobiology, 6*, 59–73.

Zecevic, N., Bourgeois, J.-P., & Rakic, P. (1989). Changes in synaptic density in motor cortex of rhesus monkey during fetal and postnatal life. *Developmental Brain Research, 50*, 11–32.

FOUR

Prenatal Risk Factors for Schizophrenia

Alan S. Brown and Ezra S. Susser

Over the past decade our research efforts have focused on the identification of prenatal risk factors for schizophrenia. In this chapter, we summarize our study designs and methods, describe our findings, discuss the implications of these findings for the field, and present our plans for future investigations. In order to provide a conceptual framework for these findings, we shall first discuss the neurodevelopmental hypothesis of schizophrenia, and briefly review previous studies by other investigators in this research domain.

NEURODEVELOPMENTAL HYPOTHESIS OF SCHIZOPHRENIA

The neurodevelopmental model of schizophrenia posits that adverse in utero events influence critical processes in the genesis of brain structures, which predispose to the emergence of schizophrenia in adulthood (Brown et al., 1999; Susser, 1999). The evidence that led to this hypothesis derives from many diverse areas of investigation; however, there appear to be three pivotal supportive findings. First, patients destined to develop schizophrenia have a tendency for diminished neurocognitive (David et al., 1997; Jones et al., 1994), neuromotor (Walker et al., 1994), and behavioral (Done et al., 1994) function. Second, patients with schizophrenia, as compared with healthy controls, have an increased frequency and severity of minor physical anomalies, particularly of the craniofacial area, which are suggestive of an in utero developmental disruption (Green et al., 1989; Waddington, 1993). Third, neuroimaging studies indicate that several of the brain abnormalities in schizophrenia, such as ventriculomegaly and diminished hippocampal volume, occur among patients in their first episode of psychosis (Bogerts et al., 1990; DeGreef et al., 1992; Nopoulos et al., 1995). Brain imaging studies have also demonstrated an increased proportion of morphologic anomalies such as cavum septum pellucidum (CSP). The *CSP* is the space between the two leaflets of the septum pellucidum, a thin sheet of cells and fibers occupying a midline position

This study is supported by NIMH grant 1K20MH 01206 (A.S.B.), a Young Investigator Award from the National Alliance for Research on Schizophrenia and Depression (NARSAD) (A.S.B.), NIMH grant 1R01MH-53147 (E.S.S.), a NARSAD Independent Investigator Award (E.S.S.), the Theodore and Vada Stanley Foundation (E.S.S.), NIMH grant 5P20MH 50727 (J.M.G.), and NIMH grant MH59342 (J.M.G.)

separating the lateral ventricles of the brain. Because the CSP normally closes within the first six months of life, its presence suggests in utero maldevelopment (Nopoulos et al., 1995).

There is little question that mutations or polymorphisms in genes responsible for critical neurodevelopmental events can explain at least some proportion of neurodevelopmental schizophrenia. For example, genetically manipulated deletions of homeobox domains (genes which specify the organization of structures throughout the body and brain) have been shown to disrupt the migration of neurons from the ventricular zone to the cortex (Anderson et al., 1997), a process that may be disturbed in schizophrenia. Nonetheless, it is our view that environmental factors, alone or in combination with genetic anomalies, play a substantial role as well. The most convincing evidence supporting this assertion derives from studies of monozygotic (MZ) twins discordant for schizophrenia. First, the rate of discordance in these twin pairs is approximately 50 percent (McGuffin et al., 1995), and some have suggested that concordance for schizophrenia in MZ twins, particularly monochorionic pairs, can be a consequence of prenatal environmental factors that affect both members of the twin pair. Supporting this notion, Davis et al. (1995) demonstrated that MZ twin pairs concordant for schizophrenia, compared to discordant MZ twin pairs, were more likely to have been monochorionic and to have shared a single placenta. Second, a landmark study of MZ twin pairs discordant for schizophrenia demonstrated that in nearly every case, the affected member of each MZ twin pair had larger cerebral ventricles and smaller hippocampi than the unaffected co-twin (Suddath et al., 1990). Since it can be presumed that these twin pairs share 100 percent of their genes, any differences in risk of illness or brain morphology can be attributed to environmental factors.

PRENATAL ENVIRONMENTAL FACTORS: REVIEW OF PREVIOUS WORK

In the search for causes of neurodevelopmental schizophrenia, investigators have therefore focused a considerable amount of attention on putative prenatal environmental factors. The relation of perinatal and neonatal complications to schizophrenia risk has also been widely investigated, although this topic is beyond the scope of the chapter.

Two well-replicated findings that provided some of the first clues as to a prenatal environmental etiology for schizophrenia concerned seasonality of birth and birth in an urban area. A large number of investigations throughout the world have consistently demonstrated a 5–15 percent excess of schizophrenic births in the late winter and early spring, and a deficiency of schizophrenia births in the summer and fall (Bradbury & Miller, 1985). Several prior studies in different countries (Lewis et al., 1992; Marcelis et al., 1998; Mortensen et al., 1999), including a recent investigation on over 2,000 schizophrenic patients, have reported that the relative risk of schizophrenia following birth in an urban area is approximately twofold. In that recent study, the population attributable risk percent of season of birth was greater than 10 percent, and the population attributable risk percent of place of birth was greater than 30 percent (Mortensen et al., 1999).

These marked differences in the magnitude of the relative and population attributable risk for both season and urbanicity of birth underscore an important distinction between these two concepts. *Relative risk* refers to the ratio of incidence rates of a disease between exposed and unexposed persons, and is therefore the usual measure for etiologic research, the purpose of which is to quantify the strength of associations between exposures and outcomes (Rothman, 1986). Put in practical terms, the comparatively small relative risks of winter or urban birth imply only modest effects of these risk factors on an exposed individual's likelihood of developing schizophrenia. The *population attributable risk percent*, on the other hand, refers to the proportion of disease occurrence in a population that potentially would be eliminated if exposure to the risk factor were prevented (Kelsey, 1996). The relatively high population attributable risk percents for both winter and urban birth suggest that identifying and lessening the exposures associated with these two variables (see next paragraph) could have important implications for the prevention of schizophrenia in the population.

Although the season of birth finding could be explained by a number of seasonally varying factors, the clear winter excess of respiratory infections suggested that a maternal viral infection, such as influenza, might account in large part for this association. A viral infection might also be a prime candidate for the urbanicity of birth finding, because more crowded living conditions can increase transmission of pathogens. In the first study on maternal influenza, Mednick et al. (1988) in Finland demonstrated an increased risk of schizophrenia after second-trimester exposure to the 1957 A2 influenza epidemic. Replications of this finding have been reported in Great Britain (Adams et al., 1993; Fahy et al., 1993; O'Callaghan et al., 1991; Takei et al., 1993), Ireland (Cannon et al., 1996), Japan (Kunugi et al., 1995), and Australia (McGrath et al., 1994). There have, however, been several failures to replicate this result, in England (Crow et al., 1991), Holland (Susser et al., 1994), the United States (Torrey et al., 1991), and Croatia (Erlenmeyer-Kimling et al., 1994). Nonetheless, studies attempting to correlate influenza epidemics over periods of many years to risk of schizophrenia have been mostly positive (Adams et al., 1993; Barr et al., 1990; Sham et al., 1992; Takei et al., 1994, 1996; Welham et al., 1993; Wright & Murray, 1995), although, again, there have been some negative studies (Grech et al., 1997; Morgan et al., 1997; Selten et al., 1998).

The potential roles of other prenatal exposures in the etiology of schizophrenia have also been examined. Hollister et al. (1996) demonstrated a significantly increased risk of schizophrenia among second- and later-born Rh incompatible offspring. Maternal stress has been associated with schizophrenia in offspring: van Os and Selten (1998) showed that the children of pregnant mothers who were in their first trimester during the 1940 invasion of the Netherlands had a significantly increased risk of schizophrenia, replicating an earlier finding by Huttunen and Niskanen (1978). Maternal pre-eclampsia (Dalman et al., 1999) and low birthweight (Hultman et al., 1999; Jones et al., 1998; McNeil & Kaij, 1978) have also been related in some studies to an increased risk of schizophrenia.

Evidence from other studies suggests that other types of psychopathology, such as affective disorders, may also originate from disturbances of early neurodevelopment. Patients with affective disorders have a tendency for developmental impairment in childhood, including low educational test scores, delayed motor milestones, and speech abnormalities (van Os et al., 1998). Other studies have suggested increased rates of winter-spring birth in subjects who subsequently developed affective disorders (Torrey et al., 1996). Moreover, some studies have suggested associations between affective disorders and both prenatal influenza exposure (Machon et al., 1997; Cannon et al., 1996) and obstetric complications (Sacker et al., 1995; Done et al., 1991). As discussed below,

Brown et al. (1995, 2000b) demonstrated a significant association between prenatal exposure to the Dutch Hunger Winter and risk of major affective disorders.

Limitations of Previous Studies

While promising, the findings reviewed above are hampered by significant limitations. The first limitation concerns documentation of the exposure. Most previous investigations relied upon data from populations rather than individuals. For example, in most of the studies on prenatal influenza, it was known that an individual was utero at the time of the epidemic, but not whether the individual's mother actually had the viral infection during pregnancy. The second limitation concerns the outcome. Most previous studies utilized clinical psychiatric diagnoses based on hospital registries or case notes, or diagnoses based on systems with relatively nonspecific criteria such as *DSM-II* (*Diagnostic and Statistical Manual of Mental Disorders*, 2nd ed.) or ICD-9, rather than research-based diagnoses generated from a direct, standardized assessments and based on modern diagnostic criteria. These two limitations predispose to misclassification of exposure and/or outcome. If the misclassification of exposure occurs independently of the outcome (nondifferential misclassification), the strength of an observed association can be blunted. If misclassification of exposure is related to the outcome (differential misclassification), then a spurious association could result. These sources of error may explain the discrepancies in findings between studies. A third limitation of previous investigations is the inability to examine the causal pathways linking the exposure to the schizophrenia outcome, due to insufficient data on relevant variables, such as aberrant maternal immune function or perinatal hypoxia.

SUMMARY OF OUR WORK ON PRENATAL RISK FACTORS FOR SCHIZOPHRENIA

Ten years ago, our group embarked upon a program of research aimed at identifying prenatal determinants of schizophrenia using more sophisticated research designs that address misclassification error, expand the range and specificity of prenatal exposures examined, and elaborate causal pathways. In this effort, we have employed two primary classes of birth cohort research designs (see Susser, 1999 for a more detailed discussion). The first has been termed the *epigenetic high-risk cohort* design. This design entails a cohort that is enriched for an environmental factor which can affect genetically programmed neurodevelopment (e.g., prenatal brain insult), and that is under observation from the in utero period until the age of risk for the disorder of interest, in our case for schizophrenia. We have conducted schizophrenia follow-up studies for two epigenetic high-risk birth cohorts: the Dutch Famine cohort and the cohort of the Rubella Birth Defects Evaluation Project (RBDEP).

The birth cohort for the second type of research design is termed the *population birth cohort*. This research design utilizes a general population of births, which are not selected for any specific exposure, and followed from birth through the risk period for schizophrenia. The prenatal exposures are gleaned from comprehensive, detailed assessments throughout pregnancy, or by accessing resources that permit the identification of prenatal etiologies in new analyses.

Below, we elaborate on our two epigenetic high-risk birth cohort studies, and on one of our population birth cohort investigations, the Prenatal Determinants of Schizophrenia (PDS) study. The methodologies corresponding to each of these investigations are summarized in Table 4.1.

Epigenetic High-Risk Studies

Dutch Famine Studies

In this section, we summarize the research design and the findings of a series of studies by our group on the relation of the Dutch Hunger Winter of 1944–1945 to adult schizophrenia and schizophrenia spectrum personality disorders. These investigations were a logical outgrowth of the original Dutch Famine Study, which aimed to relate prenatal famine to outcomes in infancy, childhood, and early adulthood, including neurocognitive development and central nervous system anomalies. We first provide an essential background by reviewing the historical circumstances of the Dutch Hunger Winter.

The Dutch Hunger Winter. The events that precipitated the Dutch Hunger Winter began in the last year of Word War II. In September 1944, a daring military operation took place, in which the Allied forces attempted a parachute drop behind Nazi lines near the city of Arnhem. Its original aim was to capture strategic bridges, facilitating a rapid invasion of Germany. Prior to the operation, the Dutch government-in-exile appealed to the people of the Netherlands to cooperate with the Allies, and they complied. Unfortunately, the operation was a complete failure for the Allied forces. Following the defeat, the Nazis imposed a total embargo on occupied Holland in retaliation for the support that the Dutch resistance gave to the Allied command.

Combined with two additional events – an unusually early winter that froze the canals traversed by barges, and the diversion of much land previously used to support agriculture – a famine was precipitated in Holland. The embargo affected the region of the Netherlands that was still under occupation; this area was known as "the West," or "famine" region. Within the West, the six largest cities – Amsterdam, Rotterdam, The Hague, Utrecht, Leiden, and Haarlem – were primarily affected. The famine progressively intensified in this region, with food rations declining to extremely low levels from February 1945 to May 1945. During these months, records indicated an official food ration below 1,000 kilocalories (kcal), the diet consisting almost exclusively of bread, potatoes, and sugar beets. In early May 1945, the West was liberated by the Allied forces, and food intake returned to levels preceding the famine period.

There were severe effects of the famine on mortality, morbidity, fertility, and reproductive outcomes (Stein et al., 1975). It is estimated that 22,000 individuals died as a result of the famine. Hunger and edema were widespread, leading to the ingestion of unusual foods, such as tulip bulbs, dogs, and cats. Nine months after the famine, the birth rate declined to less than 50 percent of baseline levels, due to decreased fertility. Exposure to the famine in the third trimester was associated with low birthweight and high infant mortality.

The Dutch Hunger Winter was one of the darker events in European history. Yet, out of this tragedy also came a unique opportunity, for it has been used by two generations of researchers as a "natural experiment" aimed at probing the role of prenatal

Table 4.1. Methodology of Birth Cohort Studies Reviewed in This Chapter

Name of Study	Type of Research Design	Sample			Exposure		Outcome		Main Analysis
		N	Year(s)	Place	Definition	Source of Data	Diagnoses	Source of Data	
Dutch Famine Study	Epigenetic high-risk birth cohort	2,327 exposed; 74,245 unexposed	1944–46	Netherlands, 6 largest cities of the West	Severe early gestational famine (<1000 kcal/day)	Monthly food rations	Schizophrenia Schizotypal personality disorder Affective psychoses	Dutch psychiatric registry diagnoses	Comparison of cumulative incidence (relative risk) of schizophrenia between cohorts exposed and unexposed to severe famine in early gestation
Rubella Birth Defects Evaluation Project (RBDEP)	Epigenetic high-risk birth cohort	70 exposed, 164 unexposed (Albany-Saratoga sample); 1,346 unexposed (ECA)*	1964	New York City	Prenatal rubella, based on clinical diagnosis of maternal rubella infection (serologic confirmation in 50% of sample)	Records of RBDEP including physician diagnoses	Nonaffective psychosis	Consensus diagnoses based on DIGS (interview)	Comparison of cumulative incidence (relative risk) of nonaffective psychosis between rubella-exposed and unexposed samples
Prenatal Determinants of Schizophrenia Study (PDS)	Population birth cohort	12,094	1959–67	Alameda County, California	1. Second trimester maternal respiratory infection 2. Maternal body-mass index	1. Obstetric/medical records 2. Maternal interview	Schizophrenia and schizophrenia spectrum disorder (SSD)	Consensus diagnoses based on DIGS and medical records	Comparison of incidence rates (rate ratio) of SSD between exposed and unexposed (proportional hazards regression)

* ECA = Epidemiological Catchment Area Sample

nutrition in health and disease. In contrast to other famines, the Dutch Hunger Winter was circumscribed in both time and place, and, as implied above, the Dutch maintained excellent documentation of its timing and severity, including its effects on health and reproductive outcomes. These attributes permitted investigators to define sequential birth cohorts exposed to the famine during specific gestational periods, and also to delineate unexposed birth cohorts. Misclassification of exposure was minimized because the famine was pervasive in the population. Furthermore, comprehensive health records generated and maintained for many years after the famine enabled the examination of in utero famine exposure in relation to neurodevelopmental and other disorders throughout the lifespan.

The Original Dutch Famine Study. In the original Dutch Famine Study, Stein et al. (1975) examined the effects of the famine on neurocognitive and other neurodevelopmental outcomes at age eighteen in military inductees, all of whom were male. Although IQ and other neurodevelopmental outcomes were found not to be affected by the famine, there was a single but salient finding: an excess of congenital anomalies of the central nervous system in the birth cohort conceived at the peak of the famine. These anomalies included spina bifida, hydrocephalus, and cerebral palsy.

The Dutch Famine and Psychiatric Outcomes. Motivated decades later by the original findings of the Dutch Famine Study, and by growing evidence of a neurodevelopmental basis to schizophrenia (see above), Susser and colleagues launched a series of investigations aimed at examining the relation of prenatal famine exposure to schizophrenia (Susser & Lin, 1992; Susser et al., 1996), schizophrenia spectrum personality disorders (Hoek et al., 1996), and affective psychoses (Brown et al., 1995; Brown et al., 2000b). We reasoned that if severe prenatal famine during conception could increase risk for congenital neural disorders, then periconceptional famine could also be a risk factor for schizophrenia, a putative neurodevelopmental disorder.

We therefore examined whether the birth cohorts conceived at the peak of the famine would have an increased risk of schizophrenia. To test this hypothesis, we capitalized upon the detailed data on famine exposure throughout gestation in the sequential birth cohorts, and a comprehensive, centralized national psychiatric registry which permitted the ascertainment of hospitalized schizophrenia cases. Using registry information on date and place of birth, each case could be assigned to the exposed or unexposed birth cohort.

Consistent with the hypothesis, we found a significant increase in risk of schizophrenia for the birth cohort conceived at the peak of the famine, as compared to the unexposed cohort [relative risk (RR) = 2.0, 95% confidence intervals (CI) = 1.2–3.4, $p < .01$]. The effect sizes were similar for men [RR = 1.9, 95% CI = 1.0–3.7, $p = .05$] and women [RR = 2.2, 95% CI = 1.0–4.7, $p = .04$]. Moreover, the risk of schizophrenia was highest in the birth cohort conceived at the peak of the famine, and was otherwise stable in the unexposed cohorts.

Using the same logic, we extended this paradigm to examine whether periconceptional exposure to the Dutch famine was associated with schizophrenia spectrum personality disorders (Hoek et al., 1996). For this purpose, we utilized data collected during a standardized examination given during military induction to virtually all Dutch men at age eighteen. These data included the ICD diagnosis of schizoid personality disorder, which included both schizoid and schizotypal personality disorders, as per ICD-10 and *DSM-IV*. Similar to our findings for schizophrenia, we demonstrated a significantly increased risk of schizoid personality disorder in the exposed birth cohort, as compared to the unexposed cohorts [RR = 2.01, 95% CI = 1.03–3.94]; and the risk of schizoid personality disorder also evidenced a substantial peak in the exposed birth cohort.

In further work, we have demonstrated that these findings are specific to schizophrenia among major hospitalized psychiatric disorders. Brown et al. (1995, 2000b) have demonstrated that early gestational famine exposure is *not* associated with an increased risk of major affective disorders. Rather, we showed that prenatal famine in later gestation increases the risk of both unipolar and bipolar affective disorders. This study may therefore have important implications for the prenatal origins of affective disorders. Interestingly, the risk of neurotic depression was not increased following prenatal exposure to the famine during any trimester.

Potential Explanations. What might explain this intriguing convergence of congenital neural defects, schizophrenia, and schizotypal personality disorder in the birth cohort conceived at the height of the Dutch Hunger Winter? This question led us to review the literature on the plausibility of prenatal nutritional deprivation on risk of schizophrenia (see Brown et al., 1996). While the most likely etiologic factor is nutritional deficiency, the fact that the famine encompassed deficiencies of many different macro- and micronutrients creates difficulty in isolating one particular class of nutrients as a causal agent. Nonetheless, the concordance between congenital neural defects, schizophrenia/spectrum disorders, and the periconceptional timing of exposure provides a potentially valuable clue. It has been established that prenatal folate deficiency during this developmental period causes neural tube defects, which comprise the bulk of the congenital neural defects in our study. Under normal circumstances, the risk of neural tube defects does not appear to co-vary with overall food intake, and the prevalence of neural tube defects manifests no clear gradient across the developed and developing world. Moreover, prenatal folate deficiency occurs commonly during pregnancy, even in industrialized countries. These facts suggest that periconceptional folate deficiency may be a risk factor for schizophrenia/spectrum disorders, even in societies in which famine is rare or nonexistent, and that the population attributable risk may be appreciable.

Nonetheless, there are other prenatal nutritional deficiencies that should be considered, as plausible candidates for schizophrenia include protein-calorie malnutrition, which has been associated with dopaminergic and glutamatergic abnormalities in adult animals (Butler et al., 1994); fatty acid deficits, which have been related to subtle neurocognitive and visual deficits in animal and some, although not all, human studies (Willatts et al., 1998; Uauy et al., 1992); and retinoid deficiency, which has well-documented teratogenic effects on fetal brain development and has been implicated in schizophrenia (Goodman, 1995; LaMantia, 1999).

The Next Generation of Dutch Famine Studies. We are presently pursuing the findings and implications of the Dutch Famine Study in ongoing investigations. Each of these studies is being led by our colleagues at the University Hospital, Utrecht, and the Hague Psychiatric Institute, in close collaboration with our group. Two important findings have emerged from these investigations thus far. First, we have confirmed a diagnosis of schizophrenia in nearly all of the famine-exposed cases, using a direct, research-based diagnostic interview (Hoek et al., unpublished data). Second, we have completed a study utilizing magnetic resonance imaging aimed at examining whether specific brain morphologic abnormalities distinguish exposed schizophrenia cases from exposed controls, unexposed schizophrenia cases, and unexposed controls (Hulshoff-Pol et al., 2000). A summary of the brain imaging findings will be reported below.

Rubella Birth Defects Evaluation Project

Our second epigenetic high-risk cohort design concerns the Rubella Birth Defects Evaluation Program (RBDEP), a birth cohort with documented prenatal exposure to rubella. This birth cohort study was initiated in New York City following the 1964 rubella epidemic. Below, we describe our rationale for investigating rubella, the details of this unique birth cohort, which has been followed longitudinally since birth, and our main findings.

Rationale for the Investigation of Rubella as a Risk Factor for Schizophrenia. Over fifty years ago, Sir Norman Gregg reported on a relation between a rubella epidemic in Australia and a markedly increased number of births of infants with congenital cataracts (Gregg, 1941). Since then, Gregg and others expanded the congenital rubella syndrome to include not only cataracts, but a number of neurodevelopmental disorders and anomalies, including hearing defects, mental retardation, cerebral palsy, and ventriculomegaly. As described below, Chess and colleagues provided suggestive evidence that prenatal rubella may also increase risk for childhood psychiatric disorders, including autism (Chess et al., 1971). Since many of these anomalies – subtle hearing deficits (David et al., 1995), a tendency for diminished neurocognitive function (David et al., 1995; Jones et al., 1994), enlarged cerebral ventricles (Pfefferbaum & Marsh, 1995), and premorbid behavioral disturbances (Done et al., 1994) – have been demonstrated in schizophrenia, this led us to hypothesize that prenatal rubella may be a risk factor for schizophrenia and other schizophrenia spectrum disorders.

Description of the Cohort. The RBDEP was established at New York University Medical Center in 1964. The primary purpose of the study was to more thoroughly delineate the clinical manifestations of congenital rubella, and to facilitate the development of management techniques for the sequelae of the infection (Cooper et al., 1969). The RBDEP enrolled mothers with a clinical diagnosis of rubella during pregnancy, and, in a smaller number, infants who were diagnosed soon after birth with congenital rubella syndrome. Serologic confirmation of infection is available for half of the mothers and infants, and nearly all of those tested were seropositive for rubella infection. The sample of the RBDEP consisted of 243 children (Chess et al., 1971).

Description of Follow-Up Studies of the RBDEP Cohort. The RBDEP cohort was administered psychiatric, intellectual, behavioral, and psychosocial evaluations during childhood, adolescence, and young adulthood. These included physical examinations, measures of IQ, temperament, behavior, and neuromotor function. These evaluations revealed several mental and physical handicaps. These included: mental retardation

(IQ < 70), deafness, blindness, and cerebral palsy. Among the 243, 137 had no mental retardation or other major physical handicaps with the exception of deafness.

Study of Nonaffective Psychosis in the RBDEP Cohort. In order to examine the relation between prenatal rubella and nonaffective psychosis, we capitalized on data collected at the young adult follow-up of the RBDEP cohort. At that time, the subjects were aged 21–23. This study is described in full in Brown et al. (2000c). At the young adult assessment, 70 subjects from this pool of 137 were located and administered a structured psychiatric diagnostic assessment, the Diagnostic Interview Schedule for Children (DISC), a comprehensive diagnostic interview which permitted *DSM-III-R* diagnoses to be made on all major psychiatric disorders. Because 59 percent of the interviewed sample was deaf, the assessment was administered on a computer, accompanied by a trained sign interpreter to assist with the interpretation of the symptom items.

For the purpose of comparison, we obtained data on two unexposed cohorts. The first was a randomly sampled cohort from a community-based study of physical and psychological health, located in Albany/Saratoga counties in New York State. This cohort was also administered the DISC. The second unexposed cohort was from the Epidemiological Catchment Area (ECA) sample, a large probability sample, which was administered the Diagnostic Interview Schedule. For brevity, we describe in full only the comparisons between the RBDEP and Albany-Saratoga cohorts. In order to equalize the period of risk for the exposed and unexposed, we restricted the age ranges for the unexposed cohorts to the same ages as for the RBDEP cohort. It should be noted that both the unexposed cohorts received an orally administered interview. Demographically, the exposed and unexposed cohorts did not differ significantly with respect to age and sex, although there was a smaller proportion of white subjects in the RBDEP as compared to the Albany/Saratoga cohort.

Our main outcome was nonaffective psychosis, which we defined as: (1) a minimum of one psychotic symptom lasting for at least 6 months; (2) no major affective disorders concurrent with the psychosis; and (3) no medical or substance use which could explain the psychosis.

We found a markedly increased risk of nonaffective psychosis in the rubella-exposed (11/70 or 15.7%). This proportion was significantly increased compared to both the Albany-Saratoga unexposed (5/164 or 3%) [RR (95% CI) = 5.2 (1.9, 14.3), $p < .001$, Fisher = s exact test] and the ECA unexposed (13/1346 or 1%) [RR (95% CI) = 16.3 (7.6–35.0), Fisher $p < .001$]. These results could not be explained by deafness or ethnicity differences, and are unlikely to be accounted for by selection bias. These findings therefore provide the first demonstration of a relation between a clearly documented prenatal viral infection and adult nonaffective psychosis.

Causal Mechanisms. Elaboration of the causal mechanisms by which prenatal rubella might lead to nonaffective psychosis are unclear; however, extensive knowledge of the teratogenic effects of this virus on brain development permits some speculations. First, it is well known that rubella infects the placenta, and that it subsequently invades the fetus, gaining access to the fetal brain. Once present in the brain, the virus is believed to impair development through two primary processes. First, rubella inhibits mitosis of neurons, leading to hypocellularity. In a recent animal model of schizophrenia, Moore et al. (1998) demonstrated that administration of the mitotoxin methylazoxymethanol acetate (MAM) (an inhibitor of mitosis) resulted in diminished thickness of prefrontal cortex in early life, and increased behavioral deficits mediated by prefrontal and temporal corticostriatal circuits, as well as deficits in sensorimotor gating in adulthood, abnormalities that have been demonstrated in schizophrenia. Second, rubella causes an encephalitis, with reactive gliosis and damage to developing neurons (South & Sever, 1985). These two mechanisms, perhaps in combination, may explain findings of marked enlargement of lateral ventricles and diminished cortical gray matter in adult subjects with congenital rubella. These morphologic abnormalities, which are among the most commonly demonstrated in schizophrenia, suggest that the above two causal mechanisms may be relevant to the increased risk of nonaffective psychosis observed in our study.

A second clue regarding pathogenesis emerged from the gestational timing of rubella infection. In nearly 80 percent of the exposed cohort, the infection occurred during the first trimester. Although the frequencies of subjects exposed to rubella in the first trimester did not differ between those with and without nonaffective psychosis, our results clearly suggest that a first-trimester viral insult can give rise to this disorder. Therefore, it is worth considering the neurodevelopmental events which occur during this gestational period. These events include neurulation, including the development of the neural tube, and neuronal proliferation (Nowakowski, 1999). Taken together with our findings regarding prenatal exposure to famine, discussed above, it appears that the first trimester may be a period of particularly high vulnerability for the development of schizophrenia and other nonaffective psychoses. It should be noted, however, that because rubella infection is known to persist during infancy and early childhood, adverse effects of the virus during these developmental periods may also contribute to the pathogenesis of nonaffective psychosis.

Columbia Rubella Study. We are presently completing work on a follow-up of the RBDEP birth cohort in mid-adulthood (age 34), the Columbia Rubella Study (CRS). The CRS is aimed at identifying new cases of schizophrenia spectrum disorders in members of this birth cohort; and improving upon the diagnostic precision through the use of a more comprehensive, orally administered interview. The CRS has confirmed the association between prenatal rubella and schizophrenia spectrum disorders (Brown et al., 2001).

Population Birth Cohort Design

A second type of research design that we have employed in the search for prenatal risk factors for schizophrenia is known as the *population birth cohort* design (Susser, 1999). In contrast to the epigenetic birth cohort studies described above, the subjects in a population birth cohort are not selected for any particular exposure. Rather, they are derived from a general population of births, in which detailed assessments are conducted during early development. Members of these birth cohorts are then followed up for the disorder of interest.

Prenatal Determinants of Schizophrenia Study
To exemplify the merits of this design, we describe in some detail one of our population-birth cohort designs, the Prenatal Determinants of Schizophrenia (PDS) study. The PDS

is a population birth cohort investigation launched by our group in 1996 (Susser, 1999). The primary purpose of the PDS is to investigate the relationship between prospectively and carefully documented prenatal, perinatal, and neonatal exposures and risk of adult schizophrenia and other schizophrenia spectrum disorders (SSD). The PDS derives from the Child Health and Development Study (CHDS), a large and highly informative population birth cohort investigation conducted from 1959 to 1966, aimed at examining the relation of pregnancy events to developmental abnormalities among the offspring. In the CHDS, nearly all pregnant women receiving routine prenatal care from the Kaiser Foundation Health Plan (KFHP) in Alameda County, California during the time frame of the study were enrolled. Their offspring, born as members of a single health plan with unified record keeping, numbered over 19,000.

The PDS study built upon this original investigation by following up the members of this birth cohort for adult SSD, defined as schizophrenia, schizoaffective disorder, psychotic disorder NOS, delusional disorder, and schizotypal personality disorder. Utilizing computerized records of KFHP, we first ascertained cohort members for both psychiatric hospitalizations and outpatient treatment. Because the computerized registries were not established until 1981, the PDS cohort consisted of the approximately 12,000 members who were KFHP members on or after that year. Ascertained potential cases were then screened for probable or possible SSD. Subjects who screened positive were located and invited for a direct diagnostic assessment, the Diagnostic Interview for Genetic Studies (DIGS). Consensus diagnoses were made in accord with *DSM-IV* criteria by a rotating group of three expert psychiatric diagnosticians. For those who could not be contacted or refused participation, psychiatric diagnoses were made by thorough review of all medical and psychiatric records.

This protocol has been completed, and has yielded a total of seventy-one cases of SSD, including forty-four diagnosed by full diagnostic assessment, and twenty-seven by chart review. Among these seventy-one, forty-three have schizophrenia and seventeen have schizoaffective disorder; the remaining eleven had other schizophrenia spectrum disorders.

Strengths of the PDS. The PDS study has several notable strengths, which represent substantial advancements over previous investigations. First, as alluded to above, detailed exposure data, including maternal characteristics prior to and during pregnancy; illnesses during pregnancy; labor and delivery complications; and neonatal events, are available from the rich CHDS database. Furthermore, maternal serum samples drawn during pregnancy and stored frozen are available, providing an unrivaled opportunity to conduct serologic assays aimed at discovering prenatal exposures of relevance to schizophrenia. In previous studies, investigators generally relied upon relatively crude prenatal exposure data, such as maternal recall of events in pregnancy, routine midwifery records, or data that applied to groups rather than individuals. Moreover, in previous studies, data were generally not available for early gestational exposures, because routine prenatal care was not initiated until mid-pregnancy or later.

Second, as described above, diagnoses were made largely by direct interview using a standardized, research-based instrument. Previous studies used clinical rather than research diagnoses, diagnoses based on systems with relatively nonspecific criteria, or diagnoses based solely on psychiatric registries or review of hospital records.

Third, the PDS study included excellent control of bias due to loss to follow-up. This strength arose from the continuous follow-up study afforded by the registries of KFHP, which provided all dates of membership and treatment for virtually all cohort members over the seventeen-year follow-up period. Using survival analysis, complete adjustment for nondifferential loss to follow-up was attained. Previous studies were hampered by incomplete adjustment for loss to follow-up, and the consequent likelihood for bias. This resulted from either lack of knowledge of the population denominator at the time of case ascertainment, so that the number of subjects leaving the population could not be enumerated; or from case ascertainment at only one point in time, prohibiting the delineation of when subjects left the cohort.

Fourth, the comprehensive database on early developmental exposures allows for good control of many potential confounding factors, and the analysis of putative causal pathways that link the primary prenatal risk factors of interest to the adult schizophrenia outcome. The scarcity of such data in previous studies did not allow for this possibility.

The PDS study therefore brings to bear an increased precision and range of prenatal data, accurate diagnoses, and sophisticated epidemiologic methodology to the investigation of prenatal exposures that may play causal roles in schizophrenia. In addition, confounding can be controlled, and causal pathways can be explored. Moreover, utilizing newly collected data on familial risk, gene-environment interactions can be elaborated. Below, we describe two initial findings which illustrate the potential of the PDS for uncovering prenatal antecedents of schizophrenia.

Research Findings from the PDS

Maternal Respiratory Infection. In this study, we examined the relation between second-trimester maternal exposure to respiratory infection and risk of SSD (Brown et al., in press). As noted earlier, previous studies on the putative association between prenatal infection and risk of schizophrenia have yielded contradictory results; and it is our view that misclassification of both exposure and outcome may explain some of these inconsistencies. Because most of these findings are confined to second-trimester prenatal influenza, we sought to test the hypothesis that respiratory infections during this gestational period might increase risk of SSD. The broader category of respiratory infections, rather than influenza alone, was used for two reasons. First, the occurrence of maternal influenza was too rare in our database to permit a meaningful analysis on its own. Second, prenatal exposure to several of these infections has yet to be examined in a study of schizophrenia.

For this purpose, we utilized a rich dataset on diagnoses of maternal medical conditions, which were prospectively diagnosed – generally by physicians – throughout pregnancy, and carefully abstracted from the gravidas' medical records. In addition to data on the presence of respiratory infection, we capitalized on the documentation of the gestational timing of infection.

The primary exposure variable was defined as all second-trimester respiratory infections in the dataset. These infections included: tuberculosis, influenza, pneumonia, pleurisy, empyema/viral respiratory infections, acute bronchitis, and upper respiratory infections. To examine whether the effect of maternal respiratory infection was specific to the second trimester, we also examined first- and third-trimester exposure to these infections. The primary outcome variable was SSD; case ascertainment, screening, and diagnosis were as described above.

In order to adjust for loss to follow-up (see above), the data were analyzed using proportional hazards regression, a method of survival analysis which accounts for different durations of follow-up among subjects. Potential confounders included maternal age, smoking, education, race, parity, alcohol use, and marital status. Among these, only maternal smoking was appreciably associated with SSD. We also controlled for maternal race and education, as previous studies have established relations between both of these demographic variables and risk of SSD.

We demonstrated that maternal exposure to respiratory infection during the second trimester was significantly associated with risk of SSD, controlling for maternal smoking, education, and race [RR = 2.13 (1.05–4.35), $X2 = 4.36$, $p = .04$]. Maternal respiratory infections during the first [RR = 0.89 (0.28–2.84), $X2 = .04$, $p = 0.84$] and the third trimesters [RR = 0.68 (0.25–1.87), $X2 = 0.56$, $p = 0.45$] were not associated with SSD. The findings were similar when the outcome was restricted to schizophrenia. A breakdown of the effects by individual infections demonstrated that upper respiratory infection accounted for much of the main result.

These findings have several potential implications for the etiopathogenesis of schizophrenia. First, they suggest that respiratory infections other than influenza may have an etiologic role, perhaps acting through a common mechanism such as maternal hyperthermia, a known teratogenic factor (Edwards, 1986) that has been related to schizophrenia (Jones et al., 1998); cold or flu medications, such as aspirin, which is associated with congenital anomalies (Lynberg et al., 1994); an excessive pro-inflammatory antibody response, which has been associated with cerebral palsy (Nelson et al., 1998); or production of a teratogenic antibody of maternal origin which disrupts fetal brain development by cross-reacting with brain antigens through molecular mimicry (Wright et al., 1999).

The second-trimester specificity of the finding provides an additional valuable clue. It has been argued previously that influenza may interfere with neuronal migration, a process that occurs mainly in the second trimester of fetal brain development (Mednick et al., 1988). It is thus conceivable that other respiratory infections, or their adverse effects on maternal or fetal physiology, may similarly disrupt the orderly migration of neurons in the fetal brain, thereby increasing vulnerability to schizophrenia in adulthood.

Maternal Pre-Pregnant Body Mass Index. The aim of this study was to investigate the relation between maternal pre-pregnant body mass index (BMI) and risk of adult schizophrenia. The study is fully described in Schaefer et al. (2000). The investigation was motivated by two lines of evidence. First, maternal malnourishment is associated with poor pregnancy outcomes, abnormal neurodevelopment, and with schizophrenia (Done et al., 1994; Susser et al., 1996). Second, *high* maternal pre-pregnant BMI has also been associated with poor pregnancy outcomes, including neural tube defects, and a recent study suggested a potential association with schizophrenia (Jones et al., 1998). In order to help resolve this question, we examined the relation of maternal pre-pregnant BMI to the development of schizophrenia and SSD. As a consequence of the previous findings, we hypothesized that BMI at the extremes of the distribution (either high or low) would be related to an increased risk of SSD.

For this purpose, we utilized reported pre-pregnant weight and height at enrollment in the CHDS from a maternal interview administered to the vast majority of gravidas. BMI was calculated as kilograms/meters^2, a reliable indicator of nutritional status and body composition. For the analysis, we divided the distribution of pre-pregant BMI into four categories, in accord with a well-established definition (Institute of Medicine, 1990).

In the main analysis, the relation of maternal pre-pregnant BMI was assessed using a multivariate proportional hazards regression model that included maternal race, a potential confounder, and sex of the offspring, a potential interaction term. We demonstrated that, compared with the offspring of mothers with average pre-pregnant BMI (20–26), the adjusted rate ratio of SSD was 1.2 (95% CI = 0.65) among offspring of mothers with low pre-pregnant BMI ($\leq$ 19), 1.8 (95% CI = 0.75–4.3) among mothers with pre-pregnant BMI of 27–30, and 2.9 (95% CI = 1.3–6.5) among mothers with pre-pregnant BMI > 30. The association occurred independently of other potential confounders, including maternal age, education, parity, and cigarette smoking. The findings were similar when the outcome was restricted to schizophrenia. There was no evidence that the association was modified by sex of the offspring, or that the relation differed between SSD cases with early versus later age of onset. Thus, these findings indicate that high, but not low, BMI may be a risk factor for SSD in a generally well-fed, middle-class, American population in the 1960s.

These results may shed light on potential causal mechanisms that may lead to schizophrenia. First, it is well documented that during the period of the study, overweight women were advised to markedly limit food intake; these restrictions could have resulted in diminished intake of micronutrients critical for proper brain development, including folic acid (MRC, 1991) or essential fatty acids (Menon & Dhopeshwarkar, 1982). In addition, amphetamines were prescribed to many of these women. These substances are potent dopamine-releasing agents and may alter the formation of dopamine neural circuitry, a phenomenon which may be relevant to the development of schizophrenia (Lyon, 1990). Another explanation for the association includes increased hemostatic factors, such as homocysteine, a sulfur-containing amino acid whose conversion to methionine is catalyzed by both folate and vitamin B12 (de Vries et al., 1997; Girling & de Swiet, 1998), which may interfere with placental blood flow, thereby compromising both fetal oxygenation and nutrition.

Moreover, these results may have important implications for the prevention of schizophrenia. Within the past twenty-five years, elevated BMI has increased significantly, affecting over 20 percent of reproductive-age women. Thus, if increased BMI is confirmed as a risk factor for schizophrenia, the attributable risk is likely to be substantial. When we understand the causal pathways (see Future Directions section), this study may ultimately translate into recommendations to obstetricians regarding optimal weight during pregnancy.

Our group is also presently pursuing studies of other population birth cohorts. The Jerusalem Perinatal Study (JPS) consists of approximately 90,000 live births with prospectively documented data on maternal/paternal demographic factors, prenatal exposures and perinatal complications. Recently, Malaspina et al. (2001) have used the JPS to demonstrate a graded association between paternal age and risk of adult schizophrenia and related disorders.

FUTURE DIRECTIONS

Identification of Risk Factors for Schizophrenia

In the upcoming years, we have an unprecedented opportunity to capitalize on the many strengths of our cohort studies to expand upon the existing literature regarding prenatal risk factors for schizophrenia. Below, we outline our future plans as they relate to the discovery of new prenatal exposures.

PDS Study

Existing Data. Using the rich existing database, and our sample of well-diagnosed SSD cases, we are presently examining several additional prenatal risk factors for this disorder. These include advanced paternal age, Rh incompatibility, maternal race and education, and unwantedness of pregnancy.

Maternal Sera. In addition, using the maternal sera, we are planning new analyses that are expected to substantially advance our knowledge of prenatal exposures in schizophrenia. These analyses provide an unprecedented opportunity to conduct examinations on risk factors which were not possible to pursue using the methodologies of earlier studies. For example, serologic assays of influenza antibody during pregnancy will provide definitive documentation of the exposure, thereby providing the best opportunity to date to test the hypothesis that prenatal influenza is a risk factor for schizophrenia.

In order to better understand our association between prenatal famine and schizophrenia, we shall explore hypotheses of specific micronutrient deficiencies as risk factors for schizophrenia by assays of micronutrients in the PDS sera. These include measures of homocysteine, an indicator of folate status, and quantification of essential fatty acids. Moreover, we can expand the range of exposures to other factors that are known to disrupt brain development, including toxins such as lead and drugs of abuse; and hormone deficiencies such as thyroid, or hormone excesses such as cortisol.

The use of these assays will also help to address many of the limitations – and extend the analysis of causal pathways – in the studies on the PDS cohort that are based on existing data, such as those described above. With regard to the maternal infection study (see above), these limitations included potential misclassification of exposure due to lack of medical attention for infection, and the lack of documentation of specific infectious agents. With respect to the study on pre-pregnant BMI, data on potential mediators – such as serum fibrinogen levels – were not available. These intervening variables could be quantified in the prenatal sera, shedding light on potential pathogenic mechanisms that underlie the association.

Collaborative Studies. Furthermore, we are presently collaborating with investigators who are following up other population birth cohorts for schizophrenia. These cohorts include the National Collaborative Perinatal Project (NCPP), a large birth cohort study with a similar research design, and conducted over the same time interval, as the PDS. Many of the same prenatal exposures were examined in the NCPP and PDS birth cohorts. In addition, similar diagnostic assessments were used in both studies to ascertain schizophrenia. The comparability of methods for identifying both prenatal exposures and schizophrenia outcomes creates the potential for pooling the cases from these two cohorts, thereby permitting the investigation of selected, rarer prenatal exposures for which larger sample sizes are necessary to ensure adequate statistical power for detecting associations.

Columbia Rubella Study. As described earlier, there were 137 cohort members of the RBDEP who were eligible for the follow-up study of schizophrenia spectrum disorders, of whom 70 were targeted for assessment at the young adult follow-up. Thus, there is the potential of identifying more cases of SSD among nearly 70 additional rubella-exposed cohort members. In future work, we plan to assess these subjects, in an attempt to replicate our finding of an increased risk of SSD. Moreover, the assessment of this sample will provide us with new cases for future neurobiologic studies discussed below.

Exploration of Genetics and Neurobiology

Genetics

Although this review has focused on prenatal environmental exposures as risk factors for schizophrenia, clearly there is strong evidence that genetic factors play an important etiologic role. Genetic defects may contribute to risk of schizophrenia by themselves, or through gene-environment interactions. Recently, several examples of this latter possibility have emerged for a number of neurodevelopmental disorders. For instance, evidence suggests that neural tube defects might arise from an interaction between a genetic abnormality that impairs homocysteine metabolism and prenatal folate deficiency. Based on our work on the Dutch Hunger Winter, in which the risk of both neural tube defects and schizophrenia were increased by periconceptional exposure to famine, we proposed that schizophrenia may develop from a similar gene-environment interaction. In another example, Wright et al. (1999) have proposed that a genetically mediated maternal autoantibody response to influenza may give rise to schizophrenia.

These findings therefore suggest a new strategy for research into the genetics of schizophrenia. If certain genes exert their effect primarily by interaction with prenatal environmental exposures, then genetic research designs aimed at isolating these genes could be greatly facilitated by employing samples enriched for the respective prenatal exposures. With regard to the example above on prenatal folate deficiency, we aim to test the hypothesis that mutations which are associated with neural tube defects, and involved in the folate metabolic cascade, play a role in schizophrenia. For this purpose, we shall quantify maternal homocysteine levels in the serum samples from the PDS birth cohort described earlier; and genotype the offspring for these mutations. We shall then examine whether the effect of prenatal folate deficiency (manifested as high homocysteine) on risk of schizophrenia is modified in the presence of these genes. Conceivably, in the absence of information on prenatal folate deficiency, these mutations would show no relation to schizophrenia. A second line of investigation may emerge from recent findings on genes that encode homeobox domain proteins, which play crucial roles in brain development, providing additional genes to be tested for interaction with prenatal exposures identified in our birth cohort studies. Moreover, the impending completion of the Human Genome Project will lead to a profusion of new candidate genes that can be investigated in relation to these prenatal factors.

Interactions between genetic mutations and prenatal environmental exposures may also have general relevance to psychopathology. For example, we previously demonstrated an association between later gestational famine and risk of major affective disorders (see The Dutch Famine and Psychiatric Outcomes). It has been well documented that affective disorders, particularly bipolar disorder, have a substantial genetic component. In addition, other evidence, reviewed above (see Prenatal Determinants of Affective Disorders), has implicated subtle neurodevelopmental perturbations in the pathogenesis of affective disorders. Thus, it will also be important in future studies to examine genetic candidates for affective disorders for potential interactions with prenatal environmental exposures. Other psychiatric/behavioral disorders can also be investigated for gene-environment interaction as vulnerability genes for these disorders are identified.

Another important purpose of genetic research is to address limitations of previous birth cohort studies of schizophrenia. For example, in our maternal respiratory infection study on the PDS cohort (see above), confounding by genetic loading for schizophrenia may have occurred, if, for example, gravidas with schizophrenia were less likely to receive prenatal care. In this case, knowledge of maternal mental illness would permit us to adjust for this potential confounding factor. Toward this end, we are presently conducting research interviews on family members of schizophrenia probands for a history of schizophrenia or spectrum disorders.

Neurobiology

Although demonstrating associations between prenatal exposures and schizophrenia is of critical importance, these studies provide limited information on pathogenesis. For this purpose, we are embarking on investigations in each of our birth cohorts aimed at delineating the causal mechanisms that mediate the relation of the prenatal exposures to the schizophrenia outcome. These investigations include neuroimaging/neuropsychologic studies and animal models.

Neuroimaging/Neuropsychology. The application of sophisticated brain imaging methods to schizophrenia research has revolutionized our understanding of the structural and functional neuropathology that underlie this illness. Magnetic resonance imaging (MRI) has revealed structural abnormalities, such as ventriculomegaly and diminished hippocampal volume. Functional neuroimaging techniques, such as positron emission tomography (PET), single photon emission computerized tomography (SPECT), and functional MRI have revealed hypometabolism in the dorsolateral prefrontal cortex during neuropsychological paradigms that activate this brain region. Despite these important advances, however, the causes of these brain abnormalities remain unknown. Utilizing the rich resources of our birth cohort studies, we have the opportunity to relate putative early developmental insults, acquired prospectively, to both structural and functional brain anomalies in well-diagnosed patients with schizophrenia.

In the PDS cohort, we are planning a study in which SSD cases and controls will receive MRI, proton (^{1}H) magnetic resonance spectroscopy (MRS), and neuropsychological testing. We hypothesize that early developmental insults will be correlated with ventriculomegaly and diminished hippocampal volume; reduced n-acetyl-aspartate (a marker of neuronal integrity) in the prefrontal cortex and hippocampus; and dysfunction in language, attention, and memory. In addition to providing validation for prenatal environmental exposures as etiologic factors in schizophrenia, these studies will shed light on pathogenesis by delineating the neural structures and functions whose development is disrupted by these exposures, and consequently give rise to schizophrenia. Furthermore, the reduction of etiologic heterogeneity attained by the use of well-characterized subjects with homogeneous early developmental exposures may have implications for neuroimaging research that extends beyond the pathogenesis of these exposures.

In the CRS study, we are presently conducting MRI and ^{1}H MRS studies on exposed cases and controls. Preliminary evidence from the MRS studies suggests that exposed cases have diminished n-acetyl-aspartate (NAA), a marker of neuronal integrity, in the prefrontal cortex and hippocampus, as compared to exposed controls (Brown et al., 1999).

In the Dutch famine cohort, we have demonstrated increased white matter hyperintensities in subjects exposed periconceptionally to the Hunger Winter, with a particular high rate in exposed schizophrenia cases (Hulshoff-Pol et al., 2000). This finding might be explained by a loss of myelin due to an inadequate supply of nutrients. In addition, we found an interaction between prenatal famine exposure and schizophrenia diagnosis in predicting diminished intracranial volume. This result suggests that diminished brain growth due to prenatal famine may have predisposed to later development of schizophrenia. It is worth noting that there were no effects of famine exposure on volumes of the total brain, lateral/third ventricle, or cerebellum.

Animal Models. The use of animal models for schizophrenia represents a promising avenue toward understanding the neurobiological effects of early developmental insults throughout the lifespan, and their relevance to clinical findings in schizophrenic patients. Animal studies permit the examination of many biological variables that are not practical or ethical to investigate in humans; and the rapid maturation of rodents permits the effects of prenatal exposures to be investigated over a much briefer time scale than studies of human populations. For example, Lipska, Weinberger, and colleagues have conducted a series of investigations using a rodent model involving a neonatal hippocampal lesion, and a variety of behavioral and neurochemical measures believed to occur in schizophrenia, such as those related to the dopamine system (see Lipska, Khaing, & Weinberger, 1999). These studies have provided some of the most persuasive evidence to date supporting the neurodevelopmental hypothesis of schizophrenia, by demonstrating excessive dopamine-mediated behaviors that are manifested in adulthood, but not in early life. Bachevalier et al. (1999) have extended this model to nonhuman primates, with many comparable findings.

By attempting to emulate early insults similar to those experienced by our birth cohort members, these types of animal models may yield significant new insights into the causal mechanisms leading to schizophrenia. For instance, our group is presently examining the behavioral and neurochemical consequences of prenatal protein deprivation in rats, in an attempt to model prenatal exposure to famine. We plan to extend these animal models to include prenatal viral exposures, and investigate new potential outcomes of relevance to schizophrenia, such as effects on the glutamatergic system.

A further question that can be addressed by the studies described above concerns the mechanisms by which diverse etiologic factors lead to the same clinical outcome.

Our work has shown that a variety of prenatal exposures, including famine (Susser et al., 1996), rubella (Brown et al., 2000c, 2001), maternal respiratory infection (Brown et al., 2000a), elevated maternal body mass index (Schaefer et al., 2000), and advanced paternal age (Brown et al., 2002; Malaspina et al., 2001) are each associated with an increased risk of schizophrenia. This suggests two distinct hypotheses. As suggested by other authors, schizophrenia is likely to be heterogeneous with regard to etiology, pathogenesis, pathophysiology, and clinical manifestations. If this is the case, then the prenatal exposures discussed above could operate through different pathogenic mechanisms, each giving rise to somewhat different pathophysiologic and clinical subtypes. Under an alternative hypothesis, schizophrenia is etiologically diverse, but these different risk factors act through a common neurobiologic mechanism to produce the adult clinical syndrome.

These two hypotheses can be tested using the methodologies proposed above. The first hypothesis would be supported if we observed that different prenatal exposures were each linked to specific structural or functional abnormalities of different brain regions, neural circuits, or variations in neurotransmitter or receptor pathology. The second hypothesis would be supported if different prenatal exposures of causal relevance to schizophrenia were associated with similar morphologic and functional abnormalities in these patients. Animal models may also help to validate this hypothesis by demonstrating similar developmental pathways arising from diverse, experimentally administered in utero exposures. One conceivable outcome of these investigations is that some combination of these two models may be present; for instance, there may be "clusters" of prenatal etiologic factors, and each cluster may operate to produce the clinical syndrome through unique pathogenic mechanisms and associated pathophysiologic processes.

Investigation of Risk Factors for Other Psychiatric Disorders

Our group is well positioned to investigate the relation of prenatal risk factors to other psychiatric disorders. As reviewed above, the affective disorders may also have prenatal origins, and thus may represent fertile ground for research on relevant prenatal determinants.

In the PDS study, we have obtained consensus diagnoses of affective disorders. This will permit us to investigate the relationship of prenatal factors to these disorders using similar methods as those used for our studies of schizophrenia. Prenatal viral infections and micronutrient deficiencies represent potentially important candidates for affective disorders. Furthermore, we have diagnosed cases of major affective disorders in subjects from the Columbia Rubella Study. The risk of these disorders, and their premorbid antecedents, will be investigated in future work. Once relationships are established, research strategies similar to those being implemented in our studies of schizophrenia, including gene-environment interaction and neuroanatomic/neuropsychologic analyses, can also be applied to the investigation of affective disorders in our cohorts. In addition, other types of psychopathology, such as suicide, anxiety disorders, or eating disorders, could also be investigated for prenatal origins in future studies of our cohorts. We also suggest that the datasets of other investigators that have proven so valuable to research on schizophrenia should be further probed for relationships between prenatal risk factors for affective disorders, and other psychopathologic outcomes.

Similar research approaches as those discussed above for schizophrenia (see Exploration of Genetics and Neurobiology) may also prove valuable in addressing the link between etiology, developmental pathways, and other forms of psychopathology. This work may help to shed light on a critical question that arises in this context: How does a specific etiologic factor lead to diverse psychopathological outcomes? Previous findings from our group on the Dutch Famine Studies, reviewed above (Brown et al., 1995; Brown et al., 2000b), suggest that the gestational timing of the insult plays a role in determining the type of psychiatric disorder which results: early gestational famine is associated with increased risk of schizophrenia, while famine exposure during later gestation is associated with an increased risk of affective disorders. This should perhaps not be surprising given profound differences in the vulnerability of the brain between early and later fetal development. The first and second gestational months are characterized by the early embryonic stages, in which cleavage and implantation, formation of the neural tube, and the formation of the major subdivisions of the brain occurs (O'Rahilly & Muller, 1999). During later gestation, the relevant developmental processes largely concern neuronal migration and differentiation of the neural elements formed during the first trimester. Thus, adverse events during early gestation, a period in which the brain is far less differentiated, are likely to have more severe and pervasive effects than developmental disruptions during later gestation. These stage-specific differences in the extent and nature of fetal developmental events are consistent with the observed clinical differences between schizophrenia and affective disorders: compared to affective disorders, schizophrenia is generally considered to be of greater severity with regard to symptomatology, course and outcome, and functional impairment.

Another important factor that can guide the developmental pathway toward one psychiatric disorder or another is genetic vulnerability. For instance, it is logical to hypothesize that the same in utero insult can lead to schizophrenia in an individual genetically predisposed to this disorder, and to affective disorder in a subject with a genetic vulnerability to that illness. The presence of affective disorder and other psychiatric diagnoses in our birth cohort studies, combined with essential clinical data on brain structure and function, genetic liability, and developmental periods of vulnerability, promise to further elaborate the underlying neurobiologic events that give rise to varying manifestations of psychopathology from a single etiologic insult.

Preventive Strategies

Another important implication of this area of work concerns the implementation of programs aimed at primary prevention. If associations between prenatal factors and risk of schizophrenia are confirmed, then this could lead to new public health recommendations and become incorporated into routine obstetric practice. This strategy is exemplified by the preventive programs instituted in many countries after rubella – one of the viruses associated with psychotic disorders in our study – was established as a teratogen. These programs, which involved routine rubella vaccinations of young children, led to a dramatic decline in cases of rubella, and the congenital rubella syndrome. As new viral risk factors for schizophrenia are identified, vaccination programs modeled on the control of rubella and other childhood illnesses may conceivably be implemented.

Prevention programs can also be established for prenatal nutritional and other exposures that are definitively shown to play an etiologic role in schizophrenia. One model for future programs, currently under way in several countries, is the routine administration of prenatal vitamins containing folic acid to pregnant women, and the supplementation of folic acid to bread and cereals. It is expected that these measures will lead to a significant decline in the risk of neural tube defects. If folate deficiency is confirmed to play a causal role in schizophrenia, such nutritional interventions may also aid in the prevention of this disorder. It must be emphasized, however, that several independent replications of our findings will be necessary before new viral or nutritional preventive strategies are considered, as there may also be potential risks associated with these interventions.

CONCLUSIONS

Despite over a century of research on schizophrenia, its origins remain unknown. The neurodevelopmental hypothesis of schizophrenia has led to a dramatic shift in our thinking regarding the etiology of this illness. One result of this new paradigm is that investigators have begun to investigate prenatal environmental factors as potential risk factors for this disorder. It has been only recently, however, that birth cohorts with prospective and well-documented gestational exposures have passed through the age of risk for schizophrenia, permitting unprecedented opportunities to examine the prenatal origins of this disorder. Research from our group on three such birth cohorts – the Dutch Hunger Winter, the Rubella Birth Defects Evaluation Project, and the Prenatal Determinants of Schizophrenia – have, respectively, yielded important findings on the potential roles of gestational nutritional deficiency, viral exposures, and pre-pregnancy body mass index in schizophrenia. Over the next several years, we anticipate that these novel research designs will yield a wealth of data which will markedly extend these findings, investigate many new prenatal exposures in the etiology of schizophrenia, and explore causal pathways between prenatal exposures and perinatal/neonatal complications. In addition, we plan to capitalize on these unique cohorts to investigate the interaction of these potential risk factors with vulnerability genes in the etiology of schizophrenia. Moreover, future brain imaging and neuropsychological studies in these cohorts, and developmental animal models, promise to elaborate the causal mechanisms by which these prenatal factors lead to schizophrenia and validate these exposures as playing an etiologic role. We are confident that this body of work will realize its potential of substantially advancing our understanding of the origins of this devastating disorder, thereby leading to important preventative and therapeutic measures.

REFERENCES

Adams, W., Kendell, R. E., Hare, E. K., & Munk-Jorgensen, P. (1993). Epidemiological evidence that maternal influenza contributes to the aetiology of schizophrenia. *British Journal of Psychiatry, 163,* 522–534.

Anderson, S. A., Eisenstat, D. D., Shi, L., & Rubenstein, L. R. (1997). Interneuron migration from basal forebrain to neocortex: dependence on Dlx genes. *Science, 278,* 474–476.

Bachevalier, J., Alvarado, M. C., & Malkova, L. (1999). Memory and socioemotional behavior in monkeys after hippocampal damage incurred in infancy or in adulthood. *Biological Psychiatry, 46,* 329–339.

Barr, C. E., Mednick, S. A., & Munk-Jorgensen, P. (1990). Exposure to influenza epidemics during gestation and adult schizophrenia. *Archives of General Psychiatry, 47,* 869–874.

Bogerts, B., Ashtari, M., DeGreef, G., Alvir, J. M. J., Bilder, R. M., & Lieberman, J. A. (1990). Reduced temporal limbic structure volumes on magnetic resonance images in first episode schizophrenia. *Psychiatry Research Neuroimage, 35,* 1–13.

Bradbury, T. N., & Miller, G. A. (1985). Season of birth in schizophrenia: A review of evidence, methodology, and etiology. *Psychological Bulletin, 3,* 569–594.

Brown, A. S. (1999). New perspectives on the neurodevelopmental hypothesis of schizophrenia. *Psychiatric Annals, 29,* 128–130.

Brown, A. S., Cohen, P., Greenwald, S., & Susser, E. (2000c). Nonaffective psychosis after prenatal exposure to rubella, *American Journal of Psychiatry, 157,* 438–443.

Brown, A. S., Cohen, P., Harkavy-Friedman, J., Malaspina, D., Gorman, J. M., & Susser, E. A. E. (2001). Bennett Research Award: Prenatal rubella, premorbid abnormalities, and adult schizophrenia. *Biological Psychiatry, 49,* 473–486.

Brown, A. S., Schaefer, C. A., Wyatt, R. J., Begg, M. D., Goetz, R., Bresnuhan, M. A., Harkavy-Friedman, J., Gorman, J. M., Malaspina, D., & Susser, E. S. (2002). Paternal age and risk of schizophrenia in adult offspring. *American Journal of Psychiatry, 159,* 1528–1533.

Brown, A. S., Schaefer, C. A., Wyatt, R. J., Goetz, R., Begg, M. D., Gorman, J. M., & Susser, E. S. (2000a). Maternal exposure to respiratory infections and adult schizophrenia spectrum disorders: a prospective birth cohort study, *Schizophrenia Bulletin, 26,* 287–295.

Brown, A. S., Susser, E. S., Butler, P. D., Richardson, A. R., Kaufmann, C. A., & Gorman, J. M. (1996). Neurobiological plausibility of prenatal nutritional deprivation as a risk factor for schizophrenia. *Journal of Nervous and Mental Disease, 184,* 71–85.

Brown, A. S., Susser, E. S., & Cohen, P. (1999). Childhood neurocognition, neuromotor function, and behavior as predictors of adult psychosis: A prospective cohort study of prenatal viral infection. Abstracts of the 7th International Congress on Schizophrenia Research, Sante Fe, New Mexico, April.

Brown, A. S., Susser, E. S., Lin, S. P., & Gorman, J. M. (1995). Affective disorders in Holland after prenatal exposure to the 1957 A2 influenza epidemic. *Biological Psychiatry, 38,* 270–273.

Brown, A. S., van Os, J., Driessens, C., Hoek, H. W., & Susser, E. S. (2000b). Further evidence of relation between prenatal famine and major affective disorder. *American Journal of Psychiatry, 157,* 190–195.

Butler, P. D., Susser, E. S., Brown, A. S., Kaufmann, C. A., & Gorman, J. M. (1994). Prenatal nutritional deprivation as a risk factor in schizophrenia: Preclinical evidence. *Neuropsychopharmacology, 11,* 227–235.

Cannon, M., Coter, D., Coffey, V. P., et al. (1996). Prenatal exposure to the 1957 influenza epidemic and adult schizophrenia: a follow-up study. *British Journal of Psychiatry, 168,* 368–371.

Chess, S., Korn, S., & Fernandez, P. (1971). *Psychiatric disorders of children with congenital rubella.* New York: Brunner/Mazel.

Cooper, L. Z., Ziring, P. R., Ockerse, A. B., Fedun, B., Kelly, B., & Krugman, S. (1969). Rubella: Clinical manifestations and management. *American Journal of Dis Child, 118,* 18–29.

Crow, T. J., Done, D. J., & Johnstone, E. C. (1991). Schizophrenia and influenza. *Lancet, 338,* 116–117.

Dalman, C., Allebeck, P., Cullberg, J., Grunewald, C., & Koster, M. (1999). Obstetric complications and the risk of schizophrenia: a longitudinal study of a national birth cohort. *Archives of General Psychiatry, 56,* 234–240.

David, A. S., Malmberg, A., Brandt, L., Allebeck, P., & Lewis, G. (1997). I.Q. and risk for schizophrenia: a population-based cohort study. *Psychological Medicine, 27,* 1311–1323.

David, A., Malmberg, A., Lewis, G., Brandt, L., Allebeck, P. (1995). Are there neurological and sensory risk factors for schizophrenia? *Schizophrenia Research, 14,* 247–251.

Davis, J. O., Puelzs, J. A., Braeua, H. S. (1995). Prenatal development of monozygotic twins and concordance for schizophrenia. *Schizophrenia Bulletin, 21,* 357–366.

DeGreef, G. M., Ashtari, B., & Bogerts, B. (1992). Volumes of ventricular system subdivisions measured from magnetic resonance images in first-episode schizophrenic patients. *Archives of General Psychiatry, 49,* 531–537.

de Vries, J. I., Dekker, G. A., Huijgens, P. C., Jakobs, C., Blomberg, B. M., & Van Geijn, H. P. (1997). Hyperhomocysteinaemia and protein S deficiency in complicated pregnancies. *British Journal of Obstetrics and Gynecology, 104,* 1248–1254.

Done, D. J., Johnston, E. C., Frith, C. D., Golding, J., Shepherd, P. M., & Crow, T. J. (1991). Complications of pregnancy and delivery in relation to psychosis in adult life: Data from the British perinatal mortality survey. *British Medical Journal, 302,* 1576–1580.

Done, D. J., Crow, T. J., Johnston, E. C., & Sacker, A. (1994). Childhood antecedents of schizophrenia and affective illness: Social adjustment at ages 7 and 11. *British Medical Journal, 309,* 699–703.

Edwards, M. J. (1986). Hyperthermia as a teratogen: A review of experimental studies and their clinical significance. *Teratogenesis, Carcinogenesis and Mutagenesis, 6,* 563–582.

Erlenmeyer-Kimling, L., Folnegovic, Z., Hrabak-Zerjavic, V., Borcic, B., Folnegovic-Smalc, V., & Susser, E. (1994). Schizophrenia and prenatal exposure to the 1957 A2 influenza epidemic in Croatia, *American Journal of Psychiatry, 151,* 1496–1498.

Fahy, T. A., Jones, P. B., & Sham, P. C. (1993). Schizophrenia in Afro-Caribbeans in the UK following prenatal exposure to the 1957 A2 influenza epidemic. *Schizophrenia Research, 6,* 98–99.

Girling, J., & de Swiet, M. (1998). Inherited thrombophilia and pregnancy. *Current Opinions in Obstetrics and Gynecology, 10,* 135–144.

Goodman, A. B. (1995). Chromosomal locations and modes of action of genes of the retinoid (vitamin A) system support their involvement in the etiology of schizophrenia. *American Journal of Med Genet, 60,* 335–348.

Grech, A., Takei, N., & Murray, R. M. (1997). Maternal exposure to influenza and paranoid schizophrenia. *Schizophrenia Research, 26,* 121–125.

Green, M. F., Satz, P., Gaier, D. J., Gancell, S., & Kharabi, F. (1989). Minor physical anomalies in schizophrenia. *Schizophrenia Bulletin, 15,* 91–99.

Gregg, N. (1941). Congenital cataract following German measles in the mother. *Trans Ophthalmol Soc, 3,* 35–45.

Hoek, H. W., & et al., unpublished data.

Hoek, H. W., Susser, E., Buck, K. A., Lumey, L. H., Liu, S. P., & Gorman, J. M. (1996). Schizoid personality disorder after prenatal exposure to famine. *American Journal of Psychiatry, 53,* 19–24.

Hoek, H. W., Brown, A. S., & Susser, E. S. (1999). The Dutch famine studies: Prenatal nutritional deficiency and schizophrenia. In E. S. Susser, A. S. Brown, & J. M. Gorman (Eds), *Prenatal exposures in schizophrenia* (pp. 135–161). Washington, D.C.: American Psychiatric Press.

Hollister, J. M., Laing, P., & Mednick, S. A. (1996). Rheusus incompatibility as a risk factor for schizophrenia in male adults. *Archives of General Psychiatry, 53,* 19–24.

Hulshoff-Pol, H. E., Hoek, H.W., Susser, E. S., Brown, A. S., Kahn, R. S., & Cispen-de Wied, C. C. (2000). Prenatal exposure to famine and brain morphology in schizophrenia. *American Journal of Psychiatry, 157,* 1170–1172.

Hultman, C. M., Ohman, A., Cnattingius, S., Wieselgren, I. M., & Lindstrom, L. H. (1997). Prenatal and neonatal risk factors for schizophrenia. *British Journal of Psychiatry, 170,* 128–133.

Hultman, C. M., Sparen, P., Takei, N., Murray, R. M., & Cnattingius, S. (1999). Prenatal and perinatal risk factors for schizophrenia, affective psychosis, and reactive psychosis of early onset: case-control study. *British Medical Journal, 318,* 421–426.

Huttunen, M. O., & Niskanen, P. (1978). Prenatal loss of father and psychiatric disorders. *Archives of General Psychiatry, 35,* 429–431.

Institute of Medicine, Committee on Nutritional Status During Pregnancy and Lactation. (1990). *Nutrition during pregnancy.* Washington, D.C.: National Academy Press.

Jones, P. B., Rantakallio, P., Hartikainen, A. L., Isohanni, M., & Sipila, P. (1998). Schizophrenia as a long-term outcome of pregnancy, delivery, and perinatal complications: A 28-year follow-up of the 1966 North Finland general population birth cohort. *American Journal of Psychiatry, 155,* 355–364.

Jones, P., Rodgers, B., Murray, R., & Marmon, M. (1994). Child developmental risk factors for adult schizophrenia in the British 1946 birth cohort. *Lancet, 344,* 1398–1402.

Kelsey, J. L. (1996). Methods in observational epidemiology. New York: Oxford University Press, pp. 37–38.

Kunugi, H., Nanko, S., Takei, N., Saito, K., Hayashi, N., & Kazamatsuri, H. (1995). Schizophrenia following in *utero* exposure to the 1957 influenza epidemics in Japan. *American Journal of Psychiatry, 152,* 450–452.

LaMantia, A. S. (1999). Forebrain induction, retinoic acid, and vulnerability to schizophrenia: insights from molecular and genetic analysis in developing mice. *Biological Psychiatry, 46,* 19–30.

Lewis,G., David, A., Andreason, S., & Allebeck, P. (1992). Schizophrenia and city life. *Lancet, 340,* 137–140.

Lipska, B. K., Khaing, Z. Z., & Weinberger, D. R. (1999). Neonatal hippocampal damage in the rat: A heuristic model of schizophrenia. *Psychiatric Annals, 29,* 157–160.

Lynberg, M. C., Khoury, M. J., Lu, X., & Cocian, T. (1994). Maternal flu, fever, and the risk of neural tube defects: A population-based case-control study. *American Journal of Epidemiology, 140,* 244–255.

Lyon, M. (1990). Animal models of mania and schizophrenia. In P. Willner (Ed.), *Behavioral models in psychopharmacology: Theoretical, industrial and clinical perspectives* (pp. 253–310). Cambridge: Cambridge University Press.

Machon, R., Mednick, S., & Huttenen, M. (1997). Adult major affective disorder after prenatal exposure to an influenza epidemic. *Archives of General Psychiatry, 54,* 322–328.

Malaspina, D., Hurlaz, S., Fennig, S., Heiman, D., Nahon, D., Feldman, D., & Susser, E. S. (2001). Advancing paternal age and the risk of schizophrenia. *Archives of General Psychiatry 58,* 361–367.

Malaspina, D., Sohler, N. L., & Susser, E. S. (1999). Interaction of genes and prenatal exposures in schizophrenia. In E. S. Susser, A. S. Brown, J. M. Gorman (Eds.), *Prenatal exposures in schizophrenia* (pp. 35–59). Washington, D.C.: American Psychiatric Press.

Marcelis, M., Navarro-Mateu, F., Murray, R., Selton, J. P., & van Os, J. (1998). Urbanization and psychosis: a study of 1942–1978 birth cohorts in The Netherlands. *Psychol Med, 28,* 871–879.

McGrath, J. J., Pemberton, M., Welham, J. L., et al. (1994). Schizophrenia and the influenza epidemics of 1954, 1957 and 1959: a Southern Hemisphere study. *Schizophrenia Research, 14,* 1–8.

McGuffin, P., Owens, M. J., & Farmer, A. E. (1995). Genetic basis of schizophrenia. *Lancet, 346,* 678–682.

McNeil, T. F., & Kaij, L. (1978). Obstetric factors in the development of schizophrenia: Complications in the birth of preschizophrenics and in reproduction by schizophrenic parents. In L. C. Wynne, R. L. Cromwell, & S. Matthysse (Eds), *The nature of schizophrenia* (pp. 401–429). New York: Wiley.

Mednick, S. A., Machon, R. A., Huttunen, M. O., et al. (1988). Adult schizophrenia following prenatal exposure to an influenza epidemic. *Archives of General Psychiatry, 45,* 189–192.

Menon, N. K., & Dhopeshwarkar, G. A. (1982). Essential fatty acid deficiency and brain development. *Prog Lipid Res, 21,* 309–326.

Morgan, V., Castle, D., Page, A., Fazio, S., Gurrin, L., Burton, P., Montgomery, P., & Jablensky, A. (1997). Influenza epidemics and incidence of schizophrenia, affective disorders and mental retardation in Western Australia: no evidence of a major effect. *Schizophrenia Research, 26,* 25–29.

Moore, H., Ghajarnia, M., & Grace, A. A. (1998). Anatomy and function of prefrontal and limbic corticostriatal circuits in a rodent model of schizophrenia, Abstracts of the 37th Annual Meeting of the American College of Neuropsychopharmacology, Las Croabas, Puerto Rico, December 14–18.

Mortensen, P. B., Pedersen, C. B., Westergaard ,T., Wohlfahrt, J., Ewald, H., Mors, O., Andersen, P. K., & Melbye, M. (1999). Effects of family history and place and season of birth on the risk of schizophrenia. *New England Journal of Medicine, 340,* 603–608.

MRC Vitamin Research Study Group. (1991). Prevention of neural tube defects: Results of the Medical Research Council Vitamin Study. *Lancet, 338,* 131–137.

Nelson, K. B., Dambrosia, J. M., Grether, J. K., & Philips, T. M. (1998). Neonatal cytokines and coagulation factors in children with cerebral palsy. *Annals of Neurology, 44,* 665–675.

Nopoulos, P., Swayze, V., Flaum, M., Ehrhardt, J. C., Yuh, W. T. C., & Andreasen, N. C. (1997). Cavum septi pellucidi in normals and patients with schizophrenia as detected by magnetic resonance imaging. *Biological Psychiatry, 41,* 1102–1108.

Nopoulos, P. I., Tores, M., Flaum, N. C., Andreasen, J. C., & Ehrhardt, Yuh, W. T. (1995). Brain morphology in first-episode schizophrenia. *American Journal of Psychiatry, 152,* 1721–1723.

Nowakowski, R. S. (1999). Prenatal development of the brain. In E. Susser, A. Brown, & J. Gorman (Eds.), *Prenatal exposure in schizophrenia* (pp. 61–85). Washington, D.C.: American Psychiatric Press.

O'Callaghan, E., Sham, P., Takei, N., Glover, G., & Murray, R. M. (1991). Schizophrenia after prenatal exposure to 1957 A2 influenza epidemic. *Lancet, 337,* 1248–1250.

O'Rahilly R., & Muller, F. (1999). *The embryonic human brain: An atlas of developmental stages, 2nd ed.* New York: Wiley, pp. 39–338.

Pfefferbaum, A., & Marsh, L. (1995). Structural brain imaging in schizophrenia. *Clinical Neuroscience, 3,* 105–111.

Richardson Andrews, R. C. (1990). Unification of the findings in schizophrenia by reference to the effects of gestational zinc deficiency. *Medical Hypotheses, 31,* 141–153.

Richardson Andrews, R. C. (1992). An update of the zinc deficiency theory of schizophrenia. Identification of the sex determining system as the site of action of reproductive zinc deficiency. *Medical Hypotheses, 38,* 284–291.

Rothman K. J. (1986). Modern epidemiology. Boston: Little Brown, pp. 36–37.

Sacker, A., Doue, D. J., Crow, T. J., & Golding, J. (1995). Antecedents of schizophrenia and affective illness. Obstetric Complications. *British Journal of Psychiatry, 166,* 734–741.

Schaefer, C., Brown, A. S., Wyatt, R. J., Kline, J., Begg, M., Bresnahan, M. A., & Susser, E. S. (2000). Maternal prepregnant body mass and risk of schizophrenia in adult offspring. *Schizophrenia Bulletin, 26,* 275–286.

Selten, P. J., Slaets, J., & Kahn, R. (1998). Prenatal exposure to influenza and schizophrenia in Surinamese and Dutch Antillean immigrants to The Netherlands. *Schizophrenia Research, 30,* 101–103.

Sham, P. C., O'Callaghan, E., Takei, N., Murray, G. K., Hare, E. H., & Murray, R. M. (1992). Schizophrenia following prenatal exposure to influenza epidemics between 1939 and 1960. *British Journal of Psychiatry, 160,* 461–466.

South, M., & Sever, J. (1985). Teratogen update: The congenital rubella syndrome. *Teratology, 31,* 297–307.

Stein, Z., Susser, M., Saenger, G., & Marolla, F. (Eds.). (1975). *Famine and human development: The Dutch Hunger Winter of 1944–1945.* New York: Oxford University Press.

Suddath, R. L., Christianson, G. W., Torrey, E. F., Casanova, M. F., & Weinberger, D. R. (1990). Anatomical abnormalities in the brains of monozygotic twins discordant for schizophrenia. *New England Journal of Medicine, 322,* 789–794.

Susser, E. S. (1999). Life course cohort studies of schizophrenia. *Psychiatric Anuals, 29,* 161–165.

Susser, E., & Lin, S. P. (1992). Schizophrenia after prenatal exposure to the Dutch Hunger Winter of 1944–45. *Archives of General Psychiatry, 49,* 983–988.

Susser, E. S., Lin, S. P., Brown, A. S., Lumey, L. H., & Erlenmeyer-Kimling, L. (1994). No relation between risk of schizophrenia and prenatal exposure to influenza in Holland. *American Journal of Psychiatry, 151,* 117–119.

Susser, E. S., Neugebauer, R., Hoek, H. W., Brown, A. S., Lin, S., Labovitz, D., & Gorman, J. M. (1996). Schizophrenia after prenatal famine. *Archives of General Psychiatry, 53,* 25–31.

Susser, E. S., Schaefer, C. A., Brown, A. S., Begg, M., & Wyatt, R. J. (2000). The design of the prenatal determinants of schizophrenia study. *Schizophrenia Bulletin, 26,* 257–273.

Takei, N., Mortensen, P. B., Klaening, U., Murray, R. M., Sham, P. C., O'Callaghan, E., & Munk-Jorgensen, P. (1996). Relationship between in *utero* exposure to influenza epidemics and risk of schizophrenia in Denmark. *Biological Psychiatry, 40*(9), 817–824.

Takei, N., O'Callaghan, E., Sham, P. C., Glover, G., & Murray, R. M. (1993). Does prenatal influenza divert susceptible females from later affective psychosis to schizophrenia? *Acta Psychiatr Scand, 88*(5), 328–336.

Takei, N., Sham, P. C., O'Callaghan, E., et al. (1994). Prenatal exposure to influenza and the development of schizophrenia: is the effect confined to females? *American Journal of Psychiatry, 151,* 117–119.

Torrey, E. F., Bowler, A. E., & Rawlings, R. (1991). An influenza epidemic and the seasonality of schizophrenic births. In E. Kurstah (Ed.), *Psychiatry and biological factors.* New York: Plenum, pp. 109–116.

Torrey, E. F., Rawlings, R. R., Ennis, J. M., Merrill, D. D., & Flores, D. S. (1996). Birth seasonality in bipolar disorder, schizophrenia, schizoaffective disorder, and stillbirth. *Schizophrenia Research, 21,* 141–149.

Uauy, R., Birch, E., Birch, D., & Peirano, P. (1992). Visual and brain function measurements in studies of n-3 fatty acid requirements of infants. *Journal of Pediatrics, 120,* S168–S180.

van Os, J., & Selten, J. P. (1998). Prenatal exposure to maternal stress and subsequent schizophrenia. The May 1940 invasion of The Netherlands. *Br J Psychiatry, 172,* 324–326.

Waddington, J. L. (1993). Neurodynamics of abnormalities in cerebral metabolism and structure in schizophrenia. *Schizophrenia Bulletin, 19,* 55–69.

Walker, E. F., Savoie, T., & Davis, D. (1994). Neuromotor precursor of schizophrenia. *Schizophrenia Bulletin, 20,* 441–451.

Welham, J. L., McGrath, J. J., & Pemberton, M. R. (1993). Schizophrenia, birthrates, and three Australian epidemics. Abstracts of the IVth International Congress on Schizophrenia Research.

Willatts, P., Forsyth, J. S., DiModugno, M. K., Varma, S., & Colvin, M. (1998). Effect of long-chain polyunsaturated fatty acids in infant formula on problem solving at 10 months of age. *Lancet, 352,* 688–691.

Wright, P., & Murray, R. M. (1995). Prenatal influenza, immunogenes and schizophrenia. In J. L. Waddington, P. F. Buckley (Eds), *The neurodevelopmental basis of schizophrenia.* Austin, Tex: RG Landes, (pp. 43–59).

Wright, P., Takei, N., Murray, R. M., & Sham, P. C. (1999). Seasonality, prenatal influenza exposure, and schizophrenia. In E. S. Susser, A. S. Brown, J. M. Gorman (Eds.), *Prenatal exposures in schizophrenia* (pp. 89–112). Washington D.C.: American Psychiatric Press.

FIVE

Obstetric Complications and Neurodevelopmental Mechanisms in Schizophrenia

Isabelle M. Rosso and Tyrone D. Cannon

Obstetric complications (OCs) are robust environmental correlates of schizophrenia (McNeil, 1988; Cannon, 1997). Deviations from the normal course of pregnancy, delivery, or early neonatal life have been associated with the development of schizophrenia in numerous studies with many different types of samples, including: adult schizophrenics and matched comparison subjects (O'Callaghan et al., 1992; Kendell, Juszczak, & Cole, 1996; Hultman, Ohman, Cnattingius, Wieselgren, & Lindstrom, 1997), siblings and twins discordant for schizophrenia (Lane & Albee, 1966; Pollack, Woerner, Goodman, & Greenberg, 1966; Pollin & Stabenau, 1968; Woerner, Pollack, & Klein, 1971; Markow & Gottesman, 1989; Eagles et al., 1990; Bracha, Torrey, Gottesman, Bigelow, & Cunniff, 1992; Günther-Genta, Bovet, & Hohlfeld, 1994; Kinney et al., 1994; Torrey et al., 1994), adopted schizophrenics (Jacobsen & Kinney, 1980), offspring of schizophrenic parents (Parnas et al., 1982; Fish, Marcus, Hans, Auerbach, & Perdue, 1992), and representative birth cohorts (Buka, Tsuang, & Lipsitt, 1993; Dalman, Allebeck, Cullberg, Grunewald, & Koster, 1999; Zornberg, Buka, & Tsuang, 2000). The two studies reporting null results are not outliers in this respect, only in that the 95 percent confidence intervals of their risk estimates included values of one (Done et al., 1991; Buka et al., 1993). One of these studies found that odds of schizophrenia were 2.6 times higher among individuals with a history of fetal hypoxia than among those without such a history ($p = .13$), but statistical power was limited by a small number of schizophrenia outcomes ($N = 8$; Buka et al., 1993). The other study found that odds of schizophrenia were 1.4 times higher among individuals exposed to complications predicting stillbirth and neonatal mortality, but this effect was not significant ($p = .51$) despite a large sample size (Done et al., 1991). The comparability of the OC measure in this latter study to those in other studies is not clear, and, curiously, cases of stillbirth and neonatal death were retained in the prediction analyses. When specific complications were examined in this cohort, bleeding during pregnancy and low birthweight were significantly related to schizophrenia (Sacker, Done, Crow, & Golding, 1995).

Because OCs suggest brain damage acquired during the pre- or perinatal period, it is reasonable to suspect that they are related to a form of schizophrenia positive for other indicators of neurodevelopmental compromise, such as delayed motor and cognitive development, poor premorbid social adjustment, and an early age at onset.

In support of this view, a recent meta-analytic study integrating individual patient data from eleven different research groups that had employed the Lewis and Murray OC scale (Lewis, Owen, & Murray, 1989) found that patients with an onset before age twenty-two were about 50 percent more likely to have a history of OCs than those with later onsets (Verdoux et al., 1997). It therefore appears that OCs, or at least some OCs, may be especially or only related to a form of schizophrenia with an early onset. If so, what is the nature of the neurally disruptive mechanism(s) by which complications during early brain development might plausibly modulate the timing of psychosis-onset several decades later?

PATHOPHYSIOLOGIC MECHANISM(S)

Most of the studies listed above employed general summary measures of OCs, making it difficult to determine whether one or more pathogenic influence(s) is (are) implicated in schizophrenia. When specific OCs have been examined, direct and indirect indicators of hypoxia emerged as prominent predictors (see McNeil, 1988 and Cannon, 1997 for reviews). Indeed, many of the individual OCs found in excess in schizophrenic samples imply either a near-certainty or a heightened probability of oxygen insufficiency. For instance, this mechanism has been clearly implicated in studies reporting a higher incidence of birth asphyxia, neonatal cyanosis, and need for resuscitation at birth in the histories of schizophrenia patients (Pollin & Stabenau, 1968; Günther-Genta et al., 1994; Verdoux et al., 1997; Dalman et al., 1999). Furthermore, obstetric research has shown that hypoxia can occur to varying degrees in association with a variety of other OCs previously associated with schizophrenia, including maternal bleeding during pregnancy (Low, Simpson, & Ramsey, 1992; Adamson et al., 1995; Low, Simpson, Tonni, & Chamberlain, 1995), preeclampsia (Low, Lindsay, & Derrick, 1997), meconium in the amniotic fluid (Low et al., 1992; Maier, Gunther, Vogel, Dudenhausn, & Obladen, 1994; Low et al., 1995, 1997), breech presentation (Low et al., 1995), umbilical cord knotting or encircling around the neck (Low et al., 1995; Salafia et al., 1995), preterm birth (Poets, Stebbens, Richard, & Southall, 1995), and placental infarction/hemorrhaging (Maier et al., 1994; Salafia et al., 1995). That most studies have found schizophrenia to be associated with an aggregation of OCs, rather than to specific ones in isolation, may therefore reflect the involvement of a single or primary mechanism (e.g., hypoxia) that is a common consequence of a number of different conditions. If hypoxia is the primary mechanism underlying the OC-schizophrenia association, the odds of schizophrenia should increase with an increasing number of hypoxia-associated OCs (i.e., these complications should aggregate together in the same patients) and complications implicating other mechanisms should show no association. Alternatively, the effects of OCs on liability for schizophrenia may be mediated by more than one obstetric mechanism. In this case, OCs reflecting different teratogenic influences should be elevated in schizophrenia, with different types of OCs appearing in different patients. Fetal underdevelopment and maternal infection during pregnancy are prominent candidates in this regard, as each has been found to be associated with schizophrenia outcome in previous studies (reviewed in Yolken & Torrey, 1995; Cannon, 1997). Further, both of these prenatal influences could at least theoretically involve a neurally disruptive mechanism other than hypoxia (e.g., reduced neuronal proliferation and interference with cell adhesion during neural migration, respectively).

ETIOLOGIC MODELS

An association with schizophrenia does not establish that OCs exert a causal influence in the disorder. Because genetic factors play a substantial role in schizophrenia (Gottesman & Moldin, 1997; Cannon, Kaprio, Lönqvist, Huttunen, & Koskenvuo, 1998), it is also possible that OCs are a consequence of genetic predisposition. For example, it has been proposed that the genes which predispose to schizophrenia may disturb neuronal migration during gestation, such that some neurons in the hippocampus and cortex are misplaced or misoriented (e.g., Cannon & Mednick, 1991; Jones & Murray, 1991). It is surmised that these "ectopic" neurons may then be compromised in their ability to elaborate appropriate synaptic connections, which in time would produce the hallucinations and delusions characteristic of schizophrenia (Weinberger, 1995). Interestingly, research with animals has shown that one of the functional consequences of experimentally induced migration disorders is neuronal hyperexcitability, which can produce spontaneous neuronal firing (epileptic activity) and cell death (Luhmann & Raabe, 1996). Abnormal neuronal migration may therefore provoke seizures, and perhaps other types of OCs, in the fetal or newborn brain. Similarly, genes predisposing to schizophrenia, if expressed in part as aberrant neuronal migration, could entail a hyperexcitability of cortical neurons which spontaneously induces OCs. In this type of scenario, OCs would be associated with schizophrenia because they are a consequence of constitutional vulnerability to the disorder, not a cause. Family studies provide a basis to test this hypothesis: If such gene-environment covariation exists, one would expect a higher rate of exposure to OCs in the nonschizophrenic first-degree relatives of schizophrenic patients than in the general population. The few studies that have investigated whether fetal underdevelopment is a cofamilial trait have generated conflicting results (Fish et al., 1992; Cannon, Mednick, Parnas, Schulsinger, Praestholm, & Vestergaards, 1993), and this question has not been addressed in regard to prenatal viral infection. In contrast, a number of studies have reported that individuals at increased genetic risk for schizophrenia do *not* have a higher likelihood of exposure to hypoxia-associated OCs (Lane & Albee, 1966; Pollack et al., 1966; Pollin & Stabenau, 1968; Woerner et al., 1971; Woerner, Pollack, & Klein, 1973; Markow & Gottesman, 1989; Eagles et al., 1990; Bracha et al., 1992; Günther-Genta et al., 1994; Kinney et al., 1994; Torrey et al., 1994; reviewed in Cannon, 1997). It therefore appears that an excess of hypoxia-associated OCs is not a consequence of genetic predisposition for schizophrenia, but rather, that fetal hypoxia may play a role in the etiology of the disorder.

If hypoxia-associated OCs do play a causal role in schizophrenia, is it the case that they can cause schizophrenia on their own? Murray and colleagues have proposed that genetic predisposition and OCs are independent etiological mechanisms, such that some cases of schizophrenia are completely genetic in origin (familial) while other cases are caused solely by OCs (sporadic) (Murray, Lewis, & Reveley, 1985; Lewis, Reveley, Reveley, Chitkara, & Murray, 1987). In support of this model, some studies have found that schizophrenic patients without affected first-degree relatives had suffered more OCs than those with a family history of schizophrenia (Reveley, Reveley, & Murray, 1984; Lewis & Murray, 1987; Schwarzkopf, Nasrallah, Olson, Coffman, & McLaughlin, 1989; Cantor-Graae, McNeil, Sjostrom, Nordstrom, & Rosenlund, 1994). However, many studies have detected no differences in rates of OCs between schizophrenics with and without an affected relative (Mirdal, Mednick, Schulsinger, & Fuchs, 1974; Hanson, Gottesman, & Heston, 1976; Rieder, Broman, & Rosenthal, 1977; Marcus, Auerbach, Wilkinson, & Burack, 1981; DeLisi, Goldin, Maxwell, Kazuba, & Gershon, 1987; Nimgaonkar, Wessely, & Murray, 1988; Foerster, Lewis, Owen, & Murray, 1991; McCreadie et al., 1992; O'Callaghan et al., 1992; Heun & Maier, 1993; Roy, Flaum, Gupta, Jaramillo, & Andreasen, 1994). These mixed findings may be at least partly attributable to methodological limitations inherent to studies using the family history design. Even if we assume that assessments of obstetric history by patient or maternal report are valid, the interpretability of such studies is severely weakened by the inadequate power of family history in modeling genetic influences in schizophrenia (i.e., both groups of patients may be at elevated risk for carrying a predisposing genotype), and by the fact that the same informants are often used to assess family and birth history. Finally, contrary to predictions of the familial-sporadic model, population-based cohort studies (Buka et al., 1993; Done et al., 1991) have found that 90 percent or more of individuals exposed to OCs (even in severe form) do not become schizophrenic, making it unlikely that they could be a major independent cause of schizophrenia.

Since the majority of individuals exposed to OCs do not become schizophrenic, other predispositional factors must be required for OCs to have schizophrenia-risk-enhancing effects in most cases. As the genetic contribution to liability to schizophrenia is on the order of 80–85 percent (Cannon, Kaprio, et al., 1998), genetic influences represent the single most important determinant of predisposition to this illness. The effects of OCs and genetic risk may therefore combine either additively or interactively in increasing disease liability. Under the simple additive model, OCs and predisposing genes would both increase risk for schizophrenia *independently* of each other, with their total effect on schizophrenia liability amounting to the sum of their individual effects. Under the gene-environment interaction model, the effects of OCs on risk for schizophrenia would *depend* on the presence of one or more predisposing genes, such that the combined effects of susceptibility genes and OCs on disease liability would exceed or otherwise differ from a simple summation of their individual effects. Returning to our earlier example, it has been hypothesized that genetic predisposition to schizophrenia is expressed in part as abnormal neuronal migration. It is possible that a unique type of migrational abnormality associated with genetic risk for schizophrenia could increase reactivity to adverse events that occur later in pregnancy (e.g., reduced tolerance to the normative hypoxic stress of labor). Thus, in this scenario, the abnormal migrational pattern produced by "schizophrenia genes" would not directly induce OCs (as do some other types of migrational abnormalities), but instead would heighten susceptibility to the effects of later-occurring OCs. Consistent with the interaction model, we have found that OCs are associated with an increased risk for schizophrenia in the offspring of affected parents but not in the offspring of normal control parents (Parnas et al., 1982; Cannon, Mednick, & Parnas, 1990). However, these high-risk studies do not exclude the possibility that OCs have a direct influence on disease liability that is simply too small to detect when liability is expressed as the presence versus absence of clinical diagnosis. Studies that employ continuous rather than categorical measures of phenotypic affection are therefore necessary to further elucidate the mode of action of OCs that cause variation in liability for schizophrenia.

In our prior work, we have found evidence supporting the gene-OC interaction model with respect to the contribution of fetal hypoxia to quantitative indicators of liability to schizophrenia. In a computed tomography study of a Danish high-risk sample, the degree of ventricular enlargement observed in the subjects as adults was predicted by the interaction of degree of genetic risk with delivery complications (Cannon et al., 1993). Among those without a history of OCs, there was a tendency for ventricular-to-brain ratio (VBR) to increase linearly with the number of parents affected (neither, one, or both), but this pattern was significantly more pronounced among those with a history of OCs. That is, the effect of delivery complications on VBR was greater among those with two affected parents compared to those with one affected parent, and greater among those with one affected compared to those with healthy parents. Notably, there was not an increase in ventricular volume among the low-risk controls as a function of OCs, implying that some degree of genetic risk was required to observe the association. This pattern of results led us to hypothesize that genetic predisposition to schizophrenia may enhance susceptibility to subcortical brain damage secondary to hypoxia, hemorrhage, or other complications during labor and delivery (Cannon et al., 1993). However, because computed tomography methods lack the sensitivity required to measure specific brain structures and to distinguish between gray and white matter, we were unable to test this hypothesis. In addition, this early study did not allow us to examine whether a specific mechanism(s) was underlying the effects of OCs on structural brain abnormalities in schizophrenia.

Our more recent work with two birth cohorts has afforded us the opportunity to address the questions outlined above. In the paragraphs that follow, we begin by briefly describing the methodology and procedures implemented in both studies. We subsequently organize the exposition of their findings concerning the role of OCs in schizophrenia, along with the hypotheses and speculations these findings have engendered, around the following questions:

- Does the OC-schizophrenia association involve one (i.e., hypoxia) or multiple neurally disruptive mechanisms?
- Are OC influences dependent on, independent of, or confounded with genetic influences in schizophrenia?
- Are OC influences relevant only to a specific developmental course of schizophrenia, that is, to an early-onset subgroup of patients?

METHOD

The Philadelphia Cohort of the Collaborative Perinatal Project (CPP)

Sample Ascertainment and Diagnostic Procedures

From 1959 to 1966, the CPP enrolled for study 9,236 offspring of 6,753 mothers who delivered at two inner-city hospital obstetric wards in Philadelphia – the Pennsylvania Hospital and the Children's Hospital of Philadelphia (Niswander & Gordon, 1972). The offspring in over 90 percent of all the deliveries at these two sites during the sampling period were enrolled. Fifty-four percent ($N = 4,956$) of the cohort members were the only children from their families enlisted in the study, and the remaining 46 percent ($N = 4,280$) were from families with two or more children participating. The recruitment sites for the Philadelphia cohort were chosen to result in a predominantly African-American cohort (88%), thus permitting ethnic balance across the CPP study sites taken together. In January 1996, we conducted a search of the Penn Longitudinal Database (Rothbard, Schinnar, Hadley, & Rovi, 1990), a citywide database for registration of contacts with public mental health facilities in Philadelphia from 1985 to 1995. This initial database search ascertained 339 (3.7%) cohort members who had ever had a psychotic disorder diagnosis (194 with schizophrenia or schizoaffective disorder and 145 with affective or drug-induced psychosis) and 858 (9.3%) who had ever had a nonpsychotic disorder diagnosis (i.e., affective, anxiety, adjustment, developmental, and substance abuse disorders). Thus, this study relied on prevalent rather than incident cases. The relatively high rate of psychotic disorders in this cohort most likely reflects that it is a predominantly low socioeconomic status population.

A random sample of 144 cases with database diagnoses of schizophrenia or other psychotic disorders were selected for a validation study based on a review of their psychiatric medical records. Diagnostic procedures followed *DSM-IV* criteria (American Psychiatric Association, 1994), using a standard coding form to record information pertinent to differential diagnosis of schizophrenia and affective disorders, age at first treatment contact, and course. Of the 144 cases whose charts were reviewed, 72 have received a *DSM-IV* diagnosis of schizophrenia or schizoaffective disorder, 41 have been diagnosed as having a psychotic form of major depressive disorder or bipolar disorder, and the remaining 31 were given a primary diagnosis of substance abuse, anxiety disorder, atypical psychosis, psychotic disorder due to a general medical condition, personality disorder, or adjustment disorder. Reliability of the diagnoses was assessed with a randomly selected sample of 94 of the cases whose charts were evaluated independently by two or more different diagnosticians. Reliability for the diagnosis of schizophrenia and schizoaffective disorder was found to be excellent ($\kappa = .85$; 93% simple agreement).

The seventy-two cases with chart-review-based *DSM-IV* diagnoses of schizophrenia or schizoaffective disorder had sixty-three nonschizophrenic siblings who were also NCPP study participants. The sixty-three siblings included seven with a history of psychiatric treatment (one with psychosis NOS, one with mental retardation, and five with affective and anxiety disorders) and fifty-six without such a history. For the normal comparison group we used the cohort members without a schizophrenic sibling and who according to our psychiatric screen had not been treated in a public mental health facility in greater Philadelphia as an adult ($N = 7,941$). Table 5.1 gives sociodemographic characteristics on the three groups of subjects: (1) cases with chart-review *DSM-IV* diagnoses of schizophrenia or schizoaffective disorder ($N = 72$), (2) nonschizophrenic siblings of the confirmed probands ($N = 63$), and (3) nonpsychiatric controls ($N = 7,941$). The median age at first treatment contact, seventeen years, was used to categorize the schizophrenia patients into those with early and later ages at onset. There was not a significant difference in age at onset between male and female patients (two-tailed t, $p = 0.6$).

Obstetric Records

A standard form was used to code information on maternal health, fetal monitoring, prenatal and perinatal complications, and neonatal conditions from the original antenatal clinic and obstetric hospital records, without knowledge of psychiatric diagnosis. Three obstetric variables were used in the analyses: fetal underdevelopment (birth weight), nonhypoxic prenatal OCs, and hypoxia-associated OCs.

Table 5.1. Demographic Characteristics by Adult Psychiatric Outcome in the CPP Cohort (Mean ± SD or N(%))

Characteristic	Category	Schizophrenia (N = 72)		Nonschizophrenic Siblings (N = 63)	No Diagnosis (N = 7,941)
		Early Onset (N = 34)	Later Onset (N = 38)		
Sex	Males	22 (64.7)	25 (65.8)	32 (50.8)	3,930 (49.5)
	Females	12 (35.3)	13 (34.2)	31 (49.2)	4,011 (50.5)
Race	Black	34 (100)	36 (97.7)	63 (100)	6910 (87.0)
	White	0 (0)	2 (5.3)	0 (0)	1031 (13.0)
Season of birth	Winter	6 (17.7)	11 (29.0)	14 (22.2)	1,975 (24.9)
	Other	28 (82.3)	27 (71.0)	49 (77.8)	5,966 (75.1)
Socioeconomic status	Mean ± SD	2.9 ± 1.8	3.0 ± 1.8	2.6 ± 2.0	3.4 ± 1.9
Mother's age	Mean ± SD	25.4 ± 7.1	23.1 ± 5.9	22.9 ± 4.8	23.8 ± 6.1
Birth order	First (%)	6 (18.2)	13 (38.2)	6 (9.5)	1,843 (24.4)
	> First (%)	27 (81.8)	21 (61.8)	57 (90.5)	5,710 (75.6)
Gestational age (wks)	Mean ± SD	39.5 ± 1.9	39.5 ± 2.1	39.3 ± 1.7	39.2 ± 2.0
Birthweight (grams)	Mean ± SD	3254 ± 447	3088 ± 525	3074 ± 544	3060 ± 557

Note: SD = standard deviation

Because we were interested in examining the rates of schizophrenia along a continuum of hypoxia severity (or likelihood), we aggregated together those complications associated with fetal hypoxia into a hypoxia-associated OC scale. We included in this scale complications considered to be direct (e.g., blue at birth, required resuscitation) or indirect (e.g., abnormalities of fetal heart rate or rhythm, meconium in amniotic fluid) indicators of fetal oxygen insufficiency. Only those indirect indicators that were predictive of the presence of one or more of the direct hypoxia indicators in the overall cohort were retained. Thus, the hypoxia-associated OC scale was comprised of eleven complications: blue at birth, required resuscitation, neonatal cyanosis, neonatal apnea, abnormalities of fetal heart rate or rhythm, umbilical cord knotted or wrapped tightly around neck, third-trimester bleeding, placental hemorrhaging or infarcts, polyhydramnios, meconium in amniotic fluid, and breech presentation. Each complication contributed 1 point to the total hypoxia-associated OC score.

The prenatal OCs scale included any maternal infection during pregnancy, as well as any maternal cardiovascular illness, pulmonary illness, hematologic illness, or maternal endocrine illness during pregnancy. Each complication contributed 1 point to the total prenatal OCs score.

Data Analysis

A logistic regression model was applied to a polytomous measure for diagnostic outcome by method of generalized logits (Proc catmod; Stokes, Davis, & Koch, 1995), a method that guards against Type I error. The outcome measure classified the cohort members into three groups: schizophrenia (N = 72), nonschizophrenic siblings of schizophrenics (N = 63), and no psychiatric diagnosis (N = 7,941). In the primary analysis, sex, race, season of birth, birth order, socioeconomic status (SES; varying on a scale of 1 [unemployed, on public assistance] to 9 [professional, upper middle class]), mother's age, birth weight, prenatal OCs, and hypoxia-associated OCs were included as predictors. Birth order, SES, mother's age, prenatal OCs, and hypoxia-associated OCs were modeled as interval variables testing for linearity in their predictive relationships with outcome. In the presence of a significant main effect of a predictor variable, odds ratios were computed contrasting each outcome (i.e., schizophrenia, sibling status) with the cohort members with no psychiatric diagnoses. To determine whether any of the predictive relationships were specific to a form of the disorder with an early age at onset, the above analyses were repeated stratifying the schizophrenia cases into those with early and later ages at onset.

Because it was possible for there to be more than one subject from the same family within an outcome group, and because the information on obstetric risk factors in such cases is not independent, we also repeated the primary analyses after averaging the obstetric measures (and covariates) within each family separately for each diagnostic group, thus preserving the assumption of independence of observations.

The 1955 Helsinki Birth Cohort

Sample Ascertainment

The sample was drawn from the total population of individuals born in Helsinki, Finland in 1955 and all of their full siblings ($N = 7,840$ and 12,796, respectively), who were screened in national case registries for psychiatric morbidity using methods previously described (Cannon, Kaprio, et al., 1998; Cannon, van Erp, et al., 1998). A total of 267 (1.3%) members of this population had a register diagnosis of 295.x (schizophrenia, schizoaffective disorder, schizophreniform disorder) according to the *Manual of the International Statistical Classification of Diseases, Injuries, and Causes of Death*, 8th edition, numbering scheme. Probands were randomly selected from this total pool and approached initially via their treating psychiatrists. Those who expressed interest in participating were contacted by project staff. Of the 106 probands who were initially approached, eighty (75%) gave informed consent to participate and met inclusion criteria for the study (i.e., a *DSM-III-R* diagnosis of schizophrenia or schizoaffective disorder on direct interview). An attempt was made to recruit at least one nonschizophrenic sibling of each studied proband, but this was possible for only sixty-two of the eighty cases. In addition, fifty-six nonschizophrenic control subjects (twenty-eight sibling pairs from twenty-eight independent families) were chosen from the same birth cohort so as to match the probands and siblings on demographic variables, after excluding any individual with a personal or family history of treated psychiatric morbidity.

Diagnostic Procedures

All subjects were interviewed using the Structured Clinical Interview for *DSM-III-R* Disorders (SCID), Patient or Non-Patient edition (Spitzer, Williams, & Gibbon, 1987). Any subject with an Axis I psychotic condition was also rated using the Scale for the Assessment of Positive Symptoms (Andreasen, 1983) and Scale for the Assessment of Negative Symptoms (Andreasen, 1984). All other subjects were interviewed and rated on the Cluster A items from the Personality Disorders Examination (Loranger, Sussman, Oldham, & Russakoff, 1985). Clinical case summaries were generated, stripped of identifying and diagnostic information, and independently evaluated by another diagnostician.

Table 5.2. Demographic Characteristics by Adult Diagnostic Outcome in the Helsinki Cohort (Mean ± SD or N(%))

| Characteristic | Category | Schizophrenia (N = 80) | | Non-Schizophrenic Siblings (N = 61) | No Diagnosis (N = 56) |
		Early Onset (N = 36)	Later Onset (N = 44)		
Sex	Males	19 (51.4)	26 (59.1)	28 (45.9)	25 (44.6)
	Females	17 (48.6)	18 (40.9)	33 (54.1)	31 (55.4)
Season of birth	Winter	3 (8.1)	9 (20.5)	8 (13.1)	36 (64.3)
	Other	33 (91.7)	35 (79.5)	53 (86.9)	20 (35.7)
Socioeconomic status	Mean ± SD	2.7 ± 1.3	2.8 ± 1.5	2.8 ± 1.5	3.5 ± 1.5
Family size	Mean ± SD	5.1 ± 1.3	5.2 ± 2.0	5.6 ± 2.1	5.1 ± 1.2
Birth order*	First (%)	12 (37.5)	14 (36.0)	9 (17.7)	23 (42.6)
	> First (%)	20 (62.5)	25 (64.1)	42 (82.3)	31 (57.4)
Mother's age**		29.1 ± 5.1	29.6 ± 5.9	30.5 ± 5.4	27.2 ± 4.5
Gestational age (wks)		37.6 ± 2.7	37.9 ± 1.3	37.8 ± 1.9	37.5 ± 2.5
Birthweight (grams)		3402 ± 594	3605 ± 466	3467 ± 516	3598 ± 516

* $p < .05$; ** $p < .01$.

Reliability of the primary diagnosis was excellent (i.e., $\kappa = .94 \pm .02$). Diagnostic disagreements were flagged, and another independent diagnostician rated those cases for consensus diagnoses.

Table 5.2 gives sociodemographic characteristics on the three groups of subjects of this study: (1) cases with *DSM-III-R* diagnoses of schizophrenia or schizoaffective disorder ($N = 80$), (2) nonschizophrenic siblings of the probands ($N = 61$), and (3) nonpsychiatric controls ($N = 56$). Age at first psychotic symptoms was used to define age at onset in this sample. Male patients had a significantly earlier age at onset than female patients: 20.1 ± 4.8 versus 22.8 ± 5.3 years, respectively (two-tailed t test, $p = 0.01$). For each gender, the median age at onset – twenty-two years for females, nineteen years for males – delimited early- and later-onset cases.

Obstetric Records

All parental demographic and obstetric data were transferred from hospital and midwife records to standardized coding forms blindly to psychiatric diagnosis. Maternal information included age, social class, marital status, weight, blood pressure, history of medical and psychiatric illnesses, and previous obstetric history. Pregnancies were monitored for the occurrence of any maternal illnesses, abnormal bleeding during pregnancy, and fetal heart rate abnormalities. Labor and delivery information included birth order, fetal presentation, placental complications (e.g., infarcts, abruption), umbilical cord complications, presence of meconium in the amniotic fluid, and skin color and muscle tone at birth. Finally, newborns' gestational age, birthweight, and early neonatal health complications (e.g., cyanosis) were also recorded. Newborns with fetal growth retardation were those whose weight was below the 10th percentile for their gestational age, whether premature, full-term, or postmature. A prenatal OCs (infection) variable was coded as either 0 or 1 depending on whether at least one of the following had been documented during pregnancy: influenza, rubella, or any other infection.

The hypoxia-associated OCs scale was derived in the same manner as described for the CPP cohort. That is, we included in this scale complications considered to be direct or indirect indicators of fetal oxygen insufficiency – retaining in the scale only indirect indicators that were predictive of direct hypoxia indicators in the overall cohort. As a result, the hypoxia-associated OC scale was comprised of eleven complications: signs of birth asphyxia, neonatal cyanosis, anorexia during pregnancy, anemia during pregnancy, third-trimester bleeding, preeclampsia, fetal distress, placental infarcts, breech presentation, prematurity, and umbilical cord knotted or tightly wrapped around the neck. Each complication contributed 1 point to the total hypoxia-associated OC score.

Data Analysis

The overall hypoxia-associated OC scale was entered into logistic regression models predicting a single, polytomous measure for diagnostic outcome by method of generalized logits (Proc Catmod; Stokes et al., 1995). The outcome measure divided subjects into four groups: early-onset schizophrenia ($N = 36$), later-onset schizophrenia ($N = 44$), nonschizophrenic siblings of schizophrenics ($N = 61$), and no psychiatric diagnosis ($N = 56$). The initial analysis considered the main effects of gender, parental social class [Rauhala scale, varying from 1–7], birth order, mother's age, prenatal infection, fetal growth retardation, hypoxia-associated OCs, and the two-way interactions of hypoxia and each of the demographic variables. Terms that failed to reach a probability criterion of $p \leq 0.10$ were excluded from the model on subsequent iterations. An adjusted odds ratio (OR) and 95 percent confidence interval (CI) were determined for each predictor, contrasting the schizophrenia and sibling groups with the nonpsychiatric comparison group. In addition, the procedure above was repeated with both a prenatal and a perinatal subscale of the hypoxia-associated OC scale to test the temporal specificity of the effects of hypoxia.

A conditional logistic regression analysis was also conducted to test the association between hypoxia-associated OCs and early-onset schizophrenia within families. This analysis was limited to families in which at least one proband and one sibling were available for analysis, and utilized family of origin as the stratification variable, thereby controlling for dependency of multiple observations per family unit.

RESULTS

The Philadelphia CPP Cohort

Table 5.3 presents the results of logistic regression analyses examining the relationship of obstetric history to adult diagnostic outcome (schizophrenia patients, unaffected siblings, nonpsychiatric controls). After accounting for demographic factors and for the nonsignificant effects of fetal underdevelopment and prenatal OCs, hypoxia-associated OCs contributed significantly to the prediction of adult diagnostic outcome. Further, when maternal infection during pregnancy was examined separately from other prenatal OCs, it was not significantly related to adult outcome ($\chi^2 = 0.8$, $df = 2$, $p = 0.68$) and controlling for it did not alter the significance of the hypoxia effect ($\chi^2 = 6.9$, $df = 2$, $p = 0.03$).

Table 5.3. Logistic Regression Results for Demographic and Obstetric Predictors of Adult Diagnostic Outcome in the CPP Cohort[1]

Source	df	X^2	p
Intercept	2	133.3	0.0000
Mother's age	2	11.9	0.0025
Sex	2	9.6	0.0081
Race[2]	1	–	–
Season of birth	2	0.0	0.9841
Birth order	2	20.3	0.0000
Socioeconomic status	2	8.9	0.0114
Birthweight	2	0.8	0.6611
Prenatal OCs	2	0.1	0.9700
Hypoxia-associated OCs	2	7.3	0.0263

[1] The likelihood ratio test for the final model showed an excellent fit ($X^2 = 1206.02$, $df = 11709$, $p = 1.0$).

[2] The overall effect of race is inestimable due to the absence of racial variation in the sibling group.

For each unit increase in hypoxia-associated OCs, risk for schizophrenia increased by 1.41 times, such that individuals with three or more hypoxia-associated complications were 3.84 times more likely to develop schizophrenia than individuals with no hypoxia-associated complications. Conversely, the odds of being an unaffected sibling of a schizophrenic were not significantly related to hypoxia-associated OCs (OR = 0.98, 95% CI = 0.74–1.28) or any of the other terms in the model.

When the schizophrenia cases were divided into those with early versus later ages at onset, the relationship between hypoxia-associated OCs and schizophrenia was found to be confined to the form with an early age at onset (OR = 1.94, 95% CI = 1.35–2.77). For each unit increase in hypoxia-associated OCs, risk for schizophrenia with an early age at onset increased by 1.94 times, such that individuals with three or more such complications were 7.30 times more likely to develop schizophrenia with an early age at onset than individuals with no such complications. In contrast, there was not a significant relationship between hypoxia-associated OCs and schizophrenia with a later age at onset (OR = 1.02, 95% CI = 0.71–1.47).

Notably, the pattern of results was the same when the odds of schizophrenia were modeled conditionally within families (i.e., only among families with one schizophrenic proband and one or more unaffected siblings). There continued to be a significant effect of hypoxia-associated OCs on risk for schizophrenia ($\chi^2 = 5.2$, df = 1, $p = 0.02$, OR = 1.36, 95% CI = 1.04–0.76) that was specific to the form with an early age at onset ($\chi^2 = 11.8$, df = 1, $p = 0.0006$, OR = 1.94, 95% CI = 1.33–2.82).

Figure 5.1 provides a graphical illustration of the linear increase in risk for schizophrenia with increasing number of hypoxia-associated OCs and the specificity of this relationship to cases with an early age at onset.

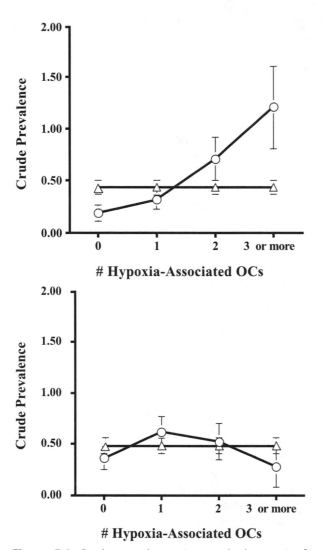

Figure 5.1. Crude prevalence (± standard errors) of schizophrenia with an early age at onset (a), schizophrenia with a later age at onset (b), and being an unaffected sibling of a schizophrenic (c) by number of hypoxia-associated obstetric complications. In each graph, the line indicated by circles gives the observed prevalence of the outcome at each degree of hypoxia exposure, and the line indicated by triangles gives the prevalence expected under the null hypothesis of no association between the risk variable and the outcome. Prevalence estimates are "crude" in this context because we can not assure that ascertainment of probands and siblings is complete. The odds of schizophrenia with an early age at onset increase by 1.94 times ($p = .001$) per unit increase in the hypoxia severity scale. There was not a significant relationship between hypoxia and schizophrenia with a later age at onset or sibling status.

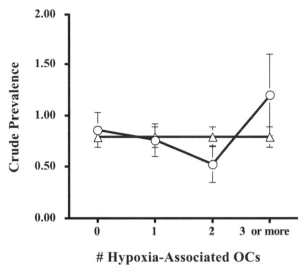

Figure 5.1. (*continued*)

The Helsinki Cohort

The pattern of results of the logistic regression analyses examining the relationship of obstetric history to adult diagnostic outcome (schizophrenia, unaffected siblings, nonpsychiatric controls) was similar to that found in the CPP cohort. In the initial regression analysis of the hypoxia-associated OC scale as a predictor of group assignment, none of the two-way interactions between hypoxia and demographic variables met the $p \leq .10$ criterion for inclusion, nor did the main effects of gender, birth order, or mother's age at birth. After excluding these variables, there was a statistically significant effect of hypoxia-associated OCs ($\chi^2 = 10.83$, df $= 3$, $p = 0.01$), after accounting for the nonsignificant effects of prenatal infection ($\chi^2 = 5.39$, df $= 3$, $p = 0.15$), and fetal growth retardation ($\chi^2 = 1.86$, df $= 3$, $p = 0.60$). Contrast analysis revealed that hypoxia-associated OCs significantly increased risk for early-onset schizophrenia ($\chi^2 = 9.27$, df $= 1$, $p = 0.002$, OR $= 2.16$, 95% CI $= 1.31$–3.53), but were not associated with later-onset schizophrenia ($\chi^2 = 0.15$, df $= 1$, $p = 0.70$, OR $= 0.89$, 95% CI $= 0.48$–1.63), or with being an unaffected sibling of a schizophrenic ($\chi^2 = 0.93$, df $= 1$, $p = 0.33$, OR $= 1.25$, 95% CI $= 0.80$–1.96). That is, odds of early-onset schizophrenia increased by 2.16 times per hypoxia-associated OC, such that those with three or more such OCs were about ten times more likely to develop early-onset schizophrenia than those with none. Further, hypoxia-associated OCs were also associated with increased risk of early-onset schizophrenia within families ($\chi^2 = 3.1$, df $= 1$, $p = 0.08$, OR $= 2.86$, 95% CI $= 0.88$–9.27).

When the previous analyses were repeated with the perinatal hypoxia subscale, there was a significant effect of perinatal hypoxia on group assignment ($\chi^2 = 10.90$, df $= 3$, $p = 0.01$) and a trend effect of social class ($\chi^2 = 6.56$, df $= 1$, $p = 0.09$), while the effects of prenatal infection ($\chi^2 = 5.44$, df $= 3$, $p = 0.15$) and fetal growth retardation ($\chi^2 = 1.52$, df $= 3$, $p = 0.70$) remained nonsignificant. Contrast analysis showed that perinatal hypoxia predicted early-onset schizophrenia ($\chi^2 = 8.06$, df $= 1$, $p = 0.005$,

OR = 2.58, 95% CI = 1.34–4.96), but not later-onset schizophrenia ($\chi^2 = 0.78$, df = 1, $p = 0.38$, OR = 0.66, 95% CI = 0.27–1.65), or unaffected sibling status ($\chi^2 = 1.84$, df = 1, $p = 0.18$, OR = 1.51, 95% CI = 0.83–2.73). Conversely, prenatal hypoxia alone was not significantly associated with group outcome ($\chi^2 = 5.05$, df = 1, $p = 0.17$) after controlling for prenatal infection ($\chi^2 = 5.89$, df = 1, $p = 0.12$) and fetal growth retardation ($\chi^2 = 1.81$, df = 1, $p = 0.61$).

DISCUSSION

Fetal Hypoxia as a Primary Obstetric Mechanism in Schizophrenia

Our findings in the Helsinki and CPP cohorts replicate those of other, smaller-scale studies (Lane & Albee, 1966; Pollack et al., 1966; Pollin & Stabenau, 1968; Woerner et al., 1971, 1973; Jacobsen & Kinney, 1980; Parnas et al., 1982; Markow & Gottesman, 1989; Eagles et al., 1990; Bracha et al., 1992; Fish et al., 1992; O'Callaghan et al., 1992; Buka et al., 1993; Günther-Genta et al., 1994; Kinney et al., 1994; Torrey et al., 1994) in showing that complications representing direct and indirect indicators of fetal hypoxia are associated with an increased risk for schizophrenia. In addition, our results extend previous findings by demonstrating that odds of schizophrenia increase linearly with an increasing number of such complications – suggesting that there is a relationship between the severity of hypoxic insult during fetal or early neonatal life and risk of developing schizophrenia in adulthood.

Our pattern of results also argues against the possibility that the effects of hypoxia-associated OCs in schizophrenia are secondary to those of nonhypoxic prenatal influences. When we modeled these latter influences directly (either in the form of an overall prenatal OCs scale or in the form of fetal underdevelopment and maternal infection during pregnancy as unique variables), they were not significantly associated with schizophrenia in either sample, and nonhypoxic OCs did not interact with or modify the significance of the hypoxia-associated OC effect. Further, because the OC-schizophrenia association has been observed in adoptees not reared in the same home as their affected relatives (Jacobsen & Kinney, 1980), we can rule out that the association is due to covariation between factors predisposing to OCs and subsequent disturbances in the rearing environment.

Evidence for Gene-Environment Interaction

Consistent with the results of all prior controlled prospective studies of individuals at genetic risk for schizophrenia (reviewed in Cannon, 1997), we found no evidence of covariation between genetic predisposition and hypoxia-associated OCs, as siblings of schizophrenics were no more likely to experience these complications than nonpsychiatric controls in either cohort. We also could detect no tendency for any of the demographic factors examined (sex, year of birth, season of birth, birth order, parental education, mother's age) to explain or qualify the hypoxia-schizophrenia association.

It would thus appear that hypoxia-associated OCs are in some manner related to the etiology of schizophrenia. Since most individuals exposed to hypoxia-associated OCs do not become schizophrenic, it is highly unlikely that they are sufficient to cause schizophrenia on their own. Other predispositional factors must therefore be required. Consistent with the results of all previous prospective studies comparing rates of OCs in schizophrenics and their unaffected siblings or co-twins (Cannon, 1997), in both cohorts the odds of schizophrenia increased with the number of hypoxia-associated OCs *within families*. Thus, given a genetic background for schizophrenia, individuals exposed to hypoxia have an increased risk for schizophrenia, and individuals without this exposure are much more likely to be unaffected. These results support a model in which the effects of fetal hypoxia interact with those of predisposing genes for schizophrenia in increasing risk for clinical manifestation of the disorder. Also consistent with this interpretation, our recent magnetic resonance study with the Helsinki sample showed that a history of fetal hypoxia predicted reduced cortical gray matter and increased sulcal cerebrospinal fluid in schizophrenic patients and their non-ill siblings, but not in controls at low genetic risk for schizophrenia (Cannon et al., 2002). It thus appears that a genetic factor in schizophrenia may render the fetal brain particularly susceptible to damage following hypoxia-ischemia.

Fetal Hypoxia and a Neurodevelopmental Model of Schizophrenia Onset

Our findings are consistent with converging epidemiologic evidence that OCs, hypoxia in particular, confer an increased risk for neurodevelopmental compromise and a form of adult schizophrenia with an early age at onset. In both cohorts, we found a robust association between fetal hypoxia and early-onset schizophrenia for both male and female patients, which strengthens the hypothesis that OCs relate specifically to a neurodevelopmental form of the disorder. In addition, our findings suggest that the specificity of the effects of hypoxia may relate in part to its time of occurrence, since perinatal but not prenatal oxygen deprivation predicted early-onset schizophrenia.

Although we can only speculate as to the mechanism(s) involved in the timing of schizophrenia onset, a likely candidate may be the rate of synaptic pruning during adolescence. Young adulthood is a time of extensive remodeling and refinement of cortical connections through a programmed elimination of synapses referred to as synaptic pruning (Hüttenlocher, 1979; Keshavan, Andersen, & Pettegrew, 1994). Interestingly, these peripubertal neurodevelopmental refinements coincide with a period of increasing risk for onset of schizophrenia. Some investigators have therefore proposed that schizophrenia arises due to an exaggeration of the normal amount of synaptic pruning, such that a reduction of neuronal synapses below a critical threshold produces psychotic symptomatology (Feinberg, 1982; Keshavan et al., 1994; McGlashan & Hofman, 2000). Individual variations in the *rate* of synaptic pruning would then vary the age of clinical onset of schizophrenia. Notably, an excess of synaptic pruning is consistent with several brain abnormalities documented in schizophrenia, including reductions in neuropil volume (Selemon, Rajkowska, & Goldman-Rakic, 1995, 1998), dendritic spine density (Glantz & Lewis, 2000; Garey et al., 1998), and synaptic protein levels (Glantz & Lewis, 1997). Further, because peripubertal pruning involves predominantly glutamatergic synapses (Smiley & Goldman-Rakic, 1993; Storm-Mathisen & Otterson, 1990), excessive cortical synaptic pruning could result in glutamate receptor hypofunction. Decreased glutamatergic function has been posited as a possible cause of excessive phasic dopaminergic activity and positive psychotic symptomatology in schizophrenia (Grace, 1991; O'Donnell & Grace, 1998).

Within this theoretical framework, how might hypoxia-associated OCs affect synaptic pruning in a way that leads to earlier onset of schizophrenia among individuals at risk? One possibility is that the neurotoxic effects of hypoxia-associated OCs might directly and immediately cause synaptic elimination and/or neuronal cell death. Preschizophrenics with a history of fetal hypoxia would then have a lower baseline number of neurons and synapses in temporal and subcortical brain regions than those without such a history. Due to this reduced neuronal and dendritic reserve, less postnatal synaptic pruning would be required to cross the psychosis threshold, resulting in an earlier age of clinical onset in individuals at genetic risk for schizophrenia. In support of this immediate-effects hypothesis, hypoxia has been shown to cause neuronal and synaptic loss within the minutes and hours immediately following the insult (Hill, 1991; Gluckman & Williams, 1992). In addition, the temporal and periventricular brain regions that are most vulnerable to the neurotoxic effects of hypoxia in the developing brain have also been consistently implicated in schizophrenia. Thus, hippocampal neurons are reduced in number and/or density following fetal hypoxia (Kuchna, 1994; Yue et al., 1997), as they appear to be in the schizophrenic brain (Falkai & Bogerts, 1986; Jeste & Lohr, 1989). Further, because the hippocampus (and cortical-temporal brain regions) send glutamatergic efferents to the nucleus accumbens, hypoxia-induced neuronal loss should reduce striatal glutamate levels and function (Csernansky & Bardgett, 1998). The resultant decreased glutamatergic modulation of striatal dopamine release may then result in excessive phasic dopaminergic activity – manifested as psychotic symptoms – at an earlier age.

An alternative, though not mutually exclusive, possibility is that hypoxia-associated OCs might lead to an earlier onset of schizophrenia by increasing the normal rate or amount of synaptic elimination that occurs during young adulthood. To our knowledge, this delayed-effects model of fetal hypoxia in schizophrenia has not been previously proposed or examined. However, we advance it here based on research findings suggesting that it is at least biologically plausible. Specifically, we propose that the immediate neurotoxic effects of hypoxia could exert a delayed influence on periadolescent synaptic rearrangement by setting up a state of glutamatergic hypofunction, whose effects would remain latent until puberty.

That glutamatergic neurotransmission might be involved in the pathogenesis of schizophrenia is supported by the observation that psychotic symptoms can be produced by phencyclidine, an antagonist of N-methyl-D-aspartate (NMDA)[1] receptor channels (Allen & Young, 1978; Jentsch & Roth, 1999). NMDA receptor antagonism also has well-established neurotoxic effects, and has been implicated in both necrotic and apoptotic neuronal cell death (Olney & Farber, 1995; Hwang, Kim, Ahn, Wie,

---

[1] Glutamate is a neurotransmitter thought to mediate the majority of excitatory synaptic transmission in the brain. NMDA receptors are a subtype of glutamate receptor. The NMDA receptor is composed of 5 protein subunits that combine to form an ion channel through the neuronal membrane. When glutamate binds to an NMDA receptor and the membrane is depolarized, the ion channel opens and permits sodium and calcium ions to flow into the neuron. The influx of calcium is thought to activate a variety of intracellular processes that alter properties of the neuron. However, an excess of intracellular calcium is toxic to neurons, and NMDA-receptor overactivation has been implicated in the pathophysiology of hypoxic-ischemic neurotoxicity (e.g., Goldberg, Weiss, Pham, & Choi, 1987).

& Koh, 1999). In addition, an optimal level of NMDA-receptor activity is critical for synaptic plasticity and for activity-dependent survival of synaptic connections in the central nervous system (McDonald & Johnston, 1990; Scheetz & Constantine-Paton, 1994). Thus, NMDA-receptor hypofunction could compromise processes of synaptic consolidation, resulting in a net loss of cortical synapses. However, the human brain appears largely insensitive to both the psychotogenic and neurotoxic effects of NMDA receptor antagonism prior to puberty (Olney & Farber, 1995). Thus, while a hypoxic insult during early brain development would be expected to result in a loss of neuronal processes carrying NMDA receptors, many of the effects of the resultant NMDA receptor hypofunction might not be "unmasked" until adolescence. In this way, fetal hypoxia might set up conditions that lead to neuronal and synaptic loss around the time of puberty.

Implications for Future Research and for the Prevention of Schizophrenia

Taken together, our cohort study findings point to oxygen deprivation as a unifying obstetric mechanism in schizophrenia, whose effects increase both the risk of its phenotypic manifestation and the severity of its associated structural brain deficits, but only among individuals with a genetic predisposition to the disorder. Our results further indicate that fetal hypoxia magnifies brain dysfunction in a manner which precipitates the onset of psychosis among preschizophrenic individuals. These findings suggest several directions for future research and for the development of preventive strategies in schizophrenia.

Prenatal Complications and Schizophrenia

It is important to note that the absence of an association between prenatal OCs and schizophrenia in the Helsinki and Philadelphia cohorts does not rule out the possibility that prenatal influences (whether hypoxic or nonhypoxic) may increase risk for schizophrenia under some circumstances. For example, we did not have sufficient power to examine whether complications occurring at different times in gestation (e.g., first vs. second vs. third trimester) might be differentially relevant to the etiology of schizophrenia. It has in fact been shown that the neural consequences of hypoxia depend in part on the developmental processes occurring in the affected brain regions at the time of insult. Studies in fetal sheep have demonstrated that hypoxia at midgestation can inhibit or delay pyramidal cell migration in the CA1 region of the hippocampus (Rees, Stringer, Juts, Hooper, & Harding, 1998; Braaksma, Douma, Nyakas, Luiten, & Aarnoudse, 1999). In contrast, neuronal migration is not affected by hypoxic insults that occur during the last third of gestation (Rees et al., 1998). There may therefore be a limited window of time in gestation (e.g., second trimester) during which hypoxic or other prenatal insults might mimic or potentiate the effects of genetic risk for schizophrenia on cortical neuronal migration. Interestingly, reported associations between viral infection and schizophrenia have been strongest when the possible viral exposure occurred between the third and seventh months of pregnancy (Yolken & Torrey, 1995). Thus, complications that occur during this "sensitive" period may have greater potential for acting as independent causal agents in schizophrenia, by virtue of their gestational timing. If these sensitive periods are very limited in duration or frequency, then an association between prenatal OCs and schizophrenia may be especially difficult to detect.

Fetal Hypoxia as a Primary Obstetric Mechanism in Schizophrenia: The Need for Direct Evidence

Evidence of an association between fetal hypoxia and schizophrenia awaits direct confirmation at the molecular level of analysis. Our epidemiologic findings suggest that OCs which share a common likelihood of causing hypoxia increase risk of developing schizophrenia in adulthood, while OCs that are unlikely to produce hypoxia do not affect schizophrenia liability. However, the conclusiveness of these findings (and of all previous studies in the field) is limited by their reliance on clinical indicators of OCs – that is, on inferred occurrences of fetal hypoxia, prenatal viral infection, and other nonhypoxic obstetric influences. These methods leave open the possibility of scoring "false positive" hypoxic or infectious events. They also make it possible to miss cases that were affected (by either hypoxia or infection) but not symptomatic, and therefore not reported in the obstetric records (e.g., mild cases of hypoxia, low-grade fevers, or acute cases whose symptoms were too transient to be noted). Thus, there is a need for the use of more sensitive, quantitative measures of adverse prenatal and perinatal influences in order to confirm and extend current understanding of obstetric risk factors for schizophrenia.

Recent methodological advances in obstetric medicine have led to the characterization of a number of direct biochemical markers of fetal hypoxia and infection, which could be applied to future research on obstetric risk factors of schizophrenia. For example, measures of umbilical cord blood pH and gas composition have been established as reliable indicators of fetal oxygenation and acid-base condition at birth, and can be obtained without risk to the fetus (Low, 1988). Blood concentrations of markers of general immune function (cytokines) and of antibodies to specific viral agents can also be assayed in umbilical cord and maternal serum samples (el-Mekki, Deverajan, Soufi, Strannegard, & al-Nakib, 1988; Lehrnbecher et al., 1996; Murtha et al., 1996). These measures would provide better estimations of the severity and duration of hypoxic and infectious events and hence permit a more sensitive test of our hypotheses. Thus, we are currently planning a biochemical screen of maternal and cord blood samples of Philadelphia cohort subjects in order to confirm and extend our findings of an association between clinical indicators of hypoxia and schizophrenia to the molecular level of analysis.

Fetal Hypoxia and Age at Onset of Schizophrenia: Mechanism(s) and Timing of the Effect

There is a compelling need for research into the mechanisms by which OCs contribute to the timing of schizophrenia onset. We have proposed that the influence of OCs on age at onset of schizophrenia might reflect the neurotoxic effects of fetal hypoxia occurring during early development and/or during the peripubertal period. Specifically, hypoxia-induced loss of neuronal processes during the perinatal period may interact with *normal* peripubertal synaptic pruning in precipitating onset, and/or may set up a silent state of NMDA-receptor hypofunction which results in *exaggerated* synaptic loss during adolescence. These immediate- and delayed-effects models present predictions that are dissociable and testable. Phosphorus magnetic resonance spectroscopy (P-MRS) can be used to measure the rate of membrane phospholipid[2] synthesis and degradation in the brain, which provides an estimate of dendritic and neuronal turnover (Pettegrew, Keshavan, & Minshaw, 1993). Prospective P-MRS studies could therefore be implemented to examine whether preschizophrenic adolescents exhibit differential amounts of synaptic and neuronal membrane loss depending on whether they have a positive or negative history of fetal hypoxia. The immediate-effects model would predict no difference in markers of synaptic turnover between preschizophrenic adolescents with and without a history of fetal hypoxia. In contrast, according to the delayed-effects model, preschizophrenic adolescents with a history positive for fetal hypoxia would exhibit higher rates, greater magnitude, and/or longer duration of synaptic and neuronal elimination than those without a history of hypoxia.

Fetal Hypoxia and Premorbid Neurobehavioral Deviance in Schizophrenia

While there is growing evidence that neurobehavioral dysfunction predates clinical onset of schizophrenia, its causes are uncertain. Studies of premorbid antecedents have demonstrated a range of functional deviance in preschizophrenic children, including cognitive, behavioral, and neuromotor deficits (Fish et al., 1992; Done et al., 1994; Jones et al., 1994; Walker et al., 1994). High-risk studies have documented similar signs of deviance in children at elevated genetic risk for schizophrenia, suggesting that some premorbid abnormalities may mark genetic predisposition to the disorder. However, there is also some evidence that nonhereditary influences may contribute to neurobehavioral precursors of schizophrenia. For example, preschizophrenic infants have higher rates of motor deficits than their healthy siblings, suggesting that nonshared environmental factors contribute to their manifestation (Walker et al., 1994). Interestingly, OCs have been shown to increase risk for childhood motor and cognitive impairment in the general population (Nelson & Ellenberg, 1984; Rantakallio & von Wendt 1986). However, the extent to which OCs contribute to neurodevelopmental precursors of schizophrenia has received comparatively little attention.

We have recently examined the contributions of hypoxia-associated OCs, prenatal OCs, and birthweight to the cognitive, motor, and behavioral functioning of the Philadelphia CPP subjects at four and seven years of age. While preschizophrenic children and their unaffected siblings had significantly worse cognitive and behavioral functioning than normal control children at both assessment points, these deficits were not significantly associated with any of the obstetric influences (for details see Bearden et al., 2000; Cannon, Bearden, et al., 2000). Thus, it does not appear that fetal hypoxia contributes to lower IQ scores or behavioral deviance among preschizophrenic children in early and middle childhood (at least, not to any greater degree than in the general

---

[2] Neurons are bounded by a plasma membrane that consists of two layers of phospholipid molecules (i.e., a lipid bilayer). One end of a phospholipid molecule is hydrophilic (i.e., water attracting), and the other end is hydrophobic (i.e., water repelling). The lipid bilayer is constructed by turning the hydrophilic ends of the phospholipid molecules in each layer toward the cell interior and the extracellular environment, while the hydrophobic ends of the molecules are facing toward the space between the layers (i.e., these ends face each other). When the membranes of neurons and dendrites are degrading, there is an increase in phospholipid break-down products that can be measured with P-MRS. During neuronal membrane synthesis, there is an increase in phospholipid precursors, which can also be measured with P-MRS.

population). In contrast, we found that hypoxia-associated OCs (and not other obstetric influences) were significantly associated with the presence of unusual movements at four years of age among preschizophrenic children, but not among their siblings or normal control subjects (Rosso, Bearden, et al., 2000). At seven years, however, a history of fetal hypoxia was no longer differentially associated with unusual movements across the three diagnostic groups. This pattern of results points to a contribution of fetal hypoxia to the excess of movement abnormalities in preschizophrenic children during early childhood. It further suggests that this contribution may be age-dependent, such that the functional manifestation of fetal hypoxic injury may include unusual movements at circumscribed period(s) of postnatal brain development. It is tempting to speculate that the effects of OCs on premorbid cognitive and behavioral functioning also depend on the maturational state of the brain. If this is the case, it may be that we did not detect these neurobehavioral effects because they do not appear until later in development. Moreover, this would be compatible with an animal model of schizophrenia by Lipska and colleagues, showing a delayed emergence of behavioral disturbances in neonatally brain-lesioned rats around the time of puberty (Lipska & Weinberger, 1993; Wood et al., 1997).

Together our findings indicate that the neurobehavioral manifestations of fetal hypoxic brain injury may vary depending on the maturational status of the brain circuits that it affects. Neurodevelopmental (and possibly neurodegenerative) changes that occur during childhood and adolescence may alter the affected brain regions' ability to compensate for the functional effects of hypoxia. Because different brain regions vary in their rate of maturation (e.g., time-course of synaptic pruning; Walker, 1994), they may also differ in the time(s) at which they unmask or release the functional effects of hypoxic injury. More longitudinal research is necessary to delineate the possible developmental changes in the premorbid neurobehavioral manifestations of OCs in schizophrenia.

Implications for Genetic Research

The growing evidence of an interaction between familial liability and fetal hypoxia suggests novel strategies for candidate gene research and preventive efforts in schizophrenia. First, our results encourage the search for genes that predispose to the disorder by creating a heightened susceptibility to the neurally disruptive effects of hypoxia. While the list of such candidates is likely to be relatively long, one prominent suspect may be genetic variations that affect NMDA receptor functioning. Several lines of research have implicated excessive activation of glutamate receptors, especially of the NMDA type, in the pathogenesis of hypoxic-ischemic neuronal injury (Choi, 1994; Volpe, 1995). Moreover, the developing brain appears to be especially vulnerable to NMDA-receptor mediated neurotoxicity (McDonald, Silverstein, & Johnston, 1988; McDonald & Johnston, 1990), such that overactivation of these receptors has more deleterious effects than in the adult brain. This enhanced susceptibility is thought to relate in part to a transient increase in NMDA receptor densities during gestation (McDonald & Johnston, 1990), and to ontogenic changes in the subunit composition of NMDA receptors during that period (Mitani, Watanabe, & Kataoka, 1998). If genetic predisposition to schizophrenia affected the number or functional subtypes of NMDA receptors expressed in developing neurons, it might therefore conceivably alter the fetal brain's capacity to withstand a hypoxic insult. Thus, an enhanced vulnerability to the effects of fetal hypoxia among individuals at risk for schizophrenia could possibly relate to genetically influenced functional changes of NMDA receptors during early brain development.

Implications for Prevention

Our findings also suggest that preventing the occurrence of fetal hypoxia, or its neurotoxic effects, might prevent or delay the development of overt schizophrenia among individuals at genetic risk for the disorder. A number of intervention or "rescue" techniques are being developed to interrupt the sequence of neurotoxic events that are set in motion by hypoxia-ischemia and that culminate in neuronal cell death (for reviews see Rosenberg, 1997; du Plessis & Johnston, 1997). Application of these techniques to newborns at combined genetic and obstetric risk for schizophrenia might conceivably reduce their lifetime risk of schizophrenia, or at least of a severe, neurodevelopmental form of schizophrenia with an early age at onset.

Alternatively, it might be possible to prevent or delay psychosis onset by pharmacologically targeting glutamate receptor dysfunction in adolescents at risk for schizophrenia. As previously discussed, a state of chronically decreased NMDA receptor functioning set up early in development (whether by genetic or obstetric factors) could predispose to excessive dopaminergic reactivity and the appearance of psychotic symptoms during young adulthood (Grace, 1991; Olney & Farber, 1995; Jentsch & Roth, 1999). As such, NMDA receptor hypofunction may be a candidate mechanism to explain (or at least contribute to) variations in age at onset of psychotic symptoms in schizophrenia. Thus, pharmacological agents which facilitate NMDA-receptor functioning (e.g., glycine, polyamines) could be investigated as therapeutic intervention strategies that might delay the clinical onset of schizophrenia among individuals deemed at risk.

REFERENCES

Adamson, S. J., Alessandri, L. M., Badawi, N., Burton, P. R., Pemberton, P. J., & Stanley, F. (1995). Predictors of neonatal encephalopathy in full-term infants. *British Medical Journal, 311,* 598–602.

Allen, M., & Young, S. (1978). Phencyclidine induced psychosis. *American Journal of Psychiatry, 135,* 1081–1084.

American Psychiatric Association. (1994). *Diagnostic and statistical manual of mental disorders* (4th ed.). Washington, D.C.: Author.

Andreasen, N. C. (1983). *The Scale for the Assessment of Negative Symptoms (SANS).* Iowa City: University of Iowa.

Andreasen, N. C. (1984). *The Scale for the Assessment of Positive Symptoms (SAPS).* Iowa City: University of Iowa.

Arnold, S. E., & Trojanowski, J. Q. (1996). Recent advances in defining the neuropathology of schizophrenia. *Acta Neuropathologica, 92,* 217–231.

Bearden, C. E., Rosso, I. M., Hollister, J. M., Sanchez, L. E., Hadley, T., & Cannon, T. D. (2000). A prospective cohort study of childhood behavioral deviance and language abnormalities as predictors of adult schizophrenia. *Schizophrenia Bulletin, 26,* 395–410.

Braaksma, M. A., Douma, B. R. K., Nyakas, C., Luiten, P. G. M., Aarnoudse, J. G. (1999). Delayed neuronal migration of protein kinase C-immunoreactive cells in hippocampal CA1 area after 48 h of moderate hypoxemia in the near term ovine fetus. *Developmental Brain Research, 114,* 253–260.

Bracha, H. S., Torrey, E. F., Gottesman, I. I., Bigelow, L. B., & Cunniff, C. (1992). Second-trimester markers of fetal size in schizophrenia: a study of monozygotic twins. *American Journal of Psychiatry, 149,* 1355–1361.

Buka, S. L., Tsuang, M. T., & Lipsitt, L. P. (1993). Pregnancy/delivery complications and psychiatric diagnosis. A prospective study. *Archives of General Psychiatry, 50,* 151–156.

Cannon, T. D. (1997). On the nature and mechanisms of obstetric influences in schizophrenia: A review and synthesis of epidemiologic studies. *International Review of Psychiatry, 9,* 387–397.

Cannon, T. D. (1998). Neurodevelopmental influences in the genesis and epigenesis of schizophrenia: An overview. *Applied & Preventive Psychology, 7,* 47–62.

Cannon, T. D., Bearden, C. E., Hollister, J. M., Rosso, I. M., Sanchez, L. E., Hadley, T. (2000). Childhood cognitive functioning in schizophrenia patients and their unaffected siblings: A prospective cohort study. *Schizophrenia Bulletin 26,* 379–394.

Cannon, T. D., Kaprio, J., Lönqvist, J., Huttunen, M. O., & Koskenvuo, M. (1998). The genetic epidemiology of schizophrenia in a Finnish twin cohort: A population-based modeling study. *Archives of General Psychiatry, 55,* 67–74.

Cannon, T. D., & Mednick, S. A. (1991). Fetal neurodevelopment and adult schizophrenia: an elaboration of the paradigm. In S. A. Mednick, T. D. Cannon, C. E. Barr, & M. Lyon (Eds.), *Fetal neural development and adult schizophrenia.* New York: Cambridge University Press.

Cannon, T. D., Mednick, S. A., & Parnas, J. (1990). Antecedents of predominantly negative- and predominantly positive-symptom schizophrenia in a high-risk population. *Archives of General Psychiatry, 47,* 622–632.

Cannon, T. D., Mednick, S. A., Parnas, J., Schulsinger, F., Praestholm, J., & Vestergaards, A. (1993). Developmental brain abnormalities in the offspring of schizophrenic mothers. I. Genetic and perinatal contributions. *Archives of General Psychiatry, 50,* 551–564.

Cannon, T. D., Rosso, I. M., Hollister, J. M., Bearden, C. E., Sanchez, L. E., & Hadley, T. (2000). A prospective cohort study of genetic and perinatal influences in the etiology of schizophrenia. *Schizophrenia Bulletin, 26,* 351–366.

Cannon, T. D., van Erp, T. G. M., Huttunen, M., Lönnqvist, J., Salonen, O., Valanne, L., Poutanen, V. P., Standertskjöld-Nordenstam, C. G., Gur, R. E, & Yan, M. (1998). Regional gray matter, white matter, and cerebrospinal fluid distributions in schizophrenic patients, their siblings, and controls. *Archives of General Psychiatry, 55,* 1084–1091.

Cannon, T. D., van Erp, T. G. M., Rosso, I. M., Huttunen, M., Lönnqvist, J., Salonen, O., Valanne, L., Poutanen, V. P., Standertskjöld-Nordenstam, C. G. (2002). Fetal hypoxia and structural brain pathology in schizophrenics, their siblings, and controls. *Archives of General Psychiatry, 59,* 35–41.

Cantor-Graae, E., McNeil, T. F., Sjostrom, K., Nordstrom, L. G., & Rosenlund, T. (1994). Obstetric complications and their relationship to other etiological risk factors in schizophrenia. A case-control study. *Journal of Nervous and Mental Disease, 182,* 645–650.

Choi, D. W. (1994) Glutamate receptors and the induction of excitotoxic neuronal death. *Progress in Brain Research, 100,* 47–51.

Csernansky, J. G., & Bardgett, M. E. (1998). Limbic-cortical neuronal damage and the pathophysiology of schizophrenia. *Schizophrenia Bulletin, 24,* 231–248.

Dalman, C., Allebeck, P., Cullberg, J., Grunewald, C., & Koster, M. (1999). Obstetric complications and the risk of schizophrenia: a longitudinal study of a national birth cohort. *Archives of General Psychiatry, 56,* 234–240.

DeLisi, L. E., Goldin, L. R., Maxwell, M. E., Kazuba, D. M., & Gershon, E. S. (1987). Clinical features of illness in siblings with schizophrenia or schizoaffective disorder. *Archives of General Psychiatry, 44,* 891–896.

Done, D. J., Crow, T. J., Johnstone, E. C., & Sacker, A. (1994). Childhood antecedents of schizophrenia and affective illness: social adjustment at ages 7 and 11 [see comments]. *BMJj (Clinical Research Ed.), 309*(6956), 699–703.

Done, D. J., Johnstone, E. C., Frith, C. D., Golding, J., Shepherd, P. M., & Crow, T. J. (1991). Complications of pregnancy and delivery in relation to psychosis in adult life: data from the British perinatal mortality survey sample. *British Medical Journal, 302,* 1576–1580.

du Plessis, A. J., & Johnston, M. V. (1997). Hypoxic-ischemic brain injury in the newborn. Cellular mechanisms and potential strategies for neuroprotection. *Clinics in Perinatology, 24*(3), 627–654.

Eagles, J. M., Gibson, I., Bremner, M. H., Clunie, F., Ebmeier, K. P., & Smith, N. C. (1990). Obstetric complications in DSM-III schizophrenics and their siblings. *Lancet, 335,* 1139–1141.

el-Mekki, A., Deverajan, L. V., Soufi, S., Strannegard, O., & al-Nakib, W. (1988). Specific and non-specific serological markers in the screening for congenital CMV infection. *Epidemiology and Infection, 101,* 495–501.

Falkai, P., & Bogerts, B. (1986). Cell loss in the hippocampus of schizophrenics. *European Archives of Psychiatry and Neurological Sciences, 236,* 154–161.

Feinberg, I. (1982). Schizophrenia: caused by a fault in programmed synaptic elimination during adolescence? *Journal of Psychiatric Research, 17,* 319–334.

Fish, B., Marcus, J., Hans, S. L., Auerbach, J. G., & Perdue, S. (1992). Infants at risk for schizophrenia: Sequelae of a genetic neurointegrative defect. *Archives of General Psychiatry, 49,* 221–235.

Foerster, A., Lewis, S. W., Owen, M. J., & Murray, R. M. (1991). Low birth weight and a family history of schizophrenia predict poor premorbid functioning in psychosis. *Schizophrenia Research, 5,* 13–20.

Garey, L. J., Ong, W. Y., Patel, T. S., Kanani, M., Davis, A., Matimer, A., Barnes, T. R., & Hirsch, S. R. (1998). Reduced dendritic spine density on cerebral cortical pyramidal neurons in schizophrenia. *J. Neurol Neurosurg Psychiatry, 65*(4), 446–453.

Glantz, L. A., & Lewis, D. A. (2000). Decreased dendritic spine density on prefrontal cortical pyramidal neurons in schizophrenia. *Archives of General Psychiatry, 57*(1), 65–73.

Glantz, L. A., & Lewis, D. A. (1997). Reduction of synaptophysin immunoreactivity in the prefrontal cortex of subjects with schizophrenia. Regional and diagnostic specificity. *Archives of General Psychiatry, 54,* 943–952.

Gluckman, P. D., & Williams, C. E. (1992). When and why do brain cells die? *Developmental Medicine and Child Neurology, 34,* 1010–1021.

Goldberg, M. P., Weiss, J. H., Pham, P. C., & Choi, D. W. (1987). N-methyl-D-aspartate receptors mediate hypoxic neuronal injury in cortical culture. *Journal of Pharmacology and Experimental Therapy, 243,* 784–791.

Gottesman, I. I., & Moldin, S. O. (1997). Schizophrenia genetics at the millenium: cautious optimism. *Clinical Genetics, 52,* 404–407.

Grace, A. A. (1991). Phasic versus tonic dopamine release and the modulation of dopamine system responsivity: schizophrenia. *Neuroscience, 41,* 1–24.

Günther-Genta, F., Bovet, P., & Hohlfeld, P. (1994). Obstetric complications and schizophrenia. A case-control study. *British Journal of Psychiatry, 164,* 165–170.

Hanson, D. R., Gottesman, I. I., & Heston, L. L. (1976). Some possible childhood indicators of adult schizophrenia inferred from children of schizophrenics. *British Journal of Psychiatry, 129,* 142–154.

Heun, R., & Maier, W. (1993). The role of obstetric complications in schizophrenia. *Journal of Nervous and Mental Disease, 181,* 220–226.

Hill, A. (1991). Current concepts of hypoxic-ischemic cerebral injury in the term newborn. *Pediatric Neurology, 7,* 317–325.

Hultman, C. M., Ohman, A., Cnattingius, S., Wieselgren, I. M., & Lindstrom, L. H. (1997). Prenatal and neonatal risk factors for schizophrenia. *British Journal of Psychiatry, 170,* 128–133.

Hüttenlocher, P. R. (1979). Synaptic density in the human frontal cortex: Developmental changes and effects of aging. *Brain Research, 163,* 195–205.

Hwang, J. Y., Kim, Y. H., Ahn, Y. H., Wie, M. B., & Koh, J. H. (1999). N-methyl-D-aspartate receptor blockade induces neuronal apoptosis in cortical culture. *Experimental Neurology, 159,* 124–130.

Jacobsen, B., & Kinney, D. K. (1980). Perinatal complications in adopted and non-adopted schizophrenics and their controls: Preliminary results. *Acta Psychiatrica Scandinavica, 285,* 337–351.

Jentsch, J. D., & Roth, R. H. (1999). The neuropsychopharmacology of phencyclidine: from NMDA receptor hypofunction to the dopamine hypothesis of schizophrenia. *Neuropsychopharmacology, 20,* 201–205.

Jeste, D. V., & Lohr, J. B. (1989). Hippocampal pathologic findings in schizophrenia. A morphometric study. *Archives of General Psychiatry, 46,* 1019–1024.

Jones, P., & Murray, R. M. (1991). The genetics of schizophrenia is the genetics of neurodevelopment. *British Journal of Psychiatry 158,* 615–623.

Jones, P., Rodgers, B., Murray, R., & Marmot, M. (1994). Child development risk factors for adult schizophrenia in the British 1946 birth cohort. *Lancet, 344*(8934), 1398–1402.

Kendell, R. E., Juszczak, E., & Cole, S. K. (1996). Obstetric complications and schizophrenia: a case control study based on standardised obstetric records. *British Journal of Psychiatry, 168,* 556–561.

Keshavan, M. S., Anderson, S., & Pettegrew, J. W. (1994). Is schizophrenia due to excessive synaptic pruning in the prefrontal cortex? The Feinberg hypothesis revisited. *Journal of Psychiatric Research, 28,* 239–265.

Kinney, D. K., Levy, D. L., Yurgelun-Todd, D. A., Medoff, D., LaJonchere, C. M., & Radford-Paregol, M. (1994). Season of birth and obstetrical complications in schizophrenics. *Journal of Psychiatric Research, 28,* 499–509.

Kraepelin, E. (1919). *Dementia Praecox*. Edinburgh: Livingstone.

Kuchna, I. (1994). Quantitative studies of human newborns' hippocampal pyramidal cells after perinatal hypoxia. *Folia Neuropathologica, 32,* 9–16.

Lane, E. A., & Albee, G. W. (1966). Comparative birth weights of schizophrenics and their siblings. *Journal of Psychology, 64,* 227–231.

Lehrnbecher, T., Schrod, L., Rutsch, P., Roos, T., Martius, J., & von Stockhausen, H. B. (1996). Immunologic parameters in cord blood indicating early-onset sepsis. *Biology of the Neonate, 4,* 206–212.

Lewis, S. W., & Murray, R. M. (1987). Obstetric complications, neurodevelopmental deviance, and risk of schizophrenia. *Journal of Psychiatric Research, 21,* 413–421.

Lewis, S. W., Owen, M. J., & Murray, R. M. (1989). Obstetric complications and schizophrenia: methodology and mechanisms. In S. C. Schulz & C. A. Tamminga (Eds.), *Schizophrenia: scientific progress* (pp. 56–68). New York: Oxford University Press.

Lewis, S. W., Reveley, A. M., Reveley, M. A., Chitkara, B., & Murray, R. M. (1987). The familial/sporadic distinction as a strategy in schizophrenia research. *British Journal of Psychiatry 151,* 306–313.

Lipska, B. K., & Weinberger, D. R. (1993). Delayed effects of neonatal hippocampal damage on haloperidol-induced catalepsy and apomorphine-induced stereotypic behaviors in the rat. *Brain Res Dev Brain Res, 75*(2), 213–222.

Loranger, A. W., Sussman, V. L., Oldham, J. M., & Russakoff, L. M. (1985). *Personality disorder examination. A structured interview for making diagnosis of DSM-IIIR personality disorders.* White Plains, N.Y.: Cornell Medical College.

Low, J. A. (1988). The role of blood gas and acid-base assessment in the diagnosis of intrapartum fetal asphyxia. *American Journal of Obstetrics and Gynecology, 159,* 1235–1240.

Low, J. A., Lindsay, B. G., & Derrick, B .A. (1997). Threshold of metabolic acidosis associated with newborn complications. *American Journal of Obstetrics and Gynecology, 177,* 1391–1394.

Low, J. A., Simpson, L. L., & Ramsey, D. A. (1992). The clinical diagnosis of asphyxia responsible for brain damage in the human fetus. *American Journal of Obstetrics and Gynecology, 167,* 11–15.

Low, J. A., Simpson, L. L., Tonni, G., & Chamberlain, S. (1995). Limitations in the clinical prediction of intrapartum fetal asphyxia. *American Journal of Obstetrics and Gynecology, 172,* 801–804.

Luhmann, H. J., & Raabe, K. (1996). Characterization of neuronal migration disorders in neocortical structures: I. Expression of epileptiform activity in an animal model. *Epilepsy Research 26,* 67–74.

Maier, R. F., Gunther, A., Vogel, M., Dudenhausen, J. W., & Obladen, M. (1994). Umbilical venous erythropoietin and umbilical arterial pH in relation to morphologic placental abnormalities. *Obstetrics and Gynecology, 84,* 81–87.

Marcus, J., Auerbach, J., Wilkinson, L., & Burack, C. M. (1981). Infants at risk for schizophrenia. The Jerusalem Infant Development Study. *Archives of General Psychiatry, 38,* 703–713.

Markow, T. A., & Gottesman, I. I. (1989). Fluctuating dermatoglyphic asymmetry in psychotic twins. *Psychiatry Research, 29,* 37–43.

McCreadie, R. G., Hall, D. J., Berry, I. J., Robertson, L. J., Ewing, J. I., & Geals, M. F. (1992). The Nithsdale schizophrenia surveys. X: Obstetric complications, family history and abnormal movements. *British Journal of Psychiatry, 160,* 799–805.

McDonald, J. W., & Johnston, M. V. (1990). Physiological and pathophysiological roles of excitatory amino acids during central nervous system development. *Brain Research Reviews, 15,* 41–70.

McDonald, J. W., Silverstein, F. S., & Johnston, M. V. (1988). Neurotoxicity of N-methyl-D-aspartate is markedly enhanced in developing rat central nervous system. *Brain Research 459*, 200–203.

McGlashan, T. H., & Hoffman, R. E. (2000). Schizophrenia as a disorder of developmentally reduced synaptic connectivity. *Archives of General Psychiatry, 57*, 637–648.

McNeil, T. F. (1988). Obstetric factors and perinatal injuries. In M. T. Tsuang & J. C. Simpson (Eds.), *Handbook of schizophrenia, vol. 3, Nosology, epidemiology and genetics* (pp. 319–343). New York: Elsevier.

Mirdal, G. K., Mednick, S. A., Schulsinger, F., & Fuchs, F. (1974). Perinatal complications in children of schizophrenic mothers. *Acta Psychiatrica Scandinavica, 50*, 553–568.

Mitani, A., Watanabe, M., & Kataoka, K. (1998). Functional change of NMDA receptors related to enhancement of susceptibility to neurotoxicity in the developing pontine nucleus. *Journal of Neuroscience, 18*, 7941–7952.

Murray, R. M., Lewis, S. W., Reveley, A. M. (1985). Towards an aetiological classification of schizophrenia. *Lancet, 1*(8436): 1023–1026.

Murtha, A. P., Greig, P. C., Jimmerson, C. E., Roitman-Johnson, B., Allen, J., & Herbert, W. N. (1996). Maternal serum interleukin-6 concentrations in patients with preterm premature rupture of membranes and evidence of infection. *American Journal of Obstetrics and Gynecology, 175*, 966–969.

Nelson, K. B., & Ellenberg, J. H. (1984). Obstetric complications as risk factors for cerebral palsy or seizure disorders. *Jama, 251*(14), 1843–1848.

Nimgaonkar, V. L., Wessely, S., & Murray, R. M. (1988). Prevalence of familiality, obstetric complications, and structural brain damage in schizophrenic patients. *British Journal of Psychiatry, 153*, 191–197.

Niswader, K. R., & Gordon, M. (1972). *The collaborative perinatal study of the National Institute of Neurological Diseases and Stroke: The women and their pregnancies.* Philadelphia: WB Saunders.

O'Callaghan, E., Gibson, T., Colohan, H. A., Buckley, P., Walshe, D. G., Larkin, C., & Waddington, J. L. (1992). Risk of schizophrenia in adults born after obstetric complications and their association with early onset of illness: a controlled study. *British Medical Journal, 305*, 1256–1259.

O'Donnell, P., & Grace, A. A. (1998). Dysfunctions in multiple interrelated systems as the neurobiological bases of schizophrenic symptoms clusters. *Schizophrenia Bulletin, 24*, 267–283.

Olney, J. W., & Farber, N. B. (1995). Glutamate receptor dysfunction and schizophrenia. *Archives of General Psychiatry, 52*, 998–1007.

Parnas, J., Schulsinger, F., Teasdale, T. W., Schulsinger, H., Feldman, P. M., & Mednick, S. A. (1982). Perinatal complications and clinical outcome within the schizophrenia spectrum. *British Journal of Psychiatry, 140*, 416–420.

Pettegrew, J. W., Keshavan, M. S., & Minshaw, N. J. (1993). 31P Nuclear magnetic resonance spectroscopy: neurodevelopment and schizophrenia. *Schizophrenia Bulletin, 19*, 35–53.

Poets, F. C., Stebbens, A. V., Richard, D., & Southall, P. D. (1995). Prolonged episodes of hypoxemia in preterm infants undetectable by cardiorespiratory monitors. *Pediatrics, 95*, 860–863.

Pollack, M., Woerner, M. G., Goodman, W., & Greenberg, I. M. (1966). Childhood development patterns of hospitalized adult schizophrenic and nonschizophrenic patients and their siblings. *American Journal of Orthopsychiatry, 36*, 510–517.

Pollin, W., & Stabenau, J. R. (1968). Biological, psychological and historical differences in a series of monozygotic twins discordant for schizophrenia. In D. Rosenthal & S. S. Kety (Eds.), *The transmission of schizophrenia* (pp. 317–332). London: Pergamon Press.

Rantakallio, P., & von Wendt, L. (1986). A prospective comparative study of the aetiology of cerebral palsy and epilepsy in a one-year birth cohort from Northern Finland. *Acta Paediatr Scand, 75*(4), 586–592.

Rees, S., Stringer, M., Just, Y., Hooper, S. B., & Harding, R. (1997). The vulnerability of the fetal sheep brain to hypoxemia at mid-gestation. *Developmental Brain Research, 103*(2), 103–118.

Rees, S., Mallard, C., Breen, S., Stringer, M., Cock, M., & Harding, R. (1998). Fetal brain injury following prolonged hypoxemia and placental insufficiency. *Comparative Biochemistry and Physiology 119A*, 653–660.

Reveley, A. M., Reveley, M. A., & Murray, R. M. (1984). Cerebral ventricular enlargement in non-genetic schizophrenia: a controlled twin study. *British Journal of Psychiatry, 144*, 89–93.

Rieder, R. O., Broman, S. H., & Rosenthal, D. (1977). The offspring of schizophrenics. II. Perinatal factors and IQ. *Archives of General Psychiatry, 34,* 789–799.

Rosenberg, P. A. (1997). Potential therapeutic intervention following hypoxic-ischemic insult. *Mental Retardation and Developmental Disabilities Research Reviews, 3,* 76–84.

Rosso, I. M., Bearden, C. E., Hollister, J. M., Gasperoni, T. L., Sanchez, L. E., Hadley, T., & Cannon, T. D. (2000). Childhood neuromotor dysfunction in schizophrenia patients and their unaffected siblings: A prospective cohort study. *Schizophrenia Bulletin 26,* 367–378.

Rosso, I. M., Cannon, T. D., Huttunen, T., Huttunen, M. O., Lönnqvist, J., & Gasperoni, T. L. (2000). Obstetric risk factors for early-onset schizophrenia in a Finnish birth cohort. *American Journal of Psychiatry 157,* 801–807.

Rothbard, A. B., Schinnar, A. P., Hadley, T. R., & Rovi, J. I. (1990). Integration of mental health data on hospital and community services. *Administrative Policy in Mental Health, 18,* 91–99.

Roy, M. A., Flaum, M. A., Gupta, S., Jaramillo, L., & Andreasen, N. C. (1994). Epidemiological and clinical correlates of familial and sporadic schizophrenia. *Acta Psychiatrica Scandinavica, 89,* 324–328.

Sacker, A., Done, D. J., Crow, T. J., & Golding, J. (1995). Antecedents of schizophrenia and affective illness. Obstetric complications. *British Journal of Psychiatry, 166,* 734–741.

Salafia, C. M., Minior, V. K., Lopez-Zeno, J. A., Whittington, S. S., Pezzullo, J. C., & Vintzileos, A. M. (1995). Relationship between placental histologic features and umbilical cord blood gases in preterm gestations. *American Journal of Obstetrics and Gynecology, 173,* 1058–1064.

Scheetz, A. J., & Constantine-Paton, M. (1994). Modulation of NMDA receptor function: implications for vertebrate neural development. *FASEB Journal, 8,* 745–752.

Schwarzkopf, S. B., Nasrallah, H. A., Olson, S. C., Coffman, J. A., & McLaughlin, J. A. (1989). Perinatal complications and genetic loading in schizophrenia: preliminary findings. *Psychiatry Research, 27,* 233–239.

Selemon, L. D., Rajkowska, G., & Goldman-Rakic, P. S. (1995). Abnormally high neuronal density in the schizophrenic cortex: A morphometric analysis of prefrontal area 9 and occipital area 17. *Archives of General Psychiatry, 52,* 805–818.

Selemon, L. D., Rajkowska, G., & Goldman-Rakic, P. S. (1998). Elevated neuronal density in prefrontal area 46 in brains from schizophrenic patients: Application of a three-dimensional, stereologic counting method. *Journal of Comparative Neurology, 392,* 402–412.

Smiley, J. F., & Goldman-Rakic, P. S. (1993). Heterogeneous targets of dopamine synapses in monkey prefrontal cortex demonstrated by serial section electron microscopy: A laminar analysis using the silver enhanced diaminobenzidine-sulfide (SEDS) immunolabeling technique. *Cerebral Cortex, 3,* 223–238.

Spitzer, R. L., Williams, J. B., & Gibbon, M. (1987). *Instruction manual for the Structured Clinical Interview for DSM-III-R (SCID).* New York: New York State Psychiatric Institute.

Stokes, M. E., Davis, C. S., & Koch, G. G. (1995). Categorical data analysis using the SAS system. Cary, N.C.: SAS Institute.

Storm-Mathisen, J., & Otterson, O. P. (1990). Immunocytochemistry of glutamate at the synaptic level. *Journal of Histochemistry and Cytochemistry, 38,* 1733–1743.

Torrey, E. F., Taylor, E. H., Bracha, H. S., Bowler, A. E., McNeil, T. F., Rawlings, R. R., Quinn, P. O., Bigelow, L. B., Rickler, K., Sjostrom, K., Higgins, E. S., & Gottesman, I. I. (1994). Prenatal origin of schizophrenia in a subgroup of discordant monozygotic twins. *Schizophrenia Bulletin, 20,* 423–432.

Verdoux, H., Geddes, J. R., Takei, N., Lawrie, S. M., Bovet, P., Eagles, J. M., Heun, R., McCreadie, R. G., McNeil, T. F., O'Callaghan, E., Stober, G., Willinger, M. U., Wright, P., & Murray, R. M. (1997). Obstetric complications and age at onset in schizophrenia: An international collaborative meta-analysis of individual patient data. *American Journal of Psychiatry, 154,* 1220–1227.

Volpe, J. J. (1995). Hypoxic-ischemic encephalopathy: neuropathology and pathogenesis. In *Neurology of the newborn,* 3rd ed. (pp. 279–312). Philadelphia: WB Saunders.

Weinberger, D. R. (1987). Implications of normal brain development for the pathogenesis of schizophrenia. *Archives of General Psychiatry, 44,* 600–669.

Walker, E. F. (1994). Developmentally moderated expressions of the neuropathology underlying schizophrenia. *Schizophrenia Bulletin, 20*(3), 453–480.

Walker, E. F., Savoie, T., & Davis, D. (1994). Neuromotor precursors of schizophrenia. *Schizophrenia Bulletin, 20*(3), 441–451.

Weinberger, D. R. (1995). Cortical maldevelopment, anti-psychotic drugs, and schizophrenia: a search for common ground. *Schizophrenia Research, 16,* 87–110.

Woerner, M. G., Pollack, M., & Klein, D. F. (1971). Birth weight and length in schizophrenics personality disorders and their siblings. *British Journal of Psychiatry, 118,* 461–464.

Woerner, M. G., Pollack, M., & Klein, D. F. (1973). Pregnancy and birth complications in psychiatric patients: a comparison of schizophrenic and personality disorder patients with their siblings. *Acta Psychiatrica Scandinavica, 49,* 712–721.

Wood, G. K., Lipska, B. K., & Weinberger, D. R. (1997). Behavioral changes in rats with early ventral hippocampal damage vary with age at damage. *Brain Res Dev Brain Res, 101*(1–2), 17–25.

World Health Organization. (1969). *Manual of the International Statistical Classification of Diseases, Injuries, and Causes of Death*, 8th ed. Geneva: WHO.

Yolken, R. H., & Torrey, E. F. (1995). Viruses, schizophrenia, and bipolar disorder. *Clinical Microbiology Reviews, 8,* 131–145.

Yue, X., Mehmet, H., Penrice, J., Cooper, C., Cady, E., Wyatt, J. S., Reynolds, E. O., Edwards, A. D., & Squier, M. V. (1997). Apoptosis and necrosis in the newborn piglet brain following transient cerebral hypoxia-ischaemia. *Neuropathology and Applied Neurobiology, 23,* 16–25.

Zornberg, G. L., Buka, S. L., & Tsuang, M. T. (2000). Hypoxic-ischemia-related fetal/neonatal complications and risk of schizophrenia and other nonaffective psychoses: A 19-year longitudinal study. *American Journal of Psychiatry 157,* 196–202.

SIX

Maternal Influences on Prenatal Neural Development Contributing to Schizophrenia

Jason Schiffman, Sarnoff A. Mednick, Ricardo Machón,
Matti Huttunen, Kay Thomas, and Seymour Levine

Research has identified disturbances in the nervous system as underlying schizophrenia since Kraepelin (1919) first proposed the term *dementia praecox*. Ample evidence now supports this earlier speculation. More recent evidence has established a neurodevelopmental basis for schizophrenia and other major mental disorders (Akbarian et al., 1993; Mednick, Cannon, Barr, & Lyon, 1991; Mednick & Hollister, 1995; Machón, Mednick, & Huttunen, 1997). In this chapter we will examine some of this evidence establishing a neurodevelopmental basis for major mental disorders, including schizophrenia, as well as propose two related mechanisms involving maternal stress and immune response processes that may mediate the maternal infection and subsequent, adult mental disorder outcome.

FETAL NEURAL DEVELOPMENT

The development of fetal neural structures is a delicate process. Neurons creating the human neocortex proliferate by the fifth month of gestation. Rapid migration and differentiation occur in the central nervous system during the second trimester (CNS; Nowakowski, 1991). The cortical subplate, essential for the formation of the cerebral cortex, also develops during the second trimester. Disruption during a critical period of proliferation may dramatically disorganize neural development leading to observable physical anomalies. Jones and Akbarian (1995) conclude, however, that the existing data suggest as "unlikely that the *proliferative* phase of forebrain ontogenesis is compromised in any major way in schizophrenia" (p. 29).

Kovelman and Scheibel (1984) suggest that disrupted neural *migration* may result in the excess of ectopic neurons found in the hippocampi of schizophrenia patients. In addition, researchers suggest that disruptions of neuronal migration account for the cytoarchitectural anomalies observed in the rostral entorhinal cortex of schizophrenia patients (Arnold, Hyman, Van Hoesen, & Damasio, 1991; Jakob & Beckman, 1986). Differentiation includes processes such as retraction of collaterals, the elimination of synapses during CNS development, and programmed pruning. A disruption of differentiation may also lead to incomplete neural formation, possibly associated with later mental disorders.

Finally, researchers have hypothesized a link between the malformation of the cortical subplate and schizophrenia. Jones and Akbarian (1995) consider the cortical plate as the foundation for the mature cerebral cortex. The subplate plays a critical role in the development of the architecture of the overarching cortex. Jones and Akbarian (1995) hypothesize that abnormal development of the cortical subplate may be responsible for the deviant distribution of neurons found in schizophrenia patients. This deviant distribution of neurons in schizophrenia may disrupt connections and increase the risk of abnormal cognitive functioning.

Disturbances in second-trimester development may compromise processes such as migration, differentiation, and cortical subplate formation. If an untimely teratogen interferes with the development of a specific brain region or structure, then that structure may be permanently maldeveloped. Additionally, brain development does not backtrack, failing to begin where development last ended. As noted, several studies implicate aberrant migration during the second trimester as a contributor to abnormal hippocampal and parahippocampal development associated with schizophrenia (Jakob & Beckmann, 1986; Kovelman & Scheibel, 1984; Scheibel & Kovelman, 1981). Akbarian and colleagues (1993) report differences in the distribution of neural density in the brains of schizophrenia patients. The authors hypothesized that impaired neural migration may account for the unusual neural density found in schizophrenia.

Using an animal model of schizophrenia, Hanlon and Sutherland (2000) report that lesioning rat brains during the equivalent of the human second trimester results in smaller amygdala and hippocampi, and larger lateral ventricles, in adult rats. These structural disruptions resemble those patterns found in patients with schizophrenia. The authors conclude that damage in the second trimester of pregnancy may contribute to later onset of schizophrenia.

SECOND-TRIMESTER TERATOGENS AND ADULT PSYCHOPATHOLOGY

It has been posited that a severe maternal stress occurring during a critical stage of neurodevelopment may adversely affect the developing fetus, elevating risk for schizophrenia in the offspring. In 1988, our group first reported an increase in the rate of adult schizophrenia diagnoses of fetuses whose mothers were exposed in their second trimester of pregnancy to the 1957 influenza virus (Mednick, Machón, Huttunen, & Bonett, 1988). Since this initial report, other groups have replicated the basic findings in a variety of national settings and cities, in both northern and southern hemispheres, and with larger cohorts. Collectively, the studies support the hypothesis that a teratogen incurred during the second trimester of fetal development increases risk for adult schizophrenia (Adams, Kendell, Hare, & Munk-Jorgensen, 1993; Fahy, Jones, Sham, Takei, & Murray, 1993; Machón & Mednick, 1994; Mednick, Machón, Huttunen, & Barr, 1990; Waddington, 1992; Welham, McGrath, & Pemberton, 1993). Fewer studies have failed to replicate the second-trimester findings (see review by Brown, 2000 for a detailed analysis of this issue).

The above findings are based on an overlap between the timing of the influenza epidemic and period of gestation based on date of birth; there is no direct evidence necessarily that the mothers were infected with influenza. However, as a follow-up to our 1988 study, we later directly accessed clinic records and documented notations of likely maternal viral infection in the obstetrical nurse records *at the time of the mother's pregnancy*. We found that 86.7 percent of schizophrenia patients whose second-trimester gestation overlapped the height of the epidemic had mothers who *actually contracted* influenza (not simply exposed) (Mednick, Huttunen, & Machón, 1994). Another research team in Germany comprised of Stober, Franzek, and Beckmann (1993) demonstrated similar, direct evidence of maternal infection and schizophrenia.

The Importance of Timing of the Teratogen and Specific Psychiatric Outcome. Timing of exposure may impact later psychopathological outcome. Five prenatal influenza infection studies similar to our own suggest that the schizophrenia-relevant teratogenic effect in the second trimester may be narrowed to the sixth month of gestation (Barr, Mednick, & Munk-Jorgensen, 1990; Kendell & Kemp, 1989; Kunugi, Nanko, & Takei, 1992; O'Callaghan et al., 1991; Sham et al., 1992).

We also have examined other psychopathologic outcomes of maternal influenza exposure (Machón, Mednick, & Huttunen, 1997; Tehrani, Brennan, Hodgins, & Mednick, 1998). Results suggest an increase in major affective disorder diagnoses among individuals exposed to the 1957 Helsinki influenza epidemic during their second trimester of gestation (Machón et al., 1997). We compared the precise timing of exposure of patients with schizophrenia to the exposure of patients with affective disorders. Approximately half of the second-trimester schizophrenia patients were exposed during the sixth month of gestation, whereas only 10 percent of the second-trimester affective disordered patients were exposed during the sixth month. The majority of second-trimester patients with affective disorders experienced influenza exposure during the fifth month of gestation (Machón, Mednick, & Huttunen, 1995).

Data from this same cohort revealed a relationship between *violent offending* and second-trimester exposure to the influenza epidemic. Mednick and Tehrani (1999) reported data suggesting that late sixth month and early seventh month exposure to the influenza epidemic increases risk for violent criminal offending. The relation seemed specific to violent offending, as we failed to detect a relationship between *property* offending and timing of exposure to the 1957 pandemic.

The Development of Drosophila as a Model for Timing of the Teratogen. The above findings suggest that the specific timing of a teratogenic event may influence the type of psychopathology that develops later. In the Helsinki study, influenza exposure in the second trimester of gestation related to adult psychopathology in the form of schizophrenia, major affective disorders, or violent offending. Within the second trimester, the exact timing of the exposure seems important to the specificity of outcome, with affective disorders associated with fifth-month exposure, schizophrenia, sixth-month exposure, and violent offending, late sixth- and early seventh-month exposure. The relative specificity of teratogenic timing related to different psychopathologic outcomes calls to mind research on the development of the drosophila (fruit fly).

Drosophila development may provide a paradigm or theoretic model for helping to understand specific timing effects of teratogens. Research shows that heat shock exposure (comprised of 35-minute heat shocks of 40.8 °C) to the drosophila pupa at the time a body part should rapidly develop appears to clearly impair or halt development of that body part. The developmental pause causes systematic structural abnormalities resembling mutant gene defects. The defects ("phenocopies") result from the interruption of gene expression during rapid development. Normal genetic expression resumes when the heat shock is withdrawn. After the shock, genetic expression continues on schedule and does not backtrack to compensate for missed growth (Petersen & Mitchell, 1982).

Each part of the body of the drosophila develops within a narrow window. For example, heat shock presented during the thirty-seventh to forty-first hours of pupal stage results in damaged, or absent, wings in the adult fruit fly. Assuming the shock remits at the forty-first hour, structures programmed to develop after the shock form normally (e.g., leg 1, 41–44 hour). The structure of the larva that develops *abnormally* depends on the structure that happens to be experiencing rapid genetic expression for development *at the time* of the heat shock.

This same critical timing is seen in mammals (e.g., rats). Rubin and associates (1999) report that an infection in a rat's first postnatal day results in different errors in development than rats infected on postnatal day 15. Those infected on postnatal day 15 "did not show signs of cerebellar hypoplasia or hyperactivity" (p. 237).

The heat shock-associated abnormalities result in phenotypes resembling genetically based abnormalities. These phenocopies do not transmit the abnormalities genetically. If we permit ourselves an analogy, we might consider the maternal influenza as an analogue to the drosophila heat shock. Thus, we might consider "maternal second-trimester influenza" schizophrenia patients as phenocopies.

SCHIZOTYPAL PERSONALITY AND SECOND-TRIMESTER DISRUPTION

In previous publications (Mednick et al., 1998), we suggested that schizophrenia is a "two-hit" disorder. The first hit is the neural developmental disorder possibly influenced by genes or prenatal environmental agents such as maternal influenza. The second hit may come in the form of unfortunate postbirth circumstances such as delivery complications, disrupted early family rearing conditions, or other environmental traumas.

We further suggest that the first hit alone, without a second hit, may increase risk for neural disorganization leading to disordered cognitive and perceptual functioning. The disordered cognitive and perceptual functioning is well depicted by the diagnosis of schizotypal personality disorder (SPD).

The Finnish Recruit Study. In the context of a database containing personality functioning data for all male conscripts in Finland, we have identified individuals who, as fetuses, were exposed to the severe 1969 Hong Kong influenza epidemic. We determined to test the hypothesis that a second-trimester maternal influenza exposure would relate to an elevation in the number of individuals with SPD characteristics. All new Finnish recruits are given the Minnesota Multiphasic Personality Inventory (MMPI) as part of a larger standardized battery of psychological measures for screening purposes. We defined a MMPI scale score pattern that would relate to an SPD diagnosis. We hypothesized that recruits exposed to an influenza epidemic during their sixth month of gestation would more often evidence a pattern of MMPI scales scores reflecting a diagnosis of SPD than nonexposed recruits. Some of these individuals will suffer a "second hit" which may increase their risk for later schizophrenia.

In 1969, a pan-epidemic of type A influenza struck Helsinki, Finland beginning the week of January 12, reaching a peak during the week of January 26, diminishing rapidly at the end of February, and ending the week of February 23. We analyzed the adult MMPI results of individuals in utero during the pan-epidemic ($N = 2,339$). As a comparison group, we examined the adult MMPI results of a non-influenza exposed group born two years later ($N = 2,151$). An individual's week of birth provided an estimate of the week of exposure to the pan-epidemic.

The literature suggests that one indicator of SPD or "schizotypy" is a 2-7-8 profile on the MMPI (Balogh, Merritt, Lennington, Fine, & Wood, 1993; Meyer, 1993; Nakano & Saccuzzo, 1985). Only scales 7 (Pt; Psychasthenia) and 8 (Sc; Schizophrenia) of the MMPI, however, had been administered to the recruits; scale 2 (D; Depression) was not administered. To provide a relative index of SPD, we thus combined scales 7 and 8 of the MMPI to construct the SPD "characteristics" scale. We hypothesized that individuals exposed to the influenza virus during the sixth month of gestation (weeks 21–24) would show elevated SPD characteristics scores as compared to control subjects born during the same weeks of the year, two years later, in an epidemic-free year. Sixth-month exposed recruits evidenced a significantly greater proportion of "elevated" (upper quartile) SPD characteristics scale scores (39%) as compared to their sixth-month controls (26%) ($p < .003$). We then examined which week (or weeks) in the sixth month accounted for this difference. The results showed that the recruits exposed in the twenty-third week of gestation had a significantly greater number of elevated (upper quartile) scores (51%) as compared to their controls (24%) ($p < .01$). For weeks 21, 22, and 24, the distribution of elevated SPD characteristics scores was similar (non-significant differences) for the exposed and control groups. In exploratory analyses, we compared the exposed and control groups' SPD characteristics scores for months 1–5 and 7–10, for which we had no hypothesis, and detected no statistically significant differences. The isolated effect of week 23 suggests the possibility of a narrow window for developmental disruptions impacting adult development of schizotypal traits.

MANIFESTATIONS OF FETAL NEURAL MALDEVELOPMENT

In this section we consider the question to what extent are the proposed disturbances in fetal neural development manifested premorbidly? We suggest that the premorbid neuromotor and neurocognitive deficits reported in the literature may reflect disruptions in fetal-neural development.

Behavioral Indicants of Fetal Brain Damage. Understanding childhood motoric deviations may inform researchers of the nature of CNS maldevelopment in adult schizophrenia. Consistent with neurodevelopmental theories of schizophrenia, we contend that the disorder begins well before psychotic symptom onset. Fetal neural brain maldevelopment may lie *clinically* dormant early in life, yet effect developing brain regions used early on for neuromotor functioning. Later (typically late teens, early twenties for males, a little later for females), when the brain matures and calls on the maldeveloped regions for more complex tasks, severe symptomatology may arise (Weinberger, 1987). In a theoretical paper on the "neurodevelopmental hypothesis" of schizophrenia, Walker (1994) emphasized the importance of investigating CNS maldevelopment resulting in neuromotor abnormalities in preschizophrenia. She suggested that subtle CNS damage corresponds to neuromotor deviance in childhood, and psychotic symptoms later in life.

Associations between markers of early life events such as second-trimester terato-gens, minor physical anomalies, dermatoglyphic abnormalities, and obstetrical com-plications with later schizophrenia support the notion that the origins of schizophrenia are established early in life. Neuromotor abnormalities in childhood also associate with adult schizophrenia, and may reflect implicated neural maldevelopment. Additionally, infants at high risk for neurological disorders, such as schizophrenia, exhibit greater numbers of attentional and cognitive deficits. Specific abnormalities in neuromotor functioning, as early as six months of age, may reflect the developmental neuropathol-ogy underlying these deficits (Hollister, Mednick, & Brennan, 1994).

Walker and colleagues examined the relation between childhood behavioral phe-nomena and adult brain morphology on MRI among schizophrenia patients (Walker, Lewine, & Neumann, 1996). Using childhood home movies as a source of data on early behavior, the authors found that neuromotor deficits and negative affect during infancy correlated with greater ventricular enlargement in adulthood. Also, parental ratings of the severity of "externalized" childhood behavior problems (likely associated with a difficult temperament) showed an inverse relation with adult cortical volume. These findings suggest that deficits in neuromotor and affective functioning predict adult brain abnormalities among premorbid children who eventually develop schizophrenia.

Schizophrenia is a disorder consistently associated with ventricular enlargement and decreased cortical volume (Harrison, 1999). Studies link prenatal and perinatal stressors to ventricular enlargement in humans (Cannon et al., 1993), and to hippocam-pal structural and cellular abnormalities in rats. As noted above, these particular brain abnormalities significantly relate to schizophrenia later in life. Additionally, Walker has noted that schizotypal adolescents with high rates of dysmorphic signs (reflect-ing prenatal stress), as well as heightened cortisol responses to stress, evidence more adjustment problems than controls (Brennan & Walker, 2001).

There is evidence suggesting that one subtype of motor abnormality, excessive in-voluntary movements (clinical and subclinical hyperkinesias or "dyskinesias"), may be uniquely linked with schizophrenia and spectrum disorders (e.g., schizotypal personal-ity disorder). Elevated rates of involuntary movements are observed in treatment-naive and medicated schizophrenia patients (Khot & Wyatt, 1991). Like adult schizophrenia patients, children who subsequently manifest the disorder show heightened involun-tary movements (e.g., hand posturing and irregular, writhing movements of the hands) as observed in home movies of preschizophrenia children from birth to two years of age (Walker, Savoie, & Davis, 1994). Further, the severity of premorbid dyskinesia is predictive of the severity of psychiatric symptoms in adulthood (Neumann & Walker, 1996).

Several studies provide prospective evidence of childhood neuromotor dysfunction in individuals who later develop schizophrenia: LaFosse (1994), Erlenmyer-Kimling and colleagues (2000), and Rosso and colleagues (2000). Using childhood neuromo-tor measures, both the LaFosse and Erlenmyer-Kimling et al. (2000) studies predicted schizophrenia in genetically at-risk samples. LaFosse reported that 40 percent of HR or Psychiatric Risk children above a severity cutoff developed schizophrenia; whereas only 7.6 percent of HR or Psychiatric Risk children below the cutoff developed schizophrenia. Similarly, Erlenmyer-Kimling and colleagues (2000) reported that 33.3 percent of HR children above a severity cutoff developed a schizophrenia spectrum disorder; whereas only 5.8 percent of HR children below the cutoff developed schizophrenia. Rosso and colleagues reported on schizophrenia patients more likely "sporadic" (presumed environmental origins) than high risk. In this sample, 3.7 percent of subjects with high unusual movements developed schizophrenia; whereas only 0.9 percent of subjects without unusual movements developed schizophrenia. These studies further support the link between childhood neuromotor dysfunction and schizophrenia, a link possibly mediated by early fetal neural maldevelopment.

WHAT MECHANISMS MEDIATE THE MATERNAL INFLUENZA-SCHIZOPHRENIA RELATIONSHIP?

In the remainder of this chapter we will consider two possible mechanisms by which maternal flu during pregnancy might result in increased risk for schizophrenia. Both of these mechanisms involve the mother's response to the infection: (1) her immune system response (cytokines), and (2) her stress response (glucocorticoids). We propose that, in at least some cases of schizophrenia, the early source of vulnerability stems from consequences of a second-trimester maternal infection or stress that results in damage to the fetal brain. We suggest that this fetal brain damage may be in part responsible for later cognitive and behavioral abnormalities and risk for major mental disorders.

Maternal Immune Response and Cytokines. There have been several attempts to link immune-system factors with risk for schizophrenia (see review by Muller et al., 2000). In our laboratory, Hollister and colleagues (1996) demonstrated that mother-infant Rh incompatibility related to increased schizophrenia in second- and third-born offspring, especially male offspring. It is possible that the mothers developed an immune response to the first-born (Rh incompatible) infant. The second- and third-born fetuses may then have been the targets of this maternal immune response. Applying this idea to the maternal influenza studies, we hypothesize that the immune response of the infected mother involves substances (cytokines such as IL-1, IL-2, IL-6, TNF-alpha, and INF-gamma) that directly (or indirectly) attack developing fetal brain systems.

Pro-inflammatory cytokines (Interleukin 1, Interleukin 6, and TNF-alpha) cause an initial acute-phase response, lasting five to seven days post-infection, characterized by fever, myalgia, headaches, cellular hypermetabolism, and multiple endocrine and enzyme responses. An increase in cytokine secretion also elicits the release of glucocorticoids, which, in turn, serves to modulate the level of cytokines (an inhibitory feedback process).

Takei and colleagues (1996) found a significant relation between exposure to influenza in the second trimester, enlarged cerebrospinal spaces (lateral and maximum third ventricles, sulcal fluid and sylvian fissure) and later development of schizophrenia. Enlargement of the ventricles raises the possibility of damaged surrounding white matter. Infection in the second trimester may trigger this process via the pro-inflammatory cytokines. It has long been known that animals infected with the Borna Disease Virus evidence numerous behavioral, emotional, and neurological abnormalities. Recent evidence, however, indicates that an immunopathological process (Hallensleben et al., 1998) mediates the neurological disorder resulting from Borna Disease Virus. No reliable trace of Borna Disease Virus has been reported in patients with schizophrenia (Czygan et al., 1999). There is a growing body of literature, however, indicating abnormalities in the immune response in schizophrenia (Gilmore & Jarskog, 1997). Akiyama

(2000) found significantly higher levels of pro-inflammatory interleukins in neurolep-tically naive patients with schizophrenia compared to controls undergoing treatment.

We hypothesize that a critical factor in fetal brain damage leading to disorders such as schizophrenia is the presence of pro-inflammatory interleukins during the second trimester of pregnancy. There is now considerable evidence that pro-inflammatory in-terleukins can contribute to the pathogenesis of neurodegeneration. Research by Yoon et al. has shown a link between pro-inflammatory interleukins and fetal white matter damage (periventricular leukomalacia, PVL) in human neonates (1996, 1997). Debillon and colleagues (2000) demonstrated a causal link between maternal infection and onset of PVL in rabbits. Inder et al. (1999) made a strong argument for diffuse white matter damage being implicated in neurological and cognitive deficits through interference with cell migration from the neural subplate and disturbance of the processes of con-nectivity in the latter part of the period of gestation.

Maternal HPA Axis Response. Not unrelated to the maternal immune system response is the stress response of the mother as she experiences an influenza infection. Cytokines produced by the mother's immune system to fight the infection also directly activate the mother's Hypothalamic-Pituitary-Adrenal (HPA) stress response. Specifically, cytokines activate the HPA axis resulting in marked increases in circulating levels of cortisol in humans and corticosterone in rodents. It is important to note that there is evidence that prenatal stress has effects on the brain; in rodents these effects have been shown to be a consequence of increased corticosterone (Keenan & Kuhn, 1999).

The immune response and the stress response are not independent. Increase in plasma level of glucocorticoids (produced by HPA axis response to stress) provides feed-back inhibition on the immune system, and limit of cytokine production. Therefore, there are several potential mechanisms whereby increased cortisol may affect the de-veloping brain in utero. First, a *deficit* in the maternal cortisol response to the influenza virus could lead to a poorly modulated increase in cytokine production, which may result in fetal brain damage (Urakubo, Jarskog, Lieberman, & Gilmore, 2001). Second, if there is an *excess* of maternal cortisol response to the infection, the high-circulating levels of glucocorticoids can have adverse effects on fetal brain development. Thus, it is conceivable that either abnormally high, or abnormally low levels of maternal cortisol could mediate fetal brain damage resulting from maternal exposure to an influenza virus (with low levels of cortisol accompanied by high levels of cytokines). In addition to the documented increases in cortisol following viral infection, there is also evidence that levels of corticotrophin-releasing hormone (CRH) emanating from the human pla-centa increase. Recent studies suggest that increases in CRH may impact some of the effects of prenatal stress on premature birth, and subsequent emotional development (Wadhwa et al., 1998).

As noted above, whether the maternal immune response or stress response will increase risk for adult schizophrenia in her offspring may depend on the timing of the infection during the pregnancy. At each stage of gestation, different areas and circuits of the fetal brain are developing rapidly. An area of the brain under rapid development may be more vulnerable to teratogenic effects. Given the established relationship between glucocorticoids and hippocampal damage (Sapolsky, 2000), one of the brain areas under rapid development during the second trimester is the hippocampus. Later in the second trimester, connections are rapidly forming between the cortex and subcortical layers.

Axon growth is a primary developmental focus. Of central interest are the connections and integration between deeper cortical layers and the thalamus and basal ganglia (Hatten, 1999; O'Leary & Koester, 1993). Disturbance of hippocampal development or of cortical-subcortical connections (by maternal immune or HPA axis factors) may be particularly relevant for the risk for schizophrenia.

Interestingly, in addition to evidence supporting developmental disruptions in offspring resulting from maternal HPA dysregulation, research also implicates dysregulated cortisol in adolescents with SPD (Weinstein, Diforio, Schiffman, Walker, & Bonsall, 1999). In a study of adolescents with SPD, Weinstein and colleagues (1999) reported higher cortisol levels in SPD adolescents than in adolescents with other psychiatric disorders, or control adolescents. The SPD adolescents also showed increased dermatoglyphic asymmetries. Dermatoglyphic asymmetries indicate fetal neural developmental disruption, possibly resulting from maternal HPA axis dysfunction. It is conceivable that maternal HPA dysfunction contributes not only to offspring brain circuitry disruption, but also to offspring HPA dysfunction related to schizotypal personality disorder.

Immune and Endocrine (HPA axis) Interactions. It is now well documented that there is an interaction between the immune system and the HPA axis. This communication between the immune system and the HPA axis is best described as bidirectional. Cytokines activate the HPA axis resulting in the neuroendocrine cascade of CRH release from the hypothalamus, ACTH from the pituitary, and glucocorticoids from the adrenal. Thus, following either bacterial or viral infections, increased cytokine levels will result in marked increases of glucocorticoids. Dunn and colleagues (1989) have shown that increased corticosterone levels persist for several days following exposure to the influenza virus in mice. These increases in glucocorticoid secretion, however, exert a feedback regulation on cytokine production, thus preventing the cytokines from "overshooting" (Turnbull & Rivier, 1999). Insofar as viral infections do result in increased HPA activity, an additional mechanism whereby prenatal exposure to influenza could influence the normal neurodevelopmental trajectory is fetal exposure to high circulating levels of cortisol during this critical period in development. There is considerable evidence that glucocorticoids influence the fetus in a variety of ways, including the developing brain (Carlson & Earls, 1997; Gunnar, Morison, Chisholm, & Schuder, 2001). In the rat, glucocorticoids appear to regulate several processes including neurogenesis, cell migration, and cell death in the neonatal hippocampus (Gould, Woolley, & McEwen, 1991). There are several reports of impaired brain development following exposure to prenatal glucocorticoid treatment. Due to the high density of glucocorticoid receptors in the hippocampus, considerable interest has been focused on the effects of glucocorticoids on the developing primate hippocampus. Inhibition of the formation of the dentate gyrus and the CA regions of the hippocampus following glucocorticoid administration was observed in 133- and 162-day-old monkey fetuses. Further MRI studies of these monkeys at twenty months of age indicated smaller hippocampal volumes (Uno et al., 1994). Numerous other effects on brain, behavior, and immune function result from antenatal steroid treatment in humans (Kay, Bird, Coe, & Dudley, 2000).

One of the unique features of human pregnancy is the existence of peptides in the placenta that are identical in structure to peptides normally found in the central nervous system. In particular, beginning at about 20–24 weeks of pregnancy there is a marked increase in placental CRH. Recently several investigators postulated that maternal-placental-fetal neuroendocrine axis, and specifically placental CRH, may mediate many of the effects of prenatal stress. Placental CRH output is responsive to stress and is induced by immune signals (IL-1). Investigators have been focusing on the birth outcomes and subsequent behavioral outcomes of increased CRH during pregnancy (Petraglia et al., 1990). Their results suggest that changes in the secretion of placental CRH (that occurs with prenatal stress) mediates premature birth, as well as temperament and behavioral reactivity, in the first three years of postnatal life. Insofar as placental CRH is readily detectable in the blood of pregnant females, we propose that a more complete assessment of the effects of infection on pregnant women and the fetus should include both cortisol and CRH determination as well as the cytokines.

FUTURE DIRECTIONS

Research to date suggests the value of a program of study examining the effects of illness during pregnancy on maternal immune reaction and HPA axis response. It is our aim to complete a prospective study of the two possible mechanisms by which we propose maternal flu during pregnancy might result in increased risk for schizophrenia. As described above, we suggest that both of these mechanisms involve the mother's response to the infection: (1) her immune system response (cytokines), and (2) her stress response (glucocorticoids). Evidence suggests that maternal influenza during the second trimester of pregnancy relates to schizophrenia in adult offspring. We hypothesize that deficits in fetal neural development are the mechanisms for this effect. The purpose of our study is to examine the role of infection and the maternal immune and stress response in this neurodevelopmental process.

The first phase of our planned project is to identify an unselected sample of women (consecutive admissions to an obstetrical clinic in Finland) experiencing serologically confirmed infections, with fever of > 37.5 °C, during their second trimester of pregnancy. Additionally, we will ascertain a sample of noninfected controls matched for stage of pregnancy at the time of the index infection. Once identified, we will obtain maternal blood at the time of admission to the clinic, several samples during the infection, and after the infection has subsided. The blood samples will provide information about the nature of the infection and the level of cytokine activity and CRH levels. We will also obtain morning and evening cortisol levels in saliva at the time of recruitment, several times during the illness, and after the infection has subsided. These saliva samples will provide information concerning circadian regulation prior to and during the infection. We will also examine the effects of the infection on levels of cortisol during pregnancy. At the time of birth we will collect placental samples to assess for further evidence of infection and ischemia and CRH.

Following delivery we intend to investigate MRI evidence of abnormalities in the infant's brain. At six months, we will examine the infant's HPA axis response to stress, the infant's temperament, and the cognitive and neuromotor development of the infants at six months of age. This will allow us the opportunity to examine the relationship between infection-induced maternal cytokine and cortisol levels during pregnancy, and the structure of the infant brain (MRI), cognitive, and temperament outcomes. We will also collect information concerning pre- and perinatal complications, and maternal self-reports of stress and depression during pregnancy, and test whether these factors mediate any relationship observed between the maternal immune/stress response and infant outcomes.

We hypothesize that pregnant women with infections will have elevated levels of pro-inflammatory cytokine activity in comparison to their pre- and post-infection levels and in comparison to noninfected controls. Further, we predict that these pregnant women with infections and fever will have elevated levels of salivary cortisol and increased plasma levels of CRH in comparison with their pre- and post-infection levels and in comparison to noninfected controls. We also hypothesize that maternal pro-inflammatory cytokine activity will correlate with MRI evidence of white matter damage in the infant; elevated maternal cortisol levels will correlate with MRI evidence of hippocampal damage and abnormal stress reactivity in the infant; and maternal cytokine, cortisol, and CRH levels will correlate with temperament, cognitive, and/or neuromotor deficits in the infant.

We plan to conduct this study in Finland; perinatal and school records are readily available. As the subjects age, we will access school records that give information on grades and test scores. In addition to the possibility of examining the academic records of these children, we also will follow their psychiatric outcome in the national registers.

CONCLUSIONS

We have examined evidence indicating that a disruption of neurodevelopmental processes at a critical period of gestation (i.e., the sixth month of the second trimester) increases the risk for later psychiatric outcome. We also have proposed two related possible mechanisms (maternal immune and maternal stress response) as mediating the maternal infection-psychiatric outcome relationship. We do not, however, ignore other possibilities. For example, immune and hormonal response may be epiphenomenal; the influenza virus may directly attack the fetal CNS. This is possible but seems unlikely. The virus is not likely to be able to pass the blood-brain barrier except under very unusual conditions.

It is also possible that the maternal infection interacts with genetic predisposition to schizophrenia, as is the case with perinatal hypoxia. We are alert to this possibility but we deem this hypothesis to be unlikely; we have examined a national sample of Finns born after the 1957 influenza epidemic and therefore exposed to infection during gestation. For all these cases we ascertained their schizophrenic first-degree relatives. We have two groups exposed to the epidemic in their second trimester, those with no first-degree relative schizophrenic and those with at least one first-degree relative schizophrenic. We found no evidence of an interaction. Those with a first-degree relative with schizophrenia evidenced no second-trimester (influenza) effect; the second-trimester effect was strong for those with no first-degree relative with schizophrenia. We interpreted this as suggesting that the genetic liability may partly consist of a disruption of neural development. In individuals who suffered this genetic disruption of development, the influenza in the second trimester had no additional effect in increasing risk for schizophrenia.

REFERENCES

Adams, W., Kendell, R.E., Hare, E.H., & Munk-Jorgensen, P. (1993). Epidemiological evidence that maternal influenza contributes to the aetiology of schizophrenia. An analysis of Scottish, English, and Danish data. *British Journal of Psychiatry, 163,* 522–534.

Akbarian, S., Vinuela, A., Kim, J.J., Potkin, S.G., Bunney, W.E., Jr., & Jones, E.G. (1993). Distorted distribution of nicotinamide-adenine dinucleotide phosphate-diaphorase neurons in temporal lobe of schizophrenics implies anomalous cortical development. *Archives of General Psychiatry, 50,* 178–187.

Akiyama, K. (2000). Serum levels of soluble IL-2 receptor alpha, IL-6 and IL-1 receptor antagonist in schizophrenia before and during neuroleptic administration. *Schizophrenia Research, 37,* 97–106.

Arnold, S.E., Hyman, B.T., Van Hoesen, G.W., & Damasio, A.R. (1991). Some cytoarchitectural abnormalities of the entorhinal cortex in schizophrenia. *Archives of General Psychiatry, 48,* 625–632.

Balogh, D.W., Merritt, R.D., Lennington, L., Fine, M., & Wood, J. (1993). Variants of the MMPI 2-7-8 code type: schizotypal correlates of high point 2, 7 and 8. *Journal of Personality Assessment, 61(3),* 474–488.

Barr, C., Mednick, S., & Munk-Jorgensen, P. (1990). Exposure to influenza epidemics during gestation and adult schizophrenia. *Archives of General Psychiatry, 47,* 869–874.

Brennan, P.A., & Walker, E.F. (2001). Vulnerability to schizophrenia: Risk factors in childhood and adolescence. In Ingram, R.E. & Price, J.M. (Eds.), *Vulnerability to psychopathology: risk across the lifespan* (pp. 329–354). New York: Guilford Press.

Brown, A.S. (2000). Prenatal infection and adult schizophrenia: A review and synthesis. *International Journal of Mental Health, 29,* 22–37.

Cannon, T.D., Mednick, S.A., Parnas, J., Schulsinger, F., Praestholm, J., & Vestergaard, A. (1993). Developmental brain abnormalities in the offspring of schizophrenic mothers. I. Contributions of genetic and perinatal factors. *Archives of General Psychiatry, 50,* 551–564.

Carlson, M., & Earls, F. (1997). Psychological and neuroendocrinological sequelae of early social deprivation in institutionalized children in Romania. *Annals of the New York Academy of Sciences, 807,* 419–428.

Czygan, M., Hallensleben, W., & Hofer, M., et al. (1999). Borna disease virus in human brains with a rare form of hippocampal degeneration but not in brains of patients with common neuropsychiatric disorders. *Journal of Infectious Disease, 180,* 1695–1699.

Debillon, T., Gras Leguen, C., Verielle, V., Winer, N., Caillon, J., Roze, J.C., & Gressens, P. (2000). Intrauterine infection induces programmed cell death in rabbit periventricular white matter. *Pediatric Research, 47,* 736–742.

Dunn, A.J., Powell, M.L., Meitin, C., & Small, P.A. (1989). Virus infection as a stressor: Influenza virus elevates plasma concentrations of corticosterone and brain concentration of MHPG, a tryptophan. *Physiology and Behavior, 45,* 591–595.

Erlenmyer-Kimling, L., Rock, D., Roberts, S.A., Janal, M., Kestenbaum, C., Cornblatt, B., Adamo, U.H., & Gottesman, I.I. (2000). Attention, memory, and motor skills as childhood predictors of schizophrenia-related psychoses: The New York High-Risk Project. *American Journal of Psychiatry, 157,* 1416–1422.

Fahy, T.A., Jones, P.B., Sham, P.C., Takei, N., & Murray, R.M. (1993). Schizophrenia in Afro-Caribbeans in the UK following prenatal exposure to the 1957 A2 influenza pandemic. *Schizophrenia Research, 9,* 132.

Gilmore, J.H., & Jarskog, L.F. (1997). Exposure to infection and brain development: Cytokines in the pathogenesis of schizophrenia. *Schizophrenia Research, 24,* 365–367.

Gould, E., Woolley, C., & McEwen, B. (1991). Adrenal steroids regulate postnatal development of the rat dentate gyrus: I. Effects of glucocorticoids on cell death. *Journal of Comparative Neurology, 313,* 479–485.

Gunnar, M., Morison, S.J., Chisholm, K., & Schuder, M. (2001). Salivary cortisol levels in children adopted from Romanian orphanages. *Development and Psychopathology, 13(3),* 611–628.

Hallensleben, W., Schwemmle, M., Hausmann, J., Stitz, L., Volk, B., Pagnstecher, A., & Staeheli, P. (1998). Borna disease virus-induced neurological disorder in mice: infection of neonates results in immunopathology. *Journal of Virology, 72,* 4379–4386.

Hanlon, F.M., & Sutherland, R.J. (2000). Changes in adult brain and behavior caused by neonatal limbic damage: Implications for the etiology of schizophrenia. *Behavioural Brain Research, 107,* 71–83.

Harrison, P.J. (1999). The neuropathology of schizophrenia. A critical review of the data and their interpretation. *Brain, 122,* 593–624.

Hatten M.B. (1999). Central nervous system neuronal migration. *Annual Review of Neuroscience, 22,* 511–539.

Hollister, J.M., Laing, P., & Mednick, S.A. (1996). Rhesus incompatibility as a risk factor for schizophrenia in male adults. *Archives of General Psychiatry, 53,* 19–24.

Hollister, M.J, Mednick, S.A., & Brennan, P.A. (1994). Impaired autonomic nervous system habituation in those at genetic risk for schizophrenia. *Archives of General Psychiatry, 51,* 552–558.

Inder, T.E., Huppi, P.S., Warfield, S., Kikinis, R., Zientara, G.P., Barnes, P.D., Jolesz, F., & Volpe, J.J. (1999). Periventricular white matter injury in the premature infant is followed by reduced cerebral cortical gray matter volume at term. *Annals of Neurology, 46,* 755–760.

Jakob, H., & Beckman, H. (1986). Prenatal development disturbances in the limbic cortex in schizophrenics. *Journal of Neural Transmitters, 65,* 303–326.

Jones, P., & Akbarian, S. (1995). Fetal viral infection and adult schizophrenia: Emipirical findings and interpretation. In Mednick, S.A. & Hollister, J.M. (Eds.), *Neural development and schizophrenia* (pp. 190–202). New York: Plenum.

Kay, H.H., Bird, I.M., Coe, C.L., & Dudley, D.J. (2000). Antenatal steroid treatment and adverse fetal effects: What is the evidence? *Journal of the Society for Gynecologic Investigation, 7,* 269–278.

Keenan, P.A., & Kuhn, T.W. (1999). Do glucocorticoids have adverse effects on brain function? *CNS Drugs, 11,* 245–251.

Kendell, R.E., & Kemp, I.W. (1989). Maternal influenza in the etiology of schizophrenia. *Archives of General Psychiatry, 46,* 878–882.

Khot, V., & Wyatt, R.J. (1991). Not all that moves is tardive dyskinesia. *American Journal of Psychiatry, 148,* 661–666.

Kovelman, J.A., & Scheibel, A.B. (1984). A neurohistological correlate of schizophrenia. *Biological Psychiatry, 19,* 1601–1621.

Kraepelin, E. (1919). *Dementia praecox and paraphrenia.* R.M. Barclay transl. 1971. Huntington, N.Y.: Robert E. Krieger Publishing.

Kunugi, H., Nanko, S., & Takei, N. (1992). Influenza and schizophrenia in Japan. *British Journal of Psychiatry, 161,* 274–275.

LaFosse, J. (1994). Motor coordination in adolescence and its relationship to adult schizophrenia. Ph.D. dissertation, University of Southern California.

Machón, R.A., & Mednick, S.A. (1994). Adult schizophrenia and early neurodevelopmental disturbances. In J. Guyotat (Ed.), *Confrontations Psychiatrigues: Epidemiologie et Psychiatrie. No. 35* (pp. 189–215). Paris: Specia Rhone-Poulenc Rore.

Machón, R.A., Mednick, S.A., & Huttunen, M.O. (1995). Fetal viral infection and adult schizophrenia: Empirical findings and interpretation. In Mednick, S.A. & Hollister, J.M. (Eds.), *Neural development and schizophrenia* (pp. 190–202). New York: Plenum.

Machón, R.A., Mednick, S.A., & Huttunen, M.O. (1997). Adult major affective disorder following prenatal exposure to an influenza epidemic. *Archives of General Psychiatry, 54,* 322–328.

Mednick, S.A., Cannon, T.D., Barr, C.E. & Lyon, M. (Eds.) (1991). *Fetal neural development and adult schizophrenia.* New York: Cambridge University Press.

Mednick, S.A., & Hollister J.M. (Eds.) (1995). *Neural development and schizophrenia: theory and research.* NATO ASI Series. Series A, Life Sciences; V. 275. New York: Plenum.

Mednick, S.A., Huttunen, M.O., & Machón, R.A. (1994). Prenatal influenza infections and adult schizophrenia. *Schizophrenia Bulletin, 20,* 263–267.

Mednick, S.A., Machón, R.A., Huttunen, M.O., & Barr, C.E. (1990). Influenza and schizophrenia: Helsinki vs. Edinburgh. *Archives of General Psychiatry, 47,* 875–876.

Mednick, S.A., Machón, R.A., Huttunen, M.O., & Bonnet, D. (1988). Adult schizophrenia following prenatal exposure to an influenza epidemic. *Archives of General Psychiatry, 45,* 189–192.

Mednick, S.A., & Tehrani, J.A. (1999). Prenatal disturbances and criminal violence. In Joshua Dressler (Ed.), *Violence in America: An Encyclopedia* (pp. 398–400). New York: Charles Scribner's Sons.

Mednick, S.A., Watson, J.B., Huttunen, M., Cannon, T.D., Katila, H., Machón, R., Mednick, B., Hollister, M., Parnas, J., Schulsinger, F, Sajaniemi, N., Voldsgaard, P., Pyhala, R., Gutkind, D., & Wang, X. (1998). A two-hit working model of the etiology of schizophrenia. In M. Lenzenweger & R.H. Dworkin (Eds.), *Origins and development of schizophrenia: advances in experimental psychopathology* (pp. 27–66). Washington, D.C.: American Psychological Association.

Meyer, R.G. (1993). *The clinician's handbook: integrated diagnostics, assessment, and intervention in adult and adolescent psychopathology*, 3rd. ed. Needham Heights, Mass.: Allyn and Bacon.

Muller, N., Riedel, M., Gruber, R., Ackenheil, M., & Schwarz, M.J. (2000). The immune system and schizophrenia. An integrative view. *Annals New York Academy of Sciences, 917*, 456–467.

Nakano, K., & Saccuzzo D.P. (1985). Schizotaxia, information processing and the MMPI 2-7-8 code type. *British Journal of Clinical Psychology, 24*, (Pt 3), 217–218.

Neumann, C.S., & Walker, E.F. (1996). Childhood neuromotor soft signs, behavior problems, and adult psychopathology. In T. Ollendick, & R. Prinz (Eds.), *Advances in clinical child psychology*, Vol. 18 (pp. 173–203). New York: Plenum.

Nowakowski, R.S. (1991). Basic processes in fetal neural development. In Mednick, S.A., Cannon, T.C., Barr, C.E., & Lyon, M. (Eds.), *Fetal neural development and adult schizophrenia* (pp. 15–40). Cambridge: Cambridge University Press.

O'Callaghan, E., Sham, P., Takei, N., Glover G., & Murray, R.M. (1991). Schizophrenia after prenatal exposure to 1957 A2 influenza epidemic. *Lancet, 337*, 1248–1250.

O'Leary, D.D.M., & Koester, S.E. (1993). Development of projection neuron types, axon pathways, and patterned connection of the mammalian cortex. *Neuron, 10*, 991–1006.

Petersen, N.S., & Mitchell, H.K. (1982). Effects of heat shock on gene expression during development: Induction and prevention of the multihair phenocopy. In M. J. Schlesinger, M. Ashburner, & A. Tissieres (Eds.), *Heat shock from bacteria to Mann* (pp. 345–352). Cold Spring Harbor, Maine: Cold Spring Harbor Laboratory.

Petraglia, F., Giardino, L., Coukos, G., Calza, L., Vale, W., & Genazzani, A.R. (1990). Corticotropin-releasing factor and parturition: plasma and amniotic fluid levels and placental binding sites. *Obstetrics and Gynecology, 75*, 784–789.

Rosso, I.M., Bearden, C.E., Hollister, J.M., Gasperoni, T.L., Sanchez, L.E., Hadley, T., & Cannon, T.D. (2000). Childhood neuromotor dysfunction in schizophrenia patients and their unaffected siblings: A prospective cohort study. *Schizophrenia Bulletin, 26*, 367–378.

Rubin, S.A., Bautista, J.R., Moran, T.H., Schwartz, G.J., & Carbone, K.M. (1999). Viral teratogenesis: Brain developmental damage associated with maturation state at time of infection. *Developmental Brain Research, 12*, 237–244.

Sapolsky, R.M. (2000). Glucocorticoids and hippocampal atrophy in neuropsychiatric disorders. *Archives of General Psychiatry, 57*, 925–935.

Scheibel, A.B., & Kovelman, J.A. (1981). Disorientation of the hippocampal and pyramidal cell and its processes in the schizophrenic patient. *Biological Psychiatry, 16*, 101–102.

Sham, P.C., O'Callaghan, E., Takei, N., Murray, G.K., Hare, F.H., & Murray, R. M. (1992). Schizophrenia following pre-natal exposure to influenza epidemics between 1939 and 1960. *British Journal of Psychiatry, 160*, 461–466.

Stober, G., Franzek, E., & Beckmann, H. (1993). Pregnancy and labor complications – their significance in the development of schizophrenic psychoses. *Fortschritte der Neurologie-Psychiatrie, 61*, 329–337.

Takei, N., Lewis, S., Jones, P., Harvey, L., & Murray, R. (1996). Prenatal exposure to influenza and increased cerebrospinal fluid spaces in schizophrenia. *Schizophrenia Bulletin, 22* (3), 521–534.

Tehrani, J.A., Brennan, P.A., Hodgins, S., & Mednick, S.A. (1998). Mental illness and criminal violence. *Social Psychiatry & Psychiatric Epidemioloy, 33* (Suppl. 1), S81–S85.

Turnbull, A.V., & Rivier, C.L. (1999). Regulation of the hypothalamic-pituitary-adrenal axis by cytokines: Actions and mechanisms of action. *Physiological Review, 79*, 1–71.

Uno, H., Eisele, S., Sakai, A., Shelton, S., Baker, E., DeJesus, O., & Holden, J. (1994). Neurotoxicity of glucocorticoids in the primate brain. *Hormones and Behavior, 28*, 336–348.

Urakubo, A., Jarskog, L.F., Lieberman, J.A., & Gilmore, J.H. (2001). Prenatal exposure to maternal infection alters cytokine expression in the placenta, amniotic fluid, and fetal brain. *Schizophrenia Research, 47,* 27–36.

Waddington, J.L. (1992). *The declining incidence of schizophrenia controversy: A new approach in a rural Irish Population.* Paper presented at the annual meeting of The Royal College of Psychiatrists, Dublin, Ireland.

Wadhwa, P.D., Porto, M., Garite, T.J., Chicz-DeMet, A., & Sandman, C.A. (1998). Maternal CRH levels in the early third trimester predict length of gestation in human pregnancy. *American Journal of Obstetrics and Gynecology, 179,* 1079–1085.

Walker, E.F. (1994). Developmentally moderated expressions of the neuropathology underlying schizophrenia. *Schizophrenia Bulletin, 20,* 453–480.

Walker, E.F., Lewine, F.J., & Neumann, C. (1996). Childhood behavioral characteristics and adult brain morphology in schizophrenia. *Schizophrenia Research, 22,* 93–101.

Walker, E.F., Savoie, T., & Davis, D. (1994). Neuromotor precursors of schizophrenia. *Schizophrenia Bulletin, 20,* 441–451.

Weinberger, D. (1987). Implications of the normal brain development for the pathogenesis of schizophrenia. *Archives of General Psychiatry, 44,* 660–669.

Weinstein, D.D., Diforio, D., Schiffman, J., Walker, E., & Bonsall, R. (1999). Minor physical anomalies, dermatoglyphic asymmetries, and cortisol levels in adolescents with schizotypal personality disorder. *American Journal of Psychiatry, 156,* 617–623.

Welham, J.L., McGrath, J.J., & Pemberton, M.R. (1993). Schizophrenia: Birthrates and three Australian epidemics. *Schizophrenia Research, 9,* 142.

Yoon, B., Romero, R., Kim, I., Koo, C.J., Choe, G., Syn, H.C., & Chi, J.G. (1997). High expression of tumor necrosis factor-alpha and interleukin-6 in periventricular leukomalacia. *American Journal of Obstetrical Gynecology, 177,* 406–412.

Yoon, B., Romero, R., Yang, S.H., Jun, J.K., Kim I., Choi J., & Syn, H.C. (1996). Interleukin-6 concentrations in umbilical cord plasma are elevated in neonates with white matter lesions associated with periventricular leukomalacia. *American Journal of Obstetrical Gynecology, 174,* 1433–1440.

PART TWO

Animal Models of Neurodevelopment and Psychopathology

SEVEN

On the Relevance of Prenatal Stress to Developmental Psychopathology

A Primate Model

Mary L. Schneider, Colleen F. Moore, and Gary W. Kraemer

In this chapter we examine the question of whether psychosocial stress during pregnancy might be one factor predisposing offspring to the development of psychopathology. We review relevant data from nonhuman primates, rodents, other mammals, and some human studies. The impetus for this chapter is derived from several sources. The first is the observation that prenatal stress effects in both humans and animals appear to share similarities with some forms of psychopathology in humans. These similarities include dysregulation of the hypothalamic-pituitary-adrenal (HPA) axis, sleep disturbances, and alterations in brain biogenic amine[1] chemical activity – disturbances that are similar to those found in humans with psychiatric disorders.

The second impetus is the recent move in the field of developmental psychopathology from a deficit model to a risk model. From the perspective of a "deficits" model, a researcher would tend to look for cause-and-effect relationships wherein a specific event, early in life, results in altered developmental outcome (Brown, 1993). Alternately, in a risk model, early life events are not viewed as singular causes of developmental outcomes, but rather they are considered as probabilistic contributors to development along with other events within a dynamic interacting complex process. Also, in a risk model, early life events are viewed as probabilistically associated with a variety of different developmental outcomes; this construct is called *multifinality*. For example, from a "deficit" viewpoint, preterm delivery can be viewed as a cause of later developmental problems, such as cerebral palsy, subtle neuromotor abnormalities, learning disabilities, and behavior problems (Goldson, 1983; Hertzig, 1981; Koops & Harmon, 1980). From a risk perspective, however, preterm delivery and *other* events, such as the extent of social,

---

[1] Biogenic amines include the neurotransmitters norepinephrine, dopamine, and serotonin. Currently, the most common treatments for clinical depression utilize drugs that increase serotonergic neurotransmission, such as Prozac (fluoxetine; see Jacobs et al., 2000, for a review).

We dedicate this chapter to Elizabeth C. Roughton, former graduate student, colleague, and treasured friend, whose generous spirit and enduring curiosity serve as a continuing inspiration to our prenatal stress work. This research was supported in part by grants from the National Institute of Alcohol Abuse and Alcoholism (AA10079), National Institute of Mental Health (MH48417), WT Grant Foundation Faculty Scholars Award, and Maternal & Child Health Bureau (MCJ009102) to MLS, and by the John D. and Catherine T. MacArthur Foundation, NIMH (MH40748 and MH60318), and NICHHD (HD 23042) to GWK.

economic, or health stress in the homes of preterm babies, are viewed as interacting to influence later outcomes. In addition, the outcomes observed are not expected in all children. The idea that multiple early events combine to influence outcomes is particularly relevant to the present research because preterm deliveries occur more frequently in families under high degrees of stress.

More recent developmental psychopathology theories have adopted a risk model, with a focus on the bidirectional transactional relationships between biological, psychological, and environmental factors that could promote or hinder positive adaptations (Boyce et al., 1998). We support this view, considering prenatal stress as one possible risk factor within an array of complex processes and mechanisms that, in combination, may underlie maladaptive development, and we reject oversimplified cause-and-effect relationships between prenatal stress and offspring outcome.

The third impetus for this chapter is related to the recent surge of interest by researchers, clinicians, and policy-makers in the effects of early environmental experiences on brain and behavioral development. Due to significant recent accomplishments in the neuroscience field, the biological aspects of early environmental influences have been the focus of much exciting research. For example, Greenough and colleagues have provided evidence that experiences during early development are assimilated into the individual's brain by altering the neural processes of the developing organism (Greenough & Black, 1992). Moreover, stressors experienced by the developing or even mature mammal can alter the expression of the genetic program and the course of neural development or remodeling (Fleming et al., 1999; Floeter & Greenough, 1979; Post, 1992). This incorporation of experience in the form of altered neural substrates then influences the way the individual experiences new events (Boyce et al., 1998; Cicchetti & Tucker, 1994; Kraemer, 1992). Thus, environmental influences on brain development are thought to have cascading effects on later functioning, which, in turn, influences brain development (Kraemer, 1986). In other words, even though early experiences are not regarded as mechanistic causes of later outcomes, such experiences do have potential to have long-lasting effects. This seeming contradiction is resolved by the fact that early alterations of brain function would be expected to alter the way later experiences are assimilated and responded to in a manner that could vary considerably across individuals and be predictable in only a probabilistic sense.

A question that naturally arises from this focus on early environmental influences on brain development concerns whether the *prenatal* environment could have effects on offspring brain development and behavior. It is commonly accepted that exposure to certain substances or events in utero, such as cigarettes, alcohol, and other drugs, can have negative effects on offspring. It is less well known, however, whether other environmental events, such as psychological stress in the pregnant mother's life, could have adverse neurodevelopmental effects. This issue is important because if a link is found between prenatal stress and vulnerability to neurodevelopmental maladaptations or developmental psychopathology, knowledge of this association could potentially influence the likelihood that vulnerable children would be referred for services early in life. Early intervention is important because it is the time of relatively high brain plasticity and behavioral flexibility, when such interventions can exert maximum benefits for the child (see Guralnick & Bennett, 1987, for a review).

A fourth impetus for this study of prenatal stress is the continuing interest in how factors related to socioeconomic status might contribute to differential vulnerability to psychopathology. A number of years ago Rutter elucidated the synergistic effect of chronic family adversity (Rutter & Quinton, 1977). Indeed, Rutter and his colleagues found that it was the *number* of risk factors that was critical, with one risk factor increasing or potentiating the effects of others. This has important implications in a society where the economically underprivileged sector is more likely to be subjected to excess uncontrollable stressors in comparison to those from a more privileged sphere of society. Because in the United States there is evidence of growing chaos and stress in the lives of families, schools, peer groups, and neighborhoods (see Bronfenbrenner, 1995), this raises concerns about the possible cascading effects of exposure to prenatal stress on development.

In discussing the issue of how prenatal stress may affect later development, we will first provide an overview of our own work on prenatal stress. We will discuss a series of four prospective longitudinal nonhuman primate studies that include both behavioral and physiological outcome measures. Next, we discuss what possible biological mechanisms for the apparent link between psychosocial stressors and vulnerability to altered development are supported by other animal research. We also briefly review prenatal stress research in humans, with a particular focus on the possible links to some forms of childhood and adult psychopathology. In the concluding section of this chapter, we discuss themes and present suggestions for future research directions.

WISCONSIN PRENATAL STRESS PRIMATE STUDIES

In this section, we describe a series of four prospective longitudinal studies examining the developmental outcomes of nonhuman primates whose mothers were exposed to stress during gestation. First, our general procedures will be described, followed by details on the methodology and results of each study. For the most part, we have studied the rhesus macaque, an Old World monkey. There are a number of reasons for the choice of this species.

First, rhesus monkeys are an excellent choice for prenatal stress studies because pregnant rhesus monkeys have been found to respond to mildly stressful manipulations, showing increased cortisol levels, yet still give birth to viable infants that are available to study into adulthood. A second reason for selecting this species concerns the richness of their behavioral and social organization and their ability to perform complex cognitive tasks. Indeed, the normative pattern of behavioral development in this species has been very well documented in the literature. Moreover, their slow-paced fetal growth rates, long gestations, single births, and relatively slow postnatal growth rates make them more similar to humans (Newell-Morris & Fahrenbruch, 1985) and allow for more extensive examination of neurobehavior during development than is possible in rapidly developing rodents (Goldman-Rakic & Brown, 1982). Thus, where the main goal of animal research is to increase our understanding of events and mechanisms that can alter the lives of humans, these characteristics of monkeys make them a much better model of behavioral development than rodents.

The study of behavioral development of rhesus monkeys in particular has an extraordinary history, which was started by Harry Harlow and his colleagues at the University of Wisconsin (Harlow, 1958; Harlow & Harlow, 1965). Harlow's seminal work set the stage for a series of studies that demonstrated the critical importance of early life experiences on a range of primate behaviors, including social behavior, complex learning capabilities, and reproductive behaviors (Sackett, 1981; Mineka & Suomi, 1978). We draw heavily from this large literature in our studies. Our work is also dependent on the extensive work that has examined the influence of psychosocial stress on physiological and behavioral systems in nonhuman primates (Coe et al., 1978). Our own unique contribution to this body of literature on the behavioral systems of the rhesus macaque includes the development of specific measures for studying, in detail, rhesus monkey neonatal neurobehavior and temperament (Schneider, Moore, Suomi, & Champoux, 1991; Schneider & Suomi, 1992). Our measures are closely analogous to those measures used with humans (Brazelton, 1984).

Our goal is to mimic recurrent daily episodic stress in order to study the effects on nonhuman primate offspring. Clearly, there is no universal definition for stress; however, most current definitions view stress as a temporary state of disharmony or threatened homeostasis (see Chrousos & Gold, 1992, for a review). This transient state triggers a network of adaptation responses to return the organism to a state of relative stability or homeostasis. Mild, brief, controllable perturbations or "stressors" can be interpreted as positive and mild stress can stimulate cognitive and emotional processes. However, severe, prolonged, and uncontrollable stress is viewed as negative, contributing to maladaptation, and ultimately to exhaustion of the animal's capacity to adapt (Selye, 1936).

This homeostatic adaptation process is a complex phenomenon involving numerous central and peripheral processes that underlie arousal, focused attention, and species-appropriate aggression, while inhibiting pathways subserving feeding and reproduction (Chrousos & Gold, 1992). Response to stress is associated with an increase in the release of corticotropin-releasing hormone (CRH), which activates the pituitary-adrenal axis. This results in the release of adrenocorticotropic hormone (ACTH) from the anterior lobe of the pituitary (see Johnson, Kamilaris, Chrousos, & Gold, 1992, for details). The release of ACTH into the bloodstream stimulates the secretion of glucocorticoids by the adrenal cortex – cortisol and 11-deoxycortisol in primates and humans, and corticosterone in rodents. A negative feedback loop exists such that circulating glucocorticoids inhibit the release of ACTH by the pituitary and also inhibit the release of CRH by the hypothalamus (Keller-Wood & Dallman, 1984). This feedback process is thought to involve the hippocampus as well, which has a high density of glucocorticoid receptor cells (Sapolsky, 1992; Sapolsky, Krey, & McEwen, 1985). Having presented this background information, we now turn to our own studies.

General Procedures

This section will focus on the overall methodology employed in four of our studies. These studies were conducted to compare the behavior and physiology of monkeys from prenatally stressed pregnancies with controls from undisturbed pregnancies. We studied these animals from infancy through adolescence. Because nonhuman primates have a condensed lifespan compared to the human, they can be studied from infancy through adolescence over a 2–4 year timespan. Two different species were used and three different stressors were employed in these studies. Overall, the effects of a noise or hormonal stressor, presented at different stages of gestation, on a variety of measures were examined. These include maternal weight gain during pregnancy, neonatal reflexes, infant temperament characteristics, and infant body weight. A variety of

Table 7.1. Conditions Employed in Prenatal Stress Studies

Study	Monkey Species	Stressor	Gestational Timing (days)	Postnatal Rearing	Sample Size
1	Rhesus	Noise	90–145	Nursery-reared	24
2	Rhesus	Noise	45–90 90–145	Mother-reared	31
3	Rhesus	ACTH	120–134	Mother-reared	12
4	Squirrel	Social relocation	Once mid-gest. vs. chronic (3x's)	Mother-reared	90

other behavioral and physiological measures obtained include measures of behavior in a novel environment, behavior during separation from an attachment figure (either mother or peers), and peer interaction social behaviors. Physiological measures of stress hormone levels (plasma cortisol and ACTH) and concentration of biogenic amines in cerebrospinal fluid were also obtained.

Table 7.1 shows the species, stressor, timing of the stressor, and the postnatal rearing condition employed in each study.

The first three studies used rhesus monkeys as subjects (Schneider, 1992a, b, c; Schneider, Coe, & Lubach, 1992; Schneider, Roughton, Koehler, & Lubach, 1999; see Table 7.1). In Studies 1 and 2, we varied the postnatal rearing conditions of the monkeys – they were nursery (hand)-reared by human caretakers in Study 1 and they were mother-reared by their own mothers in Study 2. The timing of the prenatal stressor – three noise blasts (115 dB sound at 1 m, 1,300 Hz) presented randomly during a 10-minute period to the pregnant females each day – also varied across Studies 1 and 2. In Study 1, the noise stressor was administered Monday through Friday on days 90 through 145 of a 165-day gestation period. We refer to this as "mid-late gestation" stress. In Study 2, the stressor was administered on days 45 through 90 – referred to as "early" stress – or days 90 through 145 (similar to Study 1). Note that we purposely avoided administering the stressor from conception to day 45 or from days 145 through 165 to avoid the risks of either early fetal loss or early parturition (see Schneider, 1992a; Schneider et al., 1999, for more details on the methodologies in Studies 1 and 2).

The three random noise blasts, which were administered in a darkened room, were found to significantly increase maternal cortisol levels (see details in Maternal Response to Noise Stresser). The stressor was administered five times per week at 1600 each day for females in the stress condition to mimic recurrent daily episodic stress. Controls were undisturbed during pregnancy, except for normal animal husbandry.

In Study 3, rather than using the noise stressor, pregnant rhesus monkeys were administered the pituitary hormone, ACTH, to examine maternal endocrine activation as a central mechanism underlying the prenatal stress effect. Finally, in Study 4, with a sample of squirrel monkeys, we used social relocation, or disruption of the mother's social relationships, as the prenatal stressor. Social relocation was employed either once during midgestation or three times throughout pregnancy. Studies 3 and 4 were conducted in collaboration with Christopher Coe at the Harlow Primate Laboratory (Schneider & Coe, 1993; Schneider, Coe, & Lubach, 1992).

Study 1

In Study 1, twenty-four infant rhesus monkeys (twelve prenatally stressed and twelve from undisturbed pregnancies) were separated from their mothers at birth and hand-reared by human caretakers in our laboratory primate nursery for the first thirty days of life. This extremely labor intensive and somewhat unnatural rearing condition was used in order to prevent confounding potential effects on the offspring from the prenatal stress treatment with possible effects from differential maternal treatment. The latter includes individual differences in maternal styles, and/or the possibility of differential maternal treatment due to repeated stress during pregnancy. The nursery-rearing condition also provided continuous access to the infants for repeated neurobehavioral testing. To reduce potential adverse effects from hand-rearing, individual infant cages were provided with cloth-covered heated waterbeds and movable surrogates, which provided gentle vestibular stimulation. Loops of garden hose, which served as climbing apparatuses, were also added to the cages to provide an opportunity for vestibular and proprioceptive stimulation through active sensorimotor engagement with the environment. A variety of brightly colored manipulable infant toys, which were sterilized and rotated among infants daily, were also added to the cages (see Schneider & Suomi, 1992, for details). All infants were socialized four times weekly for fifteen minutes in playgroups with other infants from similar prenatal conditions. All infants had free access to Similac infant formula. When the infants were approximately thirty days old, they were transferred from the primate nursery to the general colony and housed in mixed-sex peer groups of three infants each from the same prenatal condition according to standard protocols used at the Harlow Primate Laboratory.

Study 2

In Study 2 (Schneider et al., 1999), in order to compare the results of the hand-reared monkeys in Study 1 with a group of more typically reared monkeys, infants were reared with their mothers. As described above, we also varied the timing of the stressor. There were three groups: (1) eight infants whose mothers experienced the noise stressor during the gestational time period used in Study 1 (described above), mid-late gestation (postconception days 90 through 145); (2) ten infants whose mothers were stressed (as above) during early gestation (days 45 through 90); and (3) twelve controls from undisturbed pregnancies. Relying on Rakic's (1985, 1988, 1995) elegant studies of fetal brain development in rhesus monkeys, we regard our early-gestation stress period (day 45–90 postconception) as approximating the phase of neuronal migration while the mid-late gestation stress period (day 90–145) approximates the early portion of synaptogenesis. Rakic describes three broad phases of development: generation of neurons (days 0 through 40 postconception), neuronal migration (days 40 through 70–100), and synaptogenesis (day 112 postconception through the third month postnatally; Rakic, 1988, 1995; Zecevic & Rakic, 1991). Knowing what type of brain development is occurring at the time of the prenatal stress is important for the ultimate goal of relating the findings to human development, and also for comparing our results with those obtained with other species.

   Although most of our focus will be on Studies 1 and 2, we will also describe some of the results of Studies 3 and 4. As mentioned previously, Study 3 was conducted with rhesus monkeys, but instead of the noise stressor, pregnant monkey mothers were administered ACTH to simulate stress (Schneider, Coe, & Lubach, 1992). Study 4 was conducted with ninety squirrel monkeys whose mothers were administered a more naturalistic prenatal stressor, social relocation (Schneider & Coe, 1993). One group of pregnant females was relocated once during midgestation, while a second group experienced three changes, mimicking chronically unstable living conditions, hence, chronic prenatal stress.

Maternal Response to Noise Stressor

In Studies 1 and 2, the females were removed from the home cage and exposed to noise stress. Noise stress has also been employed as a prenatal stressor in rodent studies (Fride & Weinstock, 1988) and it has been found to be a source of psychological stress with humans (Evans, Hygge, & Bullinger, 1995; Ising, Rebentisch, Poustka, & Curio, 1990; Kryter, 1990). We found that this procedure significantly activated the hypothalamic-pituitary-adrenal (HPA) axis in the pregnant female, raising mean plasma cortisol level (baseline = 25.2 ± 2.2 μg/dl; post stress = 34.8 ± 2.4 ug/dl ($\pm$SEM).

Gestation Length and Offspring Birthweight Results

There were no effects of prenatal stress on gestation length in any of our studies, despite some evidence in human studies linking prenatal stress to preterm births (see Paarlberg, Vingerhoets, Dekker, & Van Geijn, 1995, for a review). In Study 1, the average gestation length was 171 ± 5 days for controls and 168.7 ± 5 days for mid-late gestation prenatally stressed infants. For Study 2, the average gestation length for controls was 170 ± 5 days, 169.38 ± 4.6 days for mid-late gestation stressed infants, and 167 ± 7.6 days for early-gestation stressed infants. For Study 3, the gestation lengths for control and hormone-treated pregnancies were 171.4 ± 2.9 days and 172.9 ± 6 days, respectively. Thus, in our studies, the type and intensity of prenatal stress had no detectable effect on gestation length.

Despite the lack of prenatal stress effects on length of gestation in our studies, there were effects of prenatal stress on birthweight. The birthweight effects were not, however, consistent across our studies. In Study 1, the mean birthweight (in grams) of the prenatally stressed monkeys (472 ± 16, females and 518 ± 18, males) was significantly less than controls (525 ± 19, females and 528 ± 16, males). In Study 2, the early stressed monkeys (479 ± 18, females and 468 ± 56, males) had lower birthweights than mid-late gestation stressed (595 ± 10, females and 527 ± 14, males) and controls (490 ± 19, females and 550 ± 13, males). There were no birthweight effects, however, detected in Studies 3 and 4. Thus, with regard to birthweight, we conclude from our four prenatal stress studies that the effect of prenatal stress on birthweight is probably not clinically meaningful. In other words, all of the birthweights were within two standard deviations of what is considered "normal" for rhesus monkeys, based on data for 1,270 rhesus monkeys born at the Harlow Primate Laboratory from 1973 through 1997 (478 ± 61, females and 501 ± 64, males [M $\pm$ SD]). Hence, there were no cases in our three studies of rhesus monkeys in which the infants would be categorized as having low birthweight (LBW) analogous to the clinical diagnosis of LBW in human infants.

Paarlberg and colleagues (1995) reported that the most consistent findings from research on psychosocial factors and pregnancy outcomes in humans pertained to preterm delivery. In fact, approximately 60 percent of the human studies found that prenatal stress reduced the length of the gestation period. In humans, however, other factors, such as socioeconomic status, medical problems, and other lifestyle behaviors might be mediating these effects. Because stressful conditions are associated with smoking, and consumption of alcohol and other drugs of abuse, and because smoking and consumption of other drugs are known to have negative effects on pregnancy outcomes (Brooke, Anderson, Bland, Peacock, & Stewart, 1989), it is difficult to interpret the human studies. We discussed the issue of confounding of prenatal stress with other variables in human research in more detail in Schneider and Moore (2000).

Infant Neurobehavioral Development

All infants in our studies were tested several times across the first month of life on a test battery that we previously developed to document primate infant neurobehavioral development (Schneider et al., 1991; Schneider & Suomi, 1992). Because rhesus monkey infants are strikingly similar to human neonates in terms of neuromotor abilities and temperamental behavioral styles, the test that we developed was adapted directly from human neonatal tests, primarily the Neonatal Behavioral Assessment Scale (Brazelton, 1984). In our prior studies, factor analyses were conducted using a large sample of typically developing rhesus monkey neonates. Four domains of functioning were identified, which are closely analogous to those factors recognized in human studies (see Schneider et al., 1991, for details). The four domains described, which were used in our prenatal stress studies, were as follows: Orientation, Motor Maturity, Motor Activity, and State Control. Orientation included observations of orienting reactions to visual stimuli, visual following, and duration of looking. Motor Maturity included the following items: (1) muscle tonus (antigravity flexor muscle tonus and antigravity extensor muscle tonus in neck and trunk muscles); (2) righting reactions (the ability to bring the head and neck into the vertical plane when the body was tilted 45 degrees); (3) response speed (speed of neuromotor responses to stimuli); and (4) coordination (quality of gross motor movement). Motor Activity included items measuring spontaneous movement. State Control included ratings of behavioral style throughout testing, including irritability and consolability.

Table 7.2 depicts the results for the four domains for all four studies. In Study 1, in addition to lower birthweights, the prenatally stressed monkeys had reduced scores for Motor Maturity and Motor Activity, and marginally lower scores on Orientation compared to controls. Analyses of the individual items were conducted in order to provide a more thorough understanding of these differences. It was discovered that the prenatally stressed monkeys had lower muscle tone, reduced coordination and balance scores, and slower response speeds. They were also found to be more distractible during testing and more passive as well (reduced spontaneous movements). Not surprising, they took two extra days to achieve independence in self-feeding compared to controls (Schneider, 1992a). Because the infants in Study 1 were hand-reared (to reduce potential effects from differential maternal treatment), we questioned whether these results would be observed if the monkeys were reared more normally, with their mothers. It is important to note here that hand-reared rhesus monkeys develop well physically overall; in fact, they gain weight more rapidly than their mother-reared counterparts, and score well on tests of Motor Maturity. However, because they have been shown to display behavioral abnormalities, such as excessive clinging to peers later in life (Harlow & Harlow, 1966),

Table 7.2. Neonatal Neurobehavioral Effects

Study	Conditions	Prenatal Stress Findings
1	Noise stress, rhesus, gestational days 90–145, nursery-reared	↓ birthweight ↓ motor maturity ↓ motor activity ↓ muscle tone, coordination, balance, and response speed ↑ distractibility and passivity ↑ days to independence in self feeding (Schneider, 1992a)
2	Noise stress, rhesus, gestational days 45–90 (early stress), 90–145 (mid-late stress), mother-reared	↓ birthweight (early stress) ↓ motor maturity (early stress and mid-late stress) ↓ orientation (early stress and mid-late stress) ↓ postrotary nystagmus (early stress) Early gestation is the time of greatest vulnerability to prenatal stress (Schneider et al., 1999)
3	ACTH treatment, rhesus, gestational days 120–134, mother-reared	↓ motor maturity ↓ orientation ↓ state control (Schneider, Coe, & Lubach, 1992) (Roughton et al., 1998)
4	Social relocation, squirrel, once mid-gestation vs. chronic stress, mother-reared	↓ motor maturity (chronic) ↓ motor activity (chronic) ↓ attention (chronic) ↓ muscle tone, balance, and postrotary nystagmus (chronic) (Schneider & Coe, 1993)

Note: ↓ and ↑ denote a decrease or increase, respectively, in the dependent variable compared to control animals.

our next logical step was to conduct a similar study while rearing the infants with their mothers.

The results from Study 2, conducted with the same stressor (noise stress) and a replication of the mid-late gestation timing condition, with the addition of an early-gestation stress condition, is also shown in Table 7.2. Some similarities and some differences between Studies 1 and 2 emerged. As with Study 1, Study 2 showed a birthweight effect and overall effects for Motor Maturity and Orientation. Therefore, we were able to replicate our earlier prenatal stress effects under more normal rearing conditions. Moreover, infants from *both* the mid-late gestation stress condition and the early-gestation stress condition scored lower than controls on these domains. However, an interesting finding from Study 2 was that *early* gestation emerged as a period of enhanced vulnerability for these effects. Specifically, the infants from mothers stressed during early gestation were observed to show more pervasive and more pronounced neuromotor decrements than mid-late gestation monkeys or controls (Schneider et al., 1999). They also showed reduced Motor Activity and decreased postrotary nystagmus, a measure of integrity of vestibulo-occular function that might be associated with the neuro-motor deficits noted. Also, a significant Condition X Day interaction suggested that the infants differed in their developmental trajectories. While controls exhibited the species-typical rapid developmental increases across the first month of life, early- and mid-late gestational stressed monkeys demonstrated a flat or variable developmental trajectory (see Schneider et al., 1999, for details).

In Study 3, the experiment in which pregnant rhesus monkey females were admin-istered ACTH over a two-week period during mid-late gestation (Schneider et al., 1992), a behavioral profile in infancy was found that was strikingly similar to that observed in Studies 1 and 2. Specifically, the infants from the ACTH-exposed pregnancies demon-strated a similar pattern of reduced Motor Maturity and decreased Orientation similar to that found in the offspring of noise-stressed mothers.[2] However, one striking differ-ence emerged – the infants whose mothers were treated with ACTH were rated as more irritable and more difficult to console during testing compared to controls, while the noise-stressed infants did not show this temperamental effect. It is possible that this particular discrepancy across studies might be related to the fact that the noise stressor increased cortisol levels from 25 to 34 μg/dl, on average, whereas the ACTH treatment increased maternal cortisol levels from 23 to a mean of 58.5 μg/dl. Thus, one might speculate that while mild stress might affect Motor Maturity and Orientation, a more severe perturbation, resulting from more marked elevations of cortisol levels, could also affect State Control, resulting in observation of increased irritability and inconsolability during testing.

We are extremely grateful to the late Elizabeth Roughton, a graduate student at the Harlow Primate Laboratory during this time, who collaborated with us in conducting an in-depth study of State Control in infants from ACTH-treated mothers and controls (see Roughton, Schneider, Bromley, & Coe, 1998, for details pertaining to the scoring system). In her carefully controlled study, the monkeys were videotaped immediately after they were separated from their mothers, as well as after the administration of the infant neurobehavioral assessment battery. Using a computer-assisted continuous scoring system, the amount of time spent in drowsy, alert, and irritable states was coded by testers blind to the animal's condition. Surprisingly, the infants from ACTH-treated mothers spent more time in a drowsy state compared to controls, especially during the immediate postseparation period when acute stress would presumably be the most pronounced. Conversely, the controls spent more time immediately after maternal separation in an active alert state, presumably searching for their mothers, a species-typical adaptive response to separation from their mother.

In our publication reporting this result (Roughton et al., 1998), we speculated that this finding could represent an exhaustion of the adaptation response in infants of ACTH-treated mothers. This could result in a phenomenon commonly referred to by clinicians as a "shut-down" experience. This speculation was based on the findings by Emde and colleagues (1971), who reported increased NREM sleep following cir-cumcision in human infants. Emde interpreted the increased sleep as representing a biobehavioral coping response to assist in recovery from the perturbation. Similarly,

---

[2] Although the noise stressor in Studies 1 and 2 is probably loud enough to affect the fetus directly, the consistency of the results with Study 3, which used only ACTH administered to the mother, suggests that the processes involved are related to maternal endocrine activation.

Gunnar and her colleagues (1985) reported an association between quiet sleep and the reestablishment of baseline plasma cortisol levels in human infants. In the next section, when we consider the possible mechanisms underlying prenatal stress effects, we will return to this issue of increased "drowsiness" or reduction in "active alert" state under conditions of acute stress in the Study 3 sample.

The next step in our research was to determine whether a similar pattern would emerge in a different nonhuman primate species, using a different prenatal stressor. Therefore, in Study 4, we used squirrel monkeys (*saimiri boliviensis peruviensis*), and we employed social relocation as a stressor (see Schneider & Coe, 1993, for details). Social relocation involved removing the pregnant female from her social group and putting her with unfamiliar conspecifics. This particular manipulation has been shown to cause marked changes in behavioral and endocrine system activity that persists over several weeks (Mendoza, Coe, & Levine, 1979; Kaplan, Manuck, & Gatsonis, 1990). We also varied the chronicity of the stressor, studying one group of offspring whose mothers were moved once during mid-late gestation, compared to a group of infants whose mothers were moved three times, undergoing continuously unstable living conditions. Controls, of course, were undisturbed except for the normal animal husbandry.

The findings of Study 4 are also included in Table 7.2, and indicate that the prenatally stressed squirrel monkey infants demonstrated a pattern that was strikingly similar to that found in the prenatally stressed rhesus monkey infants. Specifically, squirrel monkey infants from mothers that underwent a single move during mid-gestation stress and those that were chronically stressed showed a trend for reduced scores on Orientation, Motor Maturity, and Motor Activity and increased scores on the State Control measure (increased irritability and decreased consolability). However, the results were statistically significant only for Motor Maturity and Motor Activity for the *chronic* stress group. When individual items were examined, the infants from the chronic prenatal stress condition were found to exhibit shorter attention spans, reduced muscle tonus, reduced balance, and altered vestibular-ocular (postrotary nystagmus) responses.

Summary

Taken together, these data from four prospective nonhuman primate studies tell us several things. First, our studies reveal a specific behavioral profile associated with prenatal stress in nonhuman primates. This behavioral profile includes, most consistently, a shortened attention span and reduced neuromotor capabilities in the affected infant. This profile emerged in two different species (rhesus monkey and squirrel monkey) and under three different stress conditions (noise stress, ACTH treatment, and disruption of social relationships). Second, based on the results from Study 3, the mechanism for this effect appears to include, at least to some degree, maternal activation of the endocrine system. Furthermore, more severe endocrine activation, evidenced by higher maternal cortisol levels in Study 3, may be related to the State Control problems, as shown by more time in drowsy state, more irritability, and more difficulty consoling the infant during testing compared to controls.

Third, the early gestation period appears to be a period of increased ontogenetic vulnerability to maternal stress for neurobehavioral effects in the neonate. Thus, based on our own results, it seems to be possible that prenatal stress during the period of neuronal migration (days 40 through 70–100 postconception) may in fact be more harmful to the developing brain than stress during early synpatogenesis (day 112 post-conception through third month postnatal). This concurs with a number of studies that have suggested that the period of neuronal migration is highly sensitive to various perturbations, including toxins, viruses, and genetic mutations and may contribute to developmental dyslexia (Galaburda, Rosen, & Sherman, 1989) and schizophrenia (Kotrla, Sater, & Weinberger, 1997). Indeed, Rakic (1985) has shown that correct cell migration is critical for enabling communication between late- and early-forming neurons at important stages, before they make their synaptic connections. We will return to this important issue in our overall discussion of results.

Response to Challenges

In the previous section, we have shown that prenatally stressed infants appear to exhibit a neurobehavioral phenotype that, although it could easily be confused with genetic predilection, does appear to be at least partially due to the stressful experiences of the mothers during pregnancy. The next logical step was to examine the prenatally stressed and control monkeys themselves under stressful situations later in development. Our tests of the monkeys' responses to novelty and stress as a function of prenatal condition is based on six experiments conducted longitudinally on the prenatally stressed monkeys from Studies 1 and 2. We assessed the monkeys' behavioral responses as well as some biological variables: (1) in a primate playroom; (2) during peer separation and reunion; (3) when challenged by novelty and social separation as juveniles; (4) in the primate playroom as adolescents/young adults; (5) under new group formation; (6) and during maternal separation (see Table 7.3).

Table 7.3 reveals the common behavioral profile that is evident under this series of novelty challenges. The first evidence of the profile emerged when the nursery-reared monkeys were first tested in groups of three in the primate playroom as six-month-olds (see Schneider, 1992c, for details). It is important to note that playroom studies have been conducted for decades at the Harlow Primate Laboratory and typical responses for rhesus monkeys have been well documented. "Normal" monkeys, when placed into a novel playroom situation, initially show wariness but eventually exhibit species-typical exploration and play behavior (Harlow, Harlow, & Suomi, 1971). This is, in fact, the pattern observed in the control monkeys. In contrast, the prenatally stressed monkeys exhibited high levels of disturbance behavior (clinging to each other, self-directed behaviors) and reduced levels of exploratory behavior (such as locomotion, climbing, and exploring the environment; Schneider 1992c). Moreover, the prenatally stressed infants also exhibited a behavior that was very unexpected – 50 percent of the prenatally stressed monkeys fell asleep in the playroom, while none of the controls showed this abnormal behavioral response. Reflecting back to our previously discussed findings from the Roughton et al. (1998) study, in which increased drowsiness was detected in neonates from ACTH-treated mothers during a period of acute stress – maternal separation – our sleep data lend some support to our speculation that this might reflect an exhaustion of the stress adaptation resources of the prenatally stressed monkeys. We will return to this hypothesis later when we present physiological data on these monkeys.

The next novelty challenge, which occurred at eight months of age, was to examine prenatally stressed and control monkeys when they were separated from their cage

Table 7.3. Novelty Challenge Results for Hand-Reared Monkeys

Experiment	Novelty Challenge Test	Behavioral Findings
1	6-month playroom	↑ clinging ↑ self-directed ↑ sleep ↓ exploratory (Schneider, 1992c)
2	8-month separation/reunion	↑ clinging ↑ self-grooming ↓ locomotion, play, climb (Schneider et al., 1998)
3	18-month challenge	↑ abnormal (clinging) ↓ proximity, contact (Clarke & Schneider, 1993)
4	3–4 year playroom	↓ exploration ↑ vocalization (at first) (Clarke et al., 1996)
5	4-year new group formation	↑ self-clasping ↑ stereotypes ↑ general disturbance ↑ freezing ↓ play and exploration (Clarke et al., 1996)
6	6-month maternal separation	↑ self-grooming across days ↓ locomotion (Schneider & Moore, 2000)

Note: ↓ and ↑ denote a decrease or increase, respectively, in the dependent variable as a function of prenatal stress.

mates, housed individually for three days, and reunited. We based this study directly on the separation and reunion protocol that has been used for decades at the Harlow Primate Laboratory (Harlow & Suomi, 1974; Mineka & Suomi, 1978). Accordingly, the monkeys were separated from peers and placed in individual cages side-by-side, and observed using a computer-assisted coding system three times daily both during separation and when reunited with peers. Physiological samples were also obtained at specific times (blood and cerebral spinal fluid), which will be discussed later (Schneider et al., 1998). The behavioral data from this study indicated that, much like that reported in the playroom study, the prenatally stressed monkeys exhibited increased amounts of clinging and self-grooming and decreased amounts of locomotion, play, and climbing.

The third novelty challenge experiment was conducted when the monkeys reached what is considered the juvenile period at approximately eighteen months of age. At this time, a series of exposures to four mild stress episodes was conducted: (1) moving to a new cage; (2) moving to a new cage and exposure to the noise stressor; (3) separation from cage mates; (4) separation from cage mates and exposure to the noise stressor. These four episodes were employed randomly across individuals (see Clarke &

Schneider, 1993, for details). The results are summarized in Table 7.3, showing that pre-natally stressed monkeys showed significantly more clinging to peers (when in groups) and less proximity and contact compared to controls.

Novelty challenges in Experiments 4 and 5 were conducted when the animals were considered to be adolescents or young adults, at 3–4 years of age. In Experiments 4 and 5, they were again tested in the playroom (see Clarke, Soto, Bergholz, & Schneider, 1996, for details). Again, the pattern that emerged included *lower* levels of exploration in the prenatally stressed animals, and higher levels of vocalizations, suggesting a higher arousal level for the prenatally stressed monkeys compared to controls. Also, during new group formation, the prenatally stressed monkeys showed more disturbance behavior, such as self-clasping and stereotyped behaviors and "freezing," and less time in play and exploration.

Finally, in Experiment 6, mother-reared rhesus monkeys from Study 2 were sepa-rated from their mothers at six months of age for weaning. They were housed alone for three days prior to being placed in group housing with same-age peers. During this transition, behavioral observations were collected three times daily. Examination of the three groups of monkeys under this stressful condition showed that, for both the early and mid-late gestation stressed monkeys, *more* self-grooming was observed com-pared to controls. For locomotion, a significant Condition X Day interaction occurred, showing that while controls increased the duration of time spent in locomotor behav-ior across days, prenatally stressed monkeys showed a *decrease* in locomotor behavior across days (Schneider & Moore, 2000). Our interpretation is that the control animals were adapting to the housing change normally, whereas the prenatally stressed animals were not.

Summary

Taken together, the markedly consistent behavioral profile that was observed across the novelty challenge experiments included a *decrease* in exploration, locomotion, and play (or increased "freezing") and a striking *increase* in disturbance behavior, such as clinging and self-directed grooming or clasping in the prenatally stressed monkeys. It is interest-ing to note the well-documented view that despair or depression in rhesus monkeys is characterized by sharp decreases in play and increases in passive self-directed behaviors (Kaufman & Rosenblum, 1967; Harlow & Suomi, 1974; Kraemer & McKinney, 1979; Kraemer, 1982).

Physiological Measures during Novelty Challenge

Having described the behavioral profile that emerged repeatedly across studies of pre-natally stressed rhesus monkeys, we now shift our focus to examine the physiological data from these studies. Prior to our research, a number of rodent studies had docu-mented HPA dysregulation in prenatally stressed rodents, compared to controls. This had been reported under baseline conditions (Fride et al., 1986; Peters, 1982) and after exposure to stressful conditions – novel environments, restraint, and/or saline injec-tions, as well (Fride et al., 1986; Henry et al., 1994; McCormick, et al., 1995; Takahashi et al., 1988). Thus, we were interested in examining the HPA axis functioning in our prenatally stressed and control monkeys under baseline and stressful conditions.

Table 7.4. Physiological Findings

Manipulation	Results
Neonatal exam, short nap	↓ Cortisol during nap, females > males (Schneider & Moore, 2000)
8-month social separation	Prenatal stress > controls (change in cortisol from baseline) (Schneider et al., 1998)
6-month maternal separation	Early prenatal stress > controls (↑ ACTH levels 2 hours post separation) (Schneider & Moore, 2000)
18-month challenge	Prenatal stress > controls (↑ ACTH levels across repeated challenges) (Clarke et al., 1994)
8 + 18-month challenge	Prenatal stress > controls (MHPG & DOPAC concentration in CSF) (Schneider et al., 1998)

Note: ↓ and ↑ denotes decrease and increase respectively.

Table 7.4 shows the physiological findings. Because we had ready access to our nursery-reared monkeys in Study 1, we collected blood samples three times during the neonatal period: (1) day 3 in the nursery; (2) day 22 after a neonatal examination; and (3) day 23 after a 10-minute nap. On day 3, baseline cortisol levels were 24.3 (1.3) μg/dl, comparable to levels on day 22, after a neonatal examination, of 27.5 (2.2) μg/dl. However, cortisol values were found to fall sharply after the onset of sleep, to 12.6 (1.5) μg/dl, ($p < .001$). These data parallel findings in human newborns that show lower cortisol values as a result of sleep (Anders et al., 1970; Tennes & Carter, 1973). Sex differences were also detected, with females showing overall higher cortisol levels than males, 24.8 (2.4) compared to 19.2 (1.3) μg/dl, respectively, $p < .04$. We did not, however, find any differences between the prenatally stressed monkeys and controls at any of these time points.

We did, however, find that the nursery-reared prenatally stressed monkeys showed higher cortisol levels than controls under stressful conditions when they were eight months old. These animals were living in peer groups at the time. Social separation was found to result in a threefold increase in cortisol, 21.5 (1.3) μg/dl at baseline to 73.3 (2.7) μg/dl two hours post separation, $p = .0001$, demonstrating that social separation is a powerful psychobiological stressor for rhesus monkeys. The increase from baseline was significantly *larger* for the prenatally stressed monkeys than controls, 57 (3.9) μg/dl, increase from baseline for the prenatally stressed monkeys, and 46.4 (3.2) μg/dl for controls, $p = .05$. We reunited the monkeys on day 4 and repeated the social separation the subsequent week, replicating these effects and demonstrating intra-individual consistency of cortisol values across weeks, $r = .64$, $p < .001$.

When we used the identical separation paradigm with the mother-reared prenatally stressed monkeys from Study 2, this time separating the infants from their mothers when they were six months old, we found a significant effect on ACTH levels for early gestation stress. Moreover, the largest ACTH response at two hours postseparation was detected in the early prenatal stress group, 117 (18) μg/dl at 2-hr postseparation, compared to controls, 87.3 (27) μg/dl, and cortisol values showed a similar trend.

Next, we asked whether this altered HPA reactivity to stress would extend into the juvenile or adolescent period. We have previously described the behavioral findings observed when the monkeys were challenged at eighteen months of age in a series of stressful conditions (move to novel cage, move plus noise stressor, separation from peers, separation plus noise stressor). When we assessed the physiological data in this study, we found that the prenatal stress group showed higher ACTH concentrations than controls under these challenging conditions (see Clarke, Wittwer, Abbott, & Schneider, 1994, for details).

We also collected samples of cerebrospinal fluid (CSF) when the monkeys in Study 1 were eight and eighteen months old in order to examine biogenic amine neurotransmitter levels. These brain chemicals are considered to be important because they are related to regulation of a wide range of functions, such as emotion regulation, motor control, cognition, reward, and state regulation. We measured norepinephrine (NE), its metabolite 3-methoxy-4-hydroxyphenylglycol (MHPG), 3,4 dihydroxy-phenylacetic acid (DOPAC), the dopamine metabolite, homovanillic acid (HVA), and the serotonin metabolite 5-hydroxyindoleacetic acid (5-HIAA). Although the evidence of HPA axis alteration provided by our studies of serum cortisol and ACTH is important, because behavior necessarily involves the nervous system, studying changes in brain chemicals is even more important for explaining the behavioral alterations induced by prenatal stress.

In our prenatal stress studies, we found higher concentrations of two neurotransmitter substances known to be indicators of increased dopaminergic and adrenergic activity: MHPG and DOPAC in cerebrospinal fluid of prenatally stressed monkeys compared to controls (see Schneider et al., 1998, for details). These findings could reflect increased sympathetic nervous system activity in the prenatally stressed animals. The sympathetic nervous system is referred to as the "fight or flight" response system, that is, it is activated by stress. Similarly, a nonsignificant trend for increased NE, also an indicator of sympathetic nervous system activity, and increased HVA, a dopamine metabolite, was detected. Moreover, when we correlated the data from the eight- and eighteen-month novelty challenges, we detected marked consistency in NE ($r = .69$, $p < .05$) and MHPG ($r = .75$, $p < .02$) across ages.

Summary

Previous primate studies have shown how differential social rearing conditions can produce changes in biogenic amine system activity, and also affect learning performance (Kraemer, 1992; Kraemer & Bachavalier, 1998). Moreover, a number of human studies have been interpreted as suggesting that prior experience influences biogenic amine system functioning and may regulate neuronal plasticity, resulting in a cascade of effects that could render an individual vulnerable to psychiatric disorders. Indeed, research on humans with a variety of types of psychopathology has shown differences from controls with respect to CSF levels of neurotransmitters or metabolites and production of receptor binding sites in brain regions (Andreasen, 1997; Cowen, 1993; Holsboer & Barden, 1996; Wyatt, Apud, & Potkins, 1996). A variety of factors are potential contributors to these findings in humans: variation in genetics (Ogilvie et al., 1996; Virkkunen,

Goldman, Nielsen, & Linnoila, 1995), experience and environment or other as yet un-explained variables, which could include prenatal stress. Our results are also consistent with rodent studies that have reported differences in NE and DA concentrations in several brain areas in prenatally stressed rats compared to controls (Fride et al., 1986; Moyer, Herrenkohl, & Jacobowitz, 1978). Other studies have demonstrated altered development of serotonergic neurons in prenatally stressed rodents (Peters, 1982) and altered acetylcholine levels (Day et al., 1998).

Underlying Mechanisms

In this section, we address how maternal stress effects on fetal CNS development might be linked to behavioral reactivity and HPA-axis dysregulation of the offspring. We focus primarily on studies that employ rodent models and, to a much lesser extent, nonhuman primate studies. The first part of the discussion is based on a relatively large rodent literature, which addresses possible brain mechanisms for prenatal stress effects on offspring, including structural, functional, and biochemical processes. It is important to note, however, that the rodent prenatal stress studies vary widely in terms of the methodology employed. There are numerous differences across studies with regard to the type of stressor used, the duration for which the stressor was employed, the intensity of the stressor, and the gestation period during which it was administered. While one common method of stressing pregnant female rodents is restraint under bright lights, the stressor is administered either once or several times daily, and it is employed during a range of gestational periods (Koehl, Barbazanges, Moal, & Maccari, 1997; McCormick et al., 1995; Peters, 1990; Takahashi & Kalin, 1991; Williams, Hennessy, & Davis, 1995). Despite this variability in methodology, the results have been fairly consistent across the studies.

Hypothalamic-Pituitary-Adrenal (HPA) Axis

Earlier, we discussed the idea that prenatal stress produces a dysregulation of the HPA axis in prenatally stressed offspring. Rodent models have explored some of the mechanisms for these alterations of HPA-axis functioning. The hypothesis that appears to have the most support in the literature at the present time is the view that hormones transported from maternal blood to the placenta mediate the prenatal stress-induced HPA effects in the offspring. The overarching idea is that psychosocial stress during pregnancy alters maternal hormones circulating in the blood (primarily corticosterone and ACTH in the rodent), and that the levels of these hormones – though buffered by the active processing of the placenta – are also altered in the developing fetus. The altered levels of hormones in the fetus then affect some aspects of the developing fetal brain and hormonal feedback systems.

Studies of prenatally stressed monkeys (including our own) showed decreased exploration and locomotion, increased freezing behavior, as well as increased ACTH and cortisol responsivity to stress, compared to controls. Studies of rodents have shown that CRH not only coordinates the secretion of glucocorticoids, but also affects the behavioral responses normally observed when animals are exposed to stress, such as freezing and altered vocalizations (Sutton, Koob, Le Moal, Rivier, & Vale, 1982). Because

CRH receptor neurons are widely distributed in the brain (De Souza et al., 1985), it is hypothesized that CRH receptor cells subserve the extensive effects of CRH on behavior in rodents. This includes freezing in novel settings, increased locomotor activity in familiar settings (Sutton et al., 1982) and bizarre repetitive behavior (Koob & Bloom, 1985). Administering ACTH to rodents also results in behaviors often seen under mild stress, such as reduction of exploration in a novel environment and excessive grooming (File, 1978; Gipsen, Van der Poel, & van Wimersma Greidanus, 1973).

Prenatal Stress – Potential Mechanisms

Given this background information, we now return to our discussion of the possible underlying mechanisms for the prenatal stress effects that we have seen in our own studies. The first logical question to ask is whether hormones transported to the placenta of the pregnant female could underlie prenatal stress effects. If we look to the work of Maccari and colleagues, we find that when stress-induced glucocorticoid secretion was blocked in pregnant rodent dams that were stressed, the prenatal stress effects on the offspring were significantly reduced (Barbazanges, Piazza, Le Moal, & Maccari, 1996). Conversely, when pregnant dams were injected with CRH from day 14 through 21 of gestation, the pups were observed to show a striking resemblance to prenatally stressed pups (Williams et al., 1995). Moreover, injecting dams with ACTH during pregnancy altered the developing HPA axis – and also decreased dopaminergic activity in the pups. As described previously, in one of our own studies, in which pregnant female rhesus monkeys were injected with ACTH daily during mid-late gestation, offspring showed a behavioral profile that was markedly similar to prenatally stressed rhesus monkey offspring. Thus, experimental manipulation of the chemical events normally triggered by stress has been shown to have effects on both rodent and nonhuman primate offspring.

The next logical question is to ask how elevated maternal stress hormones might affect the developing fetal brain. In other words, is it possible for maternal stress hormones – which are released when the mother encounters a stressor – to cross the placental "barrier," and if so, how could this translate into altered behavioral and physiological development of the offspring? Unfortunately, the question of whether maternal stress hormones cross the human placenta has not been answered unequivocally. Some investigators report that maternal cortisol levels contribute to fetal concentrations levels (e.g., Schwartz, 1997), but others argue that cortisol does not cross the human placenta (Benediktsson & Seckl, 1998). It is well known that the concentration of maternal plasma ACTH rises progressively during pregnancy (Weir et al., 1971), leading to increased maternal plasma concentrations of cortisol. In fact, Rees and Lowry (1978) reported a two- or threefold increase of maternal plasma concentrations of total and unbound cortisol. Although this rise in cortisol would be thought to lead to a decrease in ACTH, through a negative feedback loop, it appears that this normal feedback loop is reduced during pregnancy (see Jacobs, 1991, for a review). In order to protect the fetus from the increased maternal cortisol, which could presumably cause early maturation of the fetus, the placenta converts cortisol to cortisone, an inactive metabolite (Murphy, 1978). Toward the latter part of pregnancy, however, the fetal metabolism shifts such that a surge in cortisol level occurs. This surge is thought to contribute to fetal lung maturation and, possibly, also to initiating the onset of labor.

Recent studies by Glover and colleagues (Gitau, Cameron, Fisk, & Glover, 1998) have measured plasma cortisol concentrations in paired maternal and fetal venous samples in humans. The samples were taken between thirteen and thirty-five weeks of gestation, and interestingly, they showed a strong linear correlation between fetal and maternal cortisol concentration ($r = .62$, $p < .001$). Thus, about 40 percent of the variance in fetal cortisol concentration appears to be due to maternal cortisol (Gitau et al., 1998). It may be that both maternal and fetal cortisol concentrations are associated with another factor, such as maternal CRH, or possibly other events that impact maternal and fetal stress systems simultaneously. Moreover, it is likely that while a portion of fetal cortisol is derived from the mother, most of the cortisol passing through the placenta is metabolized to cortisone by the placenta. However, Gitau et al. (1998) argue that even a relatively minor contribution of cortisol from the mother (10–20%), given the low levels of fetal cortisol concentration, could lead to a significant increase in fetal concentration of cortisol. In any event, the strong association between maternal and fetal cortisol concentration in humans lends support for the notion that maternal endocrine activation may be an essential mechanism for prenatal stress effects.

Fetal Neurodevelopmental Changes

The next logical question to ask is what areas of the fetal brain might be altered by increased levels of fetal cortisol concentrations. Unfortunately, there are only a few studies on this topic, and the findings are also not unequivocal. Maccari and colleagues reported decreased binding capacity of hippocampal[3] type I (mineralocorticoid) and type II (glucocorticoid) corticosteroid receptors in rodents (Barbazanges et al., 1996; Henry et al., 1994; Maccari et al., 1995). Due to the role of hippocampal glucocorticoid receptors in the negative feedback on the HPA axis in adult mammals (De Kloet & Reul, 1987), this altered hippocampal binding capacity has been hypothesized as a contributor to the HPA dysregulation seen in prenatally stressed offspring. Others have failed to find differences in the hippocampus between prenatally stressed offspring and controls. McCormick and colleagues (1995), who also reported prenatal stress effects on HPA axis stress reactivity in rats (but only in female offspring), examined glucocorticoid receptor binding in several brain structures. They failed to detect prenatal stress effects on glucocorticoid receptor density in the hypothalamus or hippocampus. They did, however, report prenatal stress effects on glucocorticoid receptor density in the frontal cortex, septum, and amygdala – the latter are interconnected structures of the limbic system involved in modulation of motivation and emotional behaviors.

Finally, there is one relevant study with prenatal hormone-treated rhesus monkeys suggesting that the fetal hippocampus may be particularly vulnerable to increased levels of maternal glucocorticoids. When Uno et al. (1990) injected pregnant rhesus monkeys with synthetic glucocorticoids (dexamethasone) daily on gestational days 120 through 132, the offspring showed reductions in neurons and irregular zonal arrangement of hippocampal neurons. Recall that days 120 to 132 would correspond to the period of synaptogenesis in the rhesus monkey.

---

[3] The hippocampus is a structure of the limbic system involved in memory, learning, and with other structures in this system (such as the amygdala), emotion regulation.

It has also been hypothesized that a hypersensitivity of cholinergic neurons (neurons that release the neurotransmitter acetylcholine) related to the septum and hippocampus may play a role in HPA axis activity in prenatally stressed rats (Day et al., 1998). This hypothesis is based on recent evidence that prenatally stressed rodents showed increased acetylcholine release in the hippocampus when tested under the stress of saline injections (Day et al., 1998). Because cholinergic neurons reportedly regulate hippocampal glucocorticoid secretion (McEwen, De Kloet, & Rostene, 1986), hypersensitivity of cholinergic neurons could be partially responsible for the HPA dysregulation seen in prenatally stressed offspring.

Similarly, a number of other neurotransmitter systems were found to be altered by prenatal stress. For example, in rats, the dopamine system has been found to be impacted (Fride et al., 1986; Henry et al., 1995). In the mammalian brain, dopamine systems play a central role in motor control, cognition, hormone release, emotional balance, and reward (Diamond, 1996). Concentrations of NE (the sympathetic neurotransmitter) and its metabolite MHPG have also found to be altered by prenatal stress (Takahashi, Turner, & Kalin, 1992). Finally, alterations of the development of serotonin neurons and decreased 5-HT levels have also been found in several brain regions of prenatally stressed rats, suggesting that mild prenatal stress affects the serotonergic system, especially in the hippocampus (Hayashi et al., 1998; Peters, 1990). Because the neurotransmitter serotonin is believed to play an important role in early brain development, facilitating synapse formation in the CNS (Lauder & Krebs, 1978), and influencing HPA axis regulation (Mitchell, Rowe, Boska, & Meaney, 1990), altered development of serotonin neurons could be related to the abnormal behavioral development associated with prenatal stress.

Is Prenatal Stress a Risk Factor for the Development of Depression or Other Forms of Psychopathology?

Given this discussion of the behavioral and physiological effects of prenatal stress, we now turn our attention to the question of whether prenatal stress might render an individual vulnerable to developmental psychopathology. The etiology and development of psychopathologies are not simple. Current theorists view multiple interacting influences as contributors to risk for psychopathology. Most approaches include social-psychological factors as interacting with genetically mediated endogenous factors in a dynamic continuously changing context (Boyce et al., 1998; Cicchetti & Tucker, 1994; Nelson & Bloom, 1997). Social contexts are thought not only to impact on psychological development but also to affect biological systems and processes. Within this framework, we believe that there are a number of reasons for including prenatal stress as a potential risk factor for the development of psychopathology.

As described previously, there are substantial data from rodent and nonhuman primate studies to support the notion that prenatally stressed individuals are more vulnerable to stressors. Because a number of psychiatric disorders are thought to be exacerbated or promoted by common stressors (Post, 1992), prenatal stress, by rendering the individual more vulnerable to common stressors, could thus be a potential contributor to a number of such disorders.

In humans, there are several retrospective correlational studies that link prenatal stress to an increased incidence of psychiatric disorders. For example, studies have linked prenatal stress to attention deficit hyperactivity disorder (ADHD) (McIntosh et al., 1995), the most common pediatric psychiatric disorder today (Swanson et al., 1995). Severe emotional disturbance (Ward, 1990), anxiety and social withdrawal (Meijer, 1985), schizophrenia and criminality (Huttunen & Niskanen, 1978) have also been linked to prenatal stress. However, these studies are retrospective and, as such, are subject to a number of methodological concerns that weaken the conclusions that can be drawn from them. These include: (1) biased reporting on pregnancy conditions, due to the mother's knowledge of an adverse outcome from the pregnancy; (2) potential confounding of prenatal and postnatal factors; and (3) the possible effects from confounding factors that often covary with prenatal stress, such as smoking, alcohol and other drug use, and nutritional factors (see Schneider & Moore, 2000, for more discussion of the literature on prenatal stress in humans).

FUTURE DIRECTIONS

It is apparent that there is much work to be done on the details of how prenatal stress impacts the stress reactivity of offspring. First, at the biochemical level, more work needs to be done on how the maternal stress hormones affect the fetal stress hormone system, and at what levels of stress. Perhaps there is a threshold beyond which the placenta is unable to process maternal CRH, ACTH, and cortisol. Knowing whether there is a threshold, and if so, what controls it, and its range of individual differences is important.

Second, because of conflicting evidence about the particular brain systems in offspring affected by prenatal stress, more work is needed to increase our understanding of how maternal stress impacts fetal brain development. Clearly, the links between processes occurring prenatally, during CNS development, and behavioral abnormalities exhibited by the offspring postnatally, are, without a doubt, exceedingly complex. In order to understand this complex relationship, it is necessary to know how prenatal stress could affect all three aspects of nervous system development: cell proliferation, cell migration, and cell differentiation (or cell death). All three aspects of nervous system development have the potential to influence the postnatal ability of the brain to process information within complex behavioral situations. A number of questions remain unanswered. What is occurring at the cellular level at the time that prenatal stress takes place? Which cell types, neurotransmitter systems, and developmental processes are affected by the prenatal stress event?

The first question is related to the timing of the prenatal stress event, and this question has been examined at the behavioral level in our primate model. The reader may recall that we reported that early gestation was a period of ontogenetic vulnerability for prenatal stress-induced neurobehavioral effects in rhesus monkey offspring (Schneider et al., 1999). As noted previously, we found that a sensitive period for prenatal stress-induced neurobehavioral effects lasts from approximately the seventh to thirteenth week of gestation. Applying information from Rakic's elegant studies of CNS development in fetal rhesus monkeys, it then appears that a period of enhanced vulnerability to prenatal stress occurs when neurons are migrating toward cerebral cortex. It is interesting to note that studies of radiation exposure in humans have found a critical period for the development of mental retardation later in life that lasted from the eighth to the fifteenth week of gestation (Otake & Schull, 1984). Moreover, research has demonstrated that if neural migration is disrupted, an aberration in cell position can result. Human abnormal neuronal migration has been associated with a number of syndromes, including dyslexia, autism, and mental retardation (Galaburda et al., 1989; Kotrla et al., 1977). Researchers believe there are several mechanisms. Abnormally positioned neurons may or may not find their normal targets, essential for normal function to be established. Alternately, the neurons might find their targets, but change their normal pathway to their targets or fail to contact the appropriate portion of the dendrites of the target cells (Caviness & Rakic, 1978; Stanfield, Caviness, & Cowan, 1979; Nowakowski & Hayes, 1999), resulting in connections that may or may not result in functional capacities that are normal (Drager, 1981; Nowakowski & Hayes, 1999).

In principle, therefore, prenatal stress could exert its CNS effects via alterations in neuronal migration, with cascading effects on CNS organization and, as a result, normal functional competence may not be maximally achieved. Specifically, abnormal networks may affect specialization of the cortex postnatally. Thus, some developmental disorders may ensue from altered "wiring," and one might expect to find common symptoms across disorders, depending on the timing of the disruption. This hypothesis has been supported by our own work, in which we found that early-gestation prenatal stress effects were similar to neurobehavioral effects resulting from early-gestation moderate-level fetal alcohol exposure (Schneider et al., 1999; Schneider, Moore, & Becker, 2001), compared to a later-occurring gestational exposure to either prenatal stress or moderate-level alcohol.

Knowing the biochemistry and neurobiological effects of prenatal stress is meaningful when those effects are linked to behavior. Thus, future studies are needed in which the timing, intensity, and duration of prenatal stress are systematically manipulated and assessments are made not only of aspects of brain function, but also of behavior. Fortunately, neuroimaging resolution has improved so that both structural and functional studies with high-resolution in vivo neuroimaging can be combined with behavioral assessments in the living subject. Neuroimaging studies of structures can now describe alterations in the size of certain structures, such as the corpus callosum, frontal lobe, and basal ganglia. However, research is needed in order to understand what changes in neurological structure and function imply for behavior. Moreover, whether other parts of the brain can compensate, and how postnatal experience affects brain development, also need to be considered.

Another complex challenge for the future is identification of the molecular basis of the role of prenatal stress in behavioral disorders. Functional neuroimaging studies are needed to describe localized areas of activity of the brain while the animal is engaged in tasks known to be affected by prenatal stress. Other procedures, such as positron emission tomography (PET) studies using radioactive ligands, while not normally suitable for experimental use with children, can be more easily employed in research with primates. For example, in our current work, we have developed a technique allowing us to examine areas of the brain rich in dopamine receptors. Our data so far suggest that prenatal stress combined with prenatal alcohol exposure results in an up-regulation of D2 receptor binding (Roberts et al., 1999), possibly due to a reduction in availability of dopamine. Studies are planned to compare early-gestation stressed monkeys with mid-late gestation prenatally stressed rhesus monkeys with regard to D2 receptor availability, presynaptic DA synthesis, and serotonergic receptor availability.

Pharmacologic challenge studies are also needed to test the behavioral reactivity of prenatal stressed and control monkeys, unmasking functional deficits that might not be apparent under the baseline conditions of laboratory housing. For example, neurotransmitter system function can be probed by administering a drug that either acts as selective receptor agonists or antagonists, evoking neurotransmitter release or inhibiting neurotransmitter synthesis or reuptake. Because alterations in the neurotransmitter dopamine (DA) are thought to underlie some long-term effects of in utero exposure to prenatal stress as well as fetal alcohol exposure, in our work, we have planned a methylphenidate (Ritalin) challenge. Methylphenidate inhibits DA uptake and raises the concentration of DA in various brain regions (Barkley, 1998; LaHoste et al., 1996).

Studies are also needed to test the current view that one event can influence two or more later-occurring developmental events, even though the later-occurring events may or may not be directly causally related (Nowakowski & Hayes, 1999). We have found that the prenatal stress treatment not only affects early attention and neuromotor function, but it also can alter maternal behavior. For example, we observed the amount of time spent in mutual-ventral contact in our mother-infant dyads on a weekly basis throughout the first six months of life (Schneider & Moore, 2000). While infants spent nearly 100 percent of their time in mutual ventral contact with their mothers during the first few weeks of life, the contact gradually declined as the control infant matured, but the prenatally stressed infants maintained high levels of contact, diverging significantly from the pattern demonstrated by control monkeys. Therefore, not only did prenatal stress disrupt early neurobehavior, but it appears to have produced cascading effects in later-occurring events, such as independence from the mother. Furthermore, the cascade view suggests that it is the combination of a number of events that ultimately influences CNS development.

If the usual transaction between mother and infant is disrupted, whether the causal sequence should be viewed as originating primarily with the infant, or with the mother, two things seem to be true theoretically. First, from the psychobiological trajectory of psychosocial development, the infant deviates from "what-it-could-have-been," in other words, what was possible under optimal circumstances. Second, it becomes difficult, if not impossible, to sort out causal sequences once the developmental process is in motion, because the mother and the infant are in a transactional process in which they affect each other's behavior over time (Kraemer, 1992; Sameroff, 1975). As individuals deviate from the optimum they will be less or more "in tune," or matched or mismatched with their immediate surroundings, and hence valued in the larger societal context. The most extreme deviations from the social context can be defined as expressions of developmental psychopathology.

From a developmental "transactional" viewpoint, all this implies that prenatally stressed infants are more likely to challenge their caregivers, and the resulting interaction may be less likely to promote optimal development. This, in turn, is likely to affect how the infant's behavior and physiology organizes its own neurobiological regulatory mechanisms. These altered regulatory mechanisms may be manifested in changes in baseline activity of neurotransmitter systems, hormonal secretions and regulation, and either exaggerated or blunted behavioral and biobehavioral responses to stressors, perhaps persisting into adolescence and adulthood.

Another fruitful area for future research will be to examine in detail the interaction of prenatal stress with postnatal environmental factors. Also, how prenatal stress interacts with teratogens, such as nicotine, alcohol, and other drug of abuse needs to be examined. It is important to investigate whether one particular variable potentiates the impact of another variable, so that the effect of the two variables together might surpass the sum of the variables (Rutter, 1983). For example, we reported some striking and rather surprising results that when monkey mothers are exposed to prenatal stress *and* consume moderate level alcohol throughout pregnancy, the incidence of fetal loss increases dramatically (there was no increase in fetal loss under conditions of alcohol alone or prenatal stress alone). Also, in male offspring, birth weight was compromised in the offspring of monkeys exposed to both prenatal stress and alcohol during pregnancy (Schneider, Roughton, & Lubach, 1997). Because prenatal stress covaries with smoking, alcohol, and other drug abuse in humans, more carefully controlled laboratory studies are needed to systematically investigate the many combinations of exposure to alcohol, drugs of abuse, and prenatal stress. Also, how such variables have different effects on certain individuals, and how one variable might have the effect of buffering or reducing the impact of another, are topics that need investigating (Rutter, 1983).

A related issue that needs further research pertains to comorbidity in developmental deficits and risk for psychopathology, such as depression. For example, in children, learning difficulties and emotional problems are commonly found together. Does this comorbidity reflect co-occurring but separate etiological factors or cascading effects of a primary perturbation? For example, animal studies suggest that prenatal stress altered offspring emotional and stress-responsive behaviors. The behavioral profile that emerged in our studies included *decreased* exploration and *increased* self-directed behaviors, similar to the behavioral profile associated with despair and depression in monkeys (Harlow, Harlow, & Suomi, 1971). Consistent with our own findings in nonhuman primates, prenatal stress in rodent studies has been associated with increased emotional behavior of pups (Alonso, Arevalo, Afonso, & Rodriguez, 1991; Fride et al., 1986; Fride, Dan, Gavish, & Weinstock, 1985; Thompson, 1957; Weinstock, 1997). For example, rat pups born to mothers that were stressed during pregnancy demonstrated a reduction of ambulatory behavior and an increase in latency to move in an open field test. Similarly, Weinstock and others reported an enhanced behavioral responsivity to stress in prenatally stressed pups evidenced by increased "defensive freezing" and altered vocalizations (see Weinstock, 1997, for a review).

The HPA-axis physiological profile associated with prenatal stress, which includes altered HPA-axis regulation – impaired feedback inhibition, especially after stress – observed in rats (Barbazanges et al., 1996; Maccari et al., 1995; Weinstock , 1997) and monkeys (Clarke et al., 1994; Schneider et al., 1998; Schneider & Moore, 2000), resembles the HPA dysregulation reported in depressed patients (Post, 1992). Also, altered neurotransmitter system activity is associated with depressive illness in humans and it was also detected in prenatally stressed monkeys (Schneider et al., 1998).

Finally, another symptom of prenatal stress that is similar to a symptom of depression in humans is the sleep disorder recently described in prenatally stressed rodents. Specifically, Dugovic et al. (1999) reported that adult rodents that had been prenatally stressed showed increased amounts of paradoxical (REM) sleep, positive correlations of REM sleep to cortisol, and increased sleep fragmentations. These kinds of sleep alterations are hallmark features of depression in humans (Kupfer, 1995).

The hypothesized mechanisms underlying the observed prenatally stress-induced sleep disorder mammals involves an alteration in serotonergic system associated with prenatal stress (Peters, 1982, 1990). Thus, alterations in the serotonergic system in prenatally stressed rodents (Peters, 1982, 1990) could interfere with regulation of both REM sleep and slow wave sleep (Sharpley, Elliot, & Attenburrow, 1994; Tortella, Echevarrua, Pastel, Cox, & Blackburn, 1989). Moreover, cholinergic and noradrenergic systems are known to interact with serotonergic systems to determine the timing and maintenance of REM sleep (Bennington & Heller, 1995). As noted previously, these systems have been shown to be altered as a consequence of prenatal stress (Day et al., 1998; Fride et al., 1986; Peters, 1982; Schneider et al., 1998). Moreover, prenatal stress effects on the HPA axis could play a role in the sleep disturbance associated with prenatal stress, given the well-documented role of the HPA axis in modulation of sleep (Opp, 1998).

Overall, a considerable amount of data at this point suggests that many psychiatric disorders are not attributable to changes in a single neurochemical or neuroendocrine system (Kraemer, 1992). For example, it is likely that depressive symptoms reflect an underlying disorganization among multiple systems. Prenatal stress would seem to have the characteristic of decreasing the organizational resilience of the neurobiological systems that normally enable individuals to adapt to common stressors. As such, it may be a risk factor for the development of later deviant or unusual behavior.

Primate studies can provide the opportunity to test possible etiological factors together and separately, and to determine behavioral and biobehavioral profiles associated with etiological factors. For example, our own studies suggest that the behavioral profile associated with prenatal stress includes attention deficits, neuromotor impairments, decreased ability to adapt to novelty but *not* hyperactivity. Offspring from prenatal alcohol exposure, on the other hand, while they do show attention and neuromotor deficits (Schneider et al., 1997), also show increased hyperactivity (unpublished data). Studies are needed to compare monkeys with and without hyperactivity with brain imaging techniques to investigate whether the distinction in behavioral profiles is reflected in brain structure and function.

Studies of the sort proposed here might ultimately have important implications for treatment and intervention programs. Better and earlier identification of at-risk children can lead to early intervention for children who show early neurobehavioral and neuromotor effects. Early treatment is especially critical for those children with unstable family environments, before these early effects translate into later behavioral problems and cognitive deficits. Intervention may be most effective when it occurs in early childhood, rather than waiting until adolescence or early adulthood (see Guralnick & Bennett, 1987, for a review).

REFERENCES

Alonso, S. J., Arevalo, R., Afonso, D., & Rodriguez, M. (1991). Effects of maternal stress during pregnancy on forced swimming test behavior of the offspring. *Physiology and Behavior, 50,* 511–517.

Alonso, S. J., Castellano, M. A., Quintero, M., & Navarro, E. (1999). Action of antidepressant drugs on maternal stress-induced hypoactivity in female rats. *Methods & Findings in Experimental & Clinical Pharmacology, 21*(4), 291–295.

Alonso, S. J., Navarro, E., Santana, C., & Rodriguez, M. (1997). Motor lateralization, behavioral despair and dopaminergic brain asymmetry after prenatal stress. *Pharmacology Biochemistry and Behavior, 58,* 443–448.

Anders, T. F., Sachar, E. J., Kream, J., Roffwarg, H. P., & Hellman, L. (1970). Behavioral state and plasma cortisol response in the human newborn. *Pediatrics, 46*(4), 532–537.

Andreasen, N. C. (1997). Linking mind and brain in the study of mental illness: A project for a scientific psychopathology. *Science, 275,* 1586–1593.

Barbazanges, A., Piazza, P. V., Le Moal, M., & Maccari, S. (1996). Maternal glucocorticoid secretion mediates long-term effects of prenatal stress. *Journal of Neuroscience, 16,* 3943–3949.

Barkley, R. A. (1998). Attention-deficit hyperactivity disorder. *Scientific American, September, 279,* 66–71.

Benediktsson, R., & Seckl, J. R. (1998). Understanding human parturition. *Lancet, 351,* 913–914.

Bennington, J. H., & Heller, H. C. (1995). Monoaminergic and cholinergic modulation of REM-sleep timing in rats. *Brain Research, 681,* 141–146.

Boyce, W. T., Frank, E., Jensen, P. S., Kessler, R. C., Nelson, C. A., Steinberg, L., & The MacArthur Foundation Research Network on Psychopathology and Development. (1998). Social context in developmental psychopathology: Recommendations for future research from the MacArthur Network on Psychopathology and Development. *Development and Psychopathology, 10,* 143–164.

Brazelton, T. B. (1984). Neonatal Behavioral Assessment Scale (2d ed.). *Clinics in developmental medicine, 88.* Philadelphia: Lippincott.

Bronfenbrenner, U. (1995). Developmental ecology through space and time: A future perspective. In P. Moen, G. H. Elder, Jr., & K. Luscher (Eds.), *Examining lives in context: Perspectives on the ecology of human development* (pp. 619–647). Washington, D.C.: American Psychological Association.

Brooke, O. G., Anderson, H. R., Bland, J. M. Peacock, J. L. & Stewart, C. M. (1989). Effects on birth weight of smoking, alcohol, caffeine, socioeconomic factors, and psychosocial stress. *British Medical Journal, 298,* 795–801.

Brown, E. R. (1993). Long-term sequelae of preterm birth. In A. Fuchs, F. Fuchs, & P. G. Stubblefield (Eds.), *Preterm birth: Causes, prevention and management* (2d ed.). New York: McGraw-Hill.

Caviness, V. S., & Rakic, P. (1978). Mechanisms of cortical development: A view from mutations in mice. *Annual Reviews of Neuroscience, I,* 297–326.

Chrousos, G. P., & Gold, P. W. (1992). The concepts of stress and stress system disorders: Overview of physical and behavioral homeostasis. *Journal of the American Medical Association, 267,* 1244–1252.

Cicchetti, D., & Tucker, D. (1994). Development and self-regulatory structures of the mind. *Development and Psychopathology, 6,* 533–549.

Clarke, A. S., & Schneider, M. L. (1993). Prenatal stress has long-term effects on behavioral responses to stress in juvenile rhesus monkeys. *Developmental Psychobiology, 26*(5), 293–304.

Clarke, A. S., Soto, A., Bergholz, T., & Schneider, M. L. (1996). Maternal gestational stress alters adaptive and social behavior in adolescent rhesus monkey offspring. *Infant Behavior and Development, 19,* 453–463.

Clarke, A. S., Wittwer, D. J., Abbott, D. H., & Schneider, M. L. (1994). Long-term effects of prenatal stress on HPA axis activity in juvenile rhesus monkeys. *Developmental Psychobiology, 27*(5), 257–269.

Coe, C. L., Mendoza, S. P., Davidson, J., Smith, E. R., Dallman, M., & Levine, S. (1978). Hormonal response to stress in the squirrel monkey. *Neuroendocrinology, 26,* 367–377.

Cowen, P. J. (1993). Serotonin receptor subtypes in depression: Evidence from studies in neuroendocrine regulation. *Clinical Neuropharmacology, 16(Suppl. 3),* S6–18.

Day, J. C., Koehl, M., Deroche, V., Le Moal, M., & Maccari, S. (1998). Prenatal stress enhances stress- and corticotropin-releasing factor-induced stimulation of hippocampal acetylcholine release in adult rats. *Journal of Neuroscience, 18*(5), 1886–1892.

De Kloet, E. R., & Reul, J. M. (1987). Feedback action and tonic influence of corticosteroids on brain function: A concept arising from the heterogeneity of brain receptor systems. *Psychoneuroendocrinology, 12,* 83–105.

De Souza, E. B., Insel, T. R., Perrin, M. H., Rivier, J., Vale, W. W., & Kuhar, M. J. (1985). Corticotropin-releasing factor receptors are widely distributed within the rat central nervous system: An autoradiographic study. *Journal of Neuroscience, 5,* 3189–3203.

Diamond, A. (1996). Evidence for the importance of dopamine for prefrontal cortex functions early in life. *Phil Trans Research Society of London, 351,* 1483–1494.

Drager, U. C. (1981). Observations on the organization of the visual cortex in the reeler mouse. *Journal of Comparative Neurology, 201,* 555–570.

Dugovic, C., Maccari, S., Weibel, L., Turek, F. W., & Van Reeth, O. (1999). High corticosterone levels in prenatally stressed rats predict persistent paradoxical sleep alterations. *Journal of Neuroscience, 19*(19), 8656–8664.

Emde, R., Harmon, R., Metcalf, D., Koenig, K., & Wagonfeld, S. (1971). Stress and neonatal sleep. *Psychosomatic Medicine, 33,* 491–497.

Evans, G. W, Hygge, S., & Bullinger, M. (1995). Chronic noise and psychological stress. *Psychological Science, 6,* 333–338.

File, S. E. (1978). ACTH but not corticosterone impairs habituation and reduces exploration. *Pharmacology, Biochemistry, and Behavior, 9,* 161–166.

Fleming, A., O'Day, D. H., & Kraemer, G. W. (1999). Neurobiology of mother-infant interactions: Experience and central nervous system plasticity across development and generations. *Neuroscience and Biobehavioral Reviews, 25,* 673–685.

Floeter, M. K., & Greenough, W. T. (1979). Cerebellar plasticity: Modification of purkinje cell structure by differential rearing in rhesus monkeys. *Science, 206,* 227–229.

Fride, E., Dan Y., Feldon, J., Halevy, G., & Weinstock, M. (1986). Effects of prenatal stress on vulnerability to stress in prepubertal and adult rats. *Physiology and Behavior, 37,* 681–687.

Fride, E., Dan, Y., Gavish, M., & Weinstock, M. (1985). Prenatal stress impairs maternal behavior in a conflict situation and reduces hippocampal benzodiazepine receptors. *Life Science, 36,* 2103–2109.

Fride, E., & Weinstock, M. (1988). Prenatal stress increases anxiety related behavior and alters cerebral lateralization of dopamine activity. *Life Science, 42,* 1059–1065.

Galaburda, A. M., Rosen, G. D., & Sherman, G. F. (1989). The neural origin of developmental dyslexia: Implications for medicine, neurology, and cognition. In A. M. Galaburda (Ed.), *From reading to neurons* (pp. 377–404). Cambridge, Mass.: MIT Press.

Gipsen, W. H., van der Poel, A., & van Wimersma Greidanus, T. (1973). Pituitary adrenal influences on behavior. Responses to test situations with or without electric footshock. *Physiology and Behavior, 10,* 345–350.

Gitau, R., Cameron, A., Fisk, N. M., & Glover, V. (1998). Fetal exposure to maternal cortisol. *The Lancet, 352*(9129), 707–708.

Goldman-Rakic, P. S., & Brown, R. M. (1982). Postnatal development of monoamine content and syntheses in the cerebral cortex of rhesus monkeys. *Developmental Brain Research, 256,* 339–349.

Goldson, E. (1983). Bronchopulmonary dysplasia: Its relation to two-year developmental functioning in the very low birthweight infant. In T. Field & A. Sostek (Eds.), *Infants born at risk* (pp. 243–250). New York: Grune & Stratton.

Greenough, W. T., & Black, J. E. (1992). Induction of brain structure by experience: Substrates for cognitive development. In M. R. Gunnar & C. A. Nelson (Eds.), *Developmental behavioral neuroscience* (Vol. 24). Hillsdale, NJ: Erlbaum.

Gunnar, M. R., Malone, S., Vance, G., & Fisch, R. O. (1985). Coping with aversive stimulation in the neonatal period: Quiet sleep and plasma cortisol levels during recovery from circumcision. *Child Development, 56,* 824–834.

Guralnick, M. J., & Bennett, F. C. (1987). A framework for early intervention. In M. J. Guralnick & F. C. Bennett (Eds.), *The effectiveness of early intervention for at-risk and handicapped children* (pp. 3–29). New York: Academic Press.

Harlow, H. F. (1958). The evolution of learning. In A. Roe & G. Simpson (Eds.), *Behavior and evolution* (pp. 269–290). New Haven: Yale University Press.

Harlow, H. F., & Harlow, M. K. (1965). The affectional systems. In H. Harlow, A. M. Schrier & F. Stollnitz (Eds.), *Behavior of nonhuman primates* (pp. 287–334). New York: Academic Press.

Harlow, H. F., & Harlow, M. (1966). Learning to love. *American Scientist, 54,* 244–272.

Harlow, H. F., Harlow, M. K., & Suomi, S. J. (1971). From thought to therapy: Lessons from a primate laboratory. *American Scientist, 59,* 538–549.

Harlow, H. F., & Suomi, S. J. (1974). Induced depression in monkeys. *Behavioral Biology, 12,* 273–296.

Hayashi, A., Nagaoka, M., Yamada, K., Ichitani, Y., Miake, Y., & Okado, N. (1998). Maternal stress induces synaptic loss and developmental disabilities of offspring. *International Journal of Developmental Neuroscience, 16*, 209–216.

Henry, C., Guegant, G., Cador, M., Arnauld, E. Arsaut, J., Le Moal, M., & Demotes-Mainard, J. (1995). Prenatal stress in rats facilitates amphetamine-induced sensitization and induces long-lasting changes in dopamine receptors in the nucleus accumbens. *Brain Research, 685*, 179–186.

Henry, C., Kabbaj, M., Simon, H., Le Moal, M., & Maccari, S. (1994). Prenatal stress increases the hypothalamo-pituitary-adrenal axis response in young and adult rats. *Journal of Neuroendocrinology, 6*, 341–345.

Hertzig, M. E. (1981). Neurological "soft" signs in low birthweight children. *Developmental Medicine & Child Neurology, 23*, 778–791.

Holsboer, F., & Barden, N. (1996). Antidepressants and hypothalamic-pituitary-adrenocortical regulation. *Endocrine Reviews, 17*(2), 187–205.

Huttunen, M. O., & Niskanen, P. (1978). Prenatal loss of father and psychiatric disorders. *Archives of General Psychiatry, 35*, 429–431.

Ising, H., Rebentisch, E., Poustka, F., & Curio, I. (1990). Annoyance and health risk caused by military low-altitude flight noise. *International Archives of Occupational and Environmental Health, 62*, 357–363.

Jacobs, B. L., van Praag, H., & Gage, F. H. (2000). Depression and the birth and death of brain cells. *American Scientist, 88*, 340–353.

Jacobs, H. S. (1991). The hypothalamus and pituitary gland. In F. Hytten & G. Chamberlain (Eds.), *Clinical physiology in obstetrics* (2d ed.). London: Blackwell Scientific.

Johnson, E. O., Kamilaris, T. C., Chrousos, G. P., & Gold, P. W. (1992). Mechanisms of stress: A dynamic overview of hormonal and behavioral homeostasis. *Neuroscience and Biobehavioral Reviews, 16*, 115–130.

Kaplan, J. R., Manuck, S. B., & Gatsonis, C. (1990). Heart rate and social status among male cynomolgus monkeys (*Macaca fascicularis*) housed in disrupted social groupings. *American Journal of Primatology, 21*, 175–187.

Kaufman, I. C., & Rosenblum, L. A. (1967). The reaction to separation in infant monkeys: Anaclitic depression and conservation-withdrawal. *Psychosomatic Medicine, 29*, 648–675.

Keller-Wood, M., & Dallman, M. (1984). Corticosteroid inhibition of ACTH secretion. *Endocrine Review, 5*, 1–24.

Koehl, M., Barbazanges, A., Moal, M. L., & Maccari, S. (1997). Prenatal stress induces a phase advance of circadian corticosterone rhythm in adult rats which is prevented by postnatal stress. *Brain Research, 759*, 317–320.

Koob, G. F., & Bloom, F. E. (1985). Corticotropin-releasing factor and behavior. *Federation Proceedings 44*, 259–263.

Koops, B. L., & Harmon R. J. (1980). Studies on longterm outcome in newborns with birthweights under 1500 g. *Advances in Behavioral Pediatrics 1*, 1–128.

Kotrla, K. J., Sater, A. K., & Weinberger, D. R. (1997). Neuropathology, neurodevelopment and schizophrenia. In M. S. Keshavan & R. B. Murray (Eds.), *Neurodevelopment & adult psychopathology* (pp. 187–198). Cambridge: Cambridge University Press.

Kraemer, G. W. (1982). Neurochemical correlates of stress and depression: Depletion or disorganization? *The Behavioral and Brain Sciences, 5*, 110.

Kraemer, G. W. (1986). Causes of changes in brain noradrenaline systems and later effects on responses to social stressors in rhesus monkeys: The Cascade Hypothesis. In *Antidepressants and receptor function (CIBA Foundation Symposium 123)* (pp. 216–233). Chichester: Wiley.

Kraemer, G. W. (1992). A psychobiological theory of attachment. *Behavioral and Brain Sciences, 15*(3), 493–511.

Kraemer, G. W., & Bachevalier, J. (1998). Cognitive changes associated with persisting behavioral effects of early psychosocial stress in rhesus monkeys: The view from psychobiology. In *Adversity, stress, and psychopathology*. Peer-reviewed monograph. Series editor B. Dohrenwend (Columbia University)(pp. 438–462). Oxford: Oxford University Press.

Kraemer, G. W., Ebert, M. H., Schmidt, D. E., & McKinney, W. T. (1989). A longitudinal study of the effects of different rearing environments on cerebrospinal fluid norepinephrine and biogenic amine metabolites in rhesus monkeys. *Neuropsychopharmacology, 2*, 175–189.

Kraemer, G. W., Ebert, M. H., Schmidt, D. E., & McKinney, W. T. (1991). Strangers in a strange land: A psychobiological study of mother-infant separation in rhesus monkeys. *Child Development, 62,* 548–566.

Kraemer, G. W., & McKinney, W. T. (1979). Interactions of pharmacological agents which alter biogenic amine metabolism and depression: An analysis of contributing factors within a primate model of depression. *Journal of Affective Disorders, 1,* 33–54.

Kryter, K. D. (1990). Aircraft noise and social factors in psychiatric hospital admission rates: A re-examination of some data. *Psychological Medicine, 20,* 395–411.

Kupfer, D. J. (1995). Sleep research in depressive illness: Clinical implications – a tasting menu. *Biological Psychiatry, 38,* 391–403.

LaHoste et al. (1996). Dopamine D4 receptor gene polymorphism is associated with Attention Deficit Hyperactivity Disorder. *Molecular Psychiatry 1,* 121–124.

Lauder, J. M., & Krebs, H. (1978). Serotonin as a differentiation signal in early neurogenesis. *Developmental Neuroscience, 1,* 15–30.

Maccari, S., Piazza, P. V., Kabbaj, M., Barbazanges, A., Simon, H., & Le Moal, M. (1995). Adoption reverses the long-term impairment in glucocorticoid feedback induced by prenatal stress. *Journal of Neuroscience, 15,* 110–115.

McCormick, C. M., Smythe, J. W., Sharma, S., & Meaney, M. J. (1995). Sex-specific effects of prenatal stress on hypothalamic-pituitary-adrenal responses to stress and brain glucocorticoid receptor density in adult rats. *Developmental Brain Research, 84,* 55–61.

McEwen, B. S., De Kloet, E. R., & Rostene, W. (1986). Adrenal steroid receptors and actions in the nervous system. *Physiology Review, 66,* 1121–1188.

McIntosh, D. E., Mulkins, R. S., & Dean, R. S. (1995). Utilization of maternal perinatal risk indicators in the differential diagnosis of ADHD and UADD children. *International Journal of Neuroscience, 81,* 35–46.

McKinney, W. T., & Bunney, W. E. (1969). Animal model of depression. I. Review of evidence: Implications for research. *Archives of General Psychiatry, 21,* 240–248.

Meijer, A. (1985). Child psychiatric sequelae of maternal war stress. *Acta Psychiatry Scandinavia, 72,* 505–511.

Mendoza, S., Coe, C. L., & Levine, S. (1979). Physiological response to group formation in the squirrel monkey. *Psychoendocrinology, 3,* 221–229.

Mineka, S., & Suomi, S. J. (1978). Social separation in monkeys. *Psychological Bulletin, 85,* 1376–1400.

Mitchell, J. B., Rowe, W., Boska, P., & Meaney, M. J. (1990). Serotonin regulates type II corticosteroid receptor binding in hippocampal cell culture. *Journal of Neuroscience, 10,* 1745–1752.

Moyer, J. A., Herrenkohl L. R., & Jacobowitz D. M. (1978). Effects of stress during pregnancy on catecholamines in discrete brain regions. *Brain Research, 121,* 385–393.

Murphy, B. E. (1978). Cortisol economy in the human fetus. In M. H. T. James, M. Serio, G. Guisli, & L. Martini (Eds.), *Endocrine function of the human adrenal cortex* (p. 509). London: Academic Press.

Murphy, B. E. (1991). Steroids and depression. *Journal of Steriod Biochem Molecular Biology, 38,* 537–559.

Murphy, B. E., & Branchaud, C. L. (1994). The fetal adrenal. In D. Tulchinsky & A. B. Little (Eds.), *Maternal-fetal endocrinology* (2d ed.) (pp. 275–295). Philadelphia: WB Saunders.

Nelson, C. A., & Bloom, F. E. (1997). Child development and neuroscience. *Child Development, 68(5),* 970–987.

Newell-Morris, L., & Fahrenbruch, C. E. (1985). Practical and evolutionary considerations for use of the nonhuman primate model in prenatal research. In E. S. Watts (Ed.), *Nonhuman primate models for human growth and development* (pp. 9–40). New York: Liss.

Nowakowski, R. S., & Hayes, N. L. (1999). CNS development: An overview. *Development and Psychopathology, 11,* 395–417.

Ogilvie, A. D., Battersby, S., Bubb, V. J., Fink, G., Harmar, A. J., Goodwin, G. M., & Smith, C. A. (1996). Polymorphism in serotonin transporter gene associated with susceptibility to major depression. *Lancet, 347,* 731–733.

Opp, M. R. (1998). Rat strain differences suggest a role for corticotropin-releasing hormone in modulating sleep. *Physiology and Behavior, 63,* 67–74.

Otake, M., & Schull, W. J. (1984). In utero exposure to A-bomb radiation and mental retardation. *British Journal of Radiology, 57,* 409–414.

Paarlberg, K. M., Vingerhoets, J. P., Dekker, G. A., & Van Geijn, H. P. (1995). Psychosocial factors and pregnancy outcome: A review with emphasis on methodological issues. *Journal of Psychosomatic Research, 39,* 563–595.

Peters, D. A. (1982). Prenatal stress effects of brain biogenic amine and plasma corticosterone levels. *Pharmacology, Biochemistry & Behavior, 17,* 721–725.

Peters, D. A. (1990). Maternal stress increases fetal brain and neonatal cerebral cortex 5-hydroxytryptamine synthesis in rats: A possible mechanism by which stress influences brain development. *Pharmacology, Biochemistry & Behavior, 35,* 943–947.

Plotsky, P. M., & Meaney, M. J. (1993). Early postnatal experience alters hypothalamic corticotropin releasing factor (CRF), mRNA, median eminence CRF content and stress-induced release in adult rats. *Molecular Brain Research, 18,* 195–200.

Post, R. M. (1992). Transduction of psychosocial stress into the neurobiology of recurrent affective disorder. *American Journal of Psychiatry, 149*(8), 999–1010.

Rakic, P. (1985). Limits of neurogenesis in primates. *Science, 227,* 154–156.

Rakic, P. (1988). Defects of neuronal migration and pathogenesis of cortical malformations. *Progressive Brain Research, 73,* 15–37.

Rakic, P. (1995). Development of cerebral cortex in human and nonhuman primates. In M. Lewis (Ed.), *Child and adolescent psychiatry,* (2d ed.) (pp. 9–29). Baltimore: Williams & Wilkins.

Rao, U., McGinty, D. J., Shinde, A., McCracken, J. T., & Poland, R. E. (1999). Prenatal stress is associated with depression-related electroencephalographic sleep changes in adult male rats: A preliminary report. *Progress in NeuroPsychopharmacology, and Biological Psychiatry, 23,* 929–939.

Rees L. H., & Lowry P. J. (1978). ACTH and related peptides. In M. H. T. James, M. Serio, G. Guisli, & L. Martini (Eds.), *Endocrine function of the human adrenal cortex* (p. 33). London: Academic Press.

Roberts, A. D., DeJesus, O. J., Schneider, M. L., Schueller, M. J., Shelton, S., & Nickles, R .J. (June, 1999). Dopamine system characterization of rhesus monkeys exposed to moderate dose alcohol in utero. *Society of Nuclear Medicine 46th Annual Meeting,* Los Angeles.

Roughton, E. C., Schneider, M. L., Bromley, L. J., & Coe, C. L. (1998). Maternal endocrine activation during pregnancy alters neurobehavioral state in primate infants. *American Journal of Occupational Therapy, 52,* 90–98.

Rutter, M. (1983). Statistical and personal interactions: Facets and perspectives. In D. Magnusson & V. Allen (Eds.), *Human development: An interactional perspective* (pp. 295–319). New York: Academic Press.

Rutter, M., & Quinton, D. (1977). Psychiatric disorder – Ecological factors and concepts of causation. In H. McGurk (Ed.), *Ecological factors in human development.* Amsterdam: North-Holland.

Sackett, G. P. (1981). A nonhuman primate model for studying causes and effects of poor pregnancy outcomes. In S. Friedman & M. Sigman (Eds.), *Preterm birth and psychological development* (pp. 41–63). New York: Academic Press.

Sameroff, A. J., (1975). Early influences on development: Fact or fancy? *Merrill-Palmer Quarterly, 21,* 267–294.

Sapolsky, R. (1992). *Stress, the aging brain, and the mechanisms of neuron death.* Cambridge, Mass.: MIT Press.

Sapolsky, R., Krey, L., & McEwen, B. (1985). Prolonged glucocorticoid exposure reduces hippocampal neural number: Implications for aging. *Journal of Neuroscience, 5,* 1222–1227.

Schneider, M. L. (1992a). The effect of mild stress during pregnancy on birth weight and neuromotor maturation in rhesus monkey infants (*Macaca mulatta*). *Infant Behavior and Development, 15,* 389–403.

Schneider, M. L. (1992b). Delayed object permanence development in prenatally stressed rhesus monkey infants (*Macaca mulatta*). *Occupational Therapy Journal of Research, 12*(2), 96–110.

Schneider, M. L. (1992c). Prenatal stress exposure alters postnatal behavioral expression under conditions of novelty challenge in rhesus monkey infants. *Developmental Psychobiology, 25*(7), 529–540.

Schneider, M. L., Clarke, A. S., Kraemer, G. W., Roughton, E. C., Lubach, G. R., Rimm-Kaufman, S. E., Schmidt, D., & Ebert, M. (1998). Prenatal stress alters brain biogenic amine levels in primates. *Development and Psychopathology, 10,* 427–440.

Schneider, M. L., & Coe, C. L. (1993). Repeated social stress during pregnancy impairs neuromotor development of the primate infant. *Journal of Developmental and Behavioral Pediatrics, 14*(2), 81–87.

Schneider, M. L., Coe, C. L., & Lubach, G. R. (1992). Endocrine activation mimics the adverse effects of prenatal stress on the neuromotor development of the infant primate. *Developmental Psychobiology, 25*(6), 427–439.

Schneider, M. L., & Moore, C. F. (2000). Effect of prenatal stress on development: A nonhuman primate model. In C. Nelson (Ed.), *Minnesota Symposium on Child Psychology* (pp. 201–243). Mahwah, NJ: Erlbaum.

Schneider, M. L., Moore, C. F., & Becker, E. F. (2001). Timing of moderate alcohol exposure during pregnancy and neonatal outcome in rhesus monkeys *(Macaca mulatta)*. *Alcoholism: Clinical and Experimental Research 25*(8), 1238–1246.

Schneider, M. L., Moore, C., Suomi, S. J., & Champoux, M. (1991). Laboratory assessment of temperament and environmental enrichment in rhesus monkey infants *(Macaca mulatta)*. *American Journal of Primatology, 25*, 137–155.

Schneider, M. L., Roughton, E. C., Koehler, A., & Lubach, G. R. (1999). Growth and development following prenatal stress in primates: An examination of ontogenetic vulnerability. *Child Development, 70*, 263–274.

Schneider, M. L., Roughton, E. C., & Lubach, G. R. (1997). Moderate alcohol consumption and psychological stress during pregnancy induces attention and neuromotor impairments in primate infants. *Child Development, 68*, 747–759.

Schneider, M. L., & Suomi, S. J. (1992). Neurobehavioral assessment in rhesus monkey neonates *(Macaca mulatta)*: Developmental changes, behavioral stability, and early experience. *Infant Behavior and Development, 15*(2), 155–177.

Schwartz L. B. (1997). Understanding human parturition. *Lancet, 350*, 1792–1793.

Seligman, M. E. P. (1975). *Helplessness: On depression, development and death.* San Francisco: W. H. Freeman.

Selye, H. (1936). A syndrome produced by severe noxious agents. *Nature (London), 138*, 32–41.

Sharpley, A. L., Elliot, J. M., & Attenburrow, M. J. (1994). Slow-wave sleep in humans: Role of 5-HT2a and 5-HT2c receptors. *Neuropharmacology, 33*, 467–471.

Stanfield, B. B., Caviness, V. S., & Cowan, W. M. (1979). The organization of certain afferents to the hippocampus and dentate gyrus in normal and reeler mice. *Journal of Comparative Neurology, 185*, 461–483.

Sutton, R. E., Koob, G. F., Le Moal, M., Rivier, J., & Vale, W. (1982). Corticotropin releasing factor (CRF) produces behavioral activation in rats. *Nature, 297*, 331–333.

Swanson, J. M., McBurnett, K., Christian, D. L., & Wigal, T. (1995). Stimulant medications and the treatment of children with ADHD. In T. H. Ollendick & J. Prinz (Eds.), *Advances in clinical child psychology* (pp. 265–315). New York: Plenum.

Takahashi, L. K., & Kalin, N. H. (1991). Early developmental and temporal characteristics of stress-induced secretion of pituitary-adrenal hormones in prenatally stressed pups. *Brain Research, 558*, 75–78.

Takahashi, L. K., Kalin, N. H., Barksdale, C. M., Vanden Burgt, J. A., & Brownfield, M. S. (1988). Stressor controllability during pregnancy influences pituitary-adrenal hormone concentrations and analgesic responsiveness in offspring. *Physiology & Behavior, 42*, 323–329.

Takahashi, L. K., Turner, J. G., & Kalin, N. H. (1992). Prenatal stress alters brain catecholaminergic activity and potentiates stress-induced behavior in adult rats. *Brain Research, 574*, 131–137.

Tennes, K., & Carter, D. (1973). Plasma cortisol levels and behavioral states in early infancy. *Psychosomatic Medicine, 35*, 121–128.

Thompson, W. R. (1957). Influence of prenatal maternal anxiety on emotionality in young rats. *Science, 15*, 698–699.

Tortella, F. C., Echevarria, E., Pastel, R. H., Cox, B., & Blackburn, T. P. (1989). Suppressant effects of selective 5-HT2 antagonists on rapid eye movement sleep in rats. *Brain Research 485*, 294–300.

Uno, H., Lohmiller, L., Thieme, C., Kemnitz, J. W., Engle, M. J., Roecker, E. B., & Farrell, P. M. (1990). Brain damage induced by prenatal exposure to dexamethasone in fetal rhesus macaques: I. Hippocampus. *Developmental Brain Research, 53*, 157–167.

Virkkunen, M., Goldman, D., Nielsen, D. A., & Linnoila, M. (1995). Low brain serotonin turnover rate (low CSF 5-HIAA) and impulsive violence. *Journal of Psychiatry & Neuroscience, 20*(4), 271–275.

Wadhwa, P. D. (1998). Prenatal stress and life-span development. In H. S. Friedman (Ed.), *Encyclopedia of Mental Health* (Vol. 3, pp. 265–280). San Diego, Calif.: Academic Press.

Wadhwa, P. D., Dunkel-Schetter, C., Chicz-DeMet, A., Porto, M., & Sandman, C. A. (1996). Prenatal psychosocial factors and the neuroendocrine axis in human pregnancy. *Psychosomatic Medicine, 58*, 432–446.

Ward, A. J. (1990). A comparison and analysis of the presence of family problems during pregnancy of mothers of "autistic" children and mothers of normal children. *Child Psychiatry and Human Development, 20*, 279–288.

Ward, A. J. (1991). Prenatal stress and childhood psychopathology. *Child Psychiatry and Human Development, 22*, 97–110.

Weinstock, M. (1997). Does prenatal stress impair coping and regulation of hypothalamic-pituitary-adrenal axis? *Neuroscience & Biobehavioral Reviews, 21*, 1–10.

Weir, R. J. Paintin, D. B., Brown, J. J., Fraser, R., Lever, A. F., Robertson, J. I., & Young, J. (1971). A serial study in pregnancy of the plasma concentration of renin, corticosteroids, electrolytes and proteins and of haematocrit and plasma volume. *Journal of Obstetrics and Gynaecology of the British Commonwealth, 78*, 590–602.

Williams, M. T., Hennessy, M. B., & Davis, H. N. (1995). CRF administered to pregnant rats alters offspring behavior and morphology. *Pharmacology Biochemistry & Behavior, 52*, 161–167.

Wyatt, R. J., Apud, J. A., & Potkins, S. (1996). New directions in the prevention and treatment of schizophrenia: A biological perspective. *Psychiatry, 59*(4), 357–370.

Zecevic, N., & Rakic, P. (1991). Synaptogenesis in monkey somatosensory cortex. *Cerebral Cortex, 1*, 510–523.

EIGHT

Nonhuman Primate Models of Developmental Psychopathology

Problems and Prospects

Dario Maestripieri and Kim Wallen

In the last two decades, research in developmental psychopathology and neuroscience has made considerable progress. Although we have learned a great deal about the time course of neural development and of psychopathology, some basic questions concerning the interaction between neurobiological and behavioral development still remain unanswered (Cicchetti, 1993). For example, we still do not know whether the emergence of a specific psychopathology requires activation of maladaptive processes during a time-critical window of vulnerability or whether simple alterations in the order or timing of neurobiological events during normal development are sufficient to induce psychopathology.

The differentiation of species, organ systems, and neural systems all involve sequencing the activation and suppression of a suite of genes and their products (Eisenberg, 1995). Changes in the endogenous timing mechanisms that regulate this programmed gene expression could affect the physical organization of the developing nervous system so that the organism's sensitivity to environmental stimuli is permanently enhanced or reduced. Altered sensitivity to the environment could then lead the organism to a developmental pathway that is atypical for the species. Alternatively, a change in timing may not be reflected in the physical organization of the developing nervous system, but advancing or delaying the deployment of a neural system could make a different system vulnerable to modification. In this view, the change in timing affects the developmental context of systems that are already in place, ultimately altering their function. Finally, changes in timing of neurobiological events early in life could create windows of vulnerability during which the developing organism may be particularly sensitive to environmental influences. Thus, temporal changes in the activation and suppression of genes regulating neural development could interact with environmental factors in the development of psychopathology.

Knowledge of the relation between neurological and behavioral development in normal and atypical populations provides the foundation for understanding the development of psychopathology (Cicchetti & Cannon, 1999). Most primate models of psychopathology, however, have been built on the simple theoretical notion that stressful events early in life can result in pathological development without precise knowledge

This work was supported by NIMH grants R01-MH57249, R01-MH62577 and K02-MH63097.

of the mechanisms through which variation in early experience normally leads individuals to follow different developmental pathways. Moreover, most of these models have not considered individual differences in vulnerability or resilience to the effects of early stress due to the presence of different risk and protective factors. Thus, the potential usefulness of primate models of developmental psychopathology has not always been fully exploited.

Similar to humans, primates have an extended period of postnatal growth and maturation in which the developing neural and neuroendocrine systems have ample opportunity to be influenced by experience (Nelson & Bloom, 1997). In addition, like humans, primate infants develop in a rich social environment where, from very early on, they experience intense and complex interactions with their caregivers and peers. These characteristics of primate development have led researchers to focus on alterations in the developing infant's social environment as possible antecedents to the development of psychopathology. Two principal manipulations have been used to alter primate development. The first deprives the developing individual, either in part or totally, of social experience, while the second alters the quality of the social experience, primarily by modifying interactions between the infant and its caregiver.

In this chapter we first review several primate paradigms involving the deprivation of early social experience, then we review a paradigm in which the quality of early social experience is altered through environmental manipulations, and finally we discuss paradigms based on naturally occurring variability in maternal behavior. For each paradigm, we discuss the possible biological mechanisms underlying pathological development and the implications of the findings for developmental psychopathology. We conclude the chapter by outlining some prospects for future research.

THE SOCIAL DEPRIVATION PARADIGMS

Mother-Infant Separation

It has long been known that the responses of monkey infants to separation from their mothers share striking similarities with children's responses to maternal separation (Bowlby, 1969). In both cases, there is an initial phase of "protest," characterized by behavioral agitation, vocalizations, and autonomic activation, followed by a phase of "despair," characterized by behavioral depression and heightened activation of the hypothalamic-pituitary-adrenal (HPA) axis. In children, the phase of despair may be followed by detachment, so that if children are reunited with their parents, they will show lack of affection and, in some cases, active avoidance. The extent to which detachment is also shown by monkey infants, however, remains unclear.

Research on mother-infant separation in monkeys has been conducted for several decades in a number of different laboratories. The scientific rationale for this research, however, has changed over the years. Early separation studies were designed to evaluate the mechanisms underlying mother-infant attachment, such as the importance of the mother as a source of contact comfort versus nutrition (Harlow, 1959). Interest in separation as a paradigm to investigate the nature of attachment has persisted over the years under the assumption that investigating the mechanisms underlying the disruption of the mother-infant bond could also provide useful information to understand the formation and maintenance of such bond (Kraemer, 1992; Reite, 1987). Some researchers, however, have challenged such assumptions and argued that responses to maternal separation are better viewed within the framework of responsiveness to stress than within the framework of attachment (Insel, 1992; Levine & Wiener, 1988). Consequently, the separation response per se has attracted a great deal of interest as a prototype of the organism's response to stress (Levine & Wiener, 1988).

Investigation of responses to maternal separation has also been stimulated by the prospect that they could provide a primate model for human clinical depression (McKinney & Bunney, 1969; Reite, 1977). Although some researchers were careful not to claim great face validity for the separation model of depression (e.g., McKinney, 1977), the primate response to separation has generally been viewed as a useful paradigm to investigate the biological correlates of depressive symptoms. In any case, whether the separation response was investigated from the perspective of attachment, stress, or as a model for clinical depression, the research has been characterized by a shift from the description of behavioral changes following separation to the investigation of a number of biological variables, including heart rate, body temperature, electroencephalogram (EEG), sleep patterns, cortisol, and immune function (e.g., Levine & Wiener, 1988; Reite, 1985).

Reviewing the studies investigating the acute responses to maternal separation is beyond the scope of this chapter because such studies generally were not conducted within a clear developmental framework (see Mineka & Suomi, 1978, for a review). More relevant to the focus of this chapter, however, is the research that has investigated the long-term developmental effects of maternal separation and other stressful early experiences. Interest in studying the long-term consequences of maternal separation for primate infant development has developed along two independent lines of research: one investigating the long-term developmental effects of short separation-reunion experiences, and the other investigating the long-term developmental effects of permanent maternal separation and social deprivation rearing.

Long-Term Effects of Short Separations

The earliest studies of the long-term effects of short separation experiences were independently conducted in Hinde's and Harlow's laboratories in the early 1970s. In one study of rhesus monkeys, Spencer-Booth and Hinde (1971) separated infants from their mothers for six or thirteen days at the age of 21–32 weeks. Infant activity and performance in a variety of tests were assessed when infants were twelve and thirty months old and compared to those of infants that had never been separated from their mothers. There were few or no behavioral differences in infant interactions with their mothers or in their tendency to approach novel objects in the home cage. When tested in a novel environment, however, the previously separated infants showed significantly greater disturbance of behavior, lower exploration, and lower manipulation of novel objects than controls. Such differences were evident at both twelve and thirty months of age, although they were less marked when the animals were older. Hinde et al. (1978) subsequently reported some other effects of a brief maternal separation on mother-infant interactions five months after the separation, and Stevenson-Hinde et al. (1980) reported some differences in subjectively assessed personality measures in the previously separated infants.

In Harlow's laboratory, the studies investigating the long-term effects of short separations involved rhesus infants that had been separated from their mothers at birth and then reared with peers. An early study by Suomi et al. (1970) reported that repetitive separations of rhesus infants from their peers resulted in severe retardation of social development. Similarly, Mineka et al. (1981) found that repetitive peer separations of juvenile and adolescent rhesus monkeys resulted in long-lasting differences in the way individuals reacted with depression to separation. Interestingly, rhesus females that had exhibited depressive reactions to repeated separations were more likely to neglect or abuse their offspring than females that had shown little or no depression in response to separation (Suomi & Ripp, 1983).

The long-term effects of brief separations from the mother were investigated by Suomi et al. (1983). In this study, four infants were subjected to repeated four-day maternal separations conducted between the third and ninth month of life. The separated infants spent more time in contact with their mothers following reunion, although the relative role played by mother and infant in maintaining contact was not assessed. Separated infants and controls showed few or no differences in response to permanent separation from their mothers, which occurred at the age of forty-three weeks, and during the subsequent seven months of peer housing. When separated infants and controls were exposed to their mothers, seven months after permanent separation, previously separated infants showed less interest in interacting with them than did controls. Thus, although the long-term effects of early separations seemed to disappear in some situations (e.g., peer housing), they were apparent in others (e.g., in the presence of mothers). The mechanisms underlying the long-term effects of peer or maternal separations remained unclear.

The only studies of the long-term effects of brief maternal separations in a species other than the rhesus monkey were conducted with pigtail macaques by Reite and colleagues. Caine et al. (1983) reported that six pigtail infants who experienced a ten-day maternal separation at 4–7 months of age did not differ in dominance rank but were rated as less sociable than controls at the age of 40.7 months. Capitanio and Reite (1984) reported that previously separated infants had fewer social contact preferences, and Capitanio et al. (1986) reported that they showed more disturbance behavior and longer latency to retrieve food (but no difference in cortisol levels) in a novel environment than controls when tested 2.5–4.9 years after the separation experience. Finally, Laudenslager et al. (1985) found that, when previously separated individuals were 4–7 years old, they showed a suppression of the in vitro lymphocyte proliferation in response to B cell and T cell mitogens, suggesting that the early separation experience resulted in altered immune function. In reviewing these studies, Reite (1987) argued that possible long-term alterations in maternal behavior following early separation and reunion may have been the mechanism underlying the developmental effects of early separation on infant behavior and physiology. Although no primate data are available to support this hypothesis, data obtained with rodents suggest that changes in maternal behavior following repeated separation from pups and pup handling result in long-term alterations in behavior and in the activity of the HPA axis in the pups (Liu et al., 1997).

Reite (1987) suggested that the early separation paradigm could provide a valid primate model for clinical problems in the failure-to-thrive area, where inadequate mothering appears to play an important role in the impairment of somatic and biobehavioral development. The lack of further research on the long-term consequences of brief separation experiences during early development, however, has prevented a comprehensive understanding of the nature of such effects as well as of their underlying mechanisms. Thus, the question of whether the effects of early separation should be viewed as the direct consequence of an acute stressful experience or as mediated by subsequent alterations in maternal behavior remains unanswered. Likewise, the usefulness of this primate paradigm for developmental psychopathology remains unclear.

Long-Term Effects of Early Social Deprivation

Although the long-term consequences of brief separation experiences have been investigated in only a few studies, a great deal more is known about the effects of permanent maternal separation. Because permanent separation between mother and infant in the laboratory is usually followed by rearing the infant in condition of total or partial social deprivation, the developmental aberrations exhibited by permanently separated infants are best viewed as the result of their rearing environment rather than of the maternal separation experience per se.

Many studies conducted in the 1960s and 1970s showed that rearing primate infants under condition of total isolation can have devastating effects on subsequent development and behavior (see Suomi, 1982, 1991 for reviews). These effects, usually subsumed under the label of "isolation syndrome," have been best studied in rhesus monkeys. At the behavioral level, they include displays of abnormal self-directed and stereotypic behavior and gross deficits in all aspects of social interactions, including affiliation, aggression, communication, mating, and parenting. Isolation effects are generally more pronounced when infants are isolated early in life and for at least six months, and when infants are denied access to any sensory stimuli from conspecifics. Denial of tactile contact appears to have more dramatic effects on infant development than denial of visual, auditory, and olfactory stimuli. Isolation rearing, however, generally involves the simultaneous deprivation of social and nonsocial sensory stimuli as well as the deprivation of different types of social stimuli.

The behavioral effects of isolation rearing generally persist into adulthood. Although some procedures, such as pairing a previously isolated infant with a nonisolated same-aged monkey "therapist," can reverse some of the social deficits displayed by isolates (Novak & Harlow, 1975; Suomi & Harlow, 1972), these individuals can rarely be successfully reintegrated into a complex social group with other mother-reared individuals (Anderson & Mason, 1974, 1978). Other environmental or pharmacological treatments may temporarily reduce abnormal behavior, but the isolation syndrome usually returns if the treatment is withdrawn (Kraemer, 1992). Recovery from isolation rearing is considerably more effective in some species of monkeys and apes than in others (Dienske & de Jonge, 1982). Although in some cases the differential effects of early isolation in different species can be accounted for by differences in life-history and social organization (e.g., the solitary orang-utans appear to be affected by social deprivation to a lesser extent than the highly social chimpanzees), in other cases the causes of interspecific differences in vulnerability to early social deprivation are less clear (e.g., in the case of closely related macaque species; Sackett et al., 1976).

In recent years, research on the long-term effects of isolation rearing has shifted its focus from behavior to physiology and neuroanatomy. This shift has been accompanied by technological advances in the assessment of brain structure and neurochemical activity. Studies of the effects of early isolation on neuroendocrine function and neuroanatomy were pioneered by Kraemer, McKinney, and their collaborators. Kraemer and colleagues reported that previously isolated rhesus monkeys showed considerable developmental variation in cerebrospinal fluid (CSF) concentrations of norepinephrine, dopamine, and serotonin metabolites relative to controls as well as lack of correlation between the different monoamine metabolites (Kraemer & McKinney, 1979; Kraemer et al., 1989). These effects persisted years after the isolation experience. Previously isolated and subsequently "rehabilitated" rhesus monkeys were also behaviorally and neurochemically hypersensitive to d-amphetamine. After the pharmacological treatment, they showed striking increases in aggressive/submissive behavior and in CSF concentrations of norepinephrine and the serotonin metabolite 5-hydroxy-indoleacetic acid (5-HIAA) (but not of the dopamine metabolite homovanilic acid, HVA; Kraemer et al., 1983, 1984). On the basis of these findings, Kraemer (1992) hypothesized that isolation rearing may produce cytoarchitectural changes in brain biogenic amine systems that result in a functional dysregulation of these systems.

Neuroanatomical alterations of isolation-reared monkeys have subsequently been reported in such brain areas as basal ganglia, hippocampus, cerebellum, corpus callosum, and neocortex. For example, isolates showed changes in dendritic branching in the neocortex (Struble & Riesen, 1978), modifications in Purkinje cell structure in the cerebellum (Floeter & Greenough, 1979), fewer tyrosine hydroxylase-immunoreactive fibers in the dopaminergic neurons of the neocortex (Morrison et al., 1990), altered chemoarchitecture of some basal ganglia regions (but not of the amygdala and other basal forebrain regions; Martin et al., 1991), cytoskeletal changes in the dentate gyrus cells of the hippocampus (Siegel et al., 1993), and reduced size of the corpus callosum (Sanchez et al., 1998). Several studies, however, reported lack of significant differences between isolates and controls in monoamine metabolite concentrations (Lewis et al., 1990), tyrosine hydroxylase- and corticotropin-releasing factor (CRF)- immunoreactive neurons in the paraventricular nucleus and arcuate nucleus of the hypothalamus (Ginsberg et al., 1993a), noradrenergic innervation density of the paraventricular nucleus of the hypothalamus (Ginsberg et al., 1993b), and overall brain volume (Sanchez et al., 1998). In some cases, long-term developmental effects of isolation rearing on brain structure or neurotransmitter systems were not directly observed but inferred from altered responses to pharmacological challenges. For example, Lewis et al. (1990) reported changes in dopamine receptor function following apomorphine challenge in previously isolated rhesus monkeys. Similarly, Coplan et al. (1992) reported differential effects of a low dose (but not of a high dose) of yohimbine in isolation-reared bonnet macaques and controls. These results were consistent with previous ones in suggesting that isolation rearing altered neurodevelopment of the noradrenergic system and/or other monoamine systems.

Further information on the long-term consequences of early social deprivation for behavioral and neuroendocrine development has been provided by studies using the peer-rearing paradigm (Chamove et al., 1973; Harlow, 1969). In this paradigm, rhesus infants are usually permanently separated from their mothers within hours after birth, hand-raised in a nursery for one or two months, and thereafter housed in small groups of same-aged infants. A longitudinal study of peer-reared versus mother-reared rhesus infants showed that, as neonates, the former were more awake, active, and irritable than the latter (Champoux et al., 1991). From one to five months of age, the peer-reared infants exhibited a greater variety of behaviors relative to the mother-reared infants, which spent most of their time in contact with their mothers. As juveniles, the two groups of individuals were indistinguishable with the exception that the peer-reared individuals showed more self-directed behaviors. Other studies have found that peer-reared juveniles showed more distress in a novel environment than mother-reared juveniles (Chamove et al., 1973; Higley, Hopkins, et al., 1992; Kraemer & McKinney, 1979; but see Shannon et al., 1998).

Research investigating the long-term consequences of peer rearing for physiological development, particularly the activity of the HPA axis, has produced some conflicting results. In various studies comparing cortisol levels, peer-reared individuals have been reported to have higher basal cortisol levels than mother-reared individuals (first month of life; Champoux et al., 1989; first 2 years of life: Higley, Suomi, et al., 1992), lower basal cortisol levels (14–30 days of age: Shannon et al., 1998), or lower basal ACTH but similar cortisol levels (1–6 months of age: Clarke, 1993). Studies comparing peer-reared and isolation-reared animals have reported higher basal cortisol levels in peer-reared animals (19 months of age: Sackett et al., 1973) or no differences in cortisol levels (4 years of age: Meyer & Bowman, 1972). When physiological responses to stressful challenges were assessed, some studies found no differences in cortisol levels between peer-reared, mother-reared, and isolation-reared monkeys (Champoux et al., 1989; Meyer & Bowman, 1972; Sackett et al., 1973), one study found that peer-reared monkeys had lower increases in ACTH and cortisol than mother-reared monkeys (Clarke, 1993), and another study reported that the cortisol levels of peer-reared monkeys were higher than those of isolation-reared monkeys but similar to those of mother-reared monkeys (Shannon et al., 1998). Shannon et al. (1998) suggested that these discrepancies in the activity of the HPA axis in relation to early rearing may have resulted from differences in the housing environment, type of stressful experiences, feeding regimen, or diurnal variation in HPA axis activity across studies. Given that prolonged cortisol elevation produces changes in central components of the HPA axis (Uno et al., 1989), persistent cortisol elevations induced by isolation rearing may be responsible for some of the behavioral and neuroanatomical alterations observed in the isolation-reared monkeys later in life. Unfortunately, the conflicting findings concerning early rearing environment and the activity of the HPA axis prevent one from making strong inferences about the possible mechanisms underlying the neuroanatomical alterations observed in socially deprived animals.

More consistent and promising findings have been obtained by studies investigating the consequences of peer-rearing for CSF concentrations of monoamine metabolites. In a study comparing rhesus monkeys that were peer-reared or mother-reared in the first six months of life, Higley et al. (1991) reported that peer-reared males but not females had higher levels of 5-HIAA at six and eighteen months than mother-reared males. Peer-reared subjects also had higher values of the noradrenaline metabolite 3-methoxy-4-hydroxyphenylglycol (MHPG; see also Higley, Suomi, et al., 1992). No rearing effects on the dopamine metabolite HVA levels were found. In a related longitudinal study, no differences in CSF concentrations of 5-HIAA were found between peer-reared and mother-reared monkeys in the first 1.5 years of life (Higley, Suomi, et al., 1992). The higher levels of MHPG in peer-reared monkeys were consistent with previous findings by Kraemer et al. (1989) in suggesting that rearing under conditions of social deprivation results in enhanced noradrenergic activity and responsivity to stress. There is some evidence, however, that early experiences interact with genetic factors in determining later CSF concentrations of monoamine metabolites (Higley et al., 1993).

In follow-up studies, peer-reared subjects exhibited lower CSF 5-HIAA concentrations at fifty months of age than mother-reared individuals (Higley, King, et al., 1996). Peer-reared subjects also consumed more alcohol than mother-reared subjects during baseline conditions. Mother-reared subjects, however, increased their rates of alcohol consumption when the CSF was obtained during a social separation experience. When peer-reared and mother-reared juveniles were observed in social groups, individuals with low CSF 5-HIAA and MHPG concentrations from both rearing groups exhibited reduced rates of social interaction and low dominance rank (Higley, Mehlman, et al., 1996). In addition, peer-reared subjects with low CSF 5-HIAA concentrations exhibited inept social behaviors and were frequently removed from their social groups for excessive aggression and deviant social behaviors. Based on these findings, Higley and colleagues suggested that the peer-rearing paradigm aggravated the negative social consequences associated with low CSF 5-HIAA and hypothesized that early experiences may generally contribute to brain serotonin changes that increase the disposition to early alcohol consumption. Consistent with this hypothesis, Heinz et al. (1998) recently reported that five-year-old rhesus monkeys that were separated from their mothers after birth showed considerable functional polymorphism of the serotonin transporter gene. In particular, there was a significant negative correlation between beta-GIT binding to serotonin transporters in the brain stem and 5-HIAA concentrations in CSF. Animals with greater beta-CIT binding and low CSF 5-HIAA concentrations displayed greater aggressiveness and were less sensitive to alcohol-induced intoxication.

Mechanisms Underlying the Effects of Social Deprivation Rearing and Relevance for Developmental Psychopathology

There is now considerable evidence that various conditions of sensory and social deprivation in early life can result in long-term alterations in behavior, neuroendocrine function, and neuroanatomy. Unfortunately, most studies in this area have not discussed the potential mechanisms underlying the observed alterations or the relevance of this research for developmental psychopathology. In most cases, authors have simply interpreted their findings as evidence that "early experience" or "environmental factors" play an important role in the development of specific neurotransmitter systems (e.g., Coplan et al., 1992; Martin et al., 1991). Early infancy in primates is a period characterized by a high degree of neuronal migration, synaptogenesis, receptor expression, and cytoarchitectonic elaboration. The brain systems that undergo the most postnatal maturation are likely to be the most vulnerable to postnatal stress. However, what aspects of the deprived rearing environment are responsible for the observed developmental alterations and the mechanisms through which such alterations occur remain unclear.

Kraemer (1992) speculated that there may be two conceptually distinct mechanisms by which early rearing can leave more mature individuals vulnerable to adverse responses to disrupted attachment. One is mediated by the effects of early maternal separation and isolation rearing on the development of brain biogenic amine systems. Assuming that the mother's presence plays an important role in regulating the infant's emotional development, isolation rearing would bring about a dysregulation of the neurochemical systems underlying the organism's responsiveness to stress. The other mechanism may be cognitive, yet, according to Kraemer (1992), it also relates to the biogenic amine component. In this view, socially deprived infants may fail to acquire critical aspects of social cognition as they develop, which would normally enable them to engage in complex social interactions and to cope with the effects of social attachment disruption.

Although Kraemer is probably correct in arguing that early social deprivation results in altered development at both the neurobiological and cognitive levels, the fact that deprivation rearing combines and confounds different forms of deprivation (e.g., motor, sensory, and social) and stress (physical and psychosocial) makes it difficult to assess the specific mechanisms and pathways through which early adverse experience alters the course of normal biobehavioral development. Similarly, the developmental effects of the peer-rearing environment are not easy to interpret. It is almost impossible to assess whether peer-reared monkeys differ from mother-reared ones because they lacked a mother, because they were hand-raised by humans in a nursery in their first month of life, or because they had the opportunity to interact with peers much earlier than the mother-reared monkeys. In fact, in developmental studies comparing peer-reared versus mother-reared monkeys, these variables are usually confounded. Unfortunately, in order for developmental psychopathology models to be useful and testable, there is a need to specify the processes through which early experience may influence the course of development (Greenberg, 1999). Therefore the relevance and usefulness of the social deprivation rearing paradigm for developmental psychopathology still remains to be established.

Some researchers who have used the isolation-rearing paradigm have acknowledged that the conditions of extreme deprivation imposed to monkey infants are rarely, if ever, experienced by humans (e.g., Reite, 1987; Rosenblum et al., 1994; Suomi, 1982). Consequently, they have argued that the usefulness of the primate isolation syndrome as a model of a specific human psychopathology is limited (e.g., Suomi, 1982). Others, however, have pointed out the behavioral similarities between the isolation syndrome and several human psychopathologies including autism, schizophrenia, antisocial personality disorder, and explosive violence syndrome (e.g., Kraemer, 1992; Kraemer et al., 1983). Higley and colleagues have argued that the peer-rearing paradigm can be useful to understand how individual genetic characteristics interact with adverse early experiences in producing the behavioral and personality characteristics (e.g., impaired impulse control and violent and antisocial behaviors) that are associated with early alcohol abuse (Heinz et al., 1998; Higley & Bennett, 1999). Coplan et al. (1995) have argued that the rearing paradigms can "provide environmental phenocopies of biologic disturbances analogous to genetically determined affective dysregulation observed in human psychopathology." Finally, some authors have suggested that the isolation-rearing paradigm, or its milder version the peer-rearing paradigm, have implications useful for understanding both normative and pathological aspects of attachment formation or disruption (e.g., Higley, Hopkins, et al., 1992; Reite & Short, 1983).

Although the findings of primate studies using the social deprivation paradigm have often been discussed using the concepts and terminology of attachment theory (Maestripieri, in press), the parallels between the environment of socially deprived monkey infants and the environment in which most human infants and children develop attachment to their caregivers and peers are not immediately apparent. More important, the living conditions and developmental experiences of socially deprived monkeys are so different from those of their free-ranging conspecifics as to question the generalizability of the findings of this research across environments, let alone across species. For example, one may argue that the early loss of the mother in the natural environment of macaque monkeys is unlikely to bring about behavioral, physiological, and neuroanatomical developmental deficits similar to those observed in the laboratory. Similarly, it is unlikely that monkey infants in their natural environment will grow up in a social environment comparable to that provided by the peer-rearing paradigm in the laboratory.

Primate research conducted with the social deprivation paradigm has undoubtedly contributed some general principles to the field of developmental psychopathology, including that (1) the early experiences that deviate greatly from the norm are those most likely to result in long-term deficits, (2) the most dramatic long-term effects will be most likely to be observed after stressful challenges, and (3) there may be considerable interindividual variability in the extent to which early experiences affect biobehavioral development (Suomi, 1991). One may question, however, whether these general principles alone warrant the further use of social deprivation paradigm, the use of any primate model of developmental psychopathology, or research with animal models in general. In fact, it may be argued that such general principles could probably be derived from developmental studies of any mammalian species, including humans. We believe, however, that research with primate models can not only contribute some general principles to the field of developmental psychopathology but also elucidate the specific mechanisms and pathways underlying psychopathological development in humans. In this regard, however, the social deprivation paradigm has already shown its limitations and other experimental paradigms are necessary.

THE FORAGING PARADIGM

The foraging paradigm was developed as a model of adverse early experience that may have long-lasting consequences for behavioral and neurobiological development without imposing the dramatic and traumatic experiences of maternal separation and social deprivation. Although the foraging paradigm is often viewed as a model of altered rearing environment, in reality the experimental manipulation involved in this paradigm occurs in a relatively short period of infant development. Therefore, the foraging paradigm may be best viewed as involving an acute stressor during development rather than a long-term manipulation of the rearing environment.

In an early study of acute food deprivation in captive pigtail and bonnet macaques, Rosenblum et al. (1969) noted that during the food deprivation period, pigtail yearlings increased the amount of time spent in contact with their mothers and decreased the frequency of play with their peers. In contrast, no effect of food deprivation was found on the behavior of bonnet infants of similar age. Based on this preliminary study and the work by Collier and colleagues with birds and rodents (e.g., Collier & Rovee-Collier, 1980), subsequent efforts were devoted to manipulating not only the amount of food available to the animals but also the difficulty of food procurement or "foraging demand."

When mother-infant pairs were first tested in the foraging paradigm by Rosenblum and Paully (1984), it was hypothesized that when food was sparse and a great deal of work was required to obtain it, mothers would encourage early independence. On the other hand, an ecologically demanding and unpredictable environment could jeopardize offspring survival and hence should result in greater maternal protectiveness. As a consequence of these conflicting demands on the mother, her ability to cope with environmental stress and mediate her infant's successful interactions with conspecifics was expected to be impaired.

These hypotheses were tested in a study in which three groups of five mother-infant pairs were each exposed to a different foraging treatment: Low Foraging Demand (LFD), High Foraging Demand (HFD), and Variable Foraging Demand (VFD). In the LFD condition, animals had access to ad libitum food, and such food could be retrieved without effort. In the HFD condition, animals had access to six times less food than the LFD animals. Finally, in the VFD condition, animals were exposed to a two-week alternation of HFD and LFD. The treatment period began when infant ages ranged from four to seventeen weeks and lasted fourteen weeks. In this study, food was provided by a foraging apparatus consisting of three rectangles of iron mesh attached to each other with their openings in line creating a series of channels. Monkeys could not see the food in the channels but could retrieve it by reaching through the mesh channels. In later studies, the HFD condition also involved digging food buried under 12 cm of woodchip bedding whereas in the LFD condition no digging was required.

Rosenblum and Paully (1984) reported that HFD mothers had daily foraging scores five times higher than those of LFD mothers, but VFD animals did not show any consistent differences in foraging activities in the LFD and HFD conditions, except for the day after the change in condition. The change from LFD to HFD, however, was associated with an increase in agonistic behavior between adults and a decrease in mother-infant contact. Mother-infant proximity, infant object exploration, and infant play also decreased to a minimum in the HFD condition. Relative to the LFD and HFD animals, the VDF adults had the highest scores of agonism and the lowest scores of affiliation. Likewise, maternal rejection and infant contacts were higher in VFD than in either HFD or LFD. Infant behavior in the VFD condition was interpreted as "disturbed" or suggestive of "anxious attachment."

Andrews and Rosenblum (1991) later replicated this study, this time using only six VFD mother-infant pairs and six LFD pairs. As in the earlier study, there were no differences in foraging between the HD and LD conditions for the VFD animals. In fact, foraging only occurred less than 10 percent of the time in both conditions. The only significant difference in mother-infant interaction was that VFD pairs were more likely to be separated during HD periods than LD periods. There were also few or no differences in mother-infant interactions between VFD and LFD animals. VFD and LFD pairs did not differ in the percentage of contacts broken by mothers, contacts made by mothers, and maternal rejections. There was no difference in total time spent out of contact, but the mean duration of the time bouts spent out of contact was shorter for the VFD pairs.

Shortly after the foraging treatments, mothers and infants were tested for one hour in a novel room for four consecutive days. Mother-infant pairs in both groups spent more time in contact in the novel room, but the increase was more marked for the VFD pairs. This difference was attributed to the finding that VFD infants broke contact with their mothers less frequently than LFD infants did. VFD infants also showed less object exploration and play. No information, however, was provided on the extent to which mothers controlled their infants' movements by restraining. Thus, it is not clear whether differences in mother-infant interactions were the result of differences in maternal behavior or infant activity, or both. After the novel environment test, three LFD infants and three VFD infants were subjected to repeated one-day separations and reunions with their mothers. No difference between groups in responses to separation or reunion was observed (Andrews & Rosenblum, 1993a). This was in contrast to an earlier finding showing that the HFD infants reacted with more depression to separation than did the LFD infants (Plimpton & Rosenblum, 1983). Another novel environment test after the separations, however, differentiated again between the two groups. As in the previous novel environment test, LFD infants made more frequent excursions from their mothers than VFD infants.

In subsequent studies, some minor modifications of the foraging paradigm were made but the basic findings were similar. For example, an attempt to manipulate the infant's motivation to be in contact with the mother prior to acute foraging task, by briefly separating infant from the mother or by feeding the infant prior to the task, had little or no effect on mother-infant interactions during the foraging task (Andrews & Rosenblum, 1992). Restriction of infants through a wire mesh so that mothers could still make contact with them but infants were denied access to the foraging area also had little or no effect on the mother's foraging activity or on mother-infant interactions (Andrews & Rosenblum, 1993b). In a final twist of the paradigm, some VFD mothers whose infants were restrained also had to solve a video task with a computer joystick to obtain their food. In the novel environment test following the foraging treatment, these mothers' infants did not break contact with them as frequently as the other infants did, although time in contact with mothers was similar. During the following mother-infant separation procedures, there were no differences in the infants' hunched posture after separation in days 1–3, but on day 5, the infants exposed to the joystick task displayed the hunched posture more frequently. One interpretation of these findings was that, following the acute foraging task, mothers and infants presumably made an effort to "compensate" for disturbance of their relationship but that the joystick task disrupted such efforts. As a result of this disruption, the mother-infant bond was "weakened" (Andrews & Rosenblum, 1994a).

The infants who were exposed with their mothers to different foraging treatments at 1–4 months of age, including those involved in the joystick task, were the subjects of another study at the age of 2.5–3.5 years, after they had been permanently separated from their mothers and housed in peer groups. Six VFD and six LFD juveniles showed no differences in behavior in their stable social groups. However, when tested in a novel environment, LFD individuals showed more affiliative behavior toward conspecifics than VFD juveniles did. Furthermore, when the LFD and VFD cohorts were merged, the LFD juveniles became dominant over the VFD juveniles (Andrews & Rosenblum, 1994b).

In subsequent studies, VFD and LFD juveniles showed differential responses to treatment with two anxiety-provoking drugs: a noradrenergic agent (yohimbine) and a serotonergic agent (mCPP). Relative to the LFD juveniles, VFD animals were hyperresponsive to yohimbine but hyporesponsive to mCPP (Rosenblum et al., 1994). VFD juveniles also exhibited higher CSF concentrations of CRF, SOM, 5-HIAA, and HVA and lower CSF concentrations of cortisol, whereas HFD and LFD juveniles did not differ in these variables (Coplan et al., 1996, 1998). However, because at the time of the study the VFD juveniles were two years old whereas the HFD and LFD juveniles were four years old, it could not be unequivocally excluded that age and not the early foraging treatment was responsible for the observed differences. Nor was it clear whether some of the observed differences reflected altered acute HPA axis responses to capture versus chronic alterations of the HPA axis activity. Finally, Smith et al. (1997) treated VFD and LFD juveniles with the alpha2-adrenoceptor agonist clonidine and found that individuals with higher baseline CSF levels of CRF showed less growth hormone secretion in response to the challenge, a finding that was interpreted as consistent with blunting of noradrenergic responsivity in these animals.

Mechanisms Underlying the Effects of the Foraging Paradigm and Relevance for Developmental Psychopathology

The interpretation and discussion of the findings obtained with the foraging paradigm mostly focused on the mothers and infants exposed to VFD treatment. The behavior of VFD infants during the novel environment test was interpreted as indicative of insecure attachment to the mother and inability to use the mother as a secure base for exploration (Andrews et al., 1993a). In this view, VFD infants did not differ from other infants in their home cage because insecure attachment and its consequences for the developing infant may remain latent until the individual's coping capacities are challenged (Andrews et al., 1993a). To account for the finding that the VFD infants did not differ from others in their response to maternal separation and reunion, it was argued that the VFD paradigm may model most accurately the affective states associated with the anticipation of separation (i.e., anxiety) rather than those associated with the experience of separation per se (e.g., depression; Coplan et al., 1995). Furthermore, it was suggested that the negative affective states in the VFD infants may have interfered with effective learning of the type of skills that would have served them in subsequent situations to which they attempted to adapt (Coplan et al., 1995).

The effects of the VFD treatment on infant behavior and neuroendocrine function were assumed to be mediated by alterations in maternal behavior. According to Rosenblum and Paully (1984), the unpredictable variability in the environment under the VFD condition created a demand that was too difficult for the mothers to master and resulted in their being unable to make rapid adjustments in foraging. Excessive maternal attentiveness to environmental factors and failure to cope with variable demands, in turn, resulted in qualitative changes in maternal interactions with infants. VFD mothers presumably became more anxious, erratic, dismissive, less responsive to their infants' signals, and less likely to engage in the "intense compensatory patterns typical of normal mothers following periods of dyadic disturbance" (Coplan et al., 1995, 1996, 1998). Such maternal behavior resulted in a diminution of the infants' perception of a security of maternal attachment (Coplan et al., 1996) so that "the development of social patterns of VFD infants was compromised despite the absence of gross behavioral pathology" (Andrews & Rosenblum, 1994a).

While the interpretation of the findings provided by Rosenblum, Coplan, and their colleagues is certainly plausible, the empirical evidence that maternal behavior was affected by the foraging treatment is weak. For example, the finding that VFD mothers showed no differences in their foraging activities between the HD and LD conditions (Andrews & Rosenblum, 1991; Rosenblum & Paully, 1984) and that, indeed, foraging only occurred in less than 10 percent of their time (Andrews & Rosenblum, 1991), may suggest that in fact the VFD treatment did not produce a conflict of demands on the mothers and that they were able to obtain the amount of food they needed without necessarily changing their foraging behavior on a biweekly basis. This interpretation is also consistent with the few differences in VFD mother-infant interactions reported by Andrews and Rosenblum (1991). Although it was reported that VFD mothers and infants pairs were more likely to be out of contact during HD periods than LD periods, VFD and LFD pairs did not differ in the total time spent out of contact, the percentage of contacts broken by mothers, contacts made by mothers, or maternal rejections (Andrews & Rosenblum, 1991). These findings are consistent with the interpretation that bi-weekly changes in foraging demand were not associated with significant changes in mother-infant interactions. Information on maternal anxiety or maternal responsiveness to infant signals was not available and therefore it is not clear whether and how these responses were affected by the foraging treatment.

If maternal behavior was not affected by the foraging treatment, it is possible that the behavioral and neuroendocrine differences between VFD and other infants pre-existed the exposure to the foraging treatment or that they were a by-product of particular experimental procedures associated with the treatment such as environmental disturbance or exposure to and contact with human caretakers. Alternatively, it is possible that differences in maternal behavior may have been present but that such differences pre-existed the foraging treatment or manifested themselves outside the foraging treatment period and independently from it. For example, it is possible that differences in mother-infant interactions between VFD and other pairs were associated with differences in the dominance rank of their mothers, which in turn resulted in the VFD individuals becoming socially subordinate to the LFD individuals. Unfortunately, without detailed information on the previous history of the subjects and their behavior before, during, and after the foraging treatment period, such alternative hypotheses cannot be adequately investigated or dismissed. Therefore, more research is needed to investigate the mechanisms by which manipulation of the foraging demand results in long-lasting alterations of infant development.

The identification of the mechanisms by which the VFD condition is associated with developmental differences in behavior and neuroendocrine function is crucial to assess the usefulness of this paradigm as a model for human developmental psychopathology. In their most recent studies, Rosenblum, Coplan, and their colleagues proposed the VFD paradigm as a model for the development of human anxiety, panic disorder, or posttraumatic stress disorder (PTSD). For example, the behavioral hyperresponsivity of VFD individuals to yohimbine was viewed as consistent with abnormal noradrenergic responses seen in patients with panic disorder or PTSD (Rosenblum et al., 1994). Similarly, the behavior of VFD infants in the novel environment test was explicitly compared to that of insecurely attached children or that of behaviorally inhibited children (Andrews & Rosenblum, 1991; Coplan et al., 1995, 1998; Rosenblum et al., 1994). According to Coplan et al. (1995), the VDF paradigm provides an opportunity to study the potential influence of disturbed early-attachment experiences on adulthood psychobiology, relatively unconfounded by the influence of heritable factors. In fact, these authors concluded that the VDF paradigm, through its emphasis on maternal-infant interaction, may model the conditions under which human anxiety is experienced during childhood more closely than isolate rearing.

Assuming that the VFD treatment actually alters mother-infant interactions and results in a condition similar to infant insecure attachment, it should be emphasized that an insecure attachment is not itself a measure of psychopathology and that insecure attachment alone is unlikely to lead to a disorder (Sroufe, 1990). Rather, in some cases an insecure attachment may set a developmental trajectory that, along with other risk factors, increases the risk for psychopathology (Greenberg, 1999). Since the foraging paradigm is aimed at modeling insecure attachment alone, without considering other risk and protective factors, and does not provide any evidence of psychopathological outcome, the relevance of this paradigm for developmental psychopathology remains unclear.

One potentially appealing characteristic of the VFD paradigm is its use of a "natural" form of environmental stress. Although it is unlikely that free-ranging primates often go through periods of time with two-week alternations in food availability and foraging demands, nevertheless the idea that mother-infant interactions may be sensitive to habitat quality and environmental change is interesting. For example, field studies of vervet monkeys have shown that poor habitat quality and low food availability are associated with higher rates of maternal rejection (Hauser & Fairbanks, 1988). Studies of maternal time budgets in gelada baboons, however, have shown that increased time in foraging is associated with reduced time spent resting and not necessarily with quantitative or qualitative changes in maternal social interactions (Dunbar & Dunbar, 1988).

Discussions of the ecological validity of the VFD paradigm have been limited. For example, Rosenblum et al. (1994) simply stated that "it is unclear what level of uncertainty may be prevalent within various natural environments in which monkeys are found. However the LFD condition represents a typically stable laboratory control environment, which has been shown to result in the development and maintenance of apparently adaptive social and reproductive patterns." Unfortunately, the extent to which the laboratory environment in question results in adaptive behavior similar to what would occur under natural conditions remains unclear. The bonnet monkeys used in the foraging studies lived in small cohorts of three mother-infant pairs and therefore in a social environment very different from that typical of macaque societies (i.e., large groups with a few unrelated males and many females with adult and immature offspring organized in matrilines; Lindburg, 1991). Moreover, the patterns of maternal behavior and infant behavior observed in the foraging studies were never directly compared to those observed in other populations of bonnet macaques living in the wild or in other captive settings. Therefore, the extent to which the findings obtained with the VFD paradigm can be generalized and extended to humans appears to be contingent upon their replicability in different environments and with different populations of primates.

PRIMATE PARADIGMS BASED ON NATURALLY OCCURRING VARIABILITY IN MATERNAL BEHAVIOR

Long-Term Effects of Naturally Occurring Variability in Parenting Styles

Primate infants spend most of their time in contact with or in close proximity to their mothers. In addition to providing nutrition and transport to their infants, primate mothers also mediate, directly or indirectly, the formation of infants' social relationships with other individuals, for example, by encouraging or discouraging interactions with specific group members. Therefore, it may be argued that developmentally meaningful variation in the primate infant's social environment is most likely to occur within the context of interactions with the mother. Unfortunately, the social deprivation paradigms involve the permanent removal of the mother after birth (thus removing the most biologically meaningful source of variability for infant development) and introduce artificial variation in the environment whose biological significance remains dubious. The foraging paradigm is based on the interesting principle of altering mother-infant relationships through modification of the physical environment, but such relationships are taken out of their social and historical context because mothers and infants live in highly artificial social environments and their previous history of interaction is not taken into consideration. Studies of attachment and developmental psychopathology in humans have increasingly focused on social systems larger than the dyad, such as those involving the family or community (Greenberg, 1999). In particular, family systems considerations are increasingly viewed as essential to understanding the role of attachment in both adaptive and maladaptive developmental processes. Thus, it is unlikely that primate paradigms that isolate the mother-infant dyad out of its normal social context will provide information directly generalizable to human research.

The relation between early experience and maladaptive developmental processes in primates can and should be studied in complex social environments. Four decades of studies of mother-infant interactions conducted in the field or in captive but socially complex environments have shown that there are striking individual differences in maternal behavior (Fairbanks, 1996). In Old World monkeys, mothers show marked individual differences in parenting style along the two orthogonal dimensions of maternal Protectiveness and Rejection (e.g., Fairbanks, 1996; Hinde & Spencer-Booth, 1971; Maestripieri, 1998a; Tanaka, 1989). The dimension of maternal Protectiveness includes variation in the degree to which the mother physically restrains infant exploration, initiates proximity and contact, and provides nurturing behaviors such as grooming. The dimension of maternal Rejection includes the degree to which the mother limits the timing and duration of suckling, carrying, and contact. These dimensions combine to make four parenting style types: mothers who are high on both dimensions are classified as Controlling; mothers low on both dimensions are classified as Laissez-Faire; mothers high on one dimension and low on the other are classified as Protective or Rejecting. Longitudinal studies have demonstrated that parenting style along these dimensions tends to be consistent over time and across infants of the same mother (Fairbanks, 1989; Berman, 1990a; Maestripieri et al., 1999).

In Old World monkeys, different parenting styles have been shown to have consequences for offspring development across the lifespan (Fairbanks & McGuire, 1988; 1993; Simpson & Datta, 1990). Moderately rejecting mothers produce infants who are more independent, more sociable, spend more time exploring the environment, and are more likely to succeed in gaining food rewards in a novel environment. During adolescence, sons of rejecting mothers respond with more boldness when confronted with a strange adult male in their group. In contrast, protective parenting produces infants who are delayed in the development of independence and are relatively fearful and cautious when faced with challenging situations. As juveniles, offspring of protective mothers are slower to approach novel objects and to explore new environments.

When daughters produce their own first infants, they usually match the maternal protectiveness, rejection, and mother-infant contact that they experienced in infancy (Fairbanks, 1989; Berman, 1990b). Thus, differences in parenting styles are transmitted across generations.

Since in humans, various forms of psychopathology are often associated with different styles of parenting experienced in childhood (as assessed retrospectively; Dozier et al., 1999), the naturally occurring variability in parenting styles could represent an excellent starting point for the development of primate models of psychopathology. Thus, one first step toward the development of such models would involve the characterization of the long-term effects of different parenting styles on behavioral, neuroendocrine, and neuroanatomical development. Research should then assess whether particular parenting styles, in combinations with specific historical and environmental circumstances, can produce significant deviations in the developmental trajectories of the offspring. In humans, specific combinations of parental rejection with overprotection or inadequate control allow some specificity in the prediction of psychological disorders (Dozier et al,. 1999). For example, affective and anxiety disorders tend to be associated most frequently with parental rejection while antisocial personality disorders are most frequently associated with harsh discipline, and inadequate control. Research with primates could further investigate the relation between early experience with different parenting styles and various forms of adaptive and maladaptive developmental outcomes by conducting longitudinal studies across the lifespan instead of relying on retrospective assessment of early experiences.

Long-Term Effects of Infant Abuse

At the extremes of the wide range of different parenting styles observed in group-living primates, there are forms of neglectful or abusive parenting that jeopardize infant survival. Infant abuse in group-living monkeys shares a number of similarities with child maltreatment including the prevalence of this phenomenon in the population, the intergenerational transmission of abuse, the relationship between infant age and vulnerability to abuse, some psychological and behavioral characteristics of abusive parents, and the role of social stress in triggering abuse (Maestripieri & Carroll, 1998a). Thus, group-living monkeys may be excellent animal models to investigate the developmental consequences of child maltreatment (Carroll & Maestripieri, 1998; Maestripieri, 1999; Maestripieri & Carroll, 1998a).

In humans, child maltreatment has been shown to pose substantial risk for disturbances in development across a broad range of domains. There is a large body of evidence indicating that maltreated children exhibit numerous difficulties in their emotional self-regulation and affective communication, insecure attachment with their caregivers, deficits in the development of their self-functioning and autonomy, delays in the perception and expression of language, limitations in their social and cognitive use of play, deficits in social information processing, and general maladjustment and incompetence in peer relations including both excessive aggressive behavior and avoidance-withdrawal (e.g., Cicchetti & Rogosch, 1994; Trickett & McBride-Chang, 1995; Wolfe, 1987). Most of these early deficits and impairments are likely to be perpetuated into later periods of development, and in some cases result in psychopathologic outcomes such as depression and attention deficit disorders, or conduct disorders ranging from drug abuse to delinquency (Cicchetti & Rogosch, 1994). Abused children are also at risk of becoming abusive parents themselves (Egeland et al., 1987).

The long-term neuroendocrine consequences of child maltreatment are only beginning to be investigated. A few recent studies have focused on the activity of the HPA axis in maltreated children (DeBellis et al., 1994; DeBellis, Baum, 1999; Hart et al., 1995; 1996; Kaufman, 1991). These studies, along with those investigating other forms of PTSD, have suggested that early child abuse may lead to an initial hyperactivity of the HPA axis, followed by a long-term dysregulation of neuroendocrine responsiveness to stress. In fact, an initial hypersecretion of CRF from the hypothalamus appears to lead to downregulation of pituitary CRF receptors, which in turn is responsible for the lower basal levels of cortisol and blunted ACTH and cortisol response to exogenous CRF observed in victims of childhood abuse or PTSD patients (Lipschitz et al., 1998; Southwick et al., 1998).

At the level of the central nervous system, the areas that are more likely to be affected by child abuse are those that are normally mobilized by fear and life-threatening situations such as the amygdala, hippocampus, corpus callosum, and prefrontal cortex (DeBellis, Keshavan, et al., 1999). Several studies using structural Magnetic Resonance Imaging (sMRI) have found reduced hippocampal volume in adult survivors of childhood physical and sexual abuse relative to controls (Bremner, 1998). Reduced hippocampal volume is most likely the result of high levels of cortisol at the time of the trauma. Because the hippocampus is thought to have an inhibitory effect on CRF release from the hypothalamus, reduced hippocampal volume and function may contribute to the elevated levels of CRF observed in victims of child abuse. Other sMRI studies have found that physical abuse and neglect, but not sexual abuse, were associated with volumetric reductions in certain regions of the corpus callosum (Teicher et al., 1997). Consistent with this finding, Teicher and colleagues (1997) found that abused children had greater EEG coherence than control subjects in left but not in the right hemisphere. Finally, studies using Positron Emission Tomography (PET) in patients with PTSD have implicated several areas including amygdala, medial prefrontal cortex, and middle temporal cortex (Rauch et al., 1996). The latter cortical areas are known to modulate emotion and fear responsiveness through inhibition of amygdala responsiveness.

In sum, several lines of behavioral, neuroendocrine, and neuroanatomical evidence indicate that child maltreatment and other traumatic experiences can have long-lasting negative consequences for affective and cognitive developmental processes. Although human research on the consequences of child maltreatment has recently made a great deal of progress, a nonhuman primate model of child maltreatment could make an important contribution to research in this area because it would allow researchers to longitudinally investigate the developmental consequences of early abuse from infancy to adulthood in a relatively short period of time and assess the neuroendocrine, neurochemical, and neuroanatomical effects of abuse with more invasive measurements than those allowed in human studies.

The natural occurrence of infant abuse in monkeys provides the opportunity to study the developmental consequences of an early adverse experience that is within the range of experience of the species and shares many similarities with child maltreatment. Although monkey infants who survive early maternal abuse appear to be less behaviorally and physically traumatized than isolation-reared monkeys, abuse perpetrated by the infant's biological mother probably entails a psychological trauma with profound negative consequences. Moreover, even if abuse is limited to the first months of infant life, continuous coexistence with the abusive mother and observation of abuse being repeated with younger siblings could contribute to reinforce and perpetuate the traumatic effects of abuse into adulthood.

Primate research investigating the consequences of early infant abuse for biobehavioral development is just beginning. Preliminary data have suggested that abused infants may be delayed in the acquisition of independence from their mothers and in the development of peer relations in the first year of life (Maestripieri & Carroll, 1998c). Abused infants also tend to have higher basal levels of ACTH and cortisol one or two months after the termination of abuse (Maestripieri & Carroll, 2000). Moreover, females who were raised by abusive mothers and have become abusive mothers themselves have higher levels of CRF, 5-HIAA, and MHPG in their CSF than do controls (Lindell et al., 2000). Thus, the neurobiological correlates of infant abuse in primates are very similar to those of child maltreatment and other forms of traumatic stress in humans. In primates, some of the neuroendocrine variables that distinguish abused from nonabused individuals also predict some aspects of social and maternal behavior in adulthood. For example, females with higher levels of CRF, 5-HIAA, or MHPG in the CSF tend to be socially isolated from their group members and reject their infants more often than other individuals (Lindell et al., 2000). The best evidence, however, that early infant abuse may result in psychopathologic outcomes is provided by the finding that female offspring born and raised by abusive monkey mothers have a high probability of becoming abusive mothers themselves (Maestripieri et al., 1997a, 1997b; Maestripieri & Carroll, 1998b).

Current research in our laboratory is further investigating the long-term consequences of early abuse for responsiveness to stress, activity of the HPA axis, and brain development in rhesus monkeys. One important contribution made by a primate model of infant abuse would be the investigation of the mechanisms underlying the transmission of abusive parenting across individuals and generations. Human research has pointed to several processes that may link early parent-child interaction to later maladaptation, including changes in cognition, emotion regulation, or motivation (Greenberg, 1999). In addition, when considering intergenerational transmission of maladaptive patterns such as abusive parenting, the possible role of genetic influence on personality or behavior cannot be ruled out (e.g., Krugman, 1997; Caspi et al., 2002). Our current research is investigating the possible role of genetic/biological traits in the transmission of abusive behavior through the use of an infant cross-fostering paradigm. With this paradigm, several female infants born to abusive mothers were fostered onto nonabusive mothers shortly after birth. Conversely, female infants born to nonabusive mothers were adopted, raised (and abused) by abusive mothers as if they were their biological offspring (Maestripieri et al., 2000). One female subject adopted and abused by an abusive mother in infancy has already produced her first offspring and displayed abusive parenting, thus suggesting that early experience rather genetic factors plays an important role in the intergenerational transmission of abuse. As soon as the other subjects reach reproductive age, more information will be available to assess the relative role of biology versus environment in the intergenerational transmission of abuse.

Attachment theory and human studies suggest that early adverse interactions with caregivers may result in later maladaptation through the construction of complementary mental representations (or internal working models) of the caregivers and the self, which would be integrated into the personality structure and later influence social interactions with other individuals. Thus, an abused child would form a representation of the caregiver, and possibly of other individuals as well, as rejecting and hostile, and of himself or herself as not worthy of help or comfort. Such representations could contribute to the perpetuation of abuse when the child finds himself or herself in the parenting role.

Monkeys are unlikely to possess the cognitive abilities necessary to form mental representations of the self or other individuals (Tomasello & Call, 1997). Therefore, the intergenerational transmission of infant abuse in monkeys, and more generally the effects of early adverse experience on later psychological functioning and behavior, must be mediated by mechanisms other than internal working models. Although complex cognitive processes certainly play an important role in the genesis and perpetuation of human psychopathologies, the primate data suggest that developmental and cross-generational consistencies in behavior may occur also in the absence of such processes.

A different mechanism that could potentially mediate the developmental and cross-generational effects of adverse early experience in both monkeys and humans involves changes in neural organization underlying emotion regulation. Although human research in this area is still speculative, it has been argued that patterns of emotion regulation established in early childhood may substantially alter both the fear-conditioning processes in the amygdala (LeDoux, 1995) and the development of connections between the limbic system and the prefrontal cortex (Schore, 1996). There may also be linkages among attachment processes, neural organization, and affective communication. Dysregulation of emotion probably plays an important role in the occurrence of abusive parenting in both humans and primates. For example, abusive mothers in monkeys have been described as hyperanxious and protective (Maestripieri, 1998b; Troisi & D'Amato, 1984) and in some cases, abuse has been observed to be temporally contiguous to stressful events (Maestripieri, 1994). Our current research on the long-term consequences of early abuse for responsiveness to stress, activity of the HPA axis, and brain development could provide information that would be important to human studies as well.

Finally, another possible mechanism mediating the developmental effects of early infant abuse could involve motivation. In this view, early experience with a caregiver could mediate, in a positive or negative way, aspects of motivation that regulate social relationships, including parenting. Experience of responsive and warm parenting in infancy could reinforce motivation to engage in affiliative and nurturing social interactions whereas experience of rejecting or abusive parenting could encourage later avoidance of social contact or hostility. Such long-term changes in motivation could result from associative processes or occur through modification of neural substrates underlying the reward mechanisms associated with social affiliation or parent-offspring attachment such as the opioid system (Graves et al., 2002). In sum, the investigation of the long-term consequences of early infant abuse in primates with longitudinal studies combining observational and manipulative techniques could provide information on the specific mechanisms and processes mediating the relation between adverse early experience and later psychopathologic outcome. Since human research has shown that attachment disorders can also develop in stable but unhealthy relationships that are not characterized by severe maltreatment (Greenberg, 1999), the study of the developmental consequences of different parenting in primates can complement research on infant abuse and elucidate the role played by forms of early adverse experience other than maltreatment in the development of maladaptive behavioral processes.

CONCLUSIONS AND FUTURE RESEARCH DIRECTIONS

Research conducted with nonhuman primates during the last four decades has made important contributions to the understanding of both normative and pathological development. Observations of mother-infant interactions and early infant development in monkeys provided the foundations upon which attachment theory was formulated (Bowlby, 1969). For example, primate studies were instrumental in developing the notion that mothers provide the primary source of comfort and protection to infants and serve as a secure base for the exploration of environment during early development (Maestripieri, in press). Primate studies of infants who were separated from their mothers and raised under conditions of social deprivation confirmed that a minimal amount of social experience is required for normal social development. Such studies, however, did not clarify whether it was the absence of a primary caregiver or the complete lack of social experience that produced the resulting psychopathology. The recognition that there is variation in early interactions with caregivers and that this variation has important consequences for infant development is a critical insight that has redirected the focus of primate studies from deprivation of early experience to altering the quality of social experience.

Although primate research has increasingly acknowledged the important role played by the quality of early experience in normal and abnormal development, primate research has yet to explore the role that the timing of experience plays in the development of psychopathology. Knowing the timing and sequence with which specific social experiences occur during development may be as important as knowing the quality of those experiences in explaining psychopathology. The more recent primate models presented here lend themselves to expanding research into models that take timing effects into account while documenting the contribution made by the quality of social relations.

The challenge to primate researchers interested in modeling human developmental psychopathology is to find experimental paradigms that reproduce events and circumstances within the normal range of experience of their species. Unfortunately, most primate researchers interested in developmental psychopathology are not interested in normative development in the natural environment and most primate researchers interested in normative development in the natural environment are not interested in psychopathological processes. For example, in primate field research, behavioral pathologies are often either denied their existence (e.g., because primate behavior is viewed as perfectly adapted to the environment) or ignored as "noise" in the system. We believe, however, that primate paradigms that are based on naturally occurring phenomena, or at least that reproduce in the laboratory phenomena that are within the range of experience of a species, hold great promise as models for developmental psychopathology.

Consistent with one of the basic principles of developmental psychopathology (Cicchetti & Cannon, 1999), we also believe that that the study of normal and abnormal development can be mutually enriching. The study of the different developmental pathways resulting from variation in early parent-offspring interactions is an important prerequisite for understanding pathological outcomes. Conversely, we may gain valuable information on normal neurobiological development by studying developmental disorders. Therefore, future research with primate models of developmental psychopathology will be fruitful if students of adaptive primate behavior in captivity or in the field pay more attention to naturally occurring behavioral pathologies while scientists interested in modeling human psychopathological phenomena pay more attention to primate behavior in natural or semi-naturalistic environments.

Future research with primates will also benefit from the incorporation of other basic principles of developmental psychopathology, such as the notions that a particular adverse event should not necessarily result in the same outcome in different individuals or circumstances, and that there may be multiple pathways to the same developmental outcome (Cicchetti, 1993). In primates just as in humans, complex pathological phenomena such as anxiety, depression, or infant abuse are unlikely to be the direct consequence of a single adverse experience. Rather, they are likely to be multiply determined and dependent on the balance of risk and protective factors. Thus, longitudinal studies of the effects of early traumatic experiences on biobehavioral development should increasingly investigate individual differences in vulnerability and resilience to the effects of such experiences and their possible biological and social correlates. If future primate research is successful in combining the use of new technologies for the study of brain-behavior relations with more ecologically valid paradigms and conceptually sophisticated explanatory frameworks, such research will likely produce exciting new information and make an important contribution to the growing discipline of developmental psychopathology.

REFERENCES

Anderson, C. O., & Mason, W. A. (1974). Early experience and complexity of social organization in groups of young rhesus monkeys. *Journal of Comparative Physiology and Psychology, 87,* 681–690.

Anderson, C. O., & Mason, W. A. (1978). Competitive social strategies in groups of deprived and experienced rhesus monkeys. *Developmental Psychobiology, 11,* 289–299.

Andrews, M. W., & Rosenblum, L. A. (1991). Attachment in monkey infants raised in variable- and low-demand environments. *Child Development, 62,* 686–693.

Andrews, M. W., & Rosenblum, L. A. (1992). Response of bonnet macaque dyads to an acute foraging task under different motivational conditions. *Developmental Psychobiology, 25,* 557–566.

Andrews, M. W., & Rosenblum, L. A. (1993a). Assessment of attachment in differentially reared infant monkeys (*Macaca radiata*): response to separation and a novel environment. *Journal of Comparative Psychology, 107,* 84–90.

Andrews, M. W., & Rosenblum, L. A. (1993b). Location-restricted dyadic interactions and maternal patterns. *American Journal of Primatology, 29,* 27–36.

Andrews, M. W., & Rosenblum, L. A. (1994a). The development of affiliative and agonistic social patterns in differentially reared monkeys. *Child Development, 65,* 1398–1404.

Andrews, M. W., & Rosenblum, L. A. (1994b). Developmental consequences of altered dyadic coping patterns in bonnet macaques. In J. J. Roeder, B. Thierry, J. R. Anderson, & N. Herrenschmidt (Eds.), *Current primatology* (pp. 265–271). Strasbourg: Universite Louis Pasteur.

Berman, C. M. (1990a). Consistency in maternal behavior within families of free-ranging rhesus monkeys: an extension of the concept of maternal style. *American Journal of Primatology, 22,* 159–169.

Berman, C. M. (1990b). Intergenerational transmission of maternal rejection rates among free-ranging rhesus monkeys. *Animal Behaviour, 39,* 329–337.

Bowlby, J. (1969). *Attachment and loss. I. Attachment.* New York: Basic Books.

Bremner, J. D. (1998). Neuroimaging of posttraumatic stress disorder. *Psychiatric Annals, 28,* 445–450.

Caine, N. G., Earle, H., & Reite, M. (1983). Personality traits of adolescent pigtailed monkeys (*Macaca nemestrina*): an analysis of social rank and early separation experience. *American Journal of Primatology, 4,* 253–260.

Capitanio, J. P., Rasmussen, K. L. R., Snyder, D. S., Laudenslager, M., & Reite, M. (1986). Long-term follow-up of previously separated pigtail macaques: group and individual differences in response to novel situations. *Journal of Child Psychology and Psychiatry, 27,* 531–538.

Capitanio, J. P., & Reite, M. (1984). The roles of early separation experience and prior familiarity in the social relations of pigtail macaques: a descriptive multivariate study. *Primates, 25,* 475–484.

Carroll, K. A., & Maestripieri, D. (1998). Infant abuse and neglect in monkeys: A discussion of definitions, epidemiology, etiology, and implications for child maltreatment. *Psychological Bulletin, 123,* 234–237.

Caspi, A., McClay, J., Moffitt, T. E., Mill, J., Martin, J., Craig, I. W., Taylor, A., & Poulton, R. (2002). Role of genotype in the cycle of violence in maltreated children. *Science, 297,* 851–854.

Chamove, A. S., Rosenblum, L. A., & Harlow, H. F. (1973). Monkeys (*Macaca mulatta*) raised with only peers: A pilot study. *Animal Behaviour, 21,* 316–325.

Champoux, M., Coe, C. L., Schanberg, S. M., Kuhn, C. M., & Suomi, S. J. (1989). Hormonal effects of early rearing conditions in the infant rhesus monkey. *American Journal of Primatology, 19,* 111–117.

Champoux, M., Metz, B., & Suomi, S. J. (1991). Behavior of nursery/peer-reared and mother-reared rhesus monkeys from birth through 2 years of age. *Primates, 32,* 509–514.

Cicchetti, D. (1993). Developmental psychopathology: Reactions, reflections, projections. *Developmental Review, 13,* 471–502.

Cicchetti, D., & Cannon, T. D. (1999). Neurodevelopmental processes in the ontogenesis and epigenesis of psychopathology. *Development & Psychopathology, 11,* 375–393.

Cicchetti D., & Rogosch, F. A. (1994). The toll of child maltreatment on the developing child. *Child and Adolescent Psychiatric Clinics of North America, 3,* 759–776.

Clarke, A. S. (1993). Social rearing effects on HPA activity over early development and in response to stress in rhesus monkeys. *Developmental Psychobiology, 26,* 433–446.

Collier, G. H., & Rovee-Collier, C. K. (1980). A comparative analysis of optimal foraging behavior: Laboratory simulations. In A. C. Kamil & T. D. Sargent (Eds.), *Foraging behavior: Ecological, ethological, and psychological approaches* (pp. 39–76). New York: Garland Press.

Coplan, J. D., Andrews, M. W., Rosenblum, L. A., Owens, M. J., Friedman, S., Gorman, J. M., & Nemeroff, C. B. (1996). Persistent elevations of cerebrospinal fluid concentrations of corticotropin-releasing factor in adult nonhuman primates exposed to early life stressors: Implications for the pathophysiology of mood and anxiety disorders. *Proceedings of the National Academy of Sciences USA, 93,* 1619–1623.

Coplan, J. D., Rosenblum, L. A., Friedman, S., Bassoff, T. B., & Gorman, J. M. (1992). Behavioral effects of oral yohimbine in differentially reared nonhuman primates. *Neuropsychopharmacology, 6,* 31–37.

Coplan, J. D., Rosenblum, L. A., & Gorman, J. M. (1995). Primate models of anxiety. Longitudinal perspectives. *Psychiatric Clinics of North America, 18,* 727–743.

Coplan, J. D., Trost, R. C., Owens, M. J., Cooper, T. B., Gorman, J. M., Nemeroff, C. B., & Rosenblum, L. A. (1998). Cerebrospinal fluid concentrations of somastotin and biogenic amines in grown primates reared by mothers exposed by manipulated foraging conditions. *Archives of General Psychiatry, 55,* 473–477.

De Bellis, M. D., Baum, A. S., Birmaher, B., Keshavan, M. S., Eccard, C. H., Boring, A. M., Jenkins, F. J., & Ryan, N. D. (1999a). Developmental traumatology. Part I: Biological stress systems. *Biological Psychiatry, 45,* 1259–1270.

De Bellis, M. D., Chrousos, G. P., Dorn, L. D., Burke, L., Helmers, K., Kling, M. A., Trickett, P., & Putnam, F. W. (1994). Adrenal axis dysregulation in sexually abused girls. *Journal of Clinical Endocrinology and Metabolism, 78,* 249–255.

De Bellis, M. D., Keshavan, M. S., Clark, D. B., Casey, B. J., Giedd, J. N., Boring, A. M., Frustaci, K., & Ryan, N. D. (1999). Developmental traumatology. Part II: Brain development. *Biological Psychiatry, 45,* 1271–1284.

Dienske, H., & de Jonge, G. (1982). A comparison of development and deprivation in non-human primates and man. *Journal of Human Evolution, 11,* 511–516.

Dozier, M., Stovall, K. C., & Albus, K. E. (1999). Attachment and psychopathology in adulthood. In J. Cassidy & P. R. Shaver (Eds.), *Handbook of attachment* (pp. 497–519). New York: Guilford Press.

Dunbar, R. I. M., & Dunbar, P. (1988). Maternal time budgets of gelada baboons. *Animal Behaviour, 36,* 970–980.

Egeland, B., Jacobvitz, D., & Papatola, K. (1987). Intergenerational continuity of abuse. In R. J. Gelles, & J. B. Lancaster (Eds.), *Child abuse and neglect. Biosocial dimensions* (pp. 255–276). New York: Aldine.

Eisenberg, L. (1995). The social construction of the human brain. *American Journal of Psychiatry, 152,* 1563–1575.

Fairbanks, L. A. (1989). Early experience and cross-generational continuity of mother-infant contact in vervet monkeys. *Developmental Psychobiology, 22,* 669–681.

Fairbanks, L. A. (1996). Individual differences in maternal styles: causes and consequences for mothers and offspring. *Advances in the Study of Behavior, 25,* 579–611.

Fairbanks, L. A., & McGuire, M. T. (1988). Long-term effects of early mothering behavior on responsiveness to the environment in vervet monkeys. *Developmental Psychobiology, 21,* 711–724.

Fairbanks, L. A., & McGuire, M. T. (1993). Maternal protectiveness and response to the unfamiliar in vervet monkeys. *American Journal of Primatology, 30,* 119–129.

Floeter, M. K., & Greenough, W. T. (1979). Cerebellar plasticity: Modification of Purkinje cell structure by differential rearing in monkeys. *Science, 206,* 227–229.

Ginsberg, S. D., Hof, P. R., McKinney, W. T., & Morrison, J. H. (1993a). Quantitative analysis of tuberoinfundibular tyrosine hydroxylase- and corticotropin-releasing factor-immunoreactive neurons in monkeys raised with differential rearing conditions. *Experimental Neurology, 120,* 95–105.

Ginsberg, S. D., Hof, P. R., McKinney, W. T., & Morrison, J. H. (1993b). The noradrenergic innervation density of the monkey paraventricular nucleus is not altered by early social deprivation. *Neuroscience Letters, 158,* 130–134.

Graves, F. C., Wallen, K., & Maestripieri, D. (2002). Opioids and attachment in rhesus macaque abusive mothers. *Behavioral Neuroscience, 116,* 489–493.

Greenberg, M. T. (1999). Attachment and psychopathology in childhood. In J. Cassidy & P. R. Shaver (Eds.), *Handbook of attachment* (pp. 469–496). New York: Guilford Press.

Harlow, H. F. (1959). Affectional response in the infant monkey. *Science, 130,* 421–432.

Harlow, H. F. (1969). Age-mate or peer affectional system. *Advances in the Study of Behavior, 2,* 333–383.

Hart, J., Gunnar, M., & Cicchetti, D. (1995). Salivary cortisol in maltreated children: evidence of relations between neuroendocrine activity and social competence. *Development and Psychopathology, 7,* 11–26.

Hart, J., Gunnar, M., & Cicchetti, D. (1996). Altered neuroendocrine activity in maltreated children related to symptoms of depression. *Development and Psychopathology, 8,* 201–214.

Hauser, M. D., & Fairbanks, L. A. (1988). Mother-offspring conflict in vervet monkeys: variation in response to ecological conditions. *Animal Behaviour, 36,* 802–813.

Heinz, A., Higley, J. D., Gorey, J. D., Saunders, R. C., Jones, D. W., Hommer, D., Zajicek, K., Suomi, S. J., Lesch, K. P., Weinsberger, D. R., & Linnoila, M. (1998). In vivo association between alcohol intoxication, aggression, and serotonin transporter availability in nonhuman primates. *American Journal of Psychiatry, 155,* 1023–1028.

Higley, J. D., & Bennett, A. J. (1999). Central nervous system serotonin and personality as variables contributing to excessive alcohol consumption in non-human primates. *Alcohol & Alcoholism, 34,* 402–418.

Higley, J. D., Hopkins, W. D., Thompson, W. W., Byrne, E. A., Hirsch, R. M., & Suomi, S. J. (1992). Peers as primary attachment sources in yearling rhesus monkeys (*Macaca mulatta*). *Developmental Psychology, 28,* 1163–1171.

Higley, J. D., King, S. T., Hasert, M. F., Champoux, M., Suomi, S. J., & Linnoila, M. (1996). Stability of interindividual differences in serotonin function and its relationship to aggressive wounding and competent social behavior in rhesus macaque females. *Neuropsychopharmacology, 14*, 67–76.

Higley, J. D., Suomi, S. J., & Linnoila, M. (1991). CSF monoamine metabolite concentrations vary according to age, rearing, and sex, and are influenced by the stressor of social separation in rhesus monkeys. *Psychopharmacology, 103*, 551–556.

Higley, J. D., Suomi, S. J., & Linnoila, M. (1992). A longitudinal assessment of CSF monoamine metabolite and plasma cortisol concentrations in young rhesus monkeys. *Biological Psychiatry, 32*, 127–145.

Higley, J. D., Mehlman, P. T., Poland, R. E., Taub, D. M., Vickers, J., Suomi, S. J., & Linnoila, M. (1996). CSF testosterone and 5-HIAA correlate with different types of aggressive behaviors. *Biological Psychiatry, 40*, 1067–1082.

Higley, J. D., Thompson, W. W., Champoux, M., Goldman, D., Hasert, M. F., Kraemer, G. W., Scanlan, J. M., Suomi, S. J., & Linnoila, M. (1993). Paternal and maternal genetic and environmental contributions to cerebrospinal fluid monoamine metabolites in rhesus monkeys (*Macaca mulatta*). *Archives of General Psychiatry, 50*, 615–623.

Hinde, R. A., Leighton-Shapiro, M. E., & McGinnis, L. (1978). Effects of various types of separation experience on rhesus monkeys five months later. *Journal of Child Psychology and Psychiatry, 19*, 199–211.

Hinde, R. A., & Spencer-Booth, Y. (1971). Towards understanding individual differences in rhesus mother-infant interaction. *Animal Behaviour, 19*, 165–173.

Insel, T. R. (1992). Oxytocin and the neurobiology of attachment. *Behavioral and Brain Sciences, 15*, 515–516.

Kaufman, J. (1991). Depressive disorders in maltreated children. *Journal of the American Academy of Child and Adolescent Psychiatry, 30*, 257–265.

Kraemer, G. W. (1992). A psychobiological theory of attachment. *Behavioral and Brain Sciences, 15*, 493–541.

Kraemer, G. W., Ebert, M. H., Lake, C. R., & McKinney, W. T. (1983). Cerebrospinal fluid measures of neurotransmitter changes associated with pharmacological alteration of the despair response to social separation in rhesus monkeys. *Psychiatry Research, 11*, 303–315.

Kraemer, G. W., Ebert, M. H., Lake, C. R., & McKinney, W. T. (1984). Hypersensitivity to d-amphetamine several years after early social deprivation in rhesus monkeys. *Psychopharmacology, 82*, 266–271.

Kraemer, G. W., Ebert, M. H., Schmidt, D. E., & McKinney, W. T. (1989). A longitudinal study of the effect of different social rearing conditions on cerebrospinal fluid norepinephrine and biogenic amine metabolites in rhesus monkeys. *Neuropsychopharmacology, 2*, 175–189.

Kraemer, G. W., & McKinney, W. T. (1979). Interactions of pharmacological agents which alter biogenic amine metabolism and depression. An analysis of contributing factors within a primate model of depression. *Journal of Affective Disorders, 1*, 33–54.

Krugman, R. D. (1997). Suppose it were a genetic disorder? *Child Abuse & Neglect, 21*, 245–246.

Laudenslager, M., Capitanio, J. P., & Reite, M. (1985). Possible effects of early separation experiences on subsequent immune function in adult macaque monkeys. *American Journal of Psychiatry, 142*, 862–864.

LeDoux, J. E. (1995). Emotion: Clues from the brain. *Annual Review of Psychology, 46*, 209–235.

Levine, S., & Wiener, S. G. (1988). Psychoendocrine aspects of mother-infant relationships in nonhuman primates. *Psychoneuroendocrinology, 13*, 143–154.

Lewis, M. H., Gluck, J. P., Beauchamp, A. J., Keresztury, M. F., & Mailman, R. B. (1990). Long-term effects of early social isolation in *Macaca mulatta*: changes in dopamine receptor function following apomorphine challenge. *Brain Research, 513*, 67–73.

Lindburg, D. G. (1991). Ecological requirements of macaques. *Laboratory Animal Science, 41*, 315–322.

Lindell, S. G., Maestripieri, D., Megna, N. L., & Higley, J. D. (2000). CSF 5-HIAA and MHPG predict infant abuse and rejection by rhesus macaque mothers. *American Journal of Primatology, 51*, 70.

Lipschitz, D. S., Rasmusson, A. M., & Southwick, S. M. (1998). Childhood posttraumatic stress disorder: A review of neurobiologic sequelae. *Psychiatric Annals, 28*, 452–457.

Liu, D., Diorio, J., Tannenbaum, B., Caldji, C., Francis, D., Freedman, A., Sharma, S., Pearson, D., Plotsky, P. M., & Meaney, M. J. (1997). Maternal care, hippocampal glucocorticoid receptors, and hypothalamic-pituitary-adrenal responses to stress. *Science, 277,* 1659–1662.

Maestripieri, D. (1994). Infant abuse associated with psychosocial stress in a group-living pigtail macaque (*Macaca nemestrina*) mother. *American Journal of Primatology, 32,* 41–49.

Maestripieri, D. (1998a). Social and demographic influences on mothering style in pigtail macaques. *Ethology, 104,* 379–385.

Maestripieri, D. (1998b). Parenting styles of abusive mothers in group-living rhesus macaques. *Animal Behaviour, 55,* 1–11.

Maestripieri, D. (1999). The biology of human parenting: Insights from nonhuman primates. *Neuroscience & Biobehavioral Reviews, 23,* 411–422.

Maestripieri, D. (in press). Attachment. In D. Maestripieri (Ed.), *Primate psychology: The mind and behavior of human and nonhuman primates.* Cambridge, Mass.: Harvard University Press.

Maestripieri, D., & Carroll, K. A. (1998a). Child abuse and neglect: Usefulness of the animal data. *Psychological Bulletin, 123,* 211–223.

Maestripieri, D., & Carroll, K. A. (1998b). Risk factors for infant abuse and neglect in group-living rhesus monkeys. *Psychological Science, 9,* 143–145.

Maestripieri, D., & Carroll, K. A. (1998c). Behavioral and environmental correlates of infant abuse in group-living pigtail macaques. *Infant Behavior & Development, 21,* 603–612.

Maestripieri, D., & Carroll, K. A. (2000). Causes and consequences of infant abuse and neglect in monkeys. *Aggression and Violent Behavior, 5,* 245–254.

Maestripieri, D., Megna, N. L., & Jovanovic, T. (2000). Adoption and maltreatment of foster infants by rhesus macaque abusive mothers. *Developmental Science, 3,* 287–293.

Maestripieri, D., Tomaszycki, M., & Carroll, K. A. (1999). Consistency and change in the behavior of rhesus macaque abusive mothers with successive infants. *Developmental Psychobiology, 34,* 29–35.

Maestripieri, D., Wallen, K., & Carroll, K. A. (1997a). Infant abuse runs in families of group-living pigtail macaques. *Child Abuse & Neglect, 21,* 465–471.

Maestripieri, D., Wallen, K., & Carroll, K. A. (1997b). Genealogical and demographic influences on infant abuse and neglect in group-living sooty mangabeys (*Cercocebus atys*). *Developmental Psychobiology, 31,* 175–180.

Martin, L. J., Spicer, D. M., Lewis, M. H., Gluck, J. P., & Cork, L. C. (1991). Social deprivation of infant rhesus monkeys alters the chemoarchitecture of the brain: I. Subcortical regions. *Journal of Neuroscience, 11,* 3344–3358.

McKinney, W. T. (1977). Animal behavioral/biological models relevant to depressive and affective disorders in humans. In J. G. Schulterbrandt & A. Raskin (Eds.), *Depression in childhood: Diagnosis, treatment, and conceptual models* (pp. 107–122). New York: Raven Press.

McKinney, W. T., & Bunney, W. E. (1969). Animal model of depression. *Archives of General Psychiatry, 21,* 240–248.

Meyer, J. S., & Bowman, R. E. (1972). Rearing experience, stress, and adrenocorticosteroids in the rhesus monkey. *Physiology and Behavior, 8,* 339–343.

Mineka, S., & Suomi, S. J. (1978). Social separation in monkeys. *Psychological Bulletin, 85,* 1376–1400.

Mineka, S., Suomi, S. J., & DeLizio, R. D. (1981). Multiple separations in adolescent monkeys: An opponent-process interpretation. *Journal of Experimental Psychology: General, 110,* 56–85.

Morrison, J. H., Hof, P. R., Janssen, W., Bassett, J. L., Foote, S. L., Kraemer, G. W., & McKinney, W. T. (1990). Quantitative neuroanatomic analyses of cerebral cortex in rhesus monkeys from different rearing conditions. *Proceedings of the Society of Neuroscience, 16,* 789.

Nelson, C. A., & Bloom, F. E. (1997). Child development and neuroscience. *Child Development, 68,* 970–987.

Novak, M. A., & Harlow, H. F. (1975). Social recovery of monkeys isolated for the first year of life: I. Rehabilitation and therapy. *Developmental Psychology, 11,* 453–465.

Plimpton, E., & Rosenblum, L. (1983). The ecological context of infant maltreatment in primates. In M. Reite & N. G. Caine (Eds.), *Child abuse: The nonhuman primate data* (pp. 103–117). New York: Alan Liss.

Rauch, S. L., van der Kolk, B. A., Fisler, R. E., Alpert, N. M., Orr, S. P., Savage, C. R., Fischman, A. J., Jenike, M. A., & Pitman, R. K. (1996). A symptom provocation study of posttraumatic stress disorder using positron emission tomography and script driven imagery. *Archives of General Psychiatry, 53,* 380–387.

Reite, M. (1977). Maternal separation in monkey infants: A model of depression. In I. Hanin & E. Usdin (Eds.), *Animal models in psychiatry and neurology* (pp. 127–139). New York: Pergamon Press.

Reite, M. (1985). Implantable biotelemetry and social separation in monkeys. In G. P. Moberg (Ed.), *Animal stress* (pp. 141–160). Bethesda, Md.: American Physiological Society.

Reite, M. (1987). Infant abuse and neglect: Lessons from the primate laboratory. *Child Abuse & Neglect, 11,* 347–355.

Reite, M., & Short, R. (1983). Maternal separation studies: rationale and methodological considerations. In K. A. Miczek (Ed.), *Ethopharmacology: Primate models of neuropsychiatric disorders* (pp. 219–253). New York: Alan Liss.

Rosenblum, L. A., Coplan, J. D., Friedman, S., Bassoff, T., Gorman, J. M., & Andrews, M. W. (1994). Adverse early experiences affect noradrenergic and serotonergic functioning in adult primates. *Biological Psychiatry, 35,* 221–227.

Rosenblum, L. A., Kaufman, I. C., & Stynes, A. J. (1969). Interspecific variations in the effects of hunger on diurnally varying behavior elements in macaques. *Brain Behavior and Evolution, 2,* 119–131.

Rosenblum, L. A., & Paully, G. S. (1984). The effects of varying environmental demands on maternal and infant behavior. *Child Development, 55,* 305–314.

Sackett, G. P., Bowman, R. E., Meyer, J. S., Tripp, R. L., & Grady, S. A. (1973). Adrenocortical and behavioral responses by differentially raised rhesus monkeys. *Physiological Psychology, 1,* 209–212.

Sackett, G. P., Holm, R. A., & Ruppenthal, G. P. (1976). Social isolation rearing: species differences in behavior of macaque monkeys. *Developmental Psychology, 12,* 283–288.

Sanchez, M. M., Hearn, E. F., Do, D., Rilling, J. K., & Herndon, J. G. (1998). Differential rearing affects corpus callosum size and cognitive function of rhesus monkeys. *Brain Research, 812,* 38–49.

Schore, A. N. (1996). The experience-dependent maturation of a regulatory system in the orbital prefrontal cortex and the origin of developmental psychopathology. *Development & Psychopathology, 8,* 59–87.

Shannon, C., Champoux, M., & Suomi, S. J. (1998). Rearing condition and plasma cortisol in rhesus monkey infants. *American Journal of Primatology, 46,* 311–321.

Siegel, S. J., Ginsberg, S. D., Hof, P. R., Foote, S. L., Young, W. G., Kraemer, G. W., McKinney, W. T., & Morrison, J. H. (1993). Effects of social deprivation in prepubescent rhesus monkeys: immunohistochemical analysis of the neurofilament protein triplet in the hippocampal formation. *Brain Research, 619,* 299–305.

Simpson, M. J. A., & Datta, S. B. (1990). Predicting infant enterprise from early relationships in rhesus macaques. *Behaviour, 116,* 42–63.

Smith, E. L. P., Coplan, J. D., Trost, R. C., Scharf, B. A., & Rosenblum, L. A. (1997). Neurobiological alterations in adult nonhuman primates exposed to unpredictable early rearing. *Annals of the New York Academy of Sciences, 821,* 545–548.

Southwick, S. M., Yehuda, R., & Wang, S. (1998). Neuroendocrine alterations in posttraumatic stress disorder. *Psychiatric Annals, 28,* 436–442.

Spencer-Booth, Y., & Hinde, R. A. (1971). Effects of brief separations from mothers during infancy on behaviour of rhesus monkeys 6–24 months later. *Journal of Child Psychology and Psychiatry, 12,* 157–172.

Sroufe, L. A. (1990). Pathways to adaptation and maladaptation: Psychopathology as developmental deviation. In D. Cicchetti (Ed.), *Rochester Symposium on Developmental Psychopathology: Vol. 1. The emergence of a discipline* (pp. 13–40). Hillsdale, N.J.: Erlbaum.

Stevenson-Hinde, J., Stillwell-Barnes, R., & Zunz, M. (1980). Subjective assessment of rhesus monkeys over four successive years. *Primates, 21,* 66–82.

Struble, R. G., & Riesen, A. H. (1978). Changes in cortical dendritic branching subsequent to partial social isolation in stumptailed monkeys. *Developmental Psychobiology, 11,* 479–486.

Suomi, S. J. (1982). Abnormal behavior and primate models of psychopathology. In J. L. Fobes & J. L. King (Eds.), *Primate behavior* (pp. 171–217). New York: Academic Press.

Suomi, S. J. (1991). Early stress and adult emotional reactivity in rhesus monkeys. In *Ciba Foundation Symposium 156 "The childhood environment and adult disease"* (pp. 171–188). Chichester: Wiley.

Suomi, S. J., & Harlow, H. F. (1972). Social rehabilitation of isolate-reared monkeys. *Developmental Psychology, 6,* 487–496.

Suomi, S. J., Harlow, H. F., & Domek, D. J. (1970). Effect of repetitive infant-infant separation in young monkeys. *Journal of Abnormal Psychology, 76,* 161–172.

Suomi, S. J., Mineka, S., & DeLizio, R. D. (1983). Short- and long-term effects of repetitive mother-infant separations on social development in rhesus monkeys. *Developmental Psychology, 19,* 770–786.

Suomi, S. J., & Ripp, C. (1983). A history of motherless mother monkey mothering at the University of Wisconsin Primate Laboratory. In M. Reite & N. G. Caine (Eds.), *Child abuse: The nonhuman primate data* (pp. 49–78). New York: Alan Liss.

Tanaka, I. (1989). Variability in the development of mother-infant relationships among free-ranging Japanese macaques. *Primates, 30,* 477–491.

Teicher, M. H., Ito, Y., Glod, C. A., Andersen, S. L., Dumont, N., & Ackerman, E. (1997). Preliminary evidence for abnormal cortical development in physically and sexually abused children using EEG coherence and MRI. *Annals of the New York Academy of Sciences, 821,* 160–175.

Tomasello, M., & Call, J. (1997). *Primate cognition.* Oxford: Oxford University Press.

Trickett, P. K., & McBride-Chang, C. (1995). The developmental impact of different forms of child abuse and neglect. *Developmental Review, 15,* 311–337.

Troisi, A., & D'Amato, F. R. (1984). Ambivalence in monkey mothering: infant abuse combined with maternal possessiveness. *Journal of Nervous and Mental Disease, 172,* 105–108.

Uno, H., Tarara, R., Else, J., Suleman, M. A., & Sapolsky, R. M. (1989). Hippocampal damage associated with prolonged and fatal stress in primates. *Journal of Neuroscience, 9,* 1705–1711.

Wolfe, D. A. (1987). *Child abuse. Implications for child development and psychopathology.* Newbury Park, Calif.: Sage Publications.

NINE

Early Orbitofrontal-Limbic Dysfunction and Autism

Jocelyne Bachevalier and Katherine A. Loveland

Only recently have researchers begun to appreciate the importance of studying the neurobiology of social cognition (Ochsner & Lieberman, 2001). This growing interest stems from evidence suggesting that dysfunction of structures within the neural network subserving social cognition may be at the origin of many neuropsychiatric disorders in humans. Reports of clinical cases with circumscribed lesions, as well as the results of neurostimulation, neurorecording, and neuroimaging of normal and impaired brain, have all provided evidence that there exists specific neural circuitry involved in the processing of social skills (for review see Adolphs, 2001). In addition, animal studies examining the neurobiology of social cognition have refined our knowledge of the brain systems that underlie such abilities and are helping us better understand how human social and emotional processes are realized (Raleigh, 1995). In this respect, nonhuman primates are undoubtedly excellent animal models, not only to investigate brain processes underlying social cognition and to determine the long-term behavioral outcomes of early dysfunction in the neural structures mediating social cognition, but also to determine the modulatory impact of perinatal experiences on brain and behavioral development (Sánchez, Ladd, & Plotsky, 2001).

Investigations of the social skills of nonhuman primates in the wild or in the laboratory have revealed that monkeys, like humans, live in social groups that are characterized by complex and dynamic social organizations maintained through a variety of specific, long-term relationships between individual group members (Cheney & Seyfarth, 1990; DeWaal, 1989). It is now clear that each member of a monkey troop establishes and maintains numerous long-term relationships with many other group members, and that the nature, intensity, and stability of each relationship varies according to the specific ages, sexes, and kinship relationship of that particular pair of monkeys. To maintain these relationships, monkeys, like humans, must perceive and use information about other individuals in the troop and adapt their behavior to function adequately within the social environment. Indeed, the presence of a stable social hierarchy within a group indicates that the individuals that make up the social group recognize one another and respond differentially depending upon with whom they are interacting. Beginning at

Research described in this chapter was supported in part by grants to the authors MH58846 (NIMH), DC00357 (NIDCD), and HD35471 (NICHD).

birth, the infant born into such a complex social group is faced with the developmental task of coming to respond differentially and appropriately to categories of social partners as well as to individuals within those categories. Thus, during development, individuals progressively learn complex rules for self-regulation of behavior that assure successful social relationships. Finally, although the ability to interpret mental states of others is still controversial in nonhuman primates (Cheney & Seyfarth, 1990), some studies have suggested that they, too, possess a rudimentary cognitive capacity for assessing intentions and motivations in others (Brothers, 1995; Byrne & Whiten, 1988). One cannot deny that the ability to communicate social intentions is likely to be far more complex in humans than in nonhuman primates. Nevertheless, it seems that the similarities between species in many phenotypic displays and basic behavioral processes outweigh the differences, suggesting that the neural mechanisms underlying social communication are likely to share common features across these species.

This chapter presents an overview of data from primate research implicating the amygdala and the orbitofrontal cortex in the regulation of social-emotional cognition and behavior. Given the importance of these brain structures in the regulation of affective states and sociality in adulthood, this neural system is likely to have a paramount role in the development of social cognition in young primates. Although research in this area has been astonishingly neglected, in this chapter we present experimental evidence indicating that this neural system appears to operate early in life and that its early dysfunction is associated with an array of heterogeneous behavioral abnormalities resembling those associated with autism. In the final part of this chapter, we relate the behavioral symptoms following early medial temporal lobe lesions in monkeys to those observed in autism and present a developmental model that may help to elucidate the neurobiology of autism within a larger framework that includes the roles of genetics and environmental experiences in bringing about the manifestations of autism.

NEURAL STRUCTURES INVOLVED IN SOCIAL-EMOTIONAL COGNITION AND BEHAVIOR

To survive, humans and other animals must navigate the species-specific social environment. Doing so requires an appreciation of the significance of others' social and emotional behavior for oneself, so that socially relevant behaviors can be appropriately self-regulated (Loveland, 1991, 2001). For example, a threat display by a rhesus monkey indicates that an approach to that individual is not welcome and is likely to result in hostilities. Another individual's behaviors not only can provide information to guide the actions appropriate to a specific instance, but can also provide more general guides to action, such as awareness of dominance relationships. Thus, social cognition (broadly construed) rests upon the ability to detect and interpret information about other individuals that is relevant to regulating one's own behavior according to the current emotional and social context. In the case of humans, the use of social information to self-regulate behavior is highly complex, reflecting not only emotional but also cognitive and cultural factors. Social cognition thus will include not only the ability to understand and reason about the cognitive mental states of other individuals, but also the ability to identify emotional states, intentions, desires, attitudes, etc., and to use this information to guide behavior.

Social cognition and social behavior are orchestrated by a complex neural network of interconnected structures, including brain regions in the ventromedial aspect of the temporal and frontal lobes, and their interconnections with the hypothalamus and brainstem (Adolphs, 2001). Within the medial temporal lobe, the amygdala comprises a set of nuclei with different connectional features (see Figure 9.1). The lateral nucleus receives an enormous array of highly processed sensory information, including visual information from faces and facial expressions, body postures and movements, as well as auditory information from specific vocal sounds and intonations, and reciprocally, via the basal nucleus, provides a route by which affective states could modulate cortical sensory stimuli. The basal nucleus in turn serves as an interface between sensory-specific cortical inputs and the central nucleus, which offers a relay to the brainstem and hypothalamus. These two neural centers are concerned with different aspects of emotional responses, including their behavioral and autonomic manifestations. Via this pathway, sensory stimuli could influence and activate emotional reactions. The basal and accessory basal nuclei project substantially to the ventral striatum, thereby offering a way by which affective states may gain access to subcortical elements of the motor system and so affect actions related to emotional responses, including the modulation of facial and vocal expressions, body postures and movements. These two amygdala nuclei are also interconnected with the anterior cingulate cortex, a cortical area implicated in the production of vocalizations in monkeys and in the initiation of speech in humans. This pathway may be crucial for the emotional modulation of vocalizations and speech. In addition, because the anterior cingulate cortex is involved in effector and executive functions, that is, in controlling visceromotor, endocrine, or skeletomotor outputs, it is likely that this area controls emotional outputs not only for speech but for all body postures and movements, and for internal emotional changes (Devinsky, Morrell, & Vogt, 1995; Vogt, Finch, & Olson, 1992). That is, as the organism evaluates the affective significance of something experienced, the anterior cingulate is involved in selecting specific responses that are consonant with the situation as evaluated (e.g., fight or flight?).

In addition, the basal nucleus of the amygdala has dense interconnections with the orbital region of the prefrontal cortex. This cortical area appears to make use of the information provided by the amygdala about emotional and affective content of things experienced and sends to the amygdala information about the social context of a situation (e.g., dominance relationships, situational features). This route may permit the modulation of emotional and social behavior according to rapid changes in a social situation. Finally, the amygdala significantly interacts with the hippocampal formation to allow affective states to act upon and modulate stored information in cortical areas (e.g., past experience with an individual).

Given the specific roles played by the amygdala and orbitofrontal cortex in the self-regulation of social-emotional behaviors, it could be argued that dysfunction of the amygdala will result in difficulty detecting information relevant to the mental states, emotions, attitudes, and intentions of others and their significance for the self, while an early dysfunction of the orbitofrontal cortex will result in a difficulty in appropriately modifying one's own behavior in response to changes in the emotional and social behavior of others. In addition, dysfunction of the hippocampal formation and of the neocortical areas interacting with it may yield difficulty in forming new memories about things experienced, as well as their emotional significance. Indeed, both nonhuman

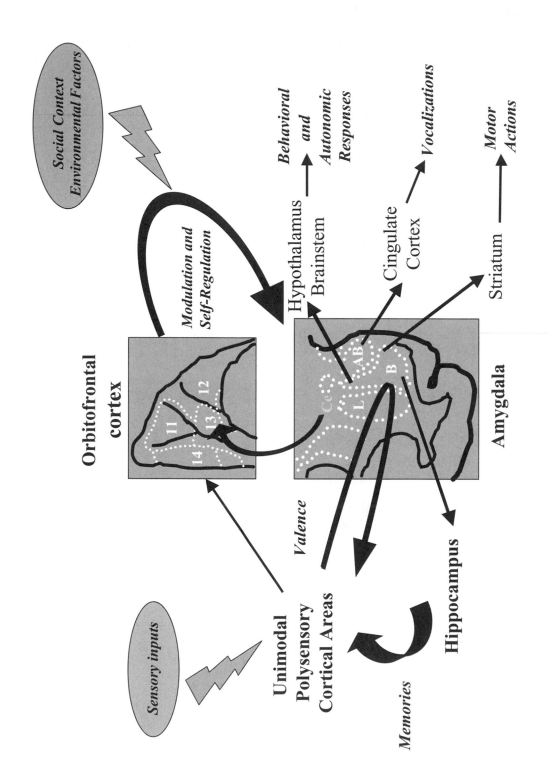

and human lesion studies have already provided strong evidence for these different possible outcomes.

However, one area of research for which data are almost totally lacking concerns the neural substrate for social cognition, and its development. Important questions in this domain are: "How does this neural circuit mature during the perinatal period and the first few years of life?" and "What is the role played by this neural network in the emergence of memories, affective states, and in the formation and maintenance of social bonds during the developmental period in primates?" In addition, given the important impacts that early environmental experiences have on the modulation and self-regulation of social cognition and its development (Sánchez et al., 2001; Schore, 1996), it seems critical to investigate how environmental experiences shape the development of these cortico-limbic structures, and to identify the different developmental windows during which environmental experiences may most significantly affect the development of this neural circuit, and thus the development of social cognition. As has been proposed by others (Cicchetti & Cannon, 1999; Schore, 1996), such a multifaceted, multidisciplinary approach will provide important information not only on the neurobiology of social development per se, but also on the origin of developmental psychopathology. As a point of departure to address these diverse questions on the neurobiology of social cognitive development, the following section will summarize studies that have examined the role played by structures within the neural circuit supporting social cognition, in the emergence of social skills in nonhuman primates.

EARLY DAMAGE TO THE MEDIAL TEMPORAL LOBE

From a neuropsychological perspective, the maturation of the neural substrate supporting social cognition can be studied via behavioral lesion experiments in the perinatal period. Thus, to investigate the role that the medial temporal lobe structures play in the development of social skills and emotional reactivity in developing monkeys, we followed the behavioral development of infant monkeys in which this neural substrate has been selectively damaged at birth. Newborn rhesus monkeys received bilateral lesions of the medial temporal lobe structures in the first few weeks of life. The development of their memory abilities, emotional reactivity, and social skills were then followed in some detail from infancy through adulthood and compared to the development of these abilities in age-matched controls. In our first group of operated animals, the lesions were relatively large, and included the amygdala, the hippocampus, and some of the adjacent medial temporal lobe cortex.

Figure 9.1. Schematic representation of the proposed orbitofrontal-amygdala circuit for the establishment, maintenance, and self-regulation of socioemotional behaviors. The two major components of this circuit are the amygdala (L: lateral nucleus, B: basal nucleus; AB: accessory basal nucleus; Ce: central nucleus) and the orbitofrontal cortex (cytoarchitectonic fields 11, 12, 13, and 14). The theoretical model suggests that, through their projectional system, the amygdala acts to detect information relevant to the mental states, emotions, attitudes, and intentions of others and their significance for the self, while the orbitofrontal cortex makes use of this information to guide goal-directed behaviors and to adjust one's own behavior in response to changes in the emotional and social behavior of others (refer to the text for a more complete description of the proposed neural circuit). It is proposed that a developmental dysfunction of this neural circuit is a biological marker for autism (from Bachevalier and Loveland, unpublished communication).

Almost immediately after the surgical removals, that is, at one month of age, memory abilities were investigated using a visual paired comparison task measuring object recognition memory. As compared to unoperated controls, infant monkeys with medial temporal lobe damage showed significant loss of object memory, and this impairment was still evident later, when the infant monkeys were tested at ten months of age in a different object recognition task (Bachevalier & Mishkin, 1994). Despite this severe recognition memory loss, monkeys with early medial temporal lobe lesions showed unimpaired abilities in mastering concurrent discrimination problems even with long intertrial intervals (Bachevalier, Brickson, Hagger, & Mishkin, 1990). Finally, the impairment in recognition memory in the operated animals persisted even when they reached adulthood and extended to tactile and spatial information as well (Málková, Mishkin, & Bachevalier, 1995). Thus, the data showed that (a) the medial temporal lobe structures operate early in life to sustain memory processes, (b) other regions of the brain cannot assume this function even when the damage occurs neonatally, and (c) recovery from early damage to this region is therefore limited at best.

To investigate the emotional and social development of infant monkeys with neonatal medial temporal lobe lesions, the social interactions between operated monkeys and their age-matched controls were analyzed at different time points in their maturation and compared to those of normal infants raised in the same conditions. Thus, unlike normal infant monkeys, those with neonatal medial temporal lobe lesions began to show numerous socioemotional abnormalities as they matured, including passivity, withdrawal from social interactions, lack of initiation of social interactions, and stereotypies. Interestingly, these striking behavioral changes were not apparent in the first two months postnatally but were present at six months (Bachevalier, Málková, & Mishkin, 2001). The results therefore indicate that the socioemotional effects of early damage to the medial temporal lobe are long-lasting, probably permanent, and if not in some way remediated, will increase in magnitude over time (i.e., they tend to "snowball" with development). Thus, these behavioral disturbances were still present when the animals reached adulthood and were greater than those observed in animals who had received the same lesions in adulthood (Málková, Mishkin, Suomi, & Bachevalier, 1997). The magnitude of difference in the social abnormalities after early or late lesions is interesting and could be due to the fact that monkeys given lesions in adulthood retained at least some skills from the socioemotional repertoire that they had acquired during maturation, whereas the neonatally operated animals never succeeded in acquiring them.

These findings demonstrate that compensatory mechanisms do not always operate to assure recovery of functions after early brain damage; indeed, in the case of socioemotional behaviors, the early medial temporal lobe lesions yielded more profound behavioral effects than late damage to the same neural system. The pattern of results thus suggests that, due to the immaturity of the brain at the time of the early medial temporal lobe lesions, the damage affected other neural systems remote from the site of the lesions. This view is indeed supported by additional studies that were performed on adult monkeys with early damage to the medial temporal lobe and their controls. First, as anticipated, the operated animals showed impairment in tasks measuring functions of the medial temporal lobe structures (recognition memory and spatial memory). However, the operated animals were unexpectedly impaired in working memory tasks, such as spatial delayed alternation, measuring dorsolateral prefrontal functions (J. Bachevalier, unpublished data). Furthermore, as compared to normal control and adult monkeys that had received the same lesions in adulthood, those with medial temporal lobe lesions in infancy showed a delayed maturation of the dorsolateral prefrontal cortex (Bertolino et al., 1997; Chlan-Fourney, Webster, Felleman, & Bachevalier, 2000), associated with a dysregulation of striatal dopaminergic neurotransmission (Heintz et al., 1999; Saunders, Kolachana, Bachevalier, & Weinberger, 1998) and increased volume of the caudate nucleus (Málková & Bachevalier, unpublished observations). Such dysregulation of prefrontal-striatal dopamine transmission could have an interesting relationship to the ritualistic and stereotyped behaviors seen in these animals, and its presence suggests that the lack of functional inputs from the medial temporal structures prevents the prefrontal cortex from undergoing proper neuronal development. More broadly, the data imply that a fixed dysfunction localized to one of the nodes of a neural circuit can influence other areas of the circuit, especially if this dysfunction occurs early in development.

In sum, the initial study demonstrated that neonatal damage to the medial temporal lobe structures in primates results in a profound loss in memory functions as well as socioemotional disturbances. But should this be regarded as a single complex syndrome, or might it be fractionated by damaging specific components of the medial temporal lobe? Further investigation of the underlying neural substrate of these behavioral disorders (Bachevalier, 1991, 1994, 2000) revealed that early damage to the amygdala yielded a pattern of socioemotional disturbances similar to that described for the large medial temporal lobe lesions, although the severity of these disturbances was much reduced. Thus, animals with neonatal amygdala lesions developed disturbances in social interactions (e.g., lack of social approaches, reduced eye contacts, low rank in dominance hierarchy) but only mild impairment in memory, most likely accounted for by damage to adjacent cortical areas (Bachevalier, Beauregard, & Alvarado, 1999). In addition, early damage to the hippocampal formation yielded severe memory deficits associated with mild changes in social interactions (e.g., withdrawals from social approaches, but maintenance of social status and normal eye contacts; Bachevalier, Alvarado, & Málková, 1999; Beauregard, Málková, & Bachevalier, 1995). Taken together, these results indicate that early damage to the amygdaloid complex and adjacent cortical areas may be more closely related to the emergence of autistic-like behaviors in monkeys than early damage to the hippocampal formation. Nevertheless, the full-fledged syndrome occurred only when damage to the amygdala was combined with damage to the hippocampus, and adjacent cortical areas.

Interestingly, there also are anecdotal reports indicating that early dysfunction of the medial temporal lobe yields significant changes in socioaffective states in children. Neuropathology in medial temporal lobe structures has been identified in several children displaying symptoms such as placidity, blunted affect, hyperorality, and aberrant sexual behavior (Caparros-Lefebvre et al., 1996; Chutorian & Antunes, 1981; Lanska & Lanska, 1993; Rossitch & Oakes, 1989; Tonsgard, Harwicke, & Levine, 1987). These findings again suggest that early insult to the medial temporal lobe in human children may yield profound changes in emotionality and social interactions. Such changes in the child's behavior may in turn lead to abnormal transactions with the environment, thereby contributing to subsequent abnormal brain development.

However, one important issue that has not been investigated is the impact of environmental experiences on an animal in which the neural circuit of social cognition

The nature of the core symptoms of ASD and their early appearance suggest that a neurobiological theory of this disorder must focus on brain systems or circuits that are implicated in the regulation of social and emotional behavior and that mature early in development. The neural network described earlier meets these criteria, and taken together with the experimental findings reported above, it can lead us to speculate about the ways in which different patterns of developmental brain dysfunction early in life might lead to different outcomes in persons with ASD. For example, dysfunction of both the amygdala and hippocampus in the first year of life, in addition to disrupting functions usually subserved by the amygdala and hippocampus, would also tend to dysregulate the orbitofrontal and dorsolateral prefrontal cortices (DLPFC), to which these structures project. A child with an early MTL dysfunction of this kind might therefore have the characteristic social-emotional deficits of ASD combined with mental retardation, most likely manifested as the more classical form of autism (e.g., Wing's Aloof category; Wing & Attwood, 1987; Wing & Gould, 1979). If instead the early brain dysfunction is restricted to the amygdala, the maturation of the orbitofrontal cortex will be adversely affected as this structure matures, but maturation of the hippocampus and DLPFC will not (or less so). Thus, severe social deficits might be manifested while intellectual functioning remains relatively unimpaired.

The observation that children with autism may have different developmental courses in early life (some manifest autism early, others appear to "regress" after a period of normal development) leads also to speculation about possible reasons for such differences. For example, if the primary dysfunction is not in the medial temporal area but in the orbitofrontal cortex, the child might not begin to manifest autistic social deficits until the second year of life, when the ventral prefrontal areas begin to mature (Schore, 1996). Subsequent development might then lead to dysregulation in the modulation of orbitofrontal-amygdala interactions. Differences in behavioral outcomes among children with autistic regression might be related to differences in the relative integrity of other brain structures, such as the dorsolateral prefrontal cortex, as well as to individual differences in experience that may further modulate brain development and learning.

The neurodevelopmental model discussed in this chapter reflects an integrated view of current ideas about the social deficits in autism, the accumulating knowledge on the neurobiology of social cognition and emotion, as well as the description of disordered patterns of behavior resulting from experimental damage to the limbic system. Because of the complexity of the clinical disorder and our incomplete knowledge of the neural system that controls and guides complex social behavior in our daily life, the model is at present oversimplified. For example, even though the amygdala and the orbitofrontal cortex are central to our neurodevelopmental model of autism, we believe that other brain structures, such as the temporal pole areas, the cingulate cortex, cerebellum, etc., and circuits in which they participate, are also likely to be involved in specific ways in this disorder. Moreover, we recognize that the neurodevelopmental model as proposed does not explain all the symptoms that can be associated with ASD, such as attention deficits, affective disorders and anxiety, repetitive behaviors, and motor differences; thus, other brain systems than those we have described may well be affected in individuals with ASD. At the present time, this neural model is offered not as a complete explanatory theory, but rather as an heuristic approach that will permit the generation of testable hypotheses about the possible outcomes that might result from early dysfunction of different portions of this neural network, under varying conditions over development of the individual.

FUTURE RESEARCH DIRECTIONS

Research in nonhuman primates has indicated that the medial temporal lobe structures play a critical role in cognitive and social development, although further research is needed to understand the specific processes by which these structures achieve their respective functions. Because of the many similarities in the perception and modulation of social signals across primates, additional developmental studies in monkeys and humans can help to elucidate the contribution of the amygdala and other related brain regions early in life, to the achievement of well-adapted social skills in adulthood. Among the most urgently needed studies to move this field forward are the following:

1. *The specific brain regions that form the neural network mediating social cognition, in both human and nonhuman primates.* It is clear that the regulation of complex social skills does not depend on one specific brain area but is subserved by a neural network specialized to support this function. Thus, studies using an array of neuropsychological and neurobiological tools should determine not only which brain structures play a critical role in social cognition but also their specific contributions to this function. Although studies in this domain have begun to appear (Adolphs, 2001), progress in our understanding of the neurobiology of social cognition remains limited.

2. *Development of the neural network subserving social cognition across the lifespan.* Because psychopathologies such as autism have their origin early in development, a better understanding is needed of the neurobiological processes by which the different brain structures related to social cognition mature and develop. Structural, metabolic, and physiological indices of primate brain development all point to a long postnatal time course of maturation that displays considerable variability from region to region and from system to system. Thus, the cytological constituents and neurochemical contents of amygdaloid nuclei and their efferent projections appear to be in place at birth (Humphrey, 1968; Kordower, Piecinski, & Rakic, 1992; Nikolic & Kostovic, 1986). However, some of the afferent projections from the temporal cortex to the amygdala continue to mature postnatally until the third month in monkeys (Webster, Ungerleider, & Bachevalier, 1991). In the hippocampus, neurons have reached their destination at birth in both humans and monkeys, but the development of dendrites and refinement of synaptic contacts continues for one to two postnatal years in monkeys and four to five years in humans (for review, see Alvarado & Bachevalier, 2000). Finally, refinement in the circuit organization of the dorsolateral prefrontal cortex undergoes substantial changes even during adolescence (i.e., two to three years in the monkeys and fourteen to seventeen years in humans, see Woo, Pucak, Kye, Matus, & Lewis, 1997). Much less is known on the maturational landmarks of the orbitofrontal cortex, however. A more detailed analysis of the major developmental stages of neural structures implicated in social cognition will not only provide information about when a specific structure is available and which specific processes it can subserve at a given time point during its maturation, but it will also provide information on critical developmental periods during which the self-reorganizing brain may allow for greater functional plasticity or more effective interventions.

3. *Interactions between brain development and risk from environmental events.* A better understanding of the neurobiological processes by which the brain structures related to social cognition develop may also provide more specific information about periods in development when greater vulnerabilities exist, such that the developing brain is more likely to be affected by adverse environmental events. Evidence from human and animal studies clearly suggests that early stressors such as those associated with inadequate caregiving, trauma, or other conditions that disrupt early social experience, are associated with differences in brain development that may have lifelong effects on the individual's emotional reactivity (Davidson, 1994; Dawson, Hessl, & Frey, 1994; Graham, Heim, Goodman, Miller, & Nemeroff, 1999; Meyer, Chrousos, & Gold, 1999; Post, Weiss, Leverich, George, Frye, & Ketter, 1996; Sánchez et al., 2001). One surprising observation is the similarities between the behavioral symptoms produced by early damage to the medial temporal lobe in primates and the symptoms following early social isolation in monkeys (see for review Sánchez et al, 2001; Bachevalier, 2000). Both experimental manipulations are associated with abnormal social skills and stereotypies resembling those seen in autism. These similarities have not only been noticed at the behavioral level but at the neural level as well. Indeed, dysregulation of prefrontal-striatal monoaminergic systems has been reported in both isolate- or peer-reared monkeys as well as in monkeys that had received neonatal damage to the medial temporal lobe (Bertolino et al., 1997, Saunders et al., 1998). This finding suggests that structures within the medial temporal lobe may be susceptible to the effects of environmental factors early in maturation, and, in turn, may initiate a cascade of neural events leading to aberrant neural circuits or structures, principally those with a protracted development, such as the prefrontal cortex. In this way, the experimental study in primates of long-term behavioral, neuroanatomical, and neurochemical effects of early damage to specific structures within the medial temporal lobe and orbitofrontal cortex is likely to yield critical information that will help elucidate the biological dysfunction involved in many developmental psychopathologies in humans.

4. *The interaction of genetic factors with experience and with brain maturation over development in autistic spectrum disorders.* Although some developmental disorders such as Down syndrome, Williams syndrome, Rett Syndrome, Prader-Willi/Angelman syndrome, and Fragile X syndrome have been found to be linked to specific genetic variations, the role of genetic factors in autism has been much less clear (Cook, Jr., 1998). At present there is much interest in uncovering genetic contributions to complex developmental and psychiatric disorders such as attention deficits, violent behavior, obsessive-compulsive disorder, depression, learning disabilities, anxiety, and autism (Asherson & Curran, 2001; Mundo, Richter, Sam, Macciardi, & Kennedy, 2001; New et al., 2001; Schmidt, Fox, Perez-Edgar, Hu, & Hamer, 2001; Yirmiya et al., 2001). Such investigations are necessary and important, for they may lead to improved understanding of risk factors for psychopathologies, as well as insights into the role of genotypes in the normal development of various areas of functioning. In particular, more information is needed about the ways in which particular genotypes may be linked to early differences in brain development that could lead to autism. However, genetic studies of autism are best viewed within the larger context of the mutual influences of genes, behavior, experience, and brain maturation (Cicchetti & Cannon, 1999; Gottlieb, 2001), rather than as a reductionistic search for the lowest possible level of explanation. Thus, at a molecular level, while genes may dictate the specific sequence and timing of brain development,

gene expression can also be modified by social and environmental factors during the postnatal period. Animal model studies have shown that genetic effects on behavior are complex and cannot always be linked to expression of specific types of behavior. Rather, genetic influences may affect how an individual is predisposed to respond in different situations and to different types of environmental challenges, such as threatening versus nonthreatening environments (Turri, Datta, DeFries, Henderson, & Flint, 2001). Tendencies to respond in certain ways (e.g., with withdrawal) may then interact with environmental experience to affect the course of development and the expression of possible psychopathology (e.g., Graham et al., 1999). For example, Post, Weiss, and Leverich (1994) have argued that in affective disorders, early stressors combined with repeated episodes of psychopathology can affect gene expression over the lifespan of the individual. One can speculate that in autistic spectrum disorders, genetic variations may affect development of the systems in the brain that subserve social cognition, affect, and self-regulation. However, the full expression of the syndrome of autism, or the extent to which it is expressed, may depend critically on the additional adverse effects of abnormal early transactions with the child's environment, which can affect both subsequent brain development and the child's learned ability to self-regulate behavior.

5. *Individual differences on the autistic spectrum of disorder.* One reason that progress has been slow in the attempt to identify neurobiological and genetic bases for autism is that the disorder is highly heterogeneous in its expression. This fact is reflected in the current, widely adopted usage, in which autism is referred to as the autistic spectrum of disorder (ASD). As was discussed earlier, individuals with ASD vary widely in areas such as the severity of social-emotional symptoms; the extent of intellectual deficits and language deficits; the extent to which associated symptoms and other psychopathologies are present; and the specific and idiosyncratic manifestations of preoccupations or repetitive behaviors (see Loveland & Tunali-Kotoski, 1997 for a review). A major challenge for any model of brain development in ASD, therefore, is to address the neural substrate for the central characteristics of the disorder, while at the same time giving an account of how variations in its expression might arise. Clearly, a simple and static unidirectional model in which a defective brain structure results in a specific behavioral deficit is not adequate for this purpose. In our model we have sought to present the basis for a more comprehensive approach, one that provides some insight into possible sources of variability linked to differences in neural development. Much further work is needed to explain how the hypothesized neural substrates for ASD, together with other brain structures likely to be involved in the disorder, reciprocally interact with both genetic and environmental influences over the life of the individual.

6. *Links between neurobiological bases and clinical manifestations of autism.* A final area that is as yet poorly understood is the relationship of hypothesized brain differences in ASD to clinical manifestations of the disorder. Although one can readily speculate about the ways that specific brain differences might be associated with behavioral manifestations in the daily lives of individuals with ASD, there is very little evidence to support such associations. Rather, the existing research has focused mostly on neuropsychological tests and laboratory experimental measures of autistic behaviors (Loveland, 2001). Moreover, there is very little known about the ways that differences in brain development in ASD are specifically related to changes in an individual's behavior over the lifespan. Studies that make testable predictions in these areas are critical to determining the validity and usefulness of brain models of ASD.

CONCLUSIONS

While the review presented here focuses on a circuit linking the amygdala and or-bitofrontal cortex, it is clear that the regulation of social cognition is orchestrated by a multitude of interconnected structures. This complexity shows how studies of non-human primates will be needed to further our understanding of the neural processes subserving social cognition. Because of the many similarities in the ways social signals are perceived and modulated across primate species, research in monkeys and humans should proceed in parallel, each informing and complementing the other with theo-retical and empirical contributions. Thus, we stress the urgent need to initiate joint clinical (human) and animal research explorations, in order to specify the contribu-tion of the amygdala and other related brain regions early in life to the achievement of well-adapted social behavior in adulthood. These clinical and experimental stud-ies will require multiple levels of analysis (brain, behavior, genetic and environmen-tal factors) given that well-adapted social skills are the results of a dynamic process linking neural maturation with environmental influences and the child's own self-regulatory activity across development (Cicchetti & Cannon, 1999; Cicchetti & Tucker, 1994; Loveland, 2001; Schore, 1996). Such a multidisciplinary research approach has the potential to revise and expand our current understanding of brain development and its relation to the development of basic behavioral processes, such as social cognition and social-emotional self-regulation. We believe that it also may offer a new foundation for determining the neuropathological bases of several developmental psychopatholo-gies in humans and, ultimately, for developing therapeutic tools to alleviate these disorders.

REFERENCES

Abell, F., Krams, M., Ashburner, J., Passingham, R., Friston, K., Frackowiak, R., Happé, F., Frith, C., & Frith, U. (1999). The neuroanatomy of autism: a voxel-based whole brain analysis of structural scans. *NeuroReport, 10,* 1647–1651.

Adolphs, R. (2001). The neurobiology of social cognition. *Current Opinion in Neurobiology, 11,* 231–239.

Alvarado, M.C., & Bachevalier, J. (2000). Revisiting the maturation of medial temporal lobe mem-ory functions in primates. *Learning & Memory, 7,* 244–256.

Asherson, P.J., & Curran, S. (2001). Approaches to gene mapping in complex disorders and their application in child psychiatry and psychology. *British Journal of Psychiatry, 179,* 122–128.

Aylward, E.H., Minshew, N.J., Goldstein, G., Honeycutt, N.A., Augustine, A.M., Yates, K.O., Barta, P.E., & Pearlson, G.D. (1999). MRI volumes of amygdala and hippocampus in non-mentally retarded autistic adolescents and adults. *Neurology, 53,* 2145–2150.

Bachevalier, J. (1991). An animal model for childhood autism: Memory loss and socioemotional disturbances following neonatal damage to the limbic system in monkeys. In C.A. Tamminga & S.C. Schulz (Eds.), *Advances in neuropsychiatry and psychopharmacology, Volume 1: schizophrenia research* (pp. 129–140). New York: Raven Press.

Bachevalier, J. (1994). Medial temporal lobe structures and autism: A review of clinical and exper-imental findings. *Neuropsychologia, 32,* 627–648.

Bachevalier, J. (2000). The amygdala, social behavior, and autism. In J.P. Aggleton (Ed.), *The amyg-dala: A functional analysis,* 2d ed. (pp. 509–544). New York: Oxford University Press.

Bachevalier, J., Alvarado, M.C., & Málková, L. (1999). Effects of early versus late damage to the hip-pocampal formation on memory and socioemotional behavior in monkeys. *Biological Psychiatry, 46,* 329–339.

Bachevalier, J., Beauregard, M., & Alvarado, M.C. (1999). Long-term effects of neonatal damage to the hippocampal formation and amygdaloid complex on object discrimination and object recognition in rhesus monkeys. *Behavioral Neuroscience, 113,* 1127–1151.

Bachevalier, J., Brickson, M., Hagger, C., & Mishkin, M. (1990). Age and sex differences in the effects of selective temporal lobe lesion on the formation of visual discrimination habits in rhesus monkeys. *Behavioral Neuroscience, 104,* 885–899.

Bachevalier, J., Málková, L., & Mishkin, M. (2001). Effects of selective neonatal medial temporal lobe lesions on socioemotional behaviors in monkeys. *Behavioral Neuroscience, 115,* 545–560.

Bachevalier J., & Mishkin M. (1994). Effects of selective neonatal temporal lobe lesions on visual recognition memory in rhesus monkeys. *Journal of Neuroscience, 14,* 2128–2139.

Bacon, A., Fein, D., Morris, R., Waterhouse, L., & Allen, D. (1998). The responses of autistic children to the distress of others. *Journal of Autism & Developmental Disorders, 28,* 129–142.

Baron-Cohen, S., Leslie, A., & Frith, U. (1985). Does the autistic child have a "theory of mind"? *Cognition, 21,* 37–46.

Baron-Cohen, S., Ring, H.A., Bullmore, E.T., Wheelwright, S., Ashwin, C., & Williams, S.C. (2000). The amygdala theory of autism. *Neuroscience and Biobehavioral Review, 24,* 355–364.

Baron-Cohen, S., Ring, H.A., Wheelwright, S., Bullmore, E.T., Brammer, M.J., Simmons, A., & Williams, S.C.R. (1999). Social intelligence in the normal and autistic brain: an fMRI study. *European Journal of Neuroscience, 11,* 1891–1898.

Bauman, M.L., & Kemper, T.L. (1993). Cytoarchitectonic changes in the brain of people with autism. In M.L. Bauman & T.L. Kemper (Eds.), *The neurobiology of autism* (pp. 119–145). Baltimore: Johns Hopkins Press.

Beauregard, M., Málková, L., & Bachevalier, J. (1995). Stereotypies and loss of social affiliation after early hippocampectomy in monkeys. *NeuroReport, 6,* 2521–2526.

Bertolino, A., Saunders, R.C., Mattay, V.S., Bachevalier, J., Frank, J.A., & Weinberger, D.R. (1997). Altered development of prefrontal neurons in rhesus monkeys with neonatal mesial temporo-limbic lesions: a proton magnetic resonance spectroscopic imaging study. *Cerebral Cortex, 7,* 740–748.

Brothers, L. (1995). Neurophysiology of the perception of intention by primates. In M.S. Gazzaniga (Ed.), *The cognitive neurosciences* (pp. 1107–1117). Cambridge, Mass.: MIT Press.

Byrne, R., & Whiten, A. (1988). *Machiavellian intelligence: Social expertise and the evolution of intellect in monkeys, apes, and humans.* Oxford: Clarendon Press.

Campbell, M., Rosenbloom, S., Perry, R., George, A.E., Kricheff, I.I., Anderson, L., Small, A.M., & Jennings, S.J. (1982). Computerized axial tomography in young autistic children. *American Journal of Psychiatry, 139,* 510–512.

Caparros-Lefebvre, D., Girard-Buttaz, I., Reboul, S., Lebert, F., Cabaret, M., Verier, A., Steinling, M., Pruvo, J.P., & Petit, H. (1996). Cognitive and psychiatric impairment in herpes simplex virus encephalitis suggest involvement of the amygdalo-frontal pathways. *Journal of Neurology, 243,* 248–256.

Capps, L., Kasari, C., Yirmiya, N., & Sigman, M. (1993). Parental perception of emotional expressiveness in children with autism. *Journal of Consulting & Clinical Psychology, 61,* 475–484.

Carper, R.A., & Courchesne, E. (2000). Inverse correlation between frontal lobe and cerebellum sizes in children with autism. *Brain, 123,* 836–844.

Cheney, D.L., & Seyfarth, R.M. (1990). *How monkeys see the world.* Chicago: University of Chicago Press.

Chlan-Fourney, J., Webster, M.J., Felleman, D.J., & Bachevalier, J. (2000). Neonatal medial temporal lobe lesions alter the distribution of tyrosine hydroxylase immunoreactive varicosities in the macaque prefrontal cortex. *Society for Neuroscience Abstract, 26,* 609.

Chutorian A.B., & Antunes J.L. (1981). Klüver-Bucy syndrome and Herpes encephalitis: Case report. *Neurosurgery, 8,* 388–390.

Cicchetti, D., & Cannon, T.D. (1999). Neurodevelopmental processes in the ontogenesis and epigenesis of psychopathology. *Development and Psychopathology, 11,* 375–393.

Cicchetti, D., & Tucker, D. (1994). Development and self-regulatory structures of the mind. *Development and Psychopathology, 6,* 533–549.

Cook, Jr., E.H. (1998). Genetics of autism. *Mental Retardation and Developmental Disabilities Research Reviews, 4,* 113–120.

Corona, R., Dissanayake, C., Arbelle, S., Wellington, P., & Sigman, M. (1998). Is affect aversive to young children with autism? Behavioral and cardiac responses to experimenter distress. *Child Development, 69,* 1494–1502.

Critchley, H.D., Daly, E.M., Bullmore, E.T., Williams, S.C., Van Amelsvoort, T., Robertson, D.M., Rowe, A., Phillips, M., McAlonan, G., Howlin, P., & Murphy, D.G. (2000). The functional neuroanatomy of social behaviour: Changes in cerebral blood flow when people with autistic disorder process facial expressions. *Brain, 123,* 2203–2212.

Damasio, A.R., Maurer, R.G., Damasio, A.R., & Chui, H. (1980). Computerized tomographic scan findings in patients with autistic behavior. *Archives of Neurology, 37,* 504–510.

Davidson, R.J. (1994). Asymmetric brain function, affective style, and psychopathology: The role of early experience and plasticity. *Development and Psychopathology, 6,* 741–758.

Dawson, G. (1996). The neuropsychology of autism. *Journal of Autism and Developmental Disorders, 26,* 179–184.

Dawson, G., Hessl, D., & Frey, K. (1994). Social influences on early-developing biological and behavioral systems related to risk for affective disorder. *Development and Psychopathology, 6,* 759–779.

DeLong, G.R. (1978). A neuropsychological interpretation of infantile autism. In E. Schopler & G.B. Mesibov (Eds.), *Autism* (pp. 207–218). New York: Plenum.

Dennis, M., Lockyer, L., & Lazenby, A.L. (2000). How high-functioning children with autism understand real and deceptive emotion. *Autism, 4,* 370–381.

Deonna, T., Ziegler, A-L., Moura-Serra, J., & Innocenti, G. (1993). Autistic regression in relation to limbic pathology and epilepsy: Report of two cases. *Developmental Medicine and Child Neurology, 35,* 166–176.

Devinsky, O., Morrell, M.J., & Vogt, B.A. (1995). Contributions of anterior cingulate cortex to behaviour. *Brain, 118,* 279–306.

DeWaal, F. (1989). *Peacemaking among primates.* Cambridge, Mass.: Harvard University Press.

Deykin, E.Y., & MacMahon, B. (1979). The incidence of seizures among children with autistic symptoms. *American Journal of Psychiatry, 136,* 860–864.

Fein, D., Pennington, B., & Waterhouse, L. (1987). Implications of social deficits in autism for neurological dysfunction. In E. Schopler & G.B. Mesibov (Eds.), *Neurobiological issues in autism* (pp. 127–144). New York: Plenum.

Filipek, P.A., Richelme, C., Kennedy, D.N., Rademacher, J., Pitcher, D.A., Zidel, S.Y., & Caviness, V.S. (1992). Morphometric analysis of the brain in developmental language disorders and autism. *Annals of Neurology, 32,* 475.

Fotheringham, J.B. (1991). Autism and its primary psychosocial and neurological deficit. *Canadian Journal of Psychiatry, 36,* 686–692.

George, M.S., Costa, D.C., Kouris, K., Ring, H.A., & Ell, P.J. (1992). Cerebral blood flow abnormalities in adults with infantile autism. *Journal of Nervous and Mental Diseases, 180,* 413–417.

Gibson, J.J. (1979). *The ecological approach to visual perception.* Boston: Houghton-Mifflin.

Gottlieb, G. (2001). A developmental psychobiological systems view: Early formulation and current status. In S. Oyama & P.E. Griffiths (Eds.), *Cycles of contingency: Developmental systems and evolution* (pp. 41–54). Cambridge, Mass.: MIT Press.

Graham, Y.P., Heim, C., Goodman, S.H., Miller, A.H., & Nemeroff, C.B. (1999). The effects of neonatal stress on brain development: Implications for psychopathology. *Development and Psychopathology, 11,* 545–565.

Grossman, J.B., Carter, A., & Volkmar, F.R. (1997). Social behavior in autism. *Annals of the New York Academy of Science, 807,* 440–454.

Hadwin, J., Baron-Cohen, S., Howlin, P., & Hill, K. (1996). Can we teach children with autism to understand emotions, belief, or pretence? *Development and Psychopathology, 8,* 345–365.

Hadwin, J., Baron-Cohen, S., Howlin, P., & Hill, K. (1997). Does teaching Theory of Mind have an effect on the ability to develop conversation in children with autism? *Journal of Autism and Developmental Disorders, 27,* 519–537.

Harrison, D.W, Demaree, H.A., Shenal, B.V., & Everhart, D.E. (1998). EEG assisted neuropsychological evaluation of autism. *International Journal of Neuroscience, 93,* 133–140.

Hashimoto, T., Sasaki, M., Fukumizu, M., Hanaoka, S., Sugai, K., & Matsuda, H. (2000). Single-photon emission computed tomography of the brain in autism: Effect of the developmental level. *Pediatric Neurology, 23,* 416–420.

Hauser, S.L., DeLong, G.R., & Rosman, N.P. (1975). Pneumoencephalographic finding in the infantile autism syndrome: A correlation with temporal lobe disease. *Brain, 98,* 667–668.

Haznedar, M.M., Buchsbaum, M.S., Wei, T-C., Hof, P.R., Cartwright, C., Bienstock, C.A., & Hollander, E. (2000). Limbic circuitry in patients with autism spectrum disorders studied with positron emission tomography and magnetic resonance imaging. *American Journal of Psychiatry, 157,* 1994–2001.

Heavey, L., Phillips, W., Baron-Cohen, S., & Rutter, M. (2000). The Awkward Moments Test: A naturalistic measure of social understanding in autism. *Journal of Autism & Developmental Disorders, 30,* 225–236.

Heintz, A., Saunders, R.C., Kolachana, B.S., Jones, D.W., Gorey, J.G., Bachevalier, J., & Weinberger, D.R. (1999). Striatal dopamine receptors and transporters in monkeys with neonatal temporal limbic damage. *Synapse, 32,* 71–79.

Hobson, R.P. (1986). The autistic child's appraisal of expressions of emotion. *Journal of Child Psychology and Psychiatry, 27,* 321–342.

Hof, P.R., Knabe, R., Bovier, P., & Bouras, C. (1991). Neuropathological observations in a case of autism presenting with self-injury behavior. *Acta Neuropathologica, 82,* 321–326.

Howard, M.A., Cowell, P.E., Boucher, J., Broks, P., Mayes, A., Farrant, A., & Roberts, N. (2000). Convergent neuroanatomical and behavioural evidence of an amygdala hypothesis of autism. *NeuroReport, 11,* 2931–2935.

Humphrey, T. (1968). The development of the human amygdala during early embryonic life. *Journal of Comparative Neurology, 132,* 135–165.

Jacobson, R., Le Couteur, A., Howlin, P., & Rutter, M. (1988). Selective subcortical abnormalities in autism. *Psychological Medicine, 18,* 39–48.

Jaedicke, S., Storoschuk, S., & Lord, C. (1994). Subjective experience and causes of affect in high-functioning children and adolescents with autism. *Development & Psychopathology. 6,* 273–284.

Jiao, Q. (2001). Research on Theory of Mind in autism [Chinese]. *Chinese Mental Health Journal, 15,* 60–62.

Joseph, R.M., & Tager-Flusberg, H. (1997). An investigation of attention and affect in children with autism and Down syndrome. *Journal of Autism & Developmental Disorders. 27,* 385–396.

Kamio, Y. (1998). Affective understanding in high-functioning autistic adolescents [Japanese]. *Japanese Journal of Child & Adolescent Psychiatry. 39,* 340–351.

Kawasaki, Y., Yokota, K., Shinomiya, M., Shimizu, Y., & Niwa, S. (1997). Electroencephalographic paroxysmal activities in the frontal area emerged in middle childhood and during adolescence in a follow-up study of autism. *Journal of Autism & Developmental Disorders, 27,* 605–620.

Klin, A.S. (2000). Attributing social meaning to ambiguous visual stimuli in higher-functioning autism and Asperger syndrome: The Social Attribution Task. *Child Psychology and Psychiatry, 41,* 831–46.

Kling, A., & Green, P.C. (1967). Effects of neonatal amygdalectomy in the maternally reared and maternally deprived macaque. *Nature, 213,* 742–743.

Kordower, J.H., Piecinski, P., & Rakic, P. (1992). Neurogenesis of the amygdaloid nuclear complex in the rhesus monkey. *Developmental Brain Research, 68,* 9–15.

Lanska, D.J., & Lanska, M.J. (1993). Klüver-Bucy syndrome in juvenile neuronal ceroid lipofuscinosis. *Journal of Child Neurology, 9,* 67–69.

Loveland, K. (1991). Social affordances and interaction: Autism and the affordances of the human environment. *Ecological Psychology, 3,* 99–119.

Loveland, K.A. (2001). Toward an ecological theory of autism. In J.A. Burack, T. Charman, N. Yirmiya, & P.R. Zelazo (Eds.), *The development of autism: Perspectives from theory and research* (pp. 17–37). Hillsdale, N.J.: Erlbaum.

Loveland, K., Pearson, D.A., Tunali-Kotoski, B., Ortegon, J., & Gibbs, M.C. (2001). Judgments of social appropriateness by children and adolescents with autism. *Journal of Autism and Developmental Disorders, 31,* 367–376.

Loveland, K., & Tunali, B. (1991). Social scripts for conversational interactions in autism and Down syndrome. *Journal of Autism and Developmental Disorders, 21,* 177–186.

Loveland, K., & Tunali-Kotoski, B. (1997). The school-aged child with autism. In Cohen, D., & Volkmar, F. (Eds.), *The handbook of autism and pervasive developmental disorders*. 2d Ed. (pp. 283–308). New York: Wiley.

Loveland, K., Tunali-Kotoski, B., Pearson, D., Brelsford, K., Ortegon, J., & Chen, R. (1994). Imitation and expression of facial affect in autism. *Development and Psychopathology, 6*, 433–444.

Loveland, K., Tunali-Kotoski, B., Pearson, D., Chen, R., Brelsford, K., & Ortegon, J. (1995). Intermodal perception of affect by persons with autism or Down syndrome. *Development and Psychopathology, 7*, 409–418.

Málková, L., Mishkin, M., & Bachevalier, J. (1995). Long-term effects of selective neonatal temporal lobe lesions on learning and memory in monkeys. *Behavioral Neuroscience, 109*, 212–226.

Málková, L., Mishkin, M., Suomi, S.J., & Bachevalier, J. (1997). Socioemotional behavior in adult rhesus monkeys after early versus late lesions of the medial temporal lobe. *Annals of the New York Academy of Science, 807*, 538–540.

McGregor, E., Whiten, A., & Blackburn, P. (1998). Teaching theory of mind by highlighting intention and illustrating thoughts: A comparison of their effectiveness with 3-year olds and autistic individuals. *British Journal of Developmental Psychology, 16*, 281–300.

Meyer, S.E., Chrousos, G.P., & Gold, P.W. (1999). Major depression and the stress system: A lifespan perspective. *Development and Psychopathology, 13*, 565–580.

Minshew, N.J., Luna, B., & Sweeney, J.A. (1999). Oculomotor evidence for neocortical systems but not cerebellar dysfunction in autism. *Neurology, 52*, 917–922.

Mundo, E., Richter, M., Sam, F., Macciardi, F., & Kennedy, J.L. (2001). "5-HT-sub(1D) function and repetitive behaviors": Reply. *American Journal of Psychiatry, 158*, 973.

New, A.S., Gelernter, J., Goodman, M, Mitropoulou, V., Koenigsberg, H., Silverman, J., & Siever, L.J. (2001). Suicide, impulsive aggression, and HTR1B genotype. *Biological Psychiatry, 50*, 62–65.

Nikolic, I., & Kostovic, I. (1986). Development of the lateral amygdaloid nucleus in the human fetus: transient presence of discrete cytoarchitectonic units. *Anatomical Embryology, 174*, 355–360.

Ochsner, K.N., & Lieberman, M.D. (2001). The emergence of social cognitive neuroscience. *American Psychologist, 56*, 717–734.

Ohnishi, T., Matsuda, H., Hashimoto, T., Kunihiro, T., Nishikawa, M., Uema, T., & Sasaki, M. (2000). Abnormal regional cerebral blood flow in childhood autism. *Brain, 123*, 1838–1844.

Payton, J.B., & Minshew, N.J. (1987). Early appearance of partial complex seizures in children with infantile autism. *Annals of Neurology, 22*, 408.

Phillips, W., Baron-Cohen, S., & Rutter, M. (1998). Understanding intention in normal development and in autism. *British Journal of Developmental Psychology, 16*, 337–348.

Pierce, K., Glad, K.S., & Schreibman, L. (1997). Social perception in children with autism: an attentional deficit? *Journal of Autism and Developmental Disorders, 27*, 265–282.

Post, R.M., Weiss, S.R.B., & Leverich, G.S. (1994). Recurrent affective disorder: Roots in developmental neurobiology and illness progression based on changes in gene expression. *Development and Psychopathology, 6*, 781–813.

Post, R.M., Weiss, S.R.B., Leverich, G.S., George, M.S., Frye, M., & Ketter, T.A. (1996). Developmental psychobiology of affective illness: Implications for early therapeutic intervention. *Development and Psychopathology, 8*, 273–305.

Prather, M.D., Lavenex, P., Mauldin-Jourdain, M.L., Mason, W.A., Capitanio, J.P., Mendoza, S.P., & Amaral, D.G. (2001). Increased social fear and decreased fear of objects in monkeys with neonatal amygdala lesions. *Neuroscience, 106*, 653–658.

Raleigh, M.J. (1995). Neural mechanisms supporting successful social decisions in simians. In Y. Christen, A. Damasion, & H. Damasio (Eds.), *Neurobiology of decision making* (pp. 63–82). Berlin: Springer.

Rieffe, C., Terwogt, M., & Stockmann, L. (2000). Understanding atypical emotions among children with autism. *Journal of Autism and Developmental Disorders, 30*, 195–203.

Rossitch, E., & Oakes, W.J. (1989). Klüver-Bucy syndrome in a child with bilateral arachnoid cysts: report of a case. *Neurosurgery, 24*, 110–112.

Sánchez, M.M., Ladd, C.O., & Plotsky, P.M. (2001). Early adverse experience as a developmental risk factor for later psychopathology: Evidence from rodent and primate models. *Development and Psychopathology, 13*, 419–449.

Saunders, R.C., Kolachana, B.S., Bachevalier, J., & Weinberger, D.R. (1998). Neonatal lesions of the medial temporal lobe disrupt prefrontal cortical regulation of striatal dopamine. *Nature, 393,* 169–171.

Schmidt, L.A., Fox, N.A., Perez-Edgar, K., Hu, S., & Hamer, D.H. (2001). Association of DRD4 with attention problems in normal childhood development. *Psychiatric Genetics, 11,* 25–29.

Schore, A.N. (1996). The experience-dependent maturation of a regulatory system in the orbital prefrontal cortex and the origin of developmental psychopathology. *Development and Psychopathology, 8,* 59–87.

Schultz, R.T., Gauthier, I., Klin, A., Fulbright, R.K., Anderson, A.W., Volkmar, F., Skudlarski, P., Lacadie, C., Cohen, D.J., & Gore, J.C. (2000). Abnormal ventral temporal cortical activity during face discrimination among individuals with autism and Asperger syndrome. *Archives of General Psychiatry, 57*(4): 331–340.

Schultz, R.T., Romanski, L.M, & Tsatsanis, K.D. (2000). Neurofunctional models of autistic disorder and Asperger syndrome: Clues from neuroimaging. In Ami Klin & Fred R. Volkmar (Eds.), *Asperger syndrome* (pp. 172–209). New York: Guilford Press.

Seegmuller, C., Gras-Vincendon, A., & Bursztejn, C. (2000). Theory of mind tasks in pervasive developmental disorders: Interest for diagnosis [French]. Original title: Intérêt diagnostique des épreuves de théorie de l'esprit dans les troubles envahissants du développement. *Annales Médico-Psychologiques, 158,* 577–580.

Serra, M., Minderaa, R.B., van Geert, P.L., & Jackson, A.E. (1999). Social-cognitive abilities in children with lesser variants of autism: skill deficits or failure to apply skills? *European Child and Adolescent Psychiatry, 8,* 301–11.

Siegel, B.V., Nuechterlein, K.H., Abel, L., Wu, J.C., & Buchsbaum, M.S. (1995). Glucose metabolic correlates of continuous performance test performance in adults with a history of infantile autism, schizophrenics, and controls. *Schizophrenia Research, 17,* 85–94.

Sigman, M.D., Kasari, C., Kwon, J.H., & Yirmiya, N. (1992). Responses to the negative emotions of others by autistic, mentally retarded, and normal children. *Child Development, 63,* 796–807.

Snow, M.E., Hertzig, M.E., & Shapiro, T. (1987). Expression of emotion in young autistic children. *Journal of the American Academy of Child and Adolescent Psychology, 26,* 836–838.

Starkstein, S.E., Vazquez, S., Vranic, D., Nanclares, V., Manes, F., Piven, J., & Plebst, C. (2000). SPECT findings in mentally retarded autistic individuals. *Journal of Neuropsychiatry and Clinical Neuroscience, 12,* 370–375.

Thompson, C.I. (1981). Long-term behavioral development of rhesus monkeys after amygdalectomy in infancy. In Y. Ben Ari (Ed.), *The amygdaloid complex* (pp. 259–270). Amsterdam: Elsevier.

Tonsgard, J.H., Harwicke, N., & Levine, S.C. (1987). Klüver-Bucy syndrome in children. *Pediatric Neurology, 3,* 162–165.

Turri, M.G., Datta, S.R., DeFries, J., Henderson, N.D., & Flint, J. (2001). QTL analysis identifies multiple behavioral dimensions in ethological tests of anxiety in laboratory mice. *Current Biology, 11,* 725–734.

Vogt, B.A., Finch, D.M., & Olson, C.R. (1992). Functional heterogeneity in cingulate cortex: The anterior executive and posterior evaluative regions. *Cerebral Cortex, 2,* 435–443.

Webster, M.J., Ungerleider, L.G., & Bachevalier, J. (1991). Connections of inferior temporal areas TE and TEO with medial temporal-lobe structures in infant and adult monkeys. *Journal of Neuroscience, 11,* 1095–1116.

Weeks, S., & Hobson, R.P. (1987). The salience of facial expression for autistic children. *Journal of Child Psychology and Psychiatry, 28,* 137–151.

Wing, L., & Attwood, A. (1987). Syndromes of autism and atypical development. In D. Cohen, A. Donellen, & R. Paul (Eds.), *Handbook of autism and pervasive developmental disorders* (pp. 3–19). New York: Wiley-Liss.

Wing, L., & Gould, J. (1979). Severe impairments of social interaction and associated abnormalities in children: Epidemiology and classification. *Journal of Autism and Developmental Disorders, 9,* 11–29.

Woo, T.U., Pucak, M.L., Kye, C.H., Matus, C.V., & Lewis, D.A. (1997). Peripubertal refinement of the intrinsic and associational circuitry in monkey prefrontal cortex. *Neuroscience, 80,* 1149–1158.

Yirmiya, N., Kasari, C., Sigman, M., & Mundy P. (1989). Facial expressions of affect in autistic, mentally retarded, and normal children. *Journal of Child Psychology and Psychiatry, 30,* 725–736.

Yirmiya, N., Pilowsky, T., Nemanov, L., Arbelle, S., Feinsilver, T., Fried, I., & Ebstein, R.P. (2001). Analysis of three coding region polymorphisms in autism: Evidence for an association with the serotonin transporter. In E. Schopler & N. Yirmiya (Eds.). *The research basis for autism intervention* (pp. 91–101). New York: Kluwer Academic/Plenum Publishers.

Yirmiya, N., Sigman, M., Kasari, C., & Mundy, P. (1992). Empathy and cognition in high-functioning children with autism. *Child Development, 63,* 150–160.

Zilbovicius, M., Garreau, B., Samson, Y., Remy, P., Barthelemy, C., Syrota, A., & Lelord, G. (1995). Delayed maturation of the frontal cortex in childhood autism. *American Journal of Psychiatry, 152,* 248–252.

PART THREE

Models of the Nature of Genetic and Environmental Influences on the Developmental Course of Psychopathology

TEN

Genetic Structure of Neurodevelopmental Traits

Implications for the Development (and Definition of) Psychopathology

Richard D. Todd and John N. Constantino

Human genetic studies over the last thirty years have demonstrated that for many be-havioral traits and most common axis I psychiatric disorders, genetic influences are on the order of 35 to 80 percent or greater (Plomin et al., 2001). These influences on com-mon traits and disorders represent the effects of numerous genes, each conferring small contributions to the phenotype of the behavior in question. These genes may interact with each other in highly complex ways which vary over the course of development and can be modulated by environmental changes. Hence, though it is straightforward to demonstrate the presence and magnitude of genetic effects contributing to traits and disorders, it remains exceedingly difficult to demonstrate which gene and neu-rodevelopmental mechanisms are involved. Further complicating the matter is that the phenotypes of many common disorders which are known to have complex genetic influences may be mimicked by rare single-gene mutations (which may provide clues to the mechanisms or pathways of these disorders). The main goals of this chapter are to review known genetic mechanisms involved in the development of psychopathology, emphasizing early onset disorders, and to demonstrate how to integrate epidemiolog-ical, clinical, and family study data to describe the genetic structure of disorders and traits. A perusal of findings from genetic studies of selected autistic syndromes illustrates the complex principles of inheritance that underlie neurodevelopmental traits.

GENETIC MECHANISMS IN SEVERE AUTISTIC SYNDROMES

Until very recently, genomic surveys looking for chromosomal locations associated with autism failed to demonstrate linkage relationships meeting conventional criteria for statistical significance (IMGSAC, 1998; Ashley-Koch et al., 1999; Auranen et al., 2000; Barrett et al., 1999; Phillippe et al., 1999; Risch et al., 1999). An analysis of data from the International Molecular Genetic Study of Autism published in September 2001 revealed strong evidence that two regions on chromosomes 2 and 7 respectively contain genes that confer susceptibility to autism (IMGSAC, 2001). Chromosome 7 has previously been associated with a variety of developmental disorders of language. Although it is likely, then, that these genes play a role in the development of autism, it is also likely that most cases of autism are a function of the effects of multiple genes operating simultaneously to produce the disorder. Model fitting estimates of the number of genes that interact to contribute to susceptibility for most cases of autism in the population range from 2–10 (Pickles et al., 1995) to 10–20 (Risch et al., 1999).

Despite this likelihood of an oligogenic mode of inheritance for most cases of categorically defined autism, some children with Fragile X syndrome, Angelman's syndrome, Tuberous Sclerosis, and Rett syndrome – all specific single-gene defects – exhibit autistic syndromes that are indistinguishable from those of autistic children without these disorders. These rare conditions represent phenocopies of the autistic syndrome, meaning that there are multiple genetic pathways to this particular clinical phenotype.

Fragile X Syndrome

One specific mechanism for mutation that has been found repeatedly in neuropsychiatric disorders is trinucleotide repeat expansion. Trinucleotide repeats consist of three nucleotides consecutively repeated (e.g., CAG CAG CAG CAG) within a region of DNA. In expansion mutations, the number of triplets in a repeat slowly increases during each meiosis until the length eventually becomes large and unstable. This represents a mechanism for variable mutations at a single locus, which can result in a wide range of phenotypic variations, particularly in terms of severity. This variability includes differences between siblings with the same disorder since different length expansions may occur during separate meioses. For example, much of the clinical variation in age of onset and severity of Huntington's Disease in a large Venezuelan family can be accounted for by earlier onset cases that have a larger expansion repeat size in the Huntington gene. Almost all of the twenty human disorders that have been attributed to trinucleotide repeat expansion mutations have involved the brain, and the central nervous system is often the primary organ system affected. Disease-causing expansion mutations may occur within genes or in intergenic DNA, in introns or in exons, in translated or nontranslated regions of DNA. Repeats are commonly found in genes that encode transcription factors (proteins that regulate the level of expression of other genes) and in genes that regulate development (Margolis et al., 1999). The specific nucleotide sequence of the repeat may, itself, have developmental implications. For example, a common feature of all CAG/glutamine expansion diseases so far studied has been the presence of inclusion bodies within neuronal nuclei and cytoplasm, formed by aggregates of mutant protein. The role of these inclusions in the development of these disorders is not yet understood.

One of the most important and prevalent trinucleotide expansion diseases affecting children is Fragile X syndrome, the most common identifiable form of hereditary mental retardation. The fragile site detectable on chromosomal analysis is attributable to a CGG expansion in the 5′ untranslated region of the fragile X mental retardation 1 (FMR1) gene (Yu et al., 1992). A small minority of cases of the disorder are caused by a nearly identical mutation (fragile X subtype E) in a separate gene, FMR2, located near FMR1 (Gecz et al., 1996), but the phenotype tends to be milder. A remarkable feature of Fragile X syndrome is the variability of its phenotypic expression. At least five factors are known to contribute to this variability, including: sex of the proband; CGG repeat length; the pattern of X-inactivation (for females); somatic cell mosaicism; and methylation status of the CpG island adjacent to the repeat. At least three pairs of monozygotic twins fully or partially discordant for Fragile X syndrome have been reported in the literature (Margolis et al., 1999).

A further aspect of trinucleotide repeats expansion with direct implications for the time course of psychopathologic development is the phenomenon of anticipation. *Anticipation* is defined as decreasing age at onset of a disease (or increasing disease severity) in affected members of successive generations of a pedigree. Two aspects of trinucleotide repeat expansion explain anticipation. First, expanded repeats are often unstably transmitted, and repeat length tends to increase in successive generations. In some cases this tendency may in part be a function of which parent is transmitting the mutation; in Fragile X syndrome, for example, expansion is primarily observed during maternal transmission. Second, longer repeat expansions are correlated with a younger age of disease onset.

A final layer of complexity involves variation in qualitative aspects of the phenotype. Although Fragile X syndrome is primarily a disorder of intellectual functioning, other organ systems are involved and other neuropsychiatric manifestations occur. For example, a significant number of males with the Fragile X mutation have autism, and many have one or more behaviors commonly observed in autism, such as hand flapping and biting, poor eye contact, or tactile defensiveness. The prevalence of autism spectrum symptoms is decreased in males who are mosaic for the expansion or in whom methylation is only partial (Margolis et al., 1999). Females with the full mutation (heterozygotes), in addition to their high rates of cognitive deficits, have high rates of anxiety symptoms, affective syndromes, and schizoid personality traits (Mazzocco et al., 1994).

What has been learned from our understanding of the trinucleotide repeat expansion diseases is that this form of genetic mutation can be responsible for variations in the timing, severity, and quality of phenotypic characteristics within a single disease entity. This becomes particularly important when considering the possibility that psychopathologic syndromes represent a confluence of disparate factors (each of which may be a function of similarly complex genetic and environmental mechanisms) which impair function by collectively eroding the normal, highly evolved compensatory mechanisms that maintain appropriate responses to the environment. Viewed this way, it seems all the more important to strive to understand each of the contributory pathways rather than to focus too exclusively on the global syndromes of destabilization that comprise our current diagnostic system.

Angelman Syndrome and Prader-Willi Syndrome

It is possible that for many neuropsychiatric disorders whose etiologies are currently unknown, the disease phenotypes are attributable to single-base (as opposed to whole-gene) mutations. Although such mutations may be nearly impossible to identify in genomic studies, single cases of disease entities associated with specific, readily identifiable cytogenetic abnormalities (such as translocation) can lead to the identification of the disease-causing gene through the identification of clones mapping to the translocation breakpoint. This permits subsequent mutation analysis of patients with no detectable cytogenetic abnormality. This was the case for Angelman syndrome (AS) and Prader-Willi syndrome (PWS), which are most often caused by deletions in the same region of chromosome 15. There is an increased incidence of autism in individuals with duplications in this region. Molecular analysis of such breakpoints has not yet led to the identification of an autism gene, although this is being pursued in several laboratories.

The key to the genetic distinction between PWS and AS is the parental origin of the chromosome containing the deletion. In PWS, the deletion is always found on the paternally donated chromosome. Conversely, in AS, the deletion is always located on the maternally donated chromosome. This discovery led to the recognition that gene expression in humans may be dictated by the chromosome on which the particular copy of that gene resides. This phenomenon is known as *genomic imprinting*. Although research on exactly how this occurs is not yet complete, one modification that is believed to play a role is the reversible addition of methyl groups to specific cytosine residues within the DNA sequence (see Rett Syndrome below for discussion of role of DNA methylation). This process occurs differently in the generation of the egg and the sperm. Genomic imprinting is considered an epigenetic phenomenon, since the gene structure (the actual sequence of nucleotides) is not affected.

Rett Syndrome

In higher organisms, such as vertebrates, a large number of genes are expressed in a tissue-specific manner or have their expression turned on or off during critical periods of development. An important mechanism for turning off DNA expression is methylation, the extent and timing of which is controlled by genes like the methyl CpG-binding proteins (Nan et al., 1997). In the case of Rett syndrome (a rare autistic syndrome primarily affecting girls, resulting in arrest of head growth and characteristic hand-wringing behavior), the affected gene encodes the methyl CpG-binding protein 2 (MeCP2) (Amir et al., 1999). Mutations in two critical domains of the protein were discovered to be present in probands affected with Rett syndrome. Mutations in MeCP2 lead either directly or indirectly to inappropriate amounts of transcription of downstream genes that MeCP2 would normally silence via DNA-methylation. Although MeCP2 is expressed in a number of tissues in the body, Rett syndrome affects primarily the central nervous system, so it is likely that the brain is particularly sensitive to disruption in the activity of this particular gene.

At the molecular level, six different types of mutations have been found in the MeCP2 among various Rett's patients (there are numerous ways in which a genetic mutation can arise and transmit itself – aside from simple nucleotide substitutions, inversions or duplications of short segments of DNA can occur, either in regions that code for proteins or in regions that regulate the expression or transcription of neighboring DNA segments; separate mutations in a single gene are termed *allelic heterogeneity*). Generally, when different regions of a single gene are mutated, they lead to the same clinical phenotype among affected individuals, but occasionally different mutations within the same gene will produce different clinical presentations. This occurs, for example, in mutations to the receptor for fibroblast growth factors, which can lead to several clinical syndromes depending on where the mutations occur.

Tuberous Sclerosis

Tuberous Sclerosis (TS) results from mutation of a gene on chromosome 9, which is inherited as an autosomal dominant trait with an estimated frequency of 1 in 30,000.

One-half of cases represent new mutations. TS is an extremely heterogeneous disease with a wide clinical spectrum that varies from severe mental retardation to an autistic syndrome to normal intelligence, even within the same family (Cheadle et al., 2000). As a rule, the younger the patient presents with symptoms and signs of TS, the greater the likelihood of developing mental retardation.

For the cases of autistic syndromes, then, it can be concluded that disparate genetic defects can lead to highly similar phenotypic traits, and that within some genetic mechanisms, there are variations that can result in nearly as wide a range of phenotypic expression as occurs between affected and unaffected individuals. This makes the search for genetic factors for a given trait highly complicated, especially when the trait is most often produced by the effects of multiple genetic factors.

IT'S NOT ALL GENETICS

Except for mutations which cause catastrophic effects, genes contribute to behavioral traits and disorders in the context of an environment which may modulate or suppress the effects of DNA mutation or genetic variation. This is most clearly seen in the addictive disorders where societal differences and trends have resulted in greatly different prevalences of alcohol and nicotine dependence between cultures and by sex. Hence, any discussion of the genetic structure or developmental course of behavioral traits and disorders must include consideration of the role of the environment.

COMMON ENVIRONMENT, UNIQUE ENVIRONMENT

Although one might argue whether two individuals ever experience the same environment, environmental effects are usually parceled into those which are thought to be common to a group of individuals under study, and those thought to be unique to a given individual (or uncorrelated among the group of individuals).

Common environmental influences may range from nuclear family factors – such as parenting style, to group factors – such as religious or cultural orientation, to factors which influence large segments of the population – such as war, famine, disease, or social revolution. Indeed, evolutionary biologists have frequently invoked common environmental factors such as climactic change or widespread famine as being the cause of genetic or cultural bottlenecks by elimination of large segments of the population. On a more microcosmic level, common environmental factors may be peer group influences or socioeconomic factors.

In contrast, unique environmental factors are those experiences that are different for different members of a sibship or a group of family members, and that operate to make family members dissimilar to one another. They may involve unique events, such as injury, illness, or other random events (experienced by one individual in a family but not by the others being studied), or may be due to different cultural factors that act as a function of age on a given individual. This latter mechanism, which cannot account for differences among twins (who are the same age), may be important in differences among nontwin siblings. Similarly, sex-based differences, which may affect boys and girls as classes, may include unique environmental experiences for opposite sex twin pairs and opposite sex nontwin siblings.

Although these examples of distinctions between common and unique environment are widely recognized, it is important to note that random errors in measurement between individuals (which, by definition, are uncorrelated) will also be parceled out as unique environmental experience. Hence, though much has been made from twin studies about the relatively large estimates of unique environment compared to common environment for many behaviors and symptoms of relevance to child psychopathology (Plomin et al., 1994), many studies either have measurement errors of similar magnitude to unique environment estimates or have no stated measurement error estimates at all. The effect of random errors in measurement is to decrease the magnitude of estimates of both genetic and common environmental factors. From this point of view, measured values of the contributions of genetic and common environmental factors should be viewed as minimal estimates.

Gene-Environment Interaction

Irrespective of the magnitude of genetic influences on a trait, the phenotypic expression of genes that influence behavior always occurs in the context of an environment, for which specific characteristics may need to be present for expression to occur. One often-cited example of gene-environment interaction is that of phenylketonuria (PKU), in which a single-gene mutation impairs the metabolism of phenylalanine, which consequently accumulates, leads to neurotoxicity, and ultimately results in mental retardation. Once the mechanism of PKU was elucidated, it became evident that removing phenylalanine from the "dietary environment" of affected individuals would prevent the phenotypic expression (mental retardation) of this genetic mutation. In this example, both the mutation and the phenylalanine containing "environment" multiply the effects of each other since the mutation in isolation has only modest effects on cognitive development.

Other evidence of gene-environment interaction in neural development comes from deprivation studies in mammals, which have convincingly demonstrated, for example, that postnatal visual input is necessary for the development of ocular dominance columns in the occipital cortex. Similarly, nonhuman primates deprived of their mothers during critical early periods sustain lifelong derangements of monoamine neurotransmitter systems in the brain which correlate with various forms of social deviance (Kraemer & Clarke, 1996). In humans, severe deprivation in the form of child abuse and neglect has been associated with a variety of psychiatric disorders (even when controlling for genetic liability to those disorders), including personality disorders (Johnson et al., 1999), major depression (Dinwiddie et al., 2000), substance abuse (Kendler et al., 2000), and autistic traits (Rutter et al., 1999). Further evidence for the role of the early environment in social development in humans comes from prospective, controlled studies demonstrating positive long-term effects of early interventions which reduce the incidence of maltreatment (Karoly et al., 1998; Olds et al., 1998). Finally, in a recent study of gene-environment interaction in antisocial development, Caspi et al. (2002) showed that maltreated children with a genotype conferring high levels of expression of monoamine oxidase A (responsible for synoptic reuptake of monoamine neurotransmitters, particularly in younger children) were substantially less likely to develop antisocial problems than were children with genotypes conferring low levels of expression of MAOA. Variations in the genotype alone were not associated with either the condition of being maltreated or the development of antisocial problems; maltreatment raised risk for antisocial outcome only in those children with the low MAOA genotype.

It is not yet known whether the association between deprivation and psychopathology is linear, sigmoidal (a function of threshold effects), or otherwise. It is most likely true that given a "good enough" environment, genetic factors operate to promote an individual's capacity to choose and construct from the environment whatever is necessary to reach his or her genetic potential for a given competency (Scarr, 1992). Regarding the question of how deficient an environment needs to be before it starts to compromise the ability of a gene to express itself, it is entirely unknown where the threshold lies for any given trait (note the persistent difficulty with establishing a scientific or legal definition of neglect for any domain of a child's environment); this constitutes an important priority for future research. It will be important for future behavioral genetic studies to completely represent the extremes of environmental variation found in nature, since failure to do so could result in underestimates of the effects of environmental influences such as deprivation (often under-represented in study samples) and variation in social conditions (often homogeneous for a specific population being studied). For example, although there may be important genetic influences on interindividual variation in homicidal behavior, genetically informative studies conducted at a single point in time would miss the fact that homicide rates increased dramatically in all major U.S. cities during the late 1980s. This phenomenon, which could not be explained by genetic influences on homicidal behavior per se, was a function of the introduction of crack cocaine to urban culture, which occurred across the U.S. during that time period. Similarly, if large-scale population-based genetic studies do not include subjects representing the entire range of environmental exposures, then the effects of extreme variation in environmental conditions can be missed, in which case trait variance attributable to genetic factors would be overestimated.

Thus, familiality of illness, which for many childhood onset disorders appears to be strong, may involve genetic or environmental factors or both. The measurement of these genetic, environmental, and gene-x-environment effects on familiality of illness is critically dependent on experimental design. As will be expanded on below, it is important to sample a range of environments before strong statements are made about the primary contributions of genes. Similarly, it is necessary to sample a range of genetic risk before concluding that a given environment is neutral, deleterious, or positive.

GENETIC DIVERSITY WITHIN AND ACROSS POPULATIONS

The sequencing of the human genome, and recent studies involving candidate genes for susceptibility to psychiatric illness, have allowed estimation of the extent to which specific gene sequences have been conserved over the course of evolution. For example, in the case of dopamine and serotonin (5-HT) receptors, which are ancient in origin (probably evolving before the divergence of vertebrate and invertebrate lineages), and for which there are many subtypes in humans, it has been learned that most variants in protein coding regions of genes with allele frequencies of 0.01 or higher involve nonconserved segments of DNA which confer functional specificity to the receptor. Most rare variants (allele frequencies lower than 0.01) are located in highly conserved segments which are important for ligand-receptor interactions. Among Caucasians, the likelihood of an individual expressing every one of the most prevalent dopamine and 5-HT receptor coding region alleles is 0.057. Therefore, 94 percent of Caucasians express at least one dopamine or serotonin receptor protein with an amino acid variation (Cravchik & Goldman, 2000).

This evolutionary diversity in neurochemical attributes may help account for the quantitative nature of many psychiatric syndromes. In general, it has been learned that genes whose function is critical may nevertheless have genetic functional variation; the frequency of such functional variants may itself vary widely among populations and may be maintained by natural selection. A case in point, the serotonin transporter (5HTT promoter) exhibits polymorphisms that account for as much as 7–9 percent of the genetic variance in anxiety-related traits (Lesch et al., 1996). The polymorphic region consists of 14 to 22 imperfect repeat units (each 20 to 23 base pairs in length) constituting 14 different alleles with substantial differences in frequencies between Caucasian and Japanese populations.

Determining the genetic architecture of basic biobehavioral traits will likely result in our knowing whether inherited psychiatric disorders are predominantly polygenic (i.e., the interaction of many alleles of small effect) or oligogenic (i.e., the product of a few major loci), whether they represent the extreme ends of continua or are determined by disease-specific alleles, and whether genetic behavioral diversity has been maintained by natural selection. The initial results from the completed sequencing of the human genome (International Human Genome Sequencing Consortium, 2001) indicate that there appear to be about 30,000–40,000 protein-coding genes in the human genome – only about twice as many as in a worm or fly. However, the genes are more complex, with more alternative splicing generating a larger number of protein products, and marked variation in the distribution of transposable elements, GC content, CpG islands, and recombination rate.

DEVELOPMENTAL SEQUENCES AND GENETIC EFFECTS

As suggested from deprivation studies of nonhuman primates, the timing of genetic and environmental influences is likely to be as important as their quality. In humans, early rearing influences appear to have a more profound influence, for example, on juvenile antisocial traits than on adult antisocial traits, despite the fact that inter-individual differences in antisocial behavior are relatively preserved over the life course. Differential heritability over the course of development is also observed for general intelligence (g) in that the magnitude of genetic influence increases steadily from infancy (20 percent) to childhood (40 percent) to adulthood (60 percent – see Plomin et al., 1997).

General intelligence is an imperfectly understood amalgam of a variety of specific cognitive abilities that are distinguishable in neuropsychological assessment. When broken down into its component parts, however, a surprising finding concerning specific cognitive abilities is that multivariate genetic analyses indicate that the same set of additive genetic factors largely influence different abilities (Plomin, 1999). These results are consistent with a model in which genetic effects on g pervade a broad range of cognitive processes. For example, the genetic effects on measures of school achievement overlap almost completely with genetic effects on g. As is true for most human behavioral traits that have been subjected to population-genetic analysis, heritability of complex dimensions such as g seems likely to be due to the additive effects of multiple genes of varying but small effect size rather than a single gene that has a major effect.

Plomin et al. (1997) conducted a 20-year longitudinal investigation of 245 children separated from their biological parents at birth and adopted in the first month of life as well as 245 matched nonadoptive (control) parents and offspring. Correlations between nonadoptive parents and children increased from less than 0.20 in infancy to about 0.40 in adolescence. The correlations between biological mothers and their adopted-away children followed a similar pattern, indicating that parent–child resemblance for g was due to genetic factors. In contrast, parent–offspring correlations for adoptive parents and their adopted children were around zero, suggesting that family environment shared by parents and offspring did not contribute importantly to parent–offspring resemblance for g.

The reasons for this apparent increase in heritability over the lifespan are not yet known. It is possible that completely new genes come to affect g as intellectual abilities mature. A well-known example of such gene switching is the transition from fetal hemoglobin to mature hemoglobin in early life. Another possibility is that relatively small genetic effects early in life "snowball" during development (Plomin, et al., 1994), creating larger and larger phenotypic effects, perhaps as individuals choose and construct from their environment what they need to support their genetic potential.

That genetic programs unfold during development has been established from other lines of research. For example, the sex of a child is determined by which sex chromosome the sperm contains. This involves the early formation of urogenital tract and other structural organ differences. Later, the activation of genes controlling sex hormone production results in the development of secondary sexual characteristics, ovulation, and spermatogenesis. The turning on and off of transcription factors which regulate the level of expression of messenger RNAs for specific combinations of genes is responsible for early differentiation of cell types and organ formation. Such genetic programs include mechanisms for regulating cell number by cell death (reviewed in Todd et al., 1995). Some of these normal developmental processes share features in common with so-called apoptotic cell death mechanisms in which an injured cell commits "suicide" by activation of specific genetic programs. These programs are sensitive to environmental insults and may help account for individual differences between identical twins.

A crucial task of behavioral genetics research is to determine how and when a given gene's effects on behavior are activated or suppressed during the course of development. Do genes that determine language delay in early childhood remain active after language has ultimately been acquired in affected individuals? Studies of animals in whom a specific gene has been experimentally mutated to render the gene inactive (e.g., knockout mice) have revealed that compensatory mechanisms frequently blunt the effects of mutations by changing the expression of other genes which operate to normalize the function altered by mutation. This has led investigators to develop "conditional knockouts": alterations of genes that increase or decrease (rather than obliterate) rates of a gene's transcription, incorporate regulators which act as a switch for turning a gene on or off, or change the expression of a gene in specific brain regions (Crusio, 1999; Plomin & Crabbe, 2000). Studies of such experimental manipulations of gene expression and their downstream consequences should lead to a more precise understanding of how gene expression is naturally turned on or off over the course of development. These techniques offer a logical way to test for neurodevelopment effects of genes and gene variations identified in human studies of traits and disease.

Personality

Basic styles of interpersonal behavior strongly influence the expression of psychopathology, or are considered pathologic when at the extremes of variation for the population. Research in normal and abnormal human populations has differentiated two dissociable domains of personality: temperament and character (Cloninger, 1987). Temperament can be defined as the automatic associative responses to basic emotional stimuli that determine habits and skills. It is traditionally conceptualized as moderately heritable. It is also conceptualized as moderately stable over time, but it is important to note that Plomin et al. (1993) found genetic influences for both continuities *and* discontinuities in early childhood temperament, as measured according to emotionality-activity-sociability (EAS) scales for temperament. In contrast to temperament, character refers to concepts about self and relations to others that develop over time and as a function of experience-dependent processes (Cloninger, Przybeck, Svrakic, & Wetzel, 1994).

The seven-factor model developed by Cloninger and colleagues (1994) identifies four dimensions of temperament that are believed (primarily from animal studies) to be influenced by disparate neuromodulatory pathways in the brain: The four dimensions of temperament in the seven-factor model are harm avoidance (HA), reward dependence (RD), novelty seeking (NS), and persistence (P). Each dimension represents a specific stimulus-response characteristic relating to initiation NS, maintenance RD, P, or inhibition HA of behavior. Genetic studies in animals and humans have found these dimensions of temperament to be moderately heritable (50–60 percent; Heath et al., 1994; Stallings et al., 1996) when individuals are reared under typical conditions for the respective species (Cloninger, 1987). Kraemer and Clarke (1996) have shown that severe perturbations in rearing conditions (e.g., maternal deprivation) are capable of resulting in derangement of the normal relationships between neuromodulators (serotonin, dopamine, and norepinephrine) believed to influence at least three of the four temperament dimensions in the seven-factor model (HA, NS, and RD, respectively).

In clinical studies of patients with personality disorders, Cloninger (1987) showed that an individual could be typed ("high" or "low") with respect to each of the four temperament dimensions, and that the resulting profile accurately predicted the specific type of personality disorder with which he or she was affected. Subsequent population-based research using Cloninger's Temperament and Character Inventory (Cloninger & Svrakic, 1997) indicated that the temperament profile alone did not predict whether or not an individual would have a personality disorder; the condition of having a personality disorder was largely determined by level of *character* development. Character development has been operationalized in the seven-factor model as the extent to which an individual is self-directed, the extent to which he or she is capable of engaging cooperatively in self-other relationships, and the extent to which he or she is capable of "transcending self" in arriving at an intuition of one's place or purpose in the larger social context. Low levels of self-directness and cooperativeness are strongly associated with clinical diagnoses of personality disorder (Cloninger & Svrakic, 1997), the type of which can be predicted by his or her temperament profile. Recently it has been shown that abuse and neglect in childhood – which represent extremes of deleterious environmental influence – predict the development of disorders of personality and social behavior even when genetic liability for psychopathology is controlled for (Caspi et al., 2000; Johnson et al., 1999).

Given what has been learned about personality from studies of the seven-factor model in adults, it is important to determine whether this model might be useful in tracing the origins of personality to early childhood. A first step is to determine whether these factors can be reliably measured in children, and whether they are associated with profiles of personality (and psychopathology) that are similar to what have been identified in adults. Some important work has already been done in this area. Tremblay et al. (1994) used twenty-eight items from the Preschool Behavior Questionnaire and ten items from the Prosocial Behavior Questionnaire to approximate dimensions of impulsivity (similar to NS), anxiety (similar to HA), and RD. They showed that the same temperament profile that predicts antisocial personality disorder in adults (i.e., high NS, low HA, low RD) could be identified in five-year-olds and predicted a dramatically increased risk of delinquency at ten-year follow-up compared to children without that profile. The implication, then, of being able to characterize temperament and character more precisely in young children is that the natural course of personality development through life can be better understood, children at risk for extremes of maladaptive personality development might be identifiable early, and efforts to promote adaptive patterns of social behavior could be channeled to those at highest risk. The utility of the seven-factor model as an empirically derived theory of personality, its precision in characterizing clinically defined personality disorder, its organization around basic stimulus-response characteristics of individuals, and its capacity to examine genetic and epigenetic contributions to personality, all make it appealing as a paradigm for tracing the origins of personality variation to early childhood.

We recently tested a preschool version of the temperament and character inventory (Constantino et al., 2002) in 305 children age 2–5 years, and found it possible to reliably measure these dimensions of personality in this age range. Future studies are warranted to test the extent to which early childhood measurements of the seven factors might predict the development of personality disorders.

THE GENETIC STRUCTURE OF CHILD PSYCHOPATHOLOGY

The review and discussion in this chapter has so far primarily focused on traits and disorders as specific conditions. Although it is convenient to think of diseases as being discrete entities with discrete identifiable etiologies, many well-defined, common disorders are extremes of continua in which clinical caseness is statistical in nature. For example, the distribution of diastolic blood pressure in the general population shows no distinct categories or groups even though we know that very high or low diastolic blood pressures are associated with serious clinical consequences. The current guidelines for determining whether an individual is hypertensive or hypotensive are based on statistical criteria which aim to minimize both the negative consequences of extremes of blood pressure as well as the potential negative consequences of treatment.

Given the probabilistic nature of defining conditions in which a range of severity exists in nature, it is helpful to take an epidemiologic perspective in investigating the etiology of such disorders. Unfortunately, few of our disorders have sufficient epidemiologic data on the presence of individual or groups of psychiatric symptoms to allow critical tests of the structure of disorders. Similarly, we lack sufficient knowledge of the environmental context of symptoms over evolutionary time periods in order to gauge whether today's problem behaviors were advantageous or neutral in the past (Thornhill & Moller, 1997). In particular, we lack sufficient data to determine whether symptom domains represent discrete disorders, continua, or some mixture of categorical and continuum entities. Similarly, whether the observed comorbidities (that is, the presence of two or more diagnostic entities in the same individual) reflect the familial aggregation of different illnesses via mechanisms such as assortative mating or reflect distinct genetic subtypes of disorders is also unclear. Obviously, these shortcomings limit our ability to define the nature and mechanism of action of genes contributing to psychopathology. These problems and their subsequent impact on the diagnosis, treatment, or investigation of our clinical entities will be highlighted by the examples of autism and attention deficit/hyperactivity disorder, which have been studied in a series of investigations in our laboratory, utilizing both clinical and epidemiologic samples of twins and singletons.

Evidence for an Autistic Continuum: Reciprocal Social Behavior (RSB) in Twins

Autism is thought to be a rare and severe early onset disorder characterized by (1) qualitative impairments in social interactions, (2) communication deficits, and (3) restricted, repetitive and stereotype patterns of behavior, interest, and activities (*DSM-IV*). Other related pervasive developmental disorders share deficits in social interactions but have variable presence of the other features of autism. A variety of twin and family studies of categorically defined illness have demonstrated that autism is largely genetically determined (Bailey et al., 1995). Interestingly, twin and family studies have also shown that the abnormal social behaviors characteristic of autism significantly aggregate in family members of autistic probands (Le Couteur et al., 1996; Piven et al., 1997; Wolff et al., 1988). Strikingly, no population-based studies have been reported regarding the prevalence of individual autism symptoms or groups of symptoms in the general population.

In the course of developing a screening instrument for the identification of pervasive developmental disorder cases for use by parents and schoolteachers, we unexpectedly found a continuous distribution of endorsement of social interaction symptoms in a random sample of students (Constantino, Przybeck et al., 2000; Constantino et al., in press). A significant fraction of these students received symptom scores overlapping with a clinic-based group of autistic and pervasive developmental disorder patients. That is, the clinic cases were at the high end of the distribution of scores in this instrument, but there was no clear dividing line between the scores of school children and clinical cases. A variety of clustering procedures was compatible with problems of social interactions being a continuous variable in this population.

This questionnaire was then completed by a parent for 232 male:male twin pairs ages 7–15 years identified through birth records of the state of Missouri. Once again, in this population-based sample of twins, social interaction problem scores appeared to be continuously distributed, as shown in Figure 10.1.

Monozygotic twin pairs had significantly higher correlations for scores than dizygotic twin pairs, consistent with the involvement of genes for this characteristic. More

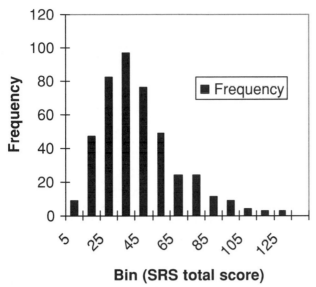

Bin (SRS total score)

Figure 10.1. Distribution of SRS scores in male twins, $n = 464$.

formal twin analyses estimated the heritability of scale scores to be 76 percent with no evidence for common environment contributions to family resemblance (Constantino & Todd, 2000). The results of these two studies taken together with previous twin and family studies of autism suggest that at least one of the core features of autism (problems with social interactions) may be continuously distributed in the population and that families of autistic individuals lie at one extreme end of this continuum. Given the reported high heritabilities of both autism and our estimates of the heritability of social problems in the general population, and given the funding that mild autistic traits aggregate in the family members of affected probands, it is possible that autism is not a rare categorical disorder as described in *DSM-IV* but is the extreme end of a population distribution with no clear division between affected and unaffected status.

The question next arose whether the strong genetic influences on subthreshold autistic traits (i.e., autistic traits that lie below the threshold for a diagnosis of autism or pervasive developmental disorder) are the same as or different from genetic influences involved in other domains of psychopathology, specifically internalizing behavior and externalizing behavior. Twin designs are capable of answering such questions about genetic overlap, as long as the various traits of interest are all measured in the individuals in a given genetically informative sample. Path models can be constructed to depict the extent to which pathways of genetic influence are shared by disparate phenotypic traits, and these models can be subjected to structural equation modeling to determine how well the models fit the data, and to generate parameter estimates quantifying the degree of genetic and environmental overlap for the best-fitting models.

Using Child Behavior Checklist (CBCL) data from the male twin pairs, structural equation modeling revealed the presence of both specific and overlapping genetic influences for autistic traits and other domains of psychopathology, as measured by the CBCL. The magnitude of genetic influence *specific* to RSB was on the order of 0.4; the remainder of genetic influences on RSB overlapped with other CBCL subdomains, primarily attention problems and thought problems.

Thus, approximately half of the (substantial) genetic influence on subthreshold autistic behavior – as measured by the Social Reciprocity Scale – is specific, that is, distinct from genetic influences on other domains of psychopathology (as measured by the CBCL). The partial causal overlap between the autistic and nonautistic symptom domains suggests that a modest proportion of the genetic influences on these disparate traits share the same genetic factors.

We have cautiously interpreted this finding to indicate the possibility that genetic factors involved in producing subthreshold manifestations of the autistic phenotype may exacerbate internalizing and externalizing traits in boys in the general population (Constantino, Hudziat et al., 2000). Since the measure of autistic traits utilized in this study (the Social Reciprocity Scale) distinguishes children with autism spectrum disorders from other psychiatric disorders (Constantino, Przybeck et al., 2000) and exhibits minimal measurement error in genetic analyses (Constantino & Todd, 2000), we do not believe that these findings can be explained away on the basis of a tendency of the instrument to measure general psychopathology (as tested in the models described earlier). Rather, it appears that subthreshold autistic deficits, which are continuously distributed in the population and exhibit a genetic structure very similar to what has previously been described for autism (Le Couteur et al., 1996), may operate to make other types of psychopathology (co-existing in a given individual) worse. Measuring such subthreshold autistic deficits may prove useful for predicting clinical course and understanding etiologic influences on a wide variety of child mental health problems.

ADHD AS A MANIFESTATION OF MULTIPLE GENETIC HETEROGENEITY

In contrast to autism, attention deficit/hyperactivity disorder (ADHD) is thought to be common and not as incapacitating as autism, though clearly associated with impairments in school, peer, or home functioning (*DSM-IV*). A variety of twin studies (whether of categorical diagnoses or symptom counts or scale measures) are compatible with ADHD having a heritability in the range of 0.6 to 0.9 (Faraone & Biederman, 1998). Under *DSM-IV* criteria, ADHD occurs in three mutually exclusive subtypes referred to as inattentive, hyperactive/impulsive, and combined. Little data have been reported on the relative heritabilities of these *DSM-IV* subtypes, but a number of studies have attempted to look independently at the heritability of inattentive and hyperactive/impulsive symptoms (Todd, 2000). Based on such analyses, several investigators have suggested that ADHD is best viewed as a continuum of problems with inattentive and hyperactive/impulsive symptoms (Hudziak et al., 1998; Levy et al., 1997). We have attempted to formally test whether ADHD is best conceived of as a categorical or continuum disorder by the application of parametric and nonparametric clustering procedures to *DSM-IV* ADHD symptom data reported by parents on their children (Neuman et al., 1999; Neuman et al., 2001; Todd et al., 2001).

Our initial results based on a sample of approximately 1,500 female twin pairs identified from birth records of the state of Missouri were interpreted as supporting a continuum position (Hudziak et al., 1998) in which there were separate continua for inattention problems, hyperactive/impulsive problems, and combined subtype problems. Similar results were found for both boys and girls in a sample of families identified through alcoholic probands (Neuman et al., 1999). Further analyses on an enlarged sample of over 2,000 female twin pairs, however, support a different model (Neuman et al., 2001; Todd et al., 2001). In a continuum model, twins in the same twin pair would be expected to lie along the same portion of the continuum but not necessarily at the same point. In contrast, if the apparent continuum represented multiple independent types of ADHD, then twin pair members would be expected to have the same type of ADHD. Analysis of within and between twin pair phenotypes using a clustering procedure referred to as latent class analysis (McCutcheon, 1987) is most compatible with there being multiple genetically independent forms of ADHD in this general population sample of female twins (Todd et al., 2001).

FUTURE DIRECTIONS

In both of these examples, careful attention to the collection and interpretation of population-based data results in models that challenge current views of the structure of these two psychopathological conditions. For autism, it is suggested that caseness represents the end of a distribution of deviance in the general population. In contrast, for ADHD there may be multiple genetically independent forms of ADHD in the general population, which only partially overlap with *DSM-IV* conceptualizations of illness. Both these findings have implications for study designs aimed at identifying genetic factors involved in these illnesses and for clinical practice. First, current estimates of the multilocus etiology of autism suggest that sufficient multiplex autism families may not exist to allow the definition of the responsible DNA elements. However, an alternate strategy for the identification of these genetic elements would be to take sibling pairs from the general population, which differ on quantitative measures of social interaction problems (a discordant quantitative trait locus [QTL] design). Specific associations found in such general population studies could then be secondarily tested in singleton and multiplex autism families.

Similarly for ADHD, linkage analysis of extended pedigrees may be inappropriate. First, if ADHD is in fact composed of multiple genetically independent forms of ADHD, then the use of extended families is likely to introduce genetic heterogeneity within single pedigrees. This greatly increases the difficulty of identifying susceptibility loci. Similarly, the use of *DSM-IV* ADHD subtypes for analysis would likely decrease the power of studies due to the mixing of different independently heritable subtypes. In the case of ADHD it may be more cost effective to focus on nuclear families with particular heritable subtypes identified through population samples as described above. Once susceptibility genes are identified, it is hoped that the identification of their function and the timing with which they express themselves over the life course will lead to the development of specific treatment strategies.

With respect to the clinical problems of who and when to treat, the results of the earlier discussions suggest these will be different for autism and ADHD. The presence of multiple genetically independent forms of ADHD may suggest specific treatments for individual subtypes. Hence, in the future it may be possible to direct pharmacological or behavioral treatments for ADHD based on either clinical or genotype information. For autism, if the true underlying problems represent a continuum, then the decision to call an individual affected or not must include risk-benefit analyses of individual treatments since the conceptualization of caseness is arbitrary.

REFERENCES

Amir, R.E., Van den Veyver, I.B., Wan, M., Tran, C.Q., Francke, U., & Zoghbi, H.Y. (1999). Rett syndrome is caused by mutation in X-linked MECP2, encoding methyl-CpG-binding protein 2. *Nature Genetics, 23,* 185–188.

Ashley-Koch, A., Wolpert, C.M., Menold, M.M., Zaeem, L., Basu, S., Donnelly, S.L., Ravan, S.A., Pwell, C.M., Qumseyeh, M.B., Aylsworth, A.S., Vance, J.M., Gilbert, J.R., et al. (1999). Genetic studies of autistic disorder and chromosome 7. *Genomics, 61,* 227–236.

Auranen, M., Nieminen, T., Majuri, S., Vanhala, R., Peltonen, L., & Jarvela, I. (2000). Analysis of autism susceptibility gene loci on chromosones 1p, 4p, 6q, 7q, 13q, 15q, 16p, 17q, 19q, and 22q in Finnish multiplex families. *Molecular Psychiatry, 5(3),* 320–322.

Bailey, A., Le Couteur, A., Gottesman, I., Bolton, P., Simonoff, E., Yuzda, E., & Rutter, M. (1995). Autism as a strongly genetic disorder: evidence from a British twin study. *Psychological Medicine, 25,* 63–77.

Barrett, S., Beck, J.C., Bernier, R., Bisson, E., Braun, T.A., Casavant, T.L., Childress, D., Folstein, S.E., Garcia, M., Gardiner, M.B., Gilman, S., Haines, J.L., Hopkins, K., Landa, R., Meyer, N.H., Mullane, J.A., Nishimura, D.Y., Palmer, P., Piven, J., Purdy, J., Santangelo, S.L., Searby, C., Sheffield, V., Singleton, J., & Slager, S. (1999). An autosomal genomic screen for autism: collaborative linkage study of autism. *American Journal of Medical Genetics, 88(6),* 609–615.

Caspi, A., McClay, J., Moffitt, T.E., Mill, J., Martin, J., Craig, I.W., Taylor, A., & Poulton R. (2002). Role of genotype in the cycle of violence in maltreated children. *Science 297,* 851–854.

Caspi, A., Taylor, A., Moffit, T.E., & Plomin, R. (2000). Neighborhood deprivation affects children's mental health; environmental risks identified in a genetic design. *Psychological Science, 11,* 338–342.

Cheadle, J.P., Reeve, M.P., Sampson, J.R., & Kwiatkowski, D.J. (2000). Molecular genetic advances in tuberous sclerosis. *Human Genetics, 107,* 97–114.

Chorney, M.J., Chorney, K., Seese, N., Owen, M.J., Daniels, J., McGuffin, P., Thompson, L.A., Detterman, D.K., Benbow, C., Lubinski, D., Eley, T., & Plomin, R. (1998). A quantitative trait locus (QTL) associated with cognitive ability in children. *Psychological Science, 9,* 159–166.

Cloninger, C.R. (1987). A systematic method for clinical description and classification of personality variants: a proposal. *Archives of General Psychiatry, 44,* 573–558.

Cloninger, C.R., Pryzbeck, T.R., Svrakic, D.M., & Wetzel, R.D. (1994). *The Temperament and Character Inventory (TCI): A guide to its development and use.* St. Louis: Washington University Center for Psychobiology of Personality.

Cloninger, C.R., & Svrakic, D.M. (1997). Integrative psychobiological approach to psychiatric assessment and treatment. *Psychiatry, 60,* 120–141.

Constantino, J.N., Cloninger, C.R., Clarke, R.A., Hashemi, B., & Przybeck, T. (2002). Application of the seven-factor model of personality to early childhood. *Psychiatry Research, 109(3),* 229–243.

Constantino, J.N., Davis, S.A., Reich, W., Schindler, M.K., Gross, M.M., Brophy, S.L., Metzger, L.M., Shoushtari, C.S., Splinter, R., & Todd, R.D. (in press). Validation of a brief quantitative genetic measure of autistic traits: Comparison of the Social Responsiveness Scale with the Autism Diagnostic Interview—Revised. *Journal of Autism and Developmental Disorders.*

Constantino, J.N., Hudziak, J.J., & Todd, R.D. (2000, October 28). Overlap of genetic influences on internalizing, externalizing and autistic traits. Presented at the Annual Meeting of the American Academy of Child and Adolescent Psychiatry, New York.

Constantino, J.N., Przybeck, T., Friesen, D., & Todd, R.D. (2000). Reciprocal social behavior in children with and without pervasive developmental disorders. *Journal of Developmental and Behavioral Pediatrics, 21,* 2–11.

Constantino, J.N., & Todd, R.D. (2000). The genetic structure of reciprocal social behavior. *American Journal of Psychiatry, 157,* 2043–2045.

Cravchik, A., & Goldman, D. (2000). Neurochemical individuality: genetic diversity among human dopamine and serotonin receptors and transporters. *Archives of General Psychiatry, 57,* 1105–1114.

Crusio, W.E. (1999). Using spontaneous and induced mutations to dissect brain and behavior genetically. *Trends in Neurosciences, 22,* 100–102.

Dinwiddie, S., Heath, A.C., Dunne, M.P., Bucholz, K.K., Madden, P.A.F., Slutske, W.S., Bierut, L.J., Statham, D.B., & Martin, N.G. (2000). Early sexual abuse and lifetime psychopathology: a co-twin-control study. *Psychological Medicine, 30,* 41–52.

Faraone, S.V., & Biederman, J. (1998). Neurobiology of attention-deficit hyperactivity disorder. *Biological Psychiatry, 44,* 951–958.

Gecz, J., Gedeon, A.K., Sutherland, G.R., & Mulley, J.C. (1996). Identification of the gene FMR2 associated with FRAXE mental retardation. *Nature Genetics, 13,* 105–108.

Heath, A.C., Cloninger, C.R., & Martin, N.G. (1994). Testing a model for the genetic structure of personality: A comparison of the personality systems of Cloninger and Eysenck. *Journal of Personality and Social Psychology 66,* 762–775.

Hudziak, J.J., Heath, A.C., Madden, P.F., Reich, W., Bucholz, K.K., Slutske, W., Bierut, L.J., Neuman, R.J., & Todd, R.D. (1998). Latent class and factor analysis of *DSM-IV* ADHD: a twin study of female adolescents. *Journal of the Amercian Academic of Child and Adolescent Psychiatry, 37,* 848–857.

International Human Genome Sequencing Consortium (2001). Initial sequencing and analysis of the human genome. *Nature, 409,* 860–921.

International Molecular Genetic Study of Autism Consortium (1998). A full genome screen for autism with evidence for linkage to a region on chromosome 7q. *Human Molecular Genetics, 7,* 571–578.

Johnson, J.J., Cohen, P., Brown, J., Smailes, E.M., & Bernstein, D.P. (1999). Childhood maltreatment increases risk for personality disorders during early adulthood. *Archives of General Psychiatry, 56,* 600–606.

Karasu, T.B. (1994). A developmental metatheory of psychopathology. *The American Journal of Psychotherapy, 48,* 581–599.

Karoly, L.A., Greenwood, P.W., Everingham, S.S., Hoube, J., Kilburn, M.R., Rydell, C.P., Sanders, M., & Chiesa, J. (1998). *Investing in our children: what we know and don't know about the costs and benefits of early childhood interventions.* Washington, D.C.: Rand Corporation.

Kendler, K.S., Bulik, C.M., Silberg, J., Hettema, J.M., Myers, J., & Prescott, C.A. (2000). Childhood sexual abuse and adult psychiatric and substance use disorders in women. *Archives of General Psychiatry, 57,* 953–959.

Kraemer, G.W., & Clarke, A.S. (1996). Social attachment, brain function and aggression. *Annals of the New York Academy of Sciences, 794,* 121–135.

Le Couteur, A., Bailey, A., Goode, S., Pickels, A., Robertson, S., Gottesman, I., & Rutter, M. (1996). A broader phenotype of autism: the clinical spectrum in twins. *Journal of Child Psychology and Psychiatry, and Allied Disciplines, 37,* 785–801.

Lesch, K.P., Bengel, D., Heils, A., Sabol, S.Z., Greenberg, B.D., Petri, S., Benjamin, J., Muller, C.R., Hamer, D.H., & Murphy, D.L. (1996). Association of anxiety-related traits with a polymorphism in the serotonin transporter gene regulatory region. *Science, 274,* 1527–1531.

Levy, F., Hay, D., McStephen, M., Wood, C., & Waldman, I. (1997). Attention-deficit hyperactivity disorder. A category or a continuum? Genetic analysis of a large-scale twin study. *Journal of the American Academy of Child and Adolescent Psychiatry, 36,* 737–744.

Margolis, R.L., McInnis, M.G., Rosenblatt, A., & Ross, C.A. (1999). Trinucleotide repeat expansion and neuropsychiatric disease. *Archives of General Psychiatry, 56,* 1019–1031.

Mazzocco, M.M., Pennington, B.F., & Hagerman, R.J. (1994). Social cognition skills among females with Fragile X. *Journal of Autism and Development Disorders, 24,* 473–485.

McCutcheon, A.L. (1987). *Latent class analysis.* Newbury Park, Calif.: Sage Publications.

Nan, X., Campoy, J., & Bird, A. (1997). MeCP2 is a transcriptional repressor with abundant binding sites in genomic chromatin. *Cell, 88,* 471–481.

Neuman, R.J., Heath, A.C., Hudziak, J.J., Reich, W., Bucholz, K.K., Madden, P.A.F., Sun, L., & Todd, R.D. (2001). Latent class analysis of ADHD and comorbid symptoms in a population sample of adolescent female twins. *Journal of Child Psychology and Psychiatry, and Allied Disciplines, 42,* 933–942.

Neuman, R.J., Todd, R.D., Heath, A.C., Reich, W., Hudziak, J.J., Bucholz, K.K., Madden, P.A., Begleiter, H., Porjesz, B., Kuperman, S., Hesselbrock, V., & Reich, T. (1999). The evaluation of ADHD typology in three contrasting samples: A latent class approach. *Journal of the American Academy of Child and Adolescent Psychiatry, 38,* 25–33.

Olds, D., Henderson, C.R., Cole, R., Eckenrode, J., Kitzman, H., Luckey, D., Pettitt, L., Sidora, K., Morris, P., & Powers, J. (1998). Long-term effects of nurse home visitation on children's criminal and antisocial behavior: 15 year outcome of a randomized controlled trial. *Journal of the American Medical Association, 280,* 1238–1244.

Philippe, A., Martinez, M., Guilloud-Bataille, M., Gillberg, C., Rastam, M., Sponheim, E., Coleman, M., Zappella, M., Aschauer, H., Van Maldergem, L., Penet, C., Feingold, J., Brice, A., & Leboyer, M. (1999). Genome-wide scan for autism susceptibility genes. *Human Molecular Genetics, 8,* 805–812.

Pickles, A., Bolton, P., Macdonald, H., Bailey, A., Le Couteur, A., Sim, C.H., & Rutter, M. (1995). Latent-class analysis of recurrence risks for complex phenotypes with selection and measurement error: a twin and family history study of autism. *American Journal of Human Genetics, 57,* 717–726.

Piven, J., Palmer, P., Jacobbi, D., Childress, D. & Arndt, S. (1997). Broader autism phenotype: evidence from a family history study of multiple-incidence autism families. *American Journal of Psychiatry, 154,* 185–190.

Plomin, R. (1999). Genetics and general cognitive ability. *Nature,* Supplement 6761, 402, C25–C29.

Plomin, R., & Crabbe J. (2000). DNA. *Psychological Bulletin, 126,* 806–828.

Plomin, R., DeFries, J.C., McClearn, G.E., & McGuffin, P. (2001). *Behavioral genetics,* 4th ed. New York: Freeman.

Plomin, R., Emde, R.N., Braungart, J.M., Campos, J., Corley, R., & Fulker, D.W. (1993). Genetic change and continuity from fourteen to twenty months: the MacArthur Longitudinal Twin Study. *Child Development, 64,* 1354–1376.

Plomin, R., Fulker, D.W., Corley, R., & DeFries, J.C. (1997). Nature, nurture and cognitive development from 1 to 16 years: a parent-offspring adoption study. *Psychological Science, 8,* 442–447.

Plomin, R., Owen, M.J., & McGuffin, P. (1994). The genetic basis of complex human behaviors. *Science, 264,* 1733–1739.

Reynolds, A.J., & Temple, J.A. (1998). Extended early childhood intervention and school achievement: age thirteen findings from the Chicago Longitudinal Study. *Child Development, 69,* 231–246.

Risch, N., Spiker, D., Lotspech, L., Nouri, N., Hinds, D., & Hallmayear, J. (1999). A genomic screen of autism: evidence for multilocus etiology. *American Journal of Human Genetics, 65,* 493–507.

Rutter, M., Andersen-Wood, L., Beckett, C., Bredenkamp, D., Castle, J., Groothues, C., Kreppner, J., Keaveney, l., Lord, C., O'Connor, T.G., & English and Romanian Adoptees (ERA) Study Team. (1999). Quasi-autistic patterns following severe early global privation. *Journal of Child Psychology and Psychiatry, 40,* 537–549.

Scarr, S. (1992). Developmental theories for the 1990s: development and individual differences. *Child Development, 63,* 1–19.

Stallings, M.C., Hewitt, J.K., Cloninger, C.R., Heath, A.C., & Eaves, L.J. (1996). Genetic and environmental structure of the Tridimensional Personality Questionnaire: three or four temperament dimensions? *Journal of Personality and Social Psychology 70,* 127–140.

Thornhill, R., & Moller, A.P. (1997). Developmental stability, disease and medicine. *Biological Reviews of the Cambridge Philosophical Society, 72,* 497–548.

Todd, R.D. (2000). Genetics of attention deficit/hyperactivity disorder: are we ready for molecular genetic studies? *American Journal of Medical Genetics, 91,* 241–243.

Todd, R.D., Rasmussen, E.K., Neuman, R.J., Reich, W., Hudziak, J.J., Bucholz, K.K., Madden, P.A.F., & Heath A. (2001). Familiality and heritability of subtypes of ADHD in a population sample of female twins. *American Journal of Psychiatry, 158,* 1891–1898.

Todd, R.D., Swarzenski, B., Giovanardi-Rossi, P., & Visconti, P. (1995). Structural and functional development of the human brain. In D. Cicchetti & D. Cohen (Eds.), *Developmental psychopathology, Vol. 1: theory and methods* (pp. 161–194). New York: Wiley.

Tremblay, R.E., Pihl, R.O., Vitaro, F., & Dobkin, P.L. (1994). Prediction early onset of male antisocial behavior from preschool behavior. *Archives of General Psychiatry 51*(9), 732–739.

Wolff, S., Narayan, S., & Moyes, B. (1988). Personality characteristics of parents of autistic children. *Journal of Child Psychology and Psychiatry, and Allied Disciplines, 29,* 143–153.

Yu, S., Pritchard, M., Kremer, E., Lynch, M., Nancarrow, J., Baker, E., Holman, K., Mulley, J.C., Warren, S.T., Schlessinger, D., Sutherland, G.R., & Richards, R.I. (1992). Fragile X genotype characterized by an unstable region of DNA. *Science, 252,* 1179–1181.

ELEVEN

Prospects and Problems in the Search for Genetic Influences on Neurodevelopment and Psychopathology

Application to Childhood Disruptive Disorders

Irwin D. Waldman

For some time, psychopathology researchers have attempted to disentangle genetic and environmental influences on psychopathology and to characterize the nature and magnitude of each of these influences. It is easy to lose sight of the fact that this represents considerable progress, as recognition of the contribution of behavior genetic approaches to understanding the etiology of psychopathology is a fairly recent event, and it was not that long ago that behavior genetic studies and findings were met with incredulity and opposition bordering on the fanatical. Nonetheless, the landmark adoption studies of the 1960s and 1970s, and the subsequent large-scale twin studies of the 1970s and 1980s, furnished strong evidence for substantial genetic influences on most forms of major adult psychopathology, including schizophrenia spectrum disorders (e.g., Kendler & Robinette, 1983; Kety, Rosenthal, Wender, & Schulsinger, 1968), bipolar and unipolar depression (Kendler et al., 1994; McGuffin, & Katz, 1989), and the anxiety disorders (Kendler et al., 1992a, 1992b). More recently, researchers have utilized molecular genetic approaches in a search for specific genes that contribute to the etiology of numerous forms of psychopathology. The recent sequencing of the human genome will only intensify this search, and brings with it considerable prospects and formidable problems.

In this chapter, I intend to briefly explicate a number of behavioral and molecular genetic research strategies that may aid in our understanding of the etiology and neurodevelopmental basis of psychopathology, particularly in the search for genetic influences and the characterization of these in terms of the neurodevelopmental mechanisms that they code for. Rather than present recent findings from my lab, as is customary in chapters such as this, I will primarily describe a number of behavioral and molecular genetic approaches that may have particular utility for elucidating the genetic influences and mediating neurodevelopmental mechanisms underlying psychopathology. I will illustrate these approaches principally with methods and findings from my main research domain, the disruptive behavior disorders of childhood, both because this research domain is the one with which I am most familiar, and because I think that some of the recently employed research designs and the findings they have yielded may offer some guidance in the search for genetic influences underlying other forms of psychopathology. Where applicable, particularly in the section on molecular genetic designs, I will also mention research designs and findings pertinent to the etiology of the schizophrenia spectrum disorders. I will also make brief mention of molecular genetic findings from studies of complex medical disorders (e.g., diabetes) and highlight their implications for finding genes that contribute to the etiology of psychopathology and its underlying neurodevelopmental mechanisms.

This chapter is composed of three major sections, the first containing a description of some developmental psychopathology concepts pertinent to behavioral genetic studies, and the second two on behavioral genetic designs themselves (i.e., one on quantitative genetic designs and the other on molecular genetic designs). The quantitative and molecular genetic sections both begin with a brief description of important background concepts and methods, then explore several research designs and the findings they have yielded, drawing implications for studies of the genetic basis of neurodevelopment and psychopathology. Each of these sections concludes with a discussion of future research directions, which have as their primary focus the extension of quantitative and molecular genetic studies of psychopathology to explicitly include neurodevelopmental mechanisms and a developmental psychopathology perspective. Despite the increasing popularity of a functional genomics approach (Plomin & Crabbe, 2000), in which brain mechanisms are considered the primary targets for investigating the expression of genes involved in both psychopathology and normal developmental outcomes, most studies of the genetics of psychopathology have not included an explicit focus on neurodevelopmental mechanisms. Similarly, despite the contributions of a developmental psychopathology perspective to understanding the etiology of both child and adult disorders, as well as their continuities and discontinuities from normal developmental outcomes, few quantitative or molecular genetic studies have incorporated developmental psychopathology concepts in their design, analysis, or interpretation of results. In this chapter, I will attempt to sketch, at least in broad brush, the appearance of future quantitative and molecular genetic studies that include measures of neurodevelopmental mechanisms along with psychopathological outcomes, as well as a developmental psychopathology perspective on the genetics of psychopathology. I believe that these two foci are necessary for quantitative and molecular genetic studies of psychopathology to advance to their next stages of development.

DEVELOPMENTAL PSYCHOPATHOLOGY CONCEPTS RELEVANT TO BEHAVIOR GENETIC STUDIES

Given the frequency with which the term *developmental psychopathology* is used as a synonym for *child psychopathology*, it is perhaps ironic that so few behavioral genetic studies include elements of a developmental psychopathology perspective, despite the obvious relevance of these elements to such studies. In this section, I briefly describe some of the elements of a developmental psychopathology perspective relevant to behavior genetic studies. This treatment will be kept brief, as it has received numerous detailed descriptions in other volumes (e.g., Cicchetti & Rogosch, 1999; Rende & Plomin, 1995). Developmental psychopathology is often mistakenly thought to be coextensive with studies of childhood psychopathology, but in reality comprises a set of principles and approaches that can be applied to studies of psychopathology and normal developmental outcomes that are either cross-sectional or longitudinal (Cicchetti, 1993). Some of the critical elements of a developmental psychopathology perspective include a focus on underlying mechanisms and processes, on continuities and discontinuities between normal and abnormal development, on individuals' developmental trajectories, on alternative pathways underlying psychopathological and normal development, and on resilience as well as risk. These will be briefly explicated in turn. I will return to these concepts in the Future Research Directions portions of both the Quantitative and Molecular Genetic sections below.

Focus on Underlying Mechanisms and Processes

Many studies of risk factors for psychopathology are limited to examining the association between a particular risk factor and a disorder. A developmental psychopathology approach attempts to transcend these simple associations in several ways. First, developmental psychopathologists strive to design their studies not only to establish an association between a disorder and one or more risk factors, but also to be informative regarding the specific causal mechanisms that underlie such associations. Hence, the emphasis of the current volume on neurodevelopmental mechanisms underlying the development of psychopathology is well in keeping with this perspective. Second, most studies of the etiology of psychopathology can be best thought of as snapshots of development, given that they characterize individual participants' outcomes at a particular developmental point in time. Even in the absence of longitudinal data, developmental psychopathologists strive to place their etiological findings in proper developmental perspective.

Focus on Continuities and Discontinuities Between Normal and Abnormal Development

Developmental psychopathologists also are quite cognizant of the fact that an individual's developmental outcome (e.g., their diagnostic status for some disorder) is not static, but can change over time and place (Cicchetti, 1993; Sroufe & Rutter, 1984). Consistent with this is the recognition that an individual's diagnostic status is somewhat arbitrary, based on surpassing a prespecified diagnostic threshold. Given what at times are only minor differences in the symptom levels of individuals above and below the diagnostic threshold, developmental psychopathologists are interested in the similarities and differences in adjustment between such individuals. This is only one example of developmental psychopathologists' interest in the continuities and discontinuities between normal and abnormal adjustment. Another example, to be discussed in further detail below, is to what extent the causes of an abnormal developmental outcome (e.g., a disorder such as Attention Deficit Hyperactivity Disorder, or ADHD) are the same or different from those of the corresponding normal range trait (e.g., the temperamental trait of activity level).

Focus on Individuals' Developmental Trajectories

Although population and group level findings may be consistent with a developmental psychopathology perspective, developmental psychopathologists are principally interested in the developmental trajectories of individuals, as has been emphasized by many researchers within this approach (Cicchetti & Rogosch, 1996, 1999; Sroufe & Rutter, 1984). Indeed, the oft-cited (e.g., Cicchetti & Rogosch, 1996, 1999) definition of developmental psychopathology bears this out, given its focus on "the origins and course of individual patterns of behavioral maladaptation ... " (Sroufe & Rutter, 1984, p.18). Thus, in research informed by a developmental psychopathology perspective, the emphasis shifts from population or group level main effects to differences at the subgroup or individual level. This shift is frequently accompanied by a concomitant shift from variable-oriented to person-oriented investigations of the course or underlying causes of disordered developmental outcomes (Cicchetti & Rogosch, 1996, 1999). This distinct emphasis often requires different analytic methods, such as latent growth models, to properly model individuals' developmental trajectories and their relations to other variables (e.g., Bryk & Raudenbush, 1992; Rogosa, 1988; Willett & Sayer, 1994).

Focus on Alternative Pathways Underlying Psychopathological and Normal Development

As described above, developmental psychopathologists are interested in characterizing individuals' developmental trajectories. As such, they distinguish among a number of alternative pathways that individuals' development may take. In particular, developmental psychopathologists make use of the terms *equifinality* and *multifinality*, developed in general systems theory (von Bertalanffy, 1968, as cited in Cicchetti & Rogosch, 1996, 1999), to refer to two general types of developmental pathways. Equifinality refers to the scenario where several distinct causes or developmental processes can eventuate in the same outcome, whereas multifinality refers to the scenario where a particular cause or developmental process can result in a multiplicity of outcomes (Cicchetti & Rogosch, 1996, 1999). Equifinality is quite similar to the concept of "final common pathway" that is discussed in many accounts of the etiology of psychopathology. Multifinality occurs when the same causal process or developmental event differs in its effects or outcome, depending on other causes, developmental contexts, or an individual's choices (Cicchetti & Rogosch, 1996). Many readers will note that multifinality can thus be construed as an example of moderation, in which the relation between a cause and some outcome varies depending on other factors, which can be studied and modeled in appropriate analyses.

Focus on Resilience as Well as Risk

While developmental psychopathologists are interested in, and frequently examine the role of, risk factors in the development of psychopathology, they are also interested in resilience. Resilience may be construed as the ability of individuals to attain adequate developmental outcomes, despite their having experienced various risk factors or adverse experiences at an earlier developmental stage. Developmental psychopathologists are thus interested in studying the pathways to adaptive outcomes of individuals at risk for psychopathology (e.g., Rolf et al., 1990) or of those who grow up in contexts that are extremely stressful or even abusive (e.g., Cicchetti, Rogosch, Lynch, & Holt, 1993; Masten & Coatsworth, 1998). Developmental psychopathologists also acknowledge that individuals may traverse developmental pathways that cycle between adaptive and maladaptive outcomes (Cicchetti & Richters, 1993), and are interested in studying the dynamic aspects of these straight and deviant pathways (Robins & Rutter, 1990). In its most basic form, the concept of resilience can thus also be construed as a form of moderation, similar to multifinality above, in which the relation between a risk factor and an outcome variable varies as a function of some protective factor.

QUANTITATIVE GENETIC DESIGNS

Among the many types of studies used to examine the etiology of disorders, behavior genetic designs (i.e., twin and adoption studies) are among the most useful, as they yield clearer causal inferences than almost any other design. Although both twin and adoption studies allow genetic and environmental influences on a trait or disorder to be disentangled, twin studies have certain advantages relative to adoption studies. These include greater accessibility and representativeness of samples to the general population, thus yielding greater generalizability of findings; contemporaneous measurement of relatives who are the same versus different ages (i.e., twin pairs versus adoptees and their biological and adoptive parents), which permits use of the same rather than different measures; and greater statistical power due both to larger sample sizes and greater genetic similarity between relatives. Twin studies examine the etiology of a trait or disorder by estimating the magnitude of genetic influences (heritability or h^2), shared environmental influences (i.e., environmental influences that are experienced in common which make family members similar to one another on the trait of interest; c^2), and nonshared environmental influences (i.e., environmental influences that are experienced uniquely which make family members different from one another on the trait of interest; e^2). These etiological influences are estimated by comparing the similarity between monozygotic (MZ) twin pairs, who are genetically identical, and fraternal or dizygotic (DZ) twin pairs, who are 50 percent genetically similar on average.

Drawing Inferences Regarding Genetic and Environmental Influences Using Twin Data

A brief description of the use of data from twins to estimate genetic and environmental influences on a trait or disorder may be helpful before presenting more complex behavior genetic models for addressing issues of comorbidity among disorders and of the overlap between disorders and the neurodevelopmental mechanisms hypothesized to underlie them. In order to estimate these influences, twin studies rely on the fact that MZ twins are identical genetically whereas DZ twins, just like nontwin siblings, are on average only 50 percent similar genetically. It also is assumed that MZ twins are no more similar than DZ twins for the *trait-relevant* aspects of the shared environment; that is, that environmental influences on the trait of interest are shared in common between members of fraternal twin pairs to the same extent as between members of identical twin pairs (this is known as the *equal environments assumption*). It also is assumed that the parents of the twins mate at random with respect to the trait being studied (i.e., that there is no *assortative mating*). Similar to the assumptions underlying other statistical analyses (e.g., normality of the residuals in a regression analysis), these assumptions are unlikely to be completely met, but quantitative genetic analyses are quite robust to minor violations of them. Given these assumptions, the correlation between identical twins comprises heritability and shared environmental influences (i.e., $r_{MZ} = h^2 + c^2$), as these are the two sets of influences that can contribute to identical twins' similarity for the trait. In contrast, the correlation between fraternal twins comprises one-half of heritability and shared environmental influences (i.e., $r_{DZ} = 1/2h^2 + c^2$), reflecting the smaller degree of genetic similarity between fraternal twins. Algebraic manipulation of the two equations for twin similarity allows one to estimate h^2, c^2, and e^2 (viz., $h^2 = 2[r_{MZ} - r_{DZ}]$, $c^2 = 2r_{DZ} - r_{MZ}$, $e^2 = 1 - r_{MZ}$).

A simple example may help to make more tangible the use of twin data to estimate heritability, shared environmental influences, and nonshared environmental influences on a trait or disorder. Imagine a twin study of symptoms of a certain disorder (e.g., ADHD) for which identical twins were correlated .70 (i.e., $r_{MZ} = .70$) and fraternal twins were correlated .35 (i.e., $r_{DZ} = .35$). Following the equations above, in this twin study heritability of the disorder would equal .70 (i.e., $h^2 = 2[.70 - .35]$), shared environmental influences would equal .0 (i.e., $c^2 = 2 * .35 - .70$), and nonshared environmental influences would equal .30 (i.e., $e^2 = 1 - .70$). In this study, the best-fitting model for the etiology of ADHD would include genetic and nonshared environmental influences, but not shared environmental influences. In contrast, imagine a second twin study of a different disorder (e.g., Conduct Disorder [CD]) for which identical twins were again correlated .70 (i.e., $r_{MZ} = .70$) but fraternal twins were correlated .50 (i.e., $r_{DZ} = .50$). Again following the equations above, heritability of this second disorder would equal .40 (i.e., $h^2 = 2[.70 - .50]$), shared environmental influences would equal .30 (i.e., $c^2 = 2 * .50 - .70$), and nonshared environmental influences would again equal .30 (i.e., $e^2 = 1 - .70$). In this study, the best-fitting model for the etiology of CD would include genetic, shared environmental, and nonshared environmental influences. While this example may be a bit simplified, it should give the reader some idea of how twin correlations are used to estimate heritability, shared environmental influences, and nonshared environmental influences, and to determine the most plausible etiological model for a given trait or disorder.

Although estimation of these influences using the twin correlations can be done simply by hand, contemporary behavior geneticists use structural equation model-fitting analytic methods that can incorporate additional information on familial relationships (e.g., correlations between nontwin siblings or parents and their children), provide statistical tests of the adequacy of these three influences (viz., h^2, c^2, and e^2) in accounting for the observed familial correlations, and test alternative models for the causal influences underlying the trait (e.g., a model including genetic and nonshared environmental influences versus a model that also includes shared environmental influences). Especially pertinent to this chapter, these analyses can be extended to examine genetic and environmental influences on the overlap or covariation among different disorders or symptom dimensions, as well as between a disorder and its hypothesized underlying neurodevelopmental mechanisms. A recent trend in quantitative genetic analyses has been to extend the investigation of genetic and environmental influences on traits considered singly (i.e., univariate behavior genetic analyses) to the case of multiple traits considered conjointly (Neale & Cardon, 1992). Multivariate behavior genetic analyses seek to explain the overlap or covariation among different traits by examining the genetic and environmental influences that they share in common. As suggested below, such analyses can shed considerable light on the classification of psychopathology and the nature of comorbidity, as well as on the explanation of psychopathological disorders in terms of their underlying neurodevelopmental mechanisms.

Before showing a more complex path model for multivariate behavior genetic analyses pertinent to comorbidity, I present a comprehensive biometric model for the genetic and environmental influences on a single trait for two twins or siblings in the path diagram in Figure 11.1. This path diagram shows the basic biometric model (Neale & Cardon, 1992) for estimating additive and dominance genetic influences, shared and

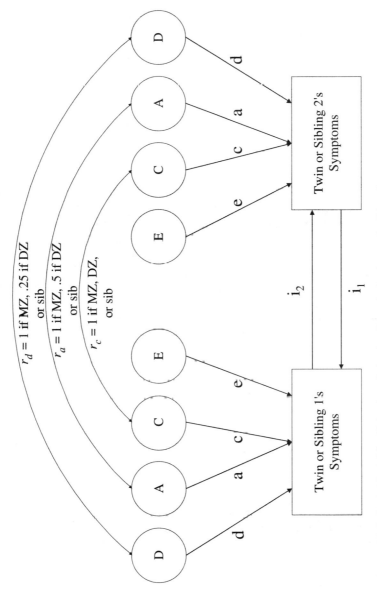

Figure 11.1. Path Model for Univariate Behavior Genetic Analyses of a Disorder

nonshared environmental influences, and the direct influence of one twin or sibling's behavior problems on their co-twin or co-sibling's behavior problems. Note that there are now two types of genetic influences, dominance and additive genetic influences, which are summed to arrive at an estimate of broad-sense heritability, or h^2. Although this path model represents the full set of potential causes on twins' behavior problems, there is not enough information in the conventional twin study design to estimate all five of these parameters simultaneously. As a consequence, contemporary twin studies present and contrast the results of a series of restricted models (i.e., models containing a subset of all potential causes) in order to find the most parsimonious model that fits the data well.

In the path diagram in Figure 11.1, D represents dominance genetic influences, A represents additive genetic influences, C represents shared environmental influences, E represents nonshared environmental influences, and i represents the direct influence of one twin's or sibling's behavior problems on their co-twin's or co-sibling's behavior problems. The circles containing these capital letters represent these latent causal genetic and environmental variables, whereas the corresponding lowercase letters (viz., d, a, c, e, and i) represent the magnitude of these influences (i.e., the parameter estimates, which are regression coefficients) on each twin or sibling's behavior problems. The square of these parameter estimates (viz., d^2, a^2, c^2, and e^2) represents the variance components corresponding to dominance and additive genetic influences, and shared and nonshared environmental influences. The three correlations in the model – r_d, r_a, and r_c – represent the similarity of particular causal influences between twins or siblings. For example, MZ and DZ twins and nontwin siblings all are correlated 1.0 for shared environmental influences (viz., r_c) consistent with the equal environments assumption. In contrast, MZ twins are correlated 1.0 for both dominance and additive genetic influences (viz., r_d and r_a), whereas DZ twins and nontwin siblings are both correlated .25 and .5 for dominance and additive genetic influences, respectively, consistent with their average level of genetic similarity.

Structural equation modeling programs such as LISREL and MX (Jöreskog & Sörbom, 1993; Neale, 1996) can iteratively fit such models to twin and sibling correlations (or variances and covariances) to provide the best estimates of the parameters; that is, parameter estimates that minimize the difference between the twin and sibling correlations implied by the model and those observed in the data. The fit of the model to the data is summarized by a χ^2 statistic, which allows both the fit of a given model and the comparative fit of alternative models to be tested statistically. This property often results in restricted models – models containing only a subset of the parameters in the full model (e.g., only a and e) – that provide an adequate fit to the data. In addition, although we presented the biometric model as applied to data from twins, the model is equally applicable to adoption study data on biologically related and adoptive siblings, and can be extended to analyze data from biologically related and adoptive parent-offspring pairs. Similarly, although we presented the biometric model for some disorder in both twins, it can be used with no loss of generality to estimate the genetic and environmental influences on a measure of the neurodevelopmental mechanisms thought to underlie psychopathology, as well as on the covariation among measures of neurodevelopmental mechanisms and symptoms of disorders (see extension below).

Twin Studies of Genetic and Environmental Influences on the Childhood Disruptive Disorders

A number of twin studies of the childhood disruptive disorders have been conducted in the past decade (see reviews by Rhee, Feigon, Bar, Hadeishi, & Waldman, 2001; Waldman & Rhee, 2002). These studies have found heritability for ADHD to be moderate to high (viz., 60%–90%) with small to moderate nonshared environmental influences and little or no shared environmental influences (Waldman & Rhee, 2002). The majority of twin studies find moderate genetic and shared and nonshared environmental influences on CD, or on related measures of childhood or adolescent antisocial behavior, though there is considerable variability in these estimates across studies (Rhee & Waldman, 2002). In a recent meta-analysis of twin and adoption studies of antisocial behavior (Rhee & Waldman, 2002), the possible moderating effects of the operationalization of antisocial behavior, assessment method, zygosity determination method, and the age and sex of the participants on genetic and environmental influences on antisocial behavior were examined. All of these variables except for participants' sex were found to moderate the genetic and environmental influences on antisocial behavior. This suggests that antisocial behavior may be a highly sensitive phenotype, such that the pattern and magnitude of genetic and environmental influences underlying this phenotype may vary depending on the operationalization and measurement of antisocial behavior, participants' characteristics, and the specific environmental contexts in which antisocial behavior is studied.

There are very few twin studies of oppositional defiant disorder (ODD), and most behavior genetic studies of ODD symptoms have treated them as part of a composite with CD symptoms. Twin studies examining the combination of ODD and CD symptoms tend to find results similar to those for CD (i.e., moderate genetic and shared and nonshared environmental influences). Those few studies that have examined ODD symptoms uniquely have yielded mixed results. One study reported moderate genetic and nonshared environmental influences, but no shared environmental influences (Eaves et al., 1997), whereas another study reported high heritability and slight nonshared environmental influences, but no shared environmental influences (Waldman, Rhee, Levy, & Hay, 2001).

Using Twin Data to Examine Genetic and Environmental Influences on the Overlap Among Disorders [and Between a Disorder and Its Putative Underlying Neurodevelopmental Mechanisms]

Multivariate behavior genetic analyses of twin study data, although not a panacea, represent state of the art methods for addressing questions of comorbidity and of the neurodevelopmental mechanisms underlying psychopathology (to be described below). Multivariate behavior genetic methods share the advantages of univariate biometric model-fitting methods mentioned above, but possess a number of additional features that make them especially useful for testing hypotheses regarding comorbidity and underlying mechanisms. First, such models seek to explain the overlap or covariation among two or more diagnostic entities, or between a disorder and its putative underlying mechanisms, in terms of their common causes by disentangling the genetic and environmental influences that contribute to such overlap. Hence, one can test alternative models for the causes of comorbidity among different disorders or for the mediational role of putative underlying mechanisms, as well as estimate the relative contribution of common genetic and environmental influences to comorbidity or mediation.

Second, univariate behavior genetic models use estimates of genetic and environmental influences to explain twin correlations (or variances and covariances) for a single trait or disorder. Hence, the data these models attempt to explain are the correlations (or variances and covariances) between twins for a single trait or disorder. Multivariate behavior genetic models are fit not only to these data, but also to the within-twin cross-trait correlations (e.g., twin 1's ADHD and CD symptoms) and the cross-twin cross-trait correlations (e.g., twin 1's ADHD symptoms and twin 2's CD symptoms). Indeed, it is these cross-twin cross-trait correlations that afford these analyses their ability to discriminate among competing models for the comorbidity among disorders because alternative models yield different expectations for the cross-twin cross-trait correlations (see Waldman & Slutske, 2000 for detailed examples). Multivariate behavior genetic models also may facilitate a stronger resolution than univariate models of the causes underlying a single disorder or trait because more information (viz., both within-twin and cross-twin cross-trait correlations) is used in analyses.

There are several multivariate behavior genetic studies of the overlap among the childhood disruptive disorders. In these studies, emphasis is placed on determining the magnitude of common and specific etiological influences on the multiple disorders. In addition, one also examines whether the common and specific etiological influences are genetic, shared environmental, or nonshared environmental in nature. The path diagram in Figure 11.2 shows a multivariate behavior genetic model for the common and specific genetic and environmental influences underlying symptoms of ADHD, ODD, and CD. Multivariate behavior genetic studies of the childhood disruptive disorders (Nadder et al., 1998; Silberg et al., 1996; Waldman et al., 2001; Willcutt et al., 1999) have found that most of the covariation among the symptoms of these disorders is due to common additive genetic influences with a moderate contribution of nonshared environmental influences. In these studies, shared environmental influences appear to contribute little, if at all, to the overlap among these disorders. In addition, one study (Waldman et al., 2001) also contrasted a series of a priori, alternative hypotheses for their fit to the data. The results indicated that a number of hypotheses regarding the comorbidity among the three disorders could be strongly rejected. Specifically, the hypotheses that genetic or nonshared environmental influences do not cause the three childhood disruptive disorders or their comorbidity, that all genetic or nonshared environmental influences act individually on the disorders without contributing to their comorbidity, that the only genetic or nonshared environmental influences on ODD and CD are those that also influence ADHD, and that the only genetic or nonshared environmental influences on ODD and CD are completely independent of ADHD, were soundly rejected. In contrast, the results suggested that the only shared environmental influences on ODD and CD are completely independent of ADHD, which is not caused by shared environmental influences.

The results of these multivariate behavior genetic analyses suggest that there is considerable overlap in the genetic and environmental influences on the three disorders. The genetic correlations in these studies suggest that most, but not all, of the genetic influences on the three disorders are shared in common, whereas the nonshared

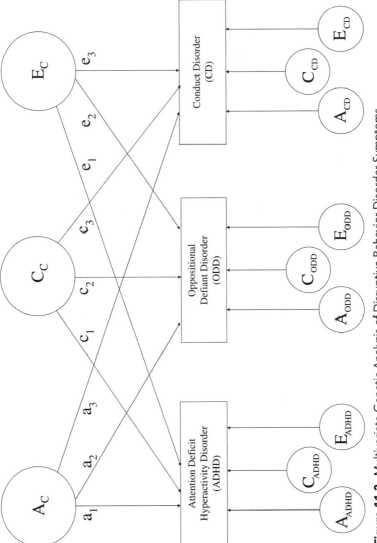

Figure 11.2. Multivariate Genetic Analysis of Disruptive Behavior Disorder Symptoms

environmental correlations suggest that a moderate amount of the nonshared environmental influences on these disorders is shared in common, but that many of these affect each disorder uniquely, albeit to a small extent. In the Waldman et al. (2001) study, for example, the majority of the overlap (93%) between ADHD on the one hand and ODD and CD on the other was due to common genetic influences, whereas the remainder (7%) was due to common nonshared environmental influences. Slightly less of the overlap between ODD and CD was due to common genetic influences (79%), with common shared and nonshared environmental influences contributing much less to their overlap (9% and 12%, respectively).

It is interesting to speculate on the meaning of these results for molecular genetic analyses of childhood disruptive disorders (to be discussed below), as well as for the neurodevelopmental mechanisms that underlie them. Given the high genetic correlations, it seems likely that most of the specific genes found to influence one of the disorders will influence the other disorders as well. These genetic correlations, and the high phenotypic correlations to which they contribute, also imply that the neurodevelopmental mechanisms underlying these three disorders are substantially shared and are themselves genetically influenced to a considerable degree. Nonetheless, it is important to recognize that while the genetic correlations among these three disorders are high, they all are less than unity. This suggests that there also will be some specific genes that influence one of the disorders and not the others, and that each of the disorders may have underlying neurodevelopmental mechanisms that are not shared with the other disorders.

FUTURE RESEARCH DIRECTIONS IN QUANTITATIVE GENETIC STUDIES OF CHILDHOOD DISRUPTIVE DISORDERS

Twin Studies of Genetic and Environmental Influences on Executive Functions and Their Covariation with Childhood Disruptive Disorders

Although there have been many large-scale univariate behavior genetic analyses of the childhood disruptive disorders over the past fifteen years, and the number of multivariate behavior genetic analyses of these disorders is increasing, there have been very few behavior genetic studies of the neurodevelopmental mechanisms that may underlie these disorders. This is ironic, given that for some time there has been considerable interest in *endophenotypes* for psychopathology, and this interest has only grown with the advent of molecular genetic studies. An endophenotype is a variable that represents a neurobiological, psychophysiological, or psychological mechanism that is thought to be centrally involved in the development of a given disorder, and to be a more proximal effect of its underlying causes. The term *endophenotype* has a number of implications, several of which can be tested using behavior genetic analyses. The first implication, a rather obvious one, is that measures of the endophenotype are related to the disorder. The second implication is that measures of the endophenotype are heritable. This implication should also be obvious given that the endophenotype must reflect the same etiology as the disorder. The third implication, which is probably not at all obvious even though it may be the most important, is that measures of the endophenotype should reflect the same genetic causes as the disorder, but to a greater degree. This is consistent with the notion of the endophenotype as a more fundamental and direct reflection of the underlying causes than is the disorder. Many readers will recognize this third implication as a *mediational* hypothesis, in that endophenotypic measures are thought to represent an intermediate phenotype that mediates – in full or in part – the causal link between the disorder and its underlying genetic influences.

Measures of executive functions such as attention, memory, impulse control, organization, and planning can be considered highly plausible candidate endophenotypes for the neurodevelopmental mechanisms that underlie the childhood disruptive disorders (see reviews by Nigg, 2001; Nigg, Blaskey, Huang-Pollock, & Rappley, in press; Pennington & Ozonoff, 1996). Nonetheless, there is a paucity of twin studies of executive functions in children, and those that have been published have included very small samples. For example, a recent twin study (Kuntsi & Stevenson, 2001) examined genetic and environmental influences on parent and teacher ratings of hyperactivity and on measures of executive functions. The sample was comprised of forty-six twin pairs in which at least one twin was hyperactive, and forty-seven control twin pairs in which neither twin was hyperactive. The executive functions assessed included measures of delay aversion, working memory, response inhibition, and response speed. Similar to previous studies (for a detailed review see Waldman & Rhee, 2002), the authors found both teacher and parent ratings of hyperactivity to be moderately to highly heritable, with the parent ratings also showing a significant rater contrast effect. The authors also found extreme levels of hyperactivity to be significantly heritable, though these were substantially lower than in previous studies (e.g., Rhee, Waldman, Hay, & Levy, 1999; Stevenson, 1992). The authors also examined to what extent the same genetic influences underlying extreme hyperactivity also underlie the executive function measures. Unfortunately, the number of twin pairs included in these analyses was very small (i.e., 18 MZ and 28 DZ pairs), and unaccountably, univariate behavior genetic analyses of the executive function measures were not conducted. Although common genetic influences were significant for extreme hyperactivity and the variability of response speed, it is difficult to know how to interpret this finding given that the magnitude of common genetic influences for several other executive function measures was quite substantial and nearly at the same level.

Clearly the study by Kuntsi and Stevenson (2001) represents a preliminary effort in this domain, and many larger twin studies of the genetic and environmental influences underlying executive function measures and their overlap with the childhood disruptive disorder symptoms are needed. What should such studies and the analyses of the data they yield look like? First, such studies should use much larger, *unselected* samples of twins, ideally several hundred pairs each of both MZ and DZ twins. Such a sample should ensure adequate statistical power to discriminate among alternative etiological models, and the unselected nature of the sample will ensure that the findings regarding genetic and environmental influences on executive function measures are generalizable to the overall population, rather than only to a clinical population of children with externalizing psychopathology. Second, a variety of executive functions should be assessed using multiple measures and these should be included along with ratings of both hyperactivity-impulsivity and inattention. This will enable the differential relations of executive function measures to the inattentive and hyperactive-impulsive dimensions of ADHD to emerge, as well as permitting multivariate behavior genetic analyses among the executive function measures and between them and the ADHD symptom dimensions. These data will help clarify the specific executive function dimensions underlying such measures and help establish their roles as distinct endophenotypes for hyperactivity-impulsivity and inattention. Third, a specific form of multivariate behavior genetic analyses should be employed, namely those that allow one to specifically address issues of mediation, as mentioned above. This analysis is known as a Cholesky decomposition, a simple example of which is shown in Figure 11.3. Rather than merely summarizing the etiology of the covariation between symptoms of a disorder and an endophenotypic measure, this model allows for specific tests of mediation of the genetic and environmental influences on the disorder via the endophenotypic measure. To illustrate, a Cholesky decomposition model for the covariation between an executive function measure and ADHD symptoms is shown in Figure 11.3. In this figure, A_1 represents additive genetic influences on the executive function measure that also influence ADHD symptoms, whereas A_2 represents additive genetic influences that are unique to ADHD symptoms (i.e., not shared in common with the executive function measure; Loehlin, 1996). Similarly, C_1 and E_1 represent shared and nonshared environmental influences on the executive function measure that also influence ADHD symptoms, whereas C_2 and E_2 represent shared and nonshared environmental influences that are unique to ADHD symptoms. If the executive function measure is truly an endophenotype for ADHD, than paths 1 and 2 – leading from the first set of additive genetic influences to the executive function measure and ADHD symptoms – should be significant and substantial in magnitude, with path 3 being smaller in magnitude (and perhaps nonsignificant) than path 2. This pattern of findings would support the executive function measure as an endophenotype for ADHD, because they are consistent with the executive function measure mediating the genetic influences on ADHD. (Note that similar findings for paths 4, 5, and 6 and for 7, 8, and 9 would support mediation of the nonshared and shared environmental influences, respectively.) Multivariate behavior genetic analyses such as these using the Cholesky decomposition model will help significantly in establishing endophenotypes for childhood disruptive disorders.

Developmental Psychopathology Approaches to Quantitative Genetic Studies of Childhood Disruptive Disorders

With rare exceptions, quantitative genetic studies of childhood disruptive disorders have not been informed by a developmental psychopathology approach (cf. Rutter et al., 1997). How would the conceptualization, design, and analysis of twin studies of childhood disruptive disorders differ if they adopted a developmental psychopathology perspective? Although a detailed answer to this question is beyond the scope of this chapter, in this section I attempt to present some brief examples of the kinds of questions and approaches that such twin studies might address and use within a developmental psychopathology perspective.

I already have discussed twin studies of neurodevelopmental mechanisms and their overlap with childhood disruptive disorders above, which are consistent with a developmental psychopathology focus on underlying mechanisms. Also consistent with a developmental psychopathology focus is an emphasis on process. Most extant twin studies appear quite fractionated in their division of genetic and environmental influences and the relative magnitudes thereof. A more integrative view, which also focuses

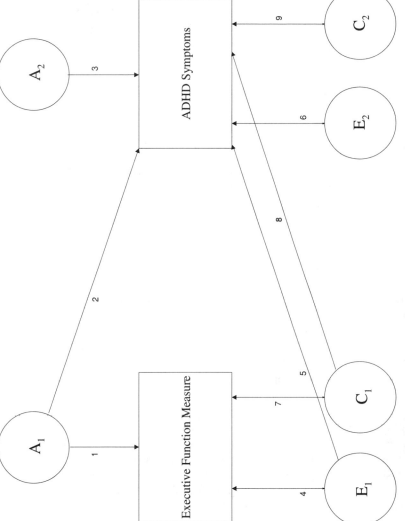

Figure 11.3. Cholesky Decomposition of Executive Function Measure and ADHD Symptoms

more strongly on process, is provided via the consideration of genotype-environment correlations and interactions (the latter will be described in more detail below). A number of recent twin and adoption studies of childhood disruptive disorders (e.g., Ge et al., 1996; Rutter et al., 1997) have moved beyond the simple decomposition of variance into genetic and environmental influences to examine the processes by which these influences act together in development. Although it is still in the early stages of such research, the investigation of genotype-environment correlations promises to provide a fuller picture of genetic and environmental influences on the development of childhood disruptive disorders.

A second aspect of a developmental psychopathology approach to quantitative genetic studies of childhood disruptive disorders involves a focus on continuities and discontinuities between normal and abnormal development. A number of twin and adoption studies of both childhood externalizing and internalizing disorders already have addressed this issue (e.g., Deater-Deckard & Plomin, 1999; Levy, Hay, McStephen, Wood, & Waldman, 1997; Rende, Plomin, Reiss, & Hetherington, 1993; Stevenson, 1992). Specifically, these studies test whether the magnitude of genetic influences on a trait or disorder is greater (or lower) at the disordered extreme than for the normal range of variation in the general population. Studies of this issue for symptoms of ADHD (Levy et al., 1997; Rhee, Waldman, Hay, & Levy, 1999; Stevenson, 1992) have found that its heritability is at least as great at the disordered extreme than for variation in the normal range, though the difference in heritabilities is frequently nonsignificant statistically, despite an appreciable difference in magnitude (Levy et al., 1997). Research on this issue is still in its toddlerhood, and future such studies would do well to use a broader diversity of analytic methods, as well as a broader conceptualization of the continuities and discontinuities between normal and abnormal development in their design and measures.

A third aspect of a developmental psychopathology perspective on quantitative genetic studies of childhood disruptive disorders involves a stronger focus on individuals' developmental trajectories than is currently the case. A number of developmental behavior genetic studies of child psychopathology have utilized longitudinal designs and the analysis of data collected at multiple timepoints. Nonetheless, the typical quantitative genetic analytic methods employed (e.g., Cholesky decompositions, genetic simplex analyses; see Neale & Cardon, 1992) are best described as variable- rather than person-centered. Recently, behavior geneticists have begun to develop hybrid analytic methods that combine the best features of latent growth curve models with a quantitative genetic approach (e.g., McArdle, 1986). These novel methods will permit the characterization of individuals' developmental trajectories while estimating the genetic and environmental influences that underlie the parameters of such trajectories (e.g., initial level, linear slope, curvilinear acceleration or deceleration). Although such methods have not yet been applied to the analysis of longitudinal data on childhood disruptive disorder symptoms, their application will aid in transforming such approaches from variable- to person-centered, and thus represent a better fit with a developmental psychopathology perspective.

A fourth aspect of a developmental psychopathology perspective on quantitative genetic studies of childhood disruptive disorders involves the use of genotype-environment (and environment-environment) interaction models to examine the forms of moderation involved in both the issues of multifinality and resilience. As mentioned above, multifinality occurs when the same causal process or developmental event differs in its effects or outcome, depending on other causes, developmental contexts, or an individuals' choices (Cicchetti & Rogosch, 1996). Also mentioned above is the concept of resilience, which may be construed as the ability of individuals to attain adequate developmental outcomes, despite their having experienced various risk factors or adverse experiences at an earlier developmental stage. Both of these developmental psychopathology concepts involve moderation because they involve differences in or deflections of individuals' developmental pathways from the trajectory that may be predicted from having, or being exposed to, a given risk factor. Some examples may help to illustrate how quantitative genetic analyses, particularly of genotype-environment and environment-environment interaction, may be used to address these developmental psychopathology issues.

An example of multifinality is provided by the following hypothetical twin study, in which a subsample of twins is reared in the normal range of neighborhood contexts, and there are two additional subsamples of twins, one reared in relatively impoverished neighborhoods characterized by very low socioeconomic status (SES), high rates of crime, and easy access to illicit drugs, the second reared in relatively privileged neighborhoods characterized by high SES, very low crime rates, and a relative dearth of illicit drugs. As presented above, multivariate behavior genetic analyses of the childhood disruptive disorders have suggested that most of the covariation between symptoms of ADHD and CD is due to common genetic influences with little or no contribution of shared environmental influences. How might the picture of the etiology of the overlap between these two disorders differ across these three environmental contexts, viewed through the analytic lens of genotype-environment (and environment-environment) interaction? One might expect the findings from the first environmental context (i.e., a normal range of neighborhood contexts) to be similar to those presented above, namely, average levels of CD symptoms in ADHD children, with the majority of the overlap between ADHD and CD being due to common genetic influences. In relatively impoverished neighborhoods, however, one might expect higher rates of CD symptoms, academic failure, and substance abuse among ADHD children, as well as some substantial proportion of the covariation between ADHD and CD symptoms to be due to common shared environmental influences. In relatively privileged neighborhoods, in stark contrast, one might expect lower rates of ADHD and especially CD, with children who are genetically predisposed to ADHD perhaps merely manifesting higher levels of activity and inattention, but not meeting diagnostic criteria or experiencing many of the sequelae of ADHD (e.g., academic failure, progression to CD) due to their receiving ancillary services (e.g., extra help from teachers, tutoring, stimulant medication) that protect against these negative outcomes. In addition, one would expect a much smaller proportion of the covariation between ADHD and CD symptoms to be due to both common genetic and shared environmental influences, given both the relative absence of some of the specific shared environmental influences thought to predispose to CD (i.e., very low SES, higher crime rates, greater availability of illicit drugs) and the likelihood that these environmental influences are also necessary for actualizing the genetic predisposition to CD. In this study, variation in neighborhood characteristics would thus emerge as specific environmental influences that lead to very different outcomes among children who are similarly predisposed toward ADHD, thus representing an example of multifinality.

An example of resilience is illustrated by the following hypothetical twin study. Imagine two subsamples of adolescent twins, one reared in the normal range of family environments, the other reared by parents who not only provide a warm, supportive environment for their children, but also are particularly adept at supervising and monitoring their teenagers' activities, friendships, and academic performance. Insofar as parenting variables such as supervision and monitoring represent a shared environmental influence on adolescent antisocial behavior, one would expect levels of antisocial behavior to be higher for the first subsample of twins than for the second. In addition, one would expect the magnitude of shared environmental influences in this twin study to be appreciable for the first subsample of twins, and much lower for the second subsample. This is due to the fact that there would be substantial variation among families in parental supervision and monitoring in the first subsample of twins, but negligible variation among families in the second subsample of twins due to the selection of parents that are high on this dimension of parenting behavior. Finally, one might also expect the heritability of antisocial behavior to be higher in the first than in the second subsample of twins, insofar as parental supervision and monitoring (or the relative lack thereof) represent aspects of the environment that are important for actualizing one's genetic predisposition for antisocial behavior. In this study, high parental supervision and monitoring would thus emerge as environmental influences that contribute to resilience among children predisposed toward manifesting high levels of antisocial behavior. These examples demonstrate how more sophisticated twin designs, namely those that transcend the simple estimation of genetic and environmental influences to examine genotype-environment and environment-environment interactions, can be used to cast quantitative genetic studies of childhood disruptive disorders within a developmental psychopathology perspective.

MOLECULAR GENETIC DESIGNS

Association and Linkage

In contrast to behavioral genetic studies, which estimate broad, abstract components of genetic and environmental variance that contribute to the liability underlying a disorder, molecular genetic studies examine the role of specific genes or genomic regions that may contribute to the etiology of a given disorder. Molecular genetic studies of disorders test for association and/or linkage between a given disorder and particular candidate genes or genomic regions. A genomic region is simply a segment of DNA of a given length and known location. Genomic regions examined in association or linkage studies may be selected due to some a priori hypothesis regarding the role in the etiology of the target disorder of one or more genes that are located in the region, or chosen more or less at random simply to provide extensive coverage of the genome in a genome scan (the more common scenario). A candidate gene is one that is hypothesized to be involved in the etiology and development of a particular disorder, given the known or plausible role of its gene product in the pathophysiology of the disorder. For example, genes that underlie various components of the dopaminergic neurotransmitter system have been hypothesized to be candidate genes for a number of psychiatric disorders (e.g., the childhood disruptive disorders, schizophrenia), given the important role that dopamine is thought to play in those disorders. Classical association studies examine the relation between the presence or absence of a disorder on the one hand, and the presence of "high-risk" versus "low-risk" forms of the gene on the other. Different forms of a gene are called "alleles," and a "high-risk" allele is a risk factor that predisposes to the disorder, whereas a "low-risk" allele can be construed as a protective factor in the sense that it is related to absence of the disorder. In association studies, the frequency of high-risk and low-risk alleles are typically contrasted in cases and controls (viz., individuals ascertained based on the presence of the target disorder versus a sample selected based on the absence of the disorder who are matched on a variety of background characteristics), with the expectation that cases will show higher frequencies of the high-risk allele than controls.

Several variations on the classic case-control association design have been developed (e.g., a comparison of symptom levels in unrelated individuals who have 0, 1, or 2 copies of the high-risk allele of a particular gene in a nonreferred sample, or in siblings that differ in the number of high-risk alleles). One very important variation is family-based association methods, such as the Haplotype-based Haplotype Relative Risk (*HHRR*, Falk & Rubinstein, 1987; Terwilliger & Ott, 1992), which contrast the alleles that are transmitted with those that are not transmitted by parents to their affected children. In this design, the nontransmitted alleles serve as controls for the transmitted alleles, which are expected to be disproportionately transmitted to the affected children if there is indeed an association between the disorder and the gene. Family-based association designs were developed to avoid the problem of population stratification that often can plague conventional case-control association studies, leading to false positive results. This problem occurs when case and control samples differ in their representation of groups of individuals (e.g., from different ethnic backgrounds) who differ in both the frequency of high- and low-risk alleles and rates (or symptom levels) of the target disorder. This mixture of subsamples that differ in both allele frequencies and symptom levels/diagnostic rates induces an association in the overall sample which may occur even in the absence of any true relation between the gene and the disorder in either of the subsamples. The most common source of population stratification is thought to be ethnic group differences, wherein ethnic groups differ both in allele frequencies and rates of disorder, although in principle stratification effects may be due to any form of population structure (e.g., differences in SES) which varies between cases and controls. Within-family association methods are thought to avoid the biasing effects of population stratification because the transmitted and nontransmitted alleles come from the same individuals within the sample of cases.

In linkage studies, typically the correlation of a disorder and anonymous DNA markers representing genomic regions is examined within family members (e.g., sibling pairs, parents and their children). In classical linkage studies, this involves examining the co-segregation of the presence or absence of the disorder with sharing particular allele(s) of a DNA marker through large family pedigrees. Note that in linkage analysis it is commonly assumed that the anonymous DNA markers are not themselves the genes contributing to the etiology of the disorder, but may be "linked" with them due to their close contiguity on the chromosome which results in their frequent co-inheritance during meiosis. In the case of strong linkage, there is a strong co-occurrence among relatives of the presence or absence of the disorder with sharing the same DNA marker allele *identical by descent (IBD)*, which means that the shared allele is not merely of the same type (i.e., *identical by state, or IBS*), but is indeed the identical allele transmitted by a common ancestor. Classical linkage analyses are commonly *model-based*, meaning that the researcher must specify a number of parameters a priori, including the base rate of the disorder, the allele frequencies, and the penetrances of the genotypes. The penetrance of a given genotype is the probability that an individual with that genotype will manifest the disorder. The investigator also can examine genetic heterogeneity by modeling the proportion of families in which the disorder is linked to the genomic region. Needless to say, in most instances the values of most if not all of these parameters would be unknown. This led statistical geneticists to develop *model-free* linkage analytic methods, which require the specification of few or no parameters a priori. Model-free analyses typically are both more flexible and less powerful than model-based linkage analyses in which values of the parameters are correctly specified. A common form of model-free linkage analysis involves estimating the proportion of alleles shared IBD among affected sibling pairs for each DNA marker examined. A departure of the proportion of alleles shared IBD from the expected Mendelian proportions (viz., .25, .50, .25, for 0, 1, and 2 alleles shared IBD, respectively) suggests that the genomic region in which that DNA marker resides is linked with the disorder.

Like association analyses, linkage analyses have undergone many important refinements. First, there has been a shift in contemporary linkage studies toward the use of many smaller family pedigrees, or large numbers of affected sibling pairs, rather than a reliance on a few very large family pedigrees. Second, linkage analyses of specific targeted candidate genes, rather than of large numbers of anonymous DNA markers, are becoming more common. One statistical genetic tool that has become quite popular for such studies is the Transmission Disequlibrium Test (*TDT*, Spielman et al., 1993). The TDT is similar to the aforementioned HHRR, in that both statistics contrast the transmitted and nontransmitted alleles from parents to their affected children. The only methodological difference between the analytic methods is that the TDT contrasts the transmitted and nontransmitted alleles from *heterozygous* parents only (i.e., parents who have one copy each of the high-risk and low-risk alleles), as opposed to contrasting the alleles transmitted by all parents as in the HHRR. Despite their apparent similarity, the TDT possesses a number of important statistical properties that distinguish it from the HHRR, including being a test of linkage as well as association, being robust to population stratification, and enabling one to include multiple affected offspring from a given family in a test of linkage. In contrast, the HHRR is a test of association only, is not completely robust to the biasing effects of population stratification, and cannot accommodate data from multiple affected offspring from the same family due to the violation of the assumption of observational independence. Given its favorable characteristics, it is little wonder that the TDT has received so much use and attention regarding its statistical properties as compared with alternative statistical genetic methods in the recent genetics literature. In addition, the TDT has recently been extended by a number of researchers (e.g., Rabinowitz, 1997; Waldman, Robinbson, & Rowe, 1999) to enable the examination of linkage between a candidate gene or DNA marker and multiple continuous as well as categorical variables (e.g., symptom levels of a disorder instead of or in addition to a diagnosis). Although linkage and association methods were originally developed to find genes for disorders and diseases, recent developments in these methods, such as the aforementioned extension of the TDT to quantitative variables, will facilitate the discovery of genes for the neurodevelopmental mechanisms underlying psychopathology. We return to this topic in some detail in the Future Research Directions section.

The Genetics of Complex Traits

A number of geneticists (e.g., Chakravarti, 1999; Lander & Schork, 1994; Risch, 2000; Risch & Merikangas, 1996) recently have highlighted important differences between the genetics of simple Mendelian diseases and of complex traits or disorders, and have focused on the special challenges posed by the search for genes that underlie the latter. These geneticists define a "complex trait" as any phenotype that does not exhibit classic Mendelian recessive or dominant inheritance attributable to a single gene locus (Lander & Schork, 1994). Complex traits and disorders have a number of features that distinguish them from Mendelian diseases. First, complex traits are thought to result from the effects of multiple genetic and environmental influences. Second, each of the multiple genes thought to underlie complex disorders likely confers only a relatively small risk for the disorder. Third, these genes are likely to have fairly low penetrance (i.e., the probability of developing the disorder given the presence of the high-risk allele or genotype) and have a relatively high allele frequency in the population. Fourth, there is likely to be genetic heterogeneity for complex traits, such that the same genotype can result in different phenotypes and different genotypes can result in the same phenotype. Note that these two forms of genetic heterogeneity parallel the developmental psychopathology concepts of multifinality and equifinality discussed above. Fifth, there is likely to be the presence of phenocopies (i.e., disorders caused by environmental influences that have the same symptom presentation as the inherited disorder) for complex disorders. Sixth, specific environmental influences are more likely to be important risk factors for complex disorders, and there may be the presence of gene- or genotype-by-environment interaction. Suffice to say, for complex traits and disorders it is most likely that the etiology and risk to relatives is composed of a multitude of susceptibility genes, each contributing only a small magnitude of the overall risk for the disorder. Indeed, most researchers consider the underlying causes of psychiatric disorders to be polygenic (i.e., influenced by many genes and environmental factors). It is an open question as to whether the neurodevelopmental mechanisms underlying psychopathology represent traits that are as complex as manifest disorders, or whether they are less complex from a genetic perspective. The issues raised above should provide some sense of the complexities inherent in finding genes that influence the development of psychopathology and its underlying neurodevelopmental mechanisms.

Candidate Gene Studies Versus Genome Scans

Broadly speaking, there are two general strategies for finding genes that contribute to the etiology of a disorder. The first is a genome scan, in which linkage is examined between a disorder and a large number of DNA markers scattered at approximately equal distances across the genome. Genome scans may be thought of as exploratory searches for putative genes that contribute to the etiology of a disorder. What makes genome scans exploratory is that neither the location of the relevant genes, nor their function or etiological relevance, is known a priori. On the other hand, the fact that major genes have been found for many medical diseases via genome scans is testament to

genes that increase the susceptibility to schizophrenia, in particular the short arm (i.e., the top portion) of chromosome 6 (i.e., 6p) and the long arm (i.e., the bottom portion) of chromosome 22 (i.e., 22q).

As difficult as it may be to obtain significant linkage findings in initial genome scans, the replication of linkage findings involves a host of additional difficulties. First, the replication of linkage findings for complex disorders such as schizophrenia appears to require samples that are much larger than the original sample (Suarez, Hampe, & Van Eerdewegh, 1994), such that true predisposing loci (i.e., specific genomic regions) often may fail to replicate even in very large samples. Second, even if one surmounts the difficulty of demonstrating statistical significance for linkage to a particular chromosomal region in a replication study, one still faces the thorny issue of deciding whether one's linkage finding is in the identical chromosomal region as the initial finding. In this sense, genetic linkage studies share much in common with real estate sales, where the mantra is "location, location, location."

Some tangible examples may be helpful for illustrating the nature and extent of these replication problems. As suggested above, there have been a number of replications of linkage between schizophrenia and DNA markers on the short arm of chromosome 6. Unfortunately, rather than being tightly clustered in a small chromosomal region, these linkage findings traverse approximately 50–60 centiMorgans, which encompasses most of the length of the short arm of this chromosome (Roberts et al., 1999). This raises the question of whether these linkage findings are converging, albeit imprecisely, on a single candidate gene for schizophrenia located somewhere in this large region, or whether the linkage findings from these studies are actually detecting multiple susceptibility loci that each happen to be located on the short arm of chromosome 6. To address this issue, Roberts et al. (1999) conducted a simulation study to examine the variability in location estimates for linkage of a DNA marker to a complex trait and thus gauge what could constitute replication across linkage studies. Using realistic conditions that would be expected to occur for a complex trait (e.g., multiple unlinked susceptibility loci, genetic heterogeneity, incomplete penetrance, and the presence of phenocopies), the authors found substantial variability in location estimates for a given linked locus across studies. The 95 percent confidence intervals for the location estimates were quite marked even with large sample sizes (e.g., 800 nuclear families) and were especially pronounced for the smaller sample sizes (e.g., 200 nuclear families) that are commonly used in psychiatric genetic studies.

Lest one be tempted to characterize this as a property of molecular genetic studies of schizophrenia, or of psychiatric disorders in general, they can be assured that this is not at all the case. One of the most exciting recent findings in psychiatric genetics is the linkage of autism to the long arm of chromosome 7 (i.e., 7q), as well as the observation that this linkage finding appeared to replicate across a few independent studies. Nonetheless, in a recent conference presentation, Santangelo et al. (2000) simultaneously analyzed the 7q linkage data from multiple samples and found little evidence to support the hypothesis of a common location across studies, thus calling into question whether this finding was indeed replicating across studies. Such questions regarding replication also are common in molecular genetic studies of complex medical diseases. For example, after a number of genome scans and candidate gene studies had identified fifteen possible susceptibility loci for insulin dependent diabetes mellitus (*IDDM*), two "second-generation" genome scans were conducted. With the exception of a previously well-established linkage to the HLA region on chromosome 6p, none of the previously reported loci were found to convincingly replicate in these studies. These findings suggest the difficulties in replicating linkage findings in general, and estimates of location in particular.

It is difficult to speculate on how this scenario would differ using neurodevelopmental mechanisms as target phenotypes or as adjuncts to psychiatric diagnoses, given the dearth of relevant studies. There are two possibilities that could increase the power and precision of linkage studies. The first is that neurodevelopmental mechanisms represent endophenotypes that are influenced more strongly and directly than manifest psychopathology. The second is that the inclusion of neurodevelopmental mechanisms along with diagnoses or symptom dimensions would refine the disorder phenotype so as to increase its validity. Either of these possibilities would strengthen the relation between the phenotype and its underlying genetic influences, which should increase both the likelihood of replication of linkage findings and the precision of location estimates.

Candidate Gene Studies of Schizophrenia and ADHD

There have been numerous candidate gene studies of schizophrenia, and more recently ADHD, in the psychiatric genetics literature. As stated above, most of the candidate genes chosen for study are genes that code for some aspect of neurotransmitter function, especially in the dopaminergic system (and to a lesser extent, the serotonergic and noradrenergic neurotransmitter systems). Additional candidate genes examined for schizophrenia are those that are important in brain development (e.g., the *BDNF* and *HOX2* genes). Unfortunately, candidate gene studies in psychiatric genetics have acquired a bad reputation in the eyes of some critics (e.g., see Crowe, 1993; Kidd, 1993), due mostly to the lack of controls for population stratification artifacts in case-control association studies (as described above) and to the failure to deal adequately with false positive findings. Nonetheless, a number of potential solutions to these problems have begun to be implemented in recent candidate gene studies of schizophrenia and ADHD. For schizophrenia, several recent meta-analyses of association findings have been published for the dopamine receptor D3 gene (*DRD3*, Williams et al., 1998) and for the serotonin receptor 2A gene (*HTR2A*, Williams et al., 1997). Although false positive results and the artifactual effects of population stratification may plague a given study, it is unlikely that these problems would bias the results of a set of studies. Indeed, these meta-analyses suggest that *DRD3* and *HTR2A*, while statistically significant across studies, are susceptibility loci that confer a slight increase (i.e., odds ratios < 1.5) in the risk of developing schizophrenia.

Although case-control studies have predominated, within-family analyses of linkage and association (e.g., using the TDT) have also been used to some extent in molecular genetic analyses of schizophrenia, and have been used extensively in studies of candidate genes and ADHD. These studies have suggested a number of candidate genes as risk factors for ADHD, including the dopamine transporter gene (*DAT1*; Cook et al., 1995; Daly et al., 1999; Gill et al., 1997; Waldman et al., 1998) and the dopamine receptor D4 and D5 genes (*DRD4* and *DRD5*; e.g., LaHoste et al., 1996; Rowe et al., 1998; Smalley et al., 1998; Swanson et al., 1998; Tahir et al., 2000). What makes these candidate gene studies of ADHD so interesting is the degree of replication of association and linkage seen across studies, in contrast to candidate gene studies of most other psychiatric disorders. For example, it is noteworthy that there is a recent meta-analysis of case-control and within-family association studies of *DRD4* and ADHD (Faraone, Doyle, & Biederman, 2001), which demonstrated a significant association for both types of studies (i.e., *case-control*: $p = .00000008$; relative risk $= 1.9, 95\%$ CI: 1.4–2.2; *within-family*: $p = .02$; relative risk $= 1.4, 95\%$ CI: 1.1–1.6).

FUTURE RESEARCH DIRECTIONS IN MOLECULAR GENETIC STUDIES OF CHILDHOOD DISRUPTIVE DISORDERS

Future Research Directions in Genome Scans

What are some of the future directions for genome scans and linkage studies that might be more fruitful? The first of these involves methods for narrowing down the chromosomal location obtained from genome scans while alleviating some of the problems mentioned at the end of the section entitled "Genome scans of schizophrenia and ADHD" above. One of the more promising methods for doing this has already borne fruit in medical genetic studies. This method is known as *linkage disequilibrium mapping* (i.e., LD mapping), which involves performing a series of TDTs over the span of the chromosomal locations yielded by genome scans or association studies. An example of the successful use of this method is for Type I diabetes, where LD mapping was used to follow up significant association findings for DNA markers on the short arm of chromosome 11 (i.e., 11p15) and to hone in on the insulin locus (*INS*) (Bennett & Todd, 1996). A variant of LD mapping applied to haplotypes (i.e., a set of closely linked alleles that tend to be co-inherited; Sudbery, 1998) was also used to demonstrate that a particular marker within the *INS* gene was indeed the functional susceptibility locus (Bennett & Todd, 1996). LD mapping also could be used profitably to follow up linkage findings, as has been done for reading disability and chromosome 15 (Morris et al., 2000), but some have raised the concern that the relation between linkage disequilibrium and genetic distance from the actual predisposing locus may degenerate over very short distances. Fortunately, these and other concerns with LD mapping are an active area being explored by statistical geneticists.

A second future direction involves the use of quantitative traits instead of or in addition to categorical diagnoses as phenotypes in genome scans and linkage analyses. This approach already has borne fruit in molecular genetic studies of schizophrenia, as two of the seven studies reporting linkage to 6p analyzed quantitative indices of schizophrenia-related traits rather than (or in addition to) the diagnosis of schizophrenia (Roberts et al., 1999). In one of these studies (Arolt et al., 1996) linkage was found with eye-tracking dysfunction – which is considered one of the primary candidate neurodevelopmental mechanisms underlying schizophrenia – whereas in the other (Brzustowicz et al., 1997), linkage was found with positive but not negative symptoms. These studies suggest that dissecting the schizophrenia phenotype into more specific components, and focusing on endophenotypes as well as the manifest diagnosis, may help significantly in finding susceptibility loci for the disorder. These suggestions are likely not specific to schizophrenia, but should hold for other psychiatric (and medical) disorders as well. Using quantitative traits in genome scans will influence issues of research design as well as of statistical analysis. A number of statistical geneticists (e.g., Cardon & Fulker, 1994; Dolan & Boomsma, 1998; Eaves & Meyer, 1994;

Gu, Todorov, & Rao, 1996; Risch & Zhang, 1995, 1996) have shown that the most powerful design for a genome scan using quantitative traits is to select a combination of sibling pairs that are highly concordant (e.g., both having scores $\geq$ the top 10% of the population) and highly discordant (e.g., one having a score $\geq$ the top 10% of the population, the other having a score $\leq$ the bottom 10% of the population) for the quantitative trait to be analyzed. This research design should provide considerable increases in statistical power for linkage studies, which would enable the detection of susceptibility loci of smaller effect size using fewer sibling pairs.

A third future direction involves the use of covariates and moderator variables in linkage analysis. Rice et al. (1999) have developed a logistic regression-based approach to sib-pair linkage analysis that allows for the incorporation of covariates, such as sex and age, as well as moderators of linkage. This analytic approach allows one to capitalize on the traditional use of covariates in analyses (i.e., to reduce error variance), while permitting explicit tests of differences in linkage as a function of moderator variables (e.g., does linkage between a DNA marker and a diagnosis or quantitative trait vary as a function of sex, age of onset, or some environmental variable). This latter feature is essential for researchers who seek to adopt a developmental psychopathology perspective on linkage studies of psychiatric disorders, given that tests of moderation are at the heart of evaluating hypotheses regarding alternative pathways and resilience (to be discussed in more detail below). Although it is just beginning to be used, this method has the potential to increase the statistical power of linkage studies, as well as facilitate the examination of more sophisticated hypotheses (e.g., gene X environment interactions) that are difficult if not impossible using more conventional linkage analytic techniques.

A fourth direction that is receiving considerable attention in the statistical genetics literature involves the search for novel susceptibility loci while conditioning on known loci. This approach came to the fore in a recent paper (Cox et al., 1999) that examined interactions between unlinked susceptibility loci in their linkage to non-insulin dependent (i.e., Type II) diabetes mellitus (NIDDM). The researchers showed increased evidence for linkage to each of two susceptibility loci when the evidence for linkage at the other locus was considered. Specifically, the evidence for linkage to a marker on chromosome 2 (i.e., *NIDDM1*) was markedly increased when the evidence for linkage to an independent marker on chromosome 15 (i.e., *CYP19*) was considered, and vice versa. Although the issues involved in statistical hypothesis testing for such methods, especially the control of Type I error rate, have yet to be fully resolved, examining interactions among susceptibility loci in genome scans represents an exciting approach for future linkage studies.

Future Research Directions in Candidate Gene Studies

There are a number of future directions that are especially promising for candidate gene studies of psychiatric disorders. First, a number of extensions of the TDT have emerged in recent years that permit the examination of linkage and association between a candidate gene and one or more quantitative and/or categorical traits, as well as moderators of linkage (e.g., Allison, 1997; Rabinowitz, 1997; Rice et al., 1995; Waldman et al., 1999). This is in contrast to the conventional TDT, which can test for linkage and association between a candidate gene and a single categorical trait only (usually a diagnosis). These methods can be used to help dissect and refine disorder phenotypes to improve the chances of finding linkage and association with candidate genes. For example, we have found that the dopamine transporter gene (*DAT1*) appears to be related to the hyperactive-impulsive symptoms of ADHD more strongly than the inattentive symptoms (Waldman et al., unpublished work), whereas the dopamine receptor D4 gene (*DRD4*) appears to be related to the inattentive symptoms but not to the hyperactive-impulsive symptoms (Rowe et al., 1998). In addition, linkage between *DAT1* and the hyperactive-impulsive symptoms was stronger for boys than girls and for older rather than younger children (Waldman et al., unpublished work). These methods also are ideal for examining linkage and association between a candidate gene and endophenotypes, although such applications have not yet been implemented.

Second, a number of researchers have begun to examine multiple markers within particular candidate genes to create haplotypes, which are likely to be more strongly linked to disorders than single markers because they allow one to more effectively converge on the functional region(s) of candidate genes. A recent example (Zhao et al., 2000) involves the controversial relation between alcoholism and the dopamine receptor D2 gene (*DRD2*), in which a haplotype constructed from several markers was linked with the disorder even though none of the individual markers in the gene showed significant linkage. This approach also has shown greater evidence for linkage between schizophrenia and the catechol-o-methyl transferase gene (*COMT*; Li et al., 2000), as well as between ADHD and *DRD4* and *DAT1* (Barr et al., 2000, 2001). Although these methods and first findings are promising, especially for honing in on the functional regions of genes, many issues remain to be resolved in the statistical analyses of haplotypes.

A third future direction that is as yet completely unexplored involves studying multiple candidate genes within a particular gene system (and eventually across multiple gene systems). For example, although multiple candidate genes have been examined for linkage and association with ADHD within the dopaminergic system, these have been studied in a piecemeal fashion, one at a time, rather than as a dopamine gene system. Finding relations between a disorder and a system of genes is in some sense more plausible than finding relations with a single gene, given that the products of such genes (i.e., the neurotransmitter transporter, receptors, precursors, and metabolic enzymes) work together as a system in the brain to influence behavior. Nonetheless, the investigation of such relations between a disorder and a system of candidate genes awaits the development of appropriate statistical genetic methods.

Developmental Psychopathology Approaches to Quantitative Genetic Studies of Childhood Disruptive Disorders

As stated above, important aspects of a developmental psychopathology perspective include a focus on underlying mechanisms and processes, on continuities and discontinuities between normal and abnormal development, on individuals' developmental trajectories, on alternative pathways underlying psychopathological and normal development, and on resilience as well as risk. I already have hinted at the first of these themes above, in my introduction of the term *endophenotypes*. There are several ways in which endophenotypic measures can serve as useful adjuncts to measures of manifest disorders. The first involves establishing association and linkage of the candidate genes related to diagnoses of psychiatric disorders (e.g., *DAT1* and *DRD4* with ADHD) with relevant neurodevelopmental measures. This is important for demonstrating that these relations are not simply limited to interviews and/or rating scales of psychopathology, but also extend to the neurodevelopmental mechanisms that are hypothesized to underlie disorders. Establishing such relations would demonstrate that they are generalizable beyond commonly used measures of psychopathology, and would begin to flesh out the neurodevelopmental mechanisms underlying psychiatric disorders. Second, if particular neurodevelopmental mechanisms are truly endophenotypes for specific disorders, they should mediate the association and linkage found between candidate genes and those disorders. This is because endophenotypes are regarded as variables that are more strongly and directly influenced by the same genes involved in the etiology of a given disorder, as explained above. Third, endophenotypic measures may help to refine psychiatric disorder phenotypes by reflecting variation relevant to the disorder that measures of manifest psychopathology (e.g., interviews and rating scales) do not capture. Thus, including relevant endophenotypic measures along with psychiatric diagnoses or symptom dimensions in molecular genetic studies should strengthen findings of association and linkage between candidate genes and psychopathology.

Up to now, very few psychiatric molecular genetic studies have included endophenotypic measures along with (or instead of) measures of manifest psychopathology. There is a considerable literature relating ADHD and schizophrenia spectrum disorders to a variety of lab measures of cognitive and neuropsychological constructs (e.g., executive functions) that are construed as neurodevelopmental mechanisms that underlie such disorders. Psychiatric geneticists are just beginning to examine these issues in studies of linkage (e.g., the aforementioned linkage study of schizophrenia that examined eye-tracking dysfunction as a phenotype; Arolt et al., 1996), as well as association (e.g., a recent study of ADHD that found association between *DRD4* and a reaction time measure of attention; Swanson et al., 2000). Needless to say, it remains for future research to include measures of the neurodevelopmental mechanisms thought to underlie psychopathology in molecular genetic studies, particularly to examine their roles as endophenotypes that mediate the relation between specific genes and disorders and that can aid in finding association and linkage with those disorders.

It will also be useful for psychiatric genetic studies to focus on both specific genes and "candidate" environmental variables in gene-environment process models. These models would focus on both gene-environment correlation and interaction. In the former set of models, the effects of specific genes on psychopathology would be examined in terms of their effects on mediating environmental variables, which would correspond to environments that individuals are exposed to or select based at least in part on their genetic predispositions. In the latter set of models, the interaction of a particular gene and a particular environmental variable would be tested in order to examine how the expression of individuals' genetic predispositions might vary according to environmental context, or how the effects of an environmental variable might differ given an individual's genetic predisposition. The difference of these *gene*-environment correlation and interaction models from corresponding *genotype*-environment correlation and interaction models that have been examined in the quantitative genetics literature (particularly in adoption studies) is that the genetic predisposition in this case would correspond to the effects of a particular gene. This is in contrast to *genotype*-environment correlation and interaction models, which infer the sum total of such

REFERENCES

Accili, D., Fishburn, C.S., Drago, J., Steiner, H., Lachowicz, J.E., Park, B.H., Gauda, E.B., Lee, E.J., Cool, M.H., Sibley, D.R., Gerfen, C.R., Westphal, H., & Fuchs, S. (1996). A targeted mutation of the D3 dopamine receptor gene is associated with hyperactivity in mice. *Proceedings of the National Academy of Sciences, 93,* 1945–1949.

Allison, D.B. (1997). Transmission Disequilibrium Tests for continuous variables. *American Journal of Human Genetics, 60,* 676–690.

Arolt, V., Lencer, R., Nolte, A., Muller-Myhsok, B., Purmann, S., Schurmann, M., Leutelt, J., Pinnow, M., & Schwinger, E. (1996). Eye tracking dysfunction is a putative phenotypic susceptibility marker of schizophrenia and maps to a locus on chromosome 6p in families with multiple occurrence of the disease. *American Journal of Medical Genetics, 67,* 564–579.

Barr, C.L., Xu, C., Kroft, J., Feng, Y., Wigg, K., Zai, G., Tannock, R., Schachar, R., Malone, M., Roberts, W., Nothen, M.M., Grunhage, F., Vandenbergh, D.J., Uhl, G., Sunohara, G., King, N., & Kennedy, J.L. (2001). Haplotype study of three polymorphisms at the dopamine transporter locus confirm linkage to attention-deficit/hyperactivity disorder. *Biological Psychiatry, 49,* 333–339.

Barr, C.L., Wigg, K.G., Bloom, S., Schachar, R., Tannock, R., Roberts, W., Malone, M., & Kennedy, J.L. (2000). Further evidence from haplotype analysis for linkage of the dopamine D4 receptor gene and attention-deficit hyperactivity disorder. *American Journal of Medical Genetics, 96,* 262–267.

Bennett, S.T., & Todd, J.A. (1996). Human type 1 diabetes and the insulin gene: Principles of mapping polygenes. *Annual Review of Genetics, 30,* 343–370.

Biederman, J., & Spencer, T. (1999). Attention-deficit/hyperactivity disorder (ADHD) as a noradrenergic disorder. *Biological Psychiatry, 46,* 1234–1242.

Bryk, A., & Raudenbush, S. (1992). *Hierarchical linear models for social and behavioral research: Applications and data analysis methods.* Newbury Park, Calif.: Sage Publications.

Brzustowicz, L.M., Honer, W.G., Chow, E.W., Hogan, J., Hodgkinson, K., & Bassett, A.S. (1997). Use of a quantitative trait to map a locus associated with severity of positive symptoms in familial schizophrenia to chromosome 6p. *American Journal of Human Genetics, 61,* 1388–1396.

Cardon, L.R., & Fulker, D.W. (1994). The power of interval mapping of quantitative trait loci, using selected sib pairs. *American Journal of Human Genetics, 55,* 825–833.

Chakravarti, A. (1999). Population genetics – making sense out of sequence. *Nature Genetics, 21,* 56–60.

Cicchetti, D. (1993). Developmental psychopathology: Reactions, reflections, projections. *Developmental Review, 13,* 471–502.

Cicchetti, D., & Richters, J.E. (1993). Developmental considerations in the investigation of conduct disorder. *Development and Psychopathology, 5,* 331–344.

Cicchetti, D., & Rogosch, F.A. (1996). Equifinality and multifinality in developmental psychopathology. *Development and Psychopathology, 8,* 597–600.

Cicchetti, D., & Rogosch, F.A. (1999). Conceptual and methodological issues in developmental psychopathology research. In P.C. Kendall, J.N. Butcher, & G.N. Holmbeck (Eds.), *Handbook of research methods in clinical psychology* (pp. 433–465). New York: Wiley.

Cicchetti, D., Rogosch, F.A., Lynch, M., & Holt, K. (1993). Resilience in maltreated children: Processes leading to adaptive outcome. *Development and Psychopathology, 5,* 629–647.

Cook, E.H. Jr., Stein, M.A., Krasowski, M.D., Cox, N.J., Olkon, D.M., Kieffer, J.E., & Leventhal, B.L. (1995). Association of Attention-Deficit Disorder and the dopamine transporter gene. *American Journal of Human Genetics, 56,* 993–998.

Cox, N.J., Frigge, M., Nicolae, D.L., Concannon, P., Hanis, C.L., Bell, G.I., & Kong, A. (1999). Loci on chromosomes 2 (NIDDM1) and 15 interact to increase susceptibility to diabetes in Mexican Americans. *Nature Genetics, 21,* 213–215.

Crowe, R.R. (1993). Candidate genes in psychiatry: an epidemiological perspective. *American Journal of Medical Genetics, 48,* 74–77.

Daly, G., Hawi, Z., Fitzgerald, M., & Gill, M. (1999). Mapping susceptibility loci in Attention Deficit Hyperactivity Disorder: Preferential transmission of parental alleles at DAT1, DBH, and DRD5 to affected children. *Molecular Psychiatry, 4,* 192–196.

Deater-Deckard, K., & Plomin, R. (1999). An adoption study of etiology of teacher and parent reports of externalizing behavior problems in middle childhood. *Child Development, 70,* 144–154.

Dolan, C.V., & Boomsma, D.I. (1998). Optimal selection of sib pairs from random samples for linkage analysis of a QTL using the EDAC test. *Behavior Genetics, 28,* 197–206.

Dulawa, S.C., Grandy, D.K., Low, M.J., Paulus, M.P., & Geyer M.A. (1999). Dopamine D4 receptor-knock-out mice exhibit reduced exploration of novel stimuli. *Journal of Neuroscience, 19,* 9550–9556.

Eaves, L.J., & Meyer, J. (1994). Locating human quantitative trait loci: Guidelines for the selection of sibling pairs for genotyping. *Behavior Genetics, 24,* 443–455.

Eaves, L.J., Silberg, J.L., Meyer, J.M., Maes, H.H., Simonoff, E., Pickles, A., Rutter, M., Neale, M.C., Reynolds, C.A., Erikson, M.T., Heath, A.C., Loeber, R., Truett, K.R., & Hewitt, J.K. (1997). Genetics and developmental psychopathology: 2. The main effects of genes and environment on behavioral problems in the Virginia Twin Study of Adolescent Behavioral Development. *Journal of Child Psychology and Psychiatry, 38,* 965–980.

Falk, C.T., & Rubenstein, P. (1987). Haplotype relative risk: an easy reliable way to construct a proper control sample for risk calculations. *Annals of Human Genetics, 51* 227–233.

Faraone, S.V., Doyle, A.E., Mick, E., & Biederman, J. (2001). Meta-analysis of the association between the 7-repeat allele of the dopamine D(4) receptor gene and attention deficit hyperactivity disorder. *American Journal of Psychiatry, 158,* 1052–1057.

Ge, X., Conger, R.D., Cadoret, R.J., Neiderhiser, J.M., et al. (1996). The developmental interface between nature and nurture: A mutual influence model of child antisocial behavior and parent behaviors. *Developmental Psychology, 32,* 574–589.

Gill, M., Daly, G., Heron, S., Hawi, Z., & Fitzgerald, M. (1997). Confirmation of association between attention deficit hyperactivity disorder and a dopamine transporter polymorphism. *Molecular Psychiatry, 2,* 311–313.

Giros, B., Jaber, M., Jones, S.R., Wightman, R.M., & Caron, M.G. (1996). Hyperlocomotion and indifference to cocaine and amphetamine in mice lacking the dopamine transporter. *Nature, 379,* 606–612.

Gu, C., Todorov, A., & Rao, D.C. (1996). Combining extremely concordant sib pairs with extremely discordant sib pairs provides a cost effective way to perform linkage analysis of quantitative trait loci. *Genetic Epidemiology, 13,* 513–533.

Jöreskog, K.G., & Sörbom, D. (1993). *LISREL VIII: User's guide.* Chicago: Scientific Software.

Kendler, K.S., Neale, M.C., Kessler, R.C., Heath, A.C., & Eaves, L.J. (1992a). Generalized anxiety disorder in women: A population-based twin study. *Archives of General Psychiatry, 49,* 267–272.

Kendler, K.S., Neale, M.C., Kessler, R.C., Heath, A.C., & Eaves, L.J. (1992b). The genetic epidemiology of phobias in women: The interrelationship of agoraphobia, situational phobia, and simple phobia. *Archives of General Psychiatry, 49,* 273–281.

Kendler, K.K., & Robinette, C.D. (1983). Schizophrenia in the National Academy of Sciences-National Research Council Twin Registry: A 16-year update. *American Journal of Psychiatry, 140,* 1551–1563.

Kendler, K.S., Walters, E.E., Truett, K.R., Heath, A.C., Neale, M.C., Martin, N.G., & Eaves, L.J. (1994). Sources of individual differences in depressive symptoms: Analysis of two samples of twins and their families. *American Journal of Psychiatry, 151,* 1605–1614.

Kety, S.S., Rosenthal, D., Wender, P.H., & Schulsinger, F. (1968). The types and prevalence of mental illness in the biological and adoptive families of adopted schizophrenics. *Journal of Psychiatric Research, 6,* 345–362.

Kidd, K.K. (1993). Associations of disease with genetic markers: deja vu all over again. *American Journal of Medical Genetics, 48,* 71–73.

Kuntsi, J., & Stevenson, J. (2001). Psychological mechanisms in hyperactivity: II. The role of genetic factors. *Journal of Child Psychology and Psychiatry, 42,* 211–219.

LaHoste, G.J., Swanson, J.M., Wigal, S.B., Glabe, C., Wigal, T., King, N., & Kennedy, J.L. (1996). Dopamine D4 receptor gene polymorphism is associated with attention deficit hyperactivity disorder. *Molecular Psychiatry, 1,* 121–124.

Lander, E.S., & Schork, N.S. (1994). Genetic dissection of complex traits. *Science, 265,* 2037–2048.

Levy, F. (1991). The dopamine theory of attention deficit hyperactivity disorder (ADHD). *Australian & New Zealand Journal of Psychiatry, 25,* 277–283.

Levy, F., Hay, D., McStephen, M., Wood, C., & Waldman, I.D. (1997). Attention-deficit hyperactivity disorder: A category or a continuum? Genetic analysis of a large-scale twin study. *Journal of the American Academy of Child and Adolescent Psychiatry, 36,* 737–744.

Li, T., Ball, D., Zhao, J., Murray, R.M., Liu, X., Sham, P.C., & Collier, D.A. (2000). Family-based linkage disequilibrium mapping using SNP marker haplotypes: application to a potential locus for schizophrenia at chromosome 22q11. *Molecular Psychiatry, 5,* 77–84.

Loehlin, J.C. (1996). The Cholesky approach: A cautionary note. *Behavior Genetics, 26,* 65–69.

Masten, A., & Coatsworth, J.D. (1998). The development of competence in favorable and unfavorable environments: Lessons from research on successful children. *American Psychologist, 53,* 205–220.

McArdle, J.J. (1986). Latent variable growth within behavior genetic models. *Behavior Genetics, 16,* 163–200.

McGuffin, P., & Katz, R. (1989). The genetics of depression and manic-depressive illness. *British Journal of Psychiatry, 155,* 294–304.

Mill, J.S., Caspi, A., McClay, J., Sugden, K., Purcell, S., Asherson, P., Craig, I., McGuffin, P., Braithwaite, A., Poulton, R., & Moffitt, T.E. (2001). The dopamine D4 receptor and the hyperactivity phenotype: A developmental-epidemiological study. Manuscript submitted for publication.

Morris, D.W., Robinson, L., Turic, D., Duke, M., Webb, V., Milham, C., Hopkin, E., Pound, K., Fernando S., Easton M., Hamshere M., Williams N., McGuffin P., Stevenson J., Krawczak M., Owen, M.J., O'Donovan, M.C., & Williams, J. (2000). Family-based association mapping provides evidence for a gene for reading disability on chromosome 15q. *Human Molecular Genetics, 9,* 843–848.

Nadder, T.S., Silberg, J.L., Eaves, L.J., Maes, H.H., & Meyer, J.M. (1998). Genetic effects on ADHD symptomatology: Results from a telephone survey. *Behavior Genetics, 28,* 83–99.

Neale, M.C. (1996). *MX Software.* Richmond: Virginia Commonwealth University.

Neale, M.C., & Cardon, L.R. (1992). *Methodology for genetic studies of twins and families.* Dordrecht: Kluwer Academic Publishers.

Nigg, J.T. (2001). Is ADHD an inhibitory disorder? *Psychological Bulletin, 127,* 571–598.

Nigg, J.T., Blaskey, L.G., Huang-Pollock, C.L., & Rappley, M.D. (in press). Neuropsychological executive functions and DSM-IV ADHD subtypes. *Journal of the American Academy of Child and Adolescent Psychiatry.*

Pennington, B.F., & Ozonoff, S. (1996). Executive functions and developmental psychopathology. *Journal of Child Psychology and Psychiatry, 37,* 51–87.

Pliszka, S.R., McCracken, J.T., & Maas, J.W. (1996). Catecholamines in attention-deficit hyperactivity disorder: current perspectives. *Journal of the American Academy of Child & Adolescent Psychiatry, 35,* 264–272.

Plomin, R., & Crabbe, J.C. (2000). DNA. *Psychological Bulletin, 126,* 806–828.

Plomin, R., & Rutter, M. (1998). Child development, molecular genetics, and what to do with genes once they are found. *Child Development, 69,* 1223–1242.

Rabinowitz, D. (1997). A transmission/disequilibrium test for quantitative trait loci. *Human Heredity, 47,* 342–350.

Rende, R., & Plomin, R. (1995). Nature, nurture, and the development of psychopathology. In D. Cicchetti & D.J. Cohen (Eds.), *Developmental psychopathology: Vol. 1. Theory and methods* (pp. 291–314). New York: Wiley.

Rende, R.D., Plomin, R., Reiss, D., & Hetherington, E.M. (1993). Genetic and environmental influences on depressive symptomatology in adolescence: Individual differences and extreme scores. *Journal of Child Psychology and Psychiatry, 34,* 1387–1398.

Rhee, S.H., Feigon, S.A., Bar, J.L., Hadeishi, Y., & Waldman, I.D. (2001). Behavior genetic approaches to psychopathology. In Adams, H. (Ed.), *Handbook of psychopathology,* 3rd ed. New York: Wiley.

Rhee, S.H., & Waldman, I.D. (2002). Genetic and environmental influences on antisocial behavior: A meta-analysis of twin and adoption studies. *Psychological Bulletin, 128,* 490–529.

Rhee, S.H., Waldman, I.D., Hay, D.A., & Levy, F. (1999). Sex differences in genetic and environmental influences on DSM-III-R Attention Deficit Hyperactivity Disorder (ADHD). *Journal of Abnormal Psychology, 108,* 24–41.

Rice, J.P., Neuman, R.J., Hoshaw, S.L., Daw, E.W., & Gu, C. (1995). TDT with covariates and genomic screens with Mod scores: Their behavior on simulated data. *Genetic Epidemiology, 12,* 659–664.

Rice, J.P., Rochberg, N., Neuman, R.J., Saccone, N.L., Liu, K-Y, Zhang, X., & Culverhouse, R. (1999). Covariates in linkage analysis. *Genetic Epidemiology, 17,* S691–S695.

Risch, N.J. (2000). Searching for genetic determinants in the new millennium. *Nature, 405,* 847–856.

Risch, N., & Merikangas, K. (1996). The future of genetic studies of complex human diseases. *Science, 273,* 1516–1517.

Risch, N.J., & Zhang, H. (1996a). Mapping quantitative trait loci with extreme discordant sib pairs: Sampling considerations. *American Journal of Human Genetics, 58,* 836–843.

Risch, N.J., & Zhang, H. (1996b). Extreme discordant sib pairs for mapping quantitative trait loci in humans. *Science, 268,* 1584–1589.

Risch, N.J., & Zhang, H. (1995). Extreme discordant sib pairs for mapping quantitative trait loci in humans. *Science, 264,* 1697–1733.

Roberts, S.B., MacLean, C.J., Neale, M.C., Eaves, L.J., & Kendler, K.S. (1999). Replication of linkage studies of complex traits: An examination of variation in location estimates. *American Journal of Human Genetics, 65,* 876–884.

Robins, L.N., & Rutter, M. (Eds.) (1990). *Straight and deviant pathways from childhood to adulthood.* New York: Cambridge University Press.

Rogosa, D.R. (1988). Myths about longitudinal research. In K.W. Schaie, R.T. Campbell, W. Meredith, & S.C. Rawlings (Eds.), *Methodological issues in aging research* (pp. 171–210). New York: Springer.

Rolf, J., Masten, A.S., Cicchetti, D., Nuechterlein, K.H., & Weintraub, S. (Eds.) (1990). *Risk and protective factors in the development of psychopathology.* New York: Cambridge University Press.

Rowe, D.C., Stever, C., Giedinghagen, L.N., Gard, J.M.C., Cleveland, H.H., Terris, S.T., Mohr, J.H., Sherman, S.L., Abramowitz, A., & Waldman, I.D. (1998). Dopamine DRD4 receptor polymorphism and attention deficit hyperactivity disorder. *Molecular Psychiatry, 3,* 419–426.

Rubinstein, M., Phillips, T.J., Bunzow, J.R., Falzone, T.L., Dziewczapolski, G., Zhang, G., Fang, Y., Larson, J.L., McDougall, J.A., Chester, J.A., Saez, C., Pugsley, T.A., Gershanik, O., Low, M.J., & Grandy, D.K. (1997). Mice lacking dopamine D4 receptors are supersensitive to ethanol, cocaine, and methylphenidate. *Cell, 90,* 991–1001.

Rutter, M., Dunn, J., Plomin, R., Simonoff, E., Pickles, A., Maugham, B., Ormel, H., Meyer, J., & Eaves, L. (1997). Integrating nature and nurture: Implications of person-environment correlations and interactions for developmental psychopathology. *Development and Psychopathology, 9,* 335–364.

Santangelo, S., Ashley-Koch, A., Pericak-Vance, M., Silverman, J., Smith, C.J., & Buxbaum, J.S.D. (2000). Combined analysis of data on chromosome 7q from three autism genome scans, *American Journal of Medical Genetics, 96.*

Seeman, P. (1995). Dopamine receptors and psychosis. *Scientific American: Science and Medicine,* 28–37.

Seeman, P., & Madras, B.K. (1998). Anti-hyperactivity medication: methylphenidate and amphetamine. *Molecular Psychiatry, 3,* 386–396.

Silberg, J., Rutter, M., Meyer, J., Maes, H., Hewitt, J., Simonoff, E., Pickles, A., Loeber, R., & Eaves, L. (1996). Genetic and environmental influences on the covariation between hyperactivity and conduct disturbance in juvenile twins. *Journal of Child Psychology and Psychiatry, 37,* 803–816.

Smalley, S.L., Bailey, J.N., Palmer, C.G., Cantwell, D.P., McGough, J.J., Del'Homme, M.A., Asarnow, J.R., Woodward, J.A., Ramsey, C., & Nelson, S.F. (1998). Evidence that the dopamine D4 receptor is a susceptibility gene in attention deficit hyperactivity disorder. *Molecular Psychiatry, 3,* 427–430.

Solanto, M.V. (1984). Neuropharmacological basis of stimulant drug action in attention deficit disorder with hyperactivity: a review and synthesis. *Psychological Bulletin, 95,* 387–409.

Spielman, R., McGinnis, J., & Ewens, W. (1993). Transmission test for linkage disequilibrium: The insulin gene region and insulin-dependent diabetes mellitus (IDDM). *American Journal of Human Genetics, 52,* 506–516.

Sroufe, L.A., & Rutter, M. (1984). The domain of developmental psychopathology. *Child Development, 55,* 17–29.

Stevenson, J. (1992). Evidence for a genetic etiology in hyperactivity in children. *Behavior Genetics*, *22*, 337–344.

Suarez, B.K., Hampe, C.L., & Van Eerdewegh, P. (1994). Problems of replicating linkage claims in psychiatry. In E. S. Gershon & C. R. Cloninger (Eds.), *Genetic approaches to mental disorders*. Washington, D.C.: American Psychiatric Press.

Sudbery, P. (1998). *Human molecular genetics*. Essex, UK: Longman.

Swanson, J., Oosterlaan, J., Murias, M., Schuck, S., Flodman, P., Spence, M.A., Wasdell, M., Ding, Y., Chi, H.C., Smith, M., Mann, M., Carlson, C., Kennedy, J.L., Sergeant, J.A., Leung, P., Zhang, Y.P., Sadeh, A., Chen, C., Whalen, C.K., Babb, K.A., Moyzis, R., & Posner M.I. (2000). Attention deficit/hyperactivity disorder children with a 7-repeat allele of the dopamine receptor D4 gene have extreme behavior but normal performance on critical neuropsychological tests of attention. *Proceedings of the National Academy of Sciences*, *97*, 4754–4759.

Swanson, J.M., Sunohara, G.A., Kennedy J.L., Regino, R., Fineberg, E., Wigal, T., Lerner, M., Williams, L., LaHoste, G.J., & Wigal, S.B. (1998). Association of the dopamine receptor D4 (DRD4) gene with a refined phenotype of attention deficit hyperactivity disorder (ADHD): A family-based approach. *Molecular Psychiatry*, *3*, 38–41.

Tahir, E., Yazgan, Y., Cirakoglu, B., Ozbay, F., Waldman, I.D., & Asherson, P.J. (2000). Association and linkage of DRD4 and DRD5 with Attention Deficit Hyperactivity Disorder (ADHD) in a sample of Turkish children. *Molecular Psychiatry*, *5*, 396–404.

Terwilliger J.D., & Ott, J. (1992). A haplotype-based haplotype relative risk statistic. *Human Heredity*, *42*, 337–346.

Waldman, I.D., & Rhee, S.H. (2002). Behavioral and molecular genetic studies of ADHD. In Sandberg, S. (Ed.), *Hyperactivity and attention disorders in childhood*, 2d ed. New York: Cambridge University Press.

Waldman, I.D., Rhee, S.H., Levy, F., & Hay, D.A. (2001). Genetic and environmental influences on the covariation among symptoms of attention deficit hyperactivity disorder, oppositional defiant disorder, and conduct disorder. In D.A. Hay & F. Levy (Eds.), *Attention, genes and ADHD*. Hillsdale, NJ: Erlbaum.

Waldman, I.D., Robinson, B.F., & Rowe, D.C. (1999). A logistic regression based extension of the TDT for continuous and categorical traits. *Annals of Human Genetics*, *63*, 329–340.

Waldman, I.D., Rowe, D.C., Abramowitz, A., Kozel, S.T., Mohr, J.H., Sherman, S.L., Cleveland, H.H., Sanders, M.L., & Stever, C. (1998). Association and linkage of the dopamine transporter gene (DAT1) and Attention Deficit Hyperactivity Disorder in children. *American Journal of Human Genetics*, *63*, 1767–1776.

Waldman, I.D., & Slutske, W.S. (2000). Antisocial behavior and alcoholism: A behavioral genetic perspective on comorbidity. *Clinical Psychology Review*, *20*, 255–287.

Willcutt, E.G., Pennington, B.F., Chhabildas, N.A., Friedman, M.C., & Alexander, J.A. (1999). Psychiatric comorbidity associated with DSM-IV ADHD in a nonreferred sample of twins. *Journal of the American Academy of Child and Adolescent Psychiatry*, *38*, 1355–1362.

Willett, J.B., & Sayer, A.G. (1994). Using covariance structure analysis to detect correlates and predictors of individual change over time. *Psychological Bulletin*, *116*, 363–381.

Williams, J., McGuffin, P., Nothen, M., & Owen, M.J. (1997). Meta-analysis of association between the 5-HT2a receptor T102C polymorphism and schizophrenia. EMASS Collaborative Group. European Multicentre Association Study of Schizophrenia. *Lancet*, *349*, 1221.

Williams, J., Spurlock, G., Holmans, P., Mant, R., Murphy, K., Jones, L., Cardno, A., Asherson, P., Blackwood, D., Muir, W., Meszaros, K., Aschauer, H., Mallet, J., Laurent, C., Pekkarinen, P., Seppala, J., Stefanis, C.N., Papadimitriou, G.N., Macciardi, F., Verga, M., Pato, C., Azevedo, H., Crocq, M.A., Gurling, H., & Owen, M.J. (1998). A meta-analysis and transmission disequilibrium study of association between the dopamine D3 receptor gene and schizophrenia. *Molecular Psychiatry*, *3*, 141–149.

Zhao, H., Zhang, S., Merikangas, K.R., Trixler, M., Wildenauer, D.B., Sun, F., & Kidd, K.K. (2000). Transmission/disequilibrium tests using multiple tightly linked markers. *American Journal of Human Genetics*, *67*, 936–946.

TWELVE

Developmental Psychoneuroimmunology

The Role of Cytokine Network Activation in the Epigenesis of Developmental Psychopathology

Douglas A. Granger, Nancy A. Dreschel, and Elizabeth A. Shirtcliff

The past three decades have witnessed exponential growth in our knowledge of the interactions among the central and peripheral nervous systems and the immune system (Ader, 1981, 2000; Ader, Felten, & Cohen, 1991). In particular, the signals and routes via which psychological and physical stressors lead to endocrine and immune responses have been studied extensively. A detailed picture of an intriguing puzzle has now begun to emerge. Theorists, applied researchers, and professionals are extrapolating these basic findings in order to consider how individual differences in psychological traits and states might be associated with immunity, illness susceptibility, and negative health outcomes (see Cohen & Herbert, 1996; Herbert & Cohen, 1993b; Kemeny & Gruenewald, 1999; Kemeny & Laudenslager, 1999; Kiecolt-Glaser & Glaser, 1995). Quite surprisingly, how such processes affect children's immunity has received scant empirical attention (e.g., Adamson-Macedo, 2000; Boyce et al., 1995; Coe, 1996, 1999). Although the field should be concerned with the ultimate impact of these phenomena for children's health, and additional research with that particular focus seems warranted, the focus of this chapter is on the implications of another leading edge of psychoneuroimmunologic research (e.g., Maier & Watkins, 1998a,b; Maier, Watkins, & Fleshner, 1994). Specifically, accumulated findings have sparked a scientific revolution regarding the direction of effects among the brain, behavior, and immunity (e.g., Blalock, 1994a; Dantzer, 2001).

Our overarching objective is to introduce a "new world of ideas" to students of child development, and to reveal how the implications of this new knowledge extend into their realm of inquiry, and may influence theories about the origins of individual differences in social behavior (Cicchetti & Lynch, 1995; Gottlieb, 1992; Sameroff, 1983). As a starting point, a historical overview of development of our understanding regarding the neuro-endocrine-immune network is provided with roadmaps to seminal papers for more interested readers. We then digress and introduce the basic features of the immune system with emphasis on cutting edge thoughts on its function as our "sixth sense." Then the concomitants and consequences of the intracellular regulatory molecules of the neuro-endocrine-immune network (e.g., cytokines) for the brain and ultimately behavior are described with direct reference to their association with developmental psychopathology. Next, we review the available evidence that supports immune system stimulated changes in central nervous and endocrine systems during were identified on lymphoid cells for a variety of the products (e.g., epinephrine, nore-pinephrine) secreted by these nerve terminals (Felten, Felten, Bellinger, & Olschowka, 1992). Additional work (see Carr, Radulescu, DeCosta, Rice, & Blalock, 1992) revealed receptors on lymphoid cells for products released by the hypothalamic-pituitary-adrenal axis (i.e., adrenocorticotropic hormone, glucocorticoids) and autonomic nervous systems (i.e., substance P, neuropeptide Y, norepinephrine). These groundbreaking studies provided the biological evidence needed to support the credibility of earlier clinical and anecdotal observations. During this period, the field of "psychoneuroimmunology" officially emerged as a discipline (Ader, 1981; Ader, Felten, & Cohen, 1991; Kiecolt-Glaser & Glaser, 1989) with a primary focus of explaining individual differences in links between stress, behavior, and health risk as mediated or moderated via the effects of psychological states on immune function. Research reports from this effort now fill the pages of health-oriented scientific journals such as *Health Psychology, Annals of Behavioral Medicine, Brain, Behavior and Immunity,* and *Psychosomatic Medicine.*

In parallel, basic research on the immune system progressed at a very rapid pace. For decades, it had been assumed that cellular communication within the immune system depended largely on physical cell-to-cell contact. This set of assumptions was challenged by experiments in the late 1960s and early 1970s (e.g., Granger & Williams, 1968; Hessinger, Daynes, & Granger, 1973) revealing that cells of the immune system secreted soluble chemical messengers of their own to initiate, maintain, and regulate cellular immune responses. These messengers were originally defined as "lymphokines" and their effects were considered to be limited within the immune system. Later it was discovered that these lymphokines (see Maier & Watkins, 1998b; Smith, 1992; Vilcek, 1998) also had effects on nonlymphoid cells at considerable distances away from the cells that secreted them. For instance, receptors for these molecules were identified on cells of the central nervous and endocrine systems (e.g., Besedovsky et al., 1983; Besedovsky & del Rey, 1989). In recognition of their functional diversity these molecules were relabeled "cytokines" in the 1970s. For psychoneuroimmunologists, this wave of new information completed a communication loop – the immune system could both receive and send biochemical signals to the CNS (see Figure 12.1). These advances stimulated a revolution of ideas regarding how the brain, behavior, and immune system influenced one another (see Maier & Watkins, 1998a,b).

Today, as we begin the twenty-first century, a new era of understanding and research on psychoneuroimmunology has evolved. The contemporary emphasis is now heavily focused within the fields of molecular biology and neuroscience (Ader, 2000; Altman, 1997). There is now unequivocal evidence that cells of the lymphoid, CNS, and endocrine systems use the same hormones, neurotransmitters, and other critical effector molecules to send and receive signals among one another. These once considered independent systems share a common set of signaling molecules and receptors and "speak" a similar chemical language (Ader et al., 1991; Blalock, 1994, 1997; Maier & Watkins, 1998a). The contemporary view is that the brain, endocrine system, and immune system constitute an interactive information network with each node capable of affecting ar d being affected by the activity of the others (Ader, 2000; Black, 1995; Cotman, Brinton, Glaburda, McEwen, & Schneider, 1987). A schematic diagram of these interactive systems with representative signaling molecules and communication routes is depicted in Figure 12.1.

THE IMMUNE SYSTEM

A basic understanding of the immune system is fundamental to thinking about its interactions with behavior and developmental psychopathology. We provide a brief overview here to highlight some of its complexities and recommend introductory texts by Janeway (2001) and Goldsby, Kindt, and Osborne (2000) for additional basic background information.

Basic Properties and Divisions. The immune system functions to protect individuals from infectious organisms, microbes, cancer, and toxins. To do this, it has the capacity to (1) distinguish between cells and molecules that belong ("self-antigens") and those that do not belong ("non-self antigens"), (2) destroy foreign antigens without doing damage to the host, and (3) record the immunologic experience so the system's response is more efficient and effective upon subsequent exposure (Clough & Roth, 1998). Immunologists divide the immune system into two functional branches: (1) innate or natural immunity and (2) specific or acquired immunity.

Innate immunity is considered a first line of defense against invading organisms. Components of the innate immune branch include physical (i.e., skin, cilia, mucous) and physiochemical barriers (e.g., gastric acid, digestive enzymes, lysosomes) and some cells (i.e., phagocytes). The most relevant component of innate immunity for this discussion are phagocytes, in particular macrophages. Macrophages are white blood cells that recognize and destroy extracellular antigens like bacteria and toxins. They identify, capture, digest, and present foreign antigens to lymphocytes (see below), as well as release a variety of intracellular messengers (cytokines such as IL-1β, IL-6, and TNF-α) that initiate and maintain inflammation.

In contrast, specific (or acquired) immunity is highly individualized in its response to antigen. The specific immune system is divided into humoral and cellular compartments. Humoral immunity is mediated by antibodies or immunoglobulins (i.e., IgA, IgG, IgM, IgD, IgE) – soluble recognition molecules secreted by B lymphocytes (B cells) that are highly specific to particular antigens. The cellular components of the specific immune system include many subtypes of lymphocytes. B cells produce and secrete immunoglobulins, record immunological memory, and present antigen to other lymphoid cells. Helper/suppressor T lymphocytes specialize in the secretion of intercellular signals that coordinate the pro- and anti-inflammatory activities of B cells, cytotoxic T cells, and macrophages. Cytotoxic T lymphocytes are mainly responsible for destroying cells that have been virally infected or have a transformed or dysregulated growth cycle (i.e., cancer cells).

Lymphocytes migrate between the lymphoid and circulatory systems. The lymphoid system is a specialized group of tissues and organs. It is made of primary lymphoid tissue (the thymus and bone marrow) where lymphocytes are produced and mature, and secondary lymphoid tissue (including lymph nodes, submucosal lymph tissue, and spleen) where antigenic stimulation causes lymphocyte proliferation and reaction. A network of lymphatic vessels connect the widely distributed parts of the lymph system with the rest of the body tissues. Lymph, a lymphocyte-rich fluid, travels from the tissue spaces through the lymphatic vessels so that most of the antigen-specific immune responses actually take place in the secondary lymphoid tissues.

Phases of the Cellular Immune Response. The complexity of the cellular immune response is phenomenal and a brief example is provided here to illustrate. The first phase is referred to as the *cognitive* phase and involves the recognition of antigen. When foreign antigen, such as bacteria, is present in the tissues or bloodstream, chemical signals are produced that attract macrophages and other phagocytes to capture and ingest the material. Inside the cell the antigen is processed with major histocompatability complex (MHC) molecules (see Janeway, 2001) and a component of the antigen is presented on the surface of the macrophage's cell membrane. Subsequently, a T helper lymphocyte binds to this complex on the surface of the macrophage. The second phase involves *differentiation* of lymphocytes specific for this antigen from a resting state to an active state. The T helper cell is activated by secretory growth factors from the macrophage. The activated T helper cell then releases other pro-inflammatory cytokines (see next section) that begin a cascade of effects. For instance, T cells specific for this antigen develop into cytotoxic cells and resting B lymphocytes develop into plasma cells that produce antibodies. Memory cells are also created so that the next time the antigen is present, the system is better prepared to quickly activate. The third phase involves the clonal expansion and *proliferation* of these activated cells. Finally, in the *effector* phase the antigen is destroyed by an "army" of specialized lymphocytes and immunoglobulins. In each phase, a cascade of cytokine signals coordinates the orchestra of cells, a process that takes hours-to-days to reach its maximum efficiency.

Our "Sixth Sense." Decoding the syntax of the neuro-endocrine-immune axis has enabled theorists to attribute new sensory and regulatory features to the immune system's extensive functional repertoire. Blalock (1994, 1997) expands the established functions of the immune system to propose that it recognizes unique environmental stimuli (i.e., viruses, bacteria, microbes) that are essentially undetectable by our classic visual, auditory, olfactory, and gustatory sensory systems. That is, one cannot see, hear, smell, taste, or feel an individual microbe. When the immune system recognizes such stimuli, the encounter is converted into a cascade of biochemical messages. These molecular signals are responsible for inducing changes in the host's metabolic, thermogenic, and behavioral states in response to infection.

The adaptive significance of the body's reaction to immune stimuli is considered to enable the host to fight pathogens efficiently. For example, increased sleepiness, reduced activity, motivation, and arousal seen with systemic infection may be an adaptive physiological mechanism to conserve energy. While it might seem paradoxical to have a decreased appetite when sick (one is sacrificing calorie and protein intake by not eating), it would be adaptive for an animal in the wild to stay in one place, conserving energy instead of risking predation (Hart, 1988). Also, fever stimulated by the immune system is a release of proinflammatory molecules (cytokines and acute phase proteins) that produce an unfavorable environment for the growth of many microbial pathogens (see Kluger, 1979). The rate of bacterial growth is consistently slower in environments with temperatures greater than 98 °F. The afflicted individual's expression of sickness behaviors (see below) also may serve to facilitate their social withdrawal, conveying benefits to the population or immediate social group by limiting the exposure of others to pathogens.

Advances in our understanding of the interactions among the immune, central nervous, and endocrine systems reveal that biobehavioral responses to infection may have even more significance than previously realized. That is, characterizing the immune system as "a sixth sense" raises the possibility that immune-to-brain communications represent a largely unexplored pathway through which biochemical signals triggered by environmental factors shape and reshape the structure and function of biological systems underlying atypical behavior. With few exceptions (e.g., Adamson-Macedo, 2000; Coe, 1996; Crnic, 1991; Shanks, Larocque, & Meaney, 1995) this set of ideas has attracted only minimal attention from developmentally oriented researchers.

CYTOKINES FOR BEHAVIORAL SCIENTISTS

In this section we describe the general properties of cytokines (the critical effector molecules thought to mediate the aforementioned sensory functions) and how peripherally activated cytokines communicate with and affect the brain, endocrine system, and behavior. Readers interested in additional detail are referred to Maier and Watkins (1998b), who present an overview of cytokines for psychologists. *The Cytokine Handbook* (Thomson, 1998), already in its third edition since its publication in 1991, provides basic detail on individual cytokines as well as on their interactions and therapeutic uses. As this is a rapidly expanding area of knowledge, interested readers may also find cutting edge information in scientific journals such as *European Cytokine Network*, *Science*, *Nature*, *Cell*, *Lancet*, *Cytokine*, *Lymphokine Research*, *Proceedings of the National Academy of Sciences*, and various immunology-related journals such as *The Journal of Immunology*, and *Journal of Neuroimmunomodulation*.

Basic Properties and Functions. Although work on lymphokines and interferons (two types of molecules now recognized to have cytokine actions) began in the 1960s, it wasn't until 1974 that the term *cytokine* was proposed to describe the entire class of molecules with these properties (Vilcek, 1998). Cytokines are small protein molecules that act as intracellular messengers (see Goldsby, Kindt, & Osborne, 2000; Thomson, 1998). They range in molecular weight from 8 to 30 KiloDaltons (kDa) and induce their effects by binding to high-affinity receptors on target cell membranes. Virtually all nucleated cells can produce cytokines, but white blood cells are the major sources. Monocytes and macrophages are especially efficient cytokine producers. Some cytokines are stored preformed in the intracellular granules for instantaneous release. However, most cytokine secretion involves *de novo* protein synthesis, a process that takes hours.

Cytokines are pleiotropic, meaning they have multiple target cells and multiple actions, and their effects are often redundant, sometimes synergistic, and less frequently antagonistic. Cytokines can be grouped according to their structure and whether they have predominantly anti-inflammatory, pro-inflammatory, or growth promoting functions. Within the immune system, interleukins (e.g., IL-1, IL-2, IL-4, IL-6, IL-10, IL-13) act as messengers between white blood cells; colony-stimulating factors (e.g., IL-3, G-CSF, m-CSF, GMCSF) promote cell proliferation; tumor necrosis factors (TNF-α, TNF-β) initiate inflammation and cause necrosis and cachexia; and interferons (e.g., INF-alpha, INF-gamma) act to interfere with viral replication. The nomenclature hints to their major functions, but most cytokines have extremely diverse effects (Clough & Roth, 1998). Some specific examples of cytokines and their main biological functions within the immune system are listed in Table 12.1.

Table 12.1. Representative Members of the Cytokine Family and Some of Their Major Biological Functions

Cytokine	Secreted by	Major Biological Activity
Interleukin-1 (IL-1α, IL-1β)	Monocytes/Macrophages	Induces synthesis of acute-phase proteins Induces fever Stimulates lymphocyte activation
Interleukin-2 (IL-2)	T Lymphocytes	Induces T lymphocyte proliferation Enhances activity of NK cells
Interleukin-4 (IL-4)	T Lymphocytes	Stimulates T and B lymphocyte proliferation Increases phagocytic (ingestive) activity of macrophage
Interleukin-6 (IL-6)	Monocytes/Macrophages	Induces synthesis of acute-phase proteins Stimulates antibody production
Interleukin-10 (IL-10)	T Lymphocytes	Suppresses macrophage cytokine secretion Down-regulates antigen presentation
Interferon gamma (IFN-γ)	NK cells/T lymphocytes	Enhances activity of macrophages Induces proliferation of B lymphocytes Inhibits viral replication
Transforming Growth Factor β (TGF-β)	Macrophages/Lymphocytes	Induces macrophage IL-1 production Limits inflammatory response and promotes wound healing
Tumor Necrosis Factor α (TNF-α)	Macrophages	Has cytotoxic (cell killing) effects Induces cytokine secretion Associated with chronic inflammation

Cytokine Regulation. Cytokines are extremely potent signaling molecules, and their presence even in very low pg/ml levels can induce substantial cellular consequences. A complex set of mechanisms exists to prevent cytokines from doing damage to the host. At least three types of endogenous cytokine inhibitors have been identified. They include: cytokine antagonists (e.g., interleukin 1 receptor antagonist IL-1ra), molecules homologous to cytokines and able to bind cytokine receptors without leading to signal transduction; shed cytokine receptors (e.g., soluble tumor necrosis factor receptors s-TNF-R type I and II), that bind cytokines in the intercellular fluid space and stop it from reaching its target cell or tissue (Gatanaga, Hwang et al., 1990; Gatanaga, Lentz et al., 1990); and other molecules that act through independent receptors that exert opposite effects on the cell (Thomson, 1998). Some cytokines also inhibit each other (e.g., IL-10 inhibits synthesis of TNF, IL-1, IL-6 and others).

The regulation of cytokines is complex and has profound consequences for the host. Inadequate production of cytokines will result in an insufficient immune response and potentially negative consequences related to pathogenesis of the microbe, bacteria, or virus (see Figure 12.2). Without medical intervention, individuals expressing consistent hypo-arousal of the cytokine network would be unlikely to survive. It is highly likely that in nature this phenotype would be removed from the gene pool within one generation as these individuals would succumb to pathogenesis (or predation). On the other hand, excessive cytokine secretion has been linked to "sickness behaviors"

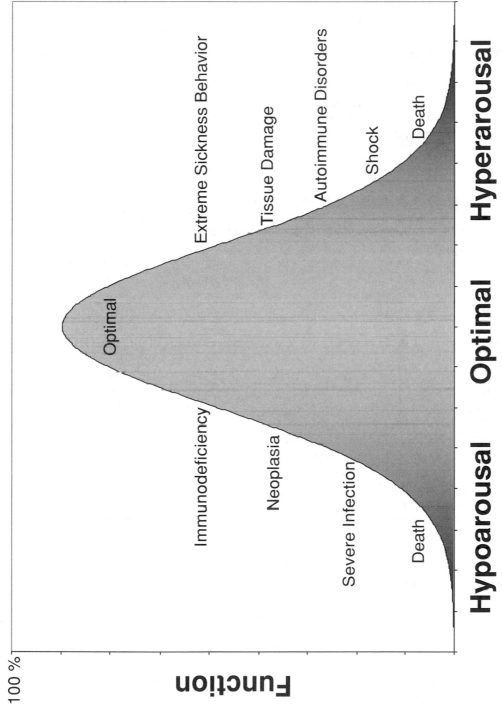

Figure 12.2. Individual differences in the activity of the cytokine network have an inverse parabolic relationship with physical and mental health. Regulation of cytokine activity within an optimal range is essential to avoid the negative biobehavioral consequences linked with either hypoarousal or hyperarousal of the immune system.

(see below), autoimmune disorders (i.e., arthritis), neurological disease (e.g., multiple sclerosis), toxic shock, and death (i.e., sepsis); see Figure 12.2. It is plausible that in populations under selective pressure, individuals expressing hyper-arousal of the cytokine network would also be removed from the gene pool. That is, when challenged by immune stimuli these individuals would experience severe fatigue, fever, loss of appetite, inactivity, social withdrawal, weight loss, and cognitive slowing which significantly increase risk of predation. Thus, in the wild, selective pressure from microorganisms and predators may serve to regulate the gene pool such that reproductively fit individuals have cytokine networks that operate within an optimal range of function (see Figure 12.2).

How Peripherally Activated Cytokines Talk to the Brain. The most well characterized pathway through which peripheral immunological stimuli signal changes in the brain begins with the macrophage. When activated, macrophages secrete a cascade of cytokines and other chemical messengers (see Figure 12.1). Importantly, it is the cytokine products released in response to immune stimulation, not the direct effect of the immunological stimulus (e.g., bacterial or viral pathogenesis), that are thought to mediate many of the resulting changes in the brain (Dantzer, Bluthe, & Goodall, 1993; Dinarello, 1984a,b). Molecular, cellular, and *in vivo* evidence suggests that macrophage-derived interleukin-1 (IL-1) has the most systemic and hormonal-type effects of the cytokines (Smith, 1992) with widespread consequences for the brain (Weiss, Quan, & Sundar, 1994). Two forms of IL-1 exist, α and β (Dinarello, 1988, 1992). IL-1β is the dominant soluble biologically active form in the circulation and brain (Benveniste, 1992b; Chensue, Shmyre-Forsch, Otterness, & Kunkel, 1989; Smith, 1992). Peripheral administration of nanogram (ng) amounts of IL-1β stimulates corticotropin-releasing factor (CRF) release from hypothalamic neurons (Harbuz & Lightman, 1992; Sapolsky, Rivier, Yamamoto, Plotsky, & Vale, 1987; Woolski, Smith, Meyer, Fuller, & Blalock, 1985) resulting in increased circulating levels of ACTH and corticosterone (Dunn, 1988, 1990). Interestingly, reports by Berkenbosch (Berkenbosch, de Goeij, Rey, & Besedovsky, 1989; Berkenbosch, de Rijk, Del Rey, & Besedovsky, 1990; Berkenbosch, Van Dam, DeRijk, & Schotanus, 1992) and Dunn (e.g., Chuluyan, Saphier, Rohn, & Dunn, 1992; Dunn, 1992a,b) demonstrate that peripheral administration of IL-1β may also potentiate the HPA axis response to environmental challenge.

Cytokines have a variety of effects on cerebral neurotransmission (see Dunn & Wang, 1995; Dunn, Wang, & Ando, 1999). IL-1β acts to stimulate cerebral norepinephrine (NE) metabolism, probably reflecting increased synaptic release. IL-1, IL-6, and TNF also stimulate indoleamine metabolism of tryptophan and decrease the concentration of serotonin (5-HT). Through their action on indoleamines, cytokines also affect the synthesis of quinolinic (QUIN) and kynurenic acid (see Figure 12.3). QUIN is an agonist of the N-methyl-d-aspartate (NMDA) receptor and other excitatory amino acid receptors. These receptors mediate excitatory amino acid neurotransmission within the hippocampus, basal ganglia, and cerebral cortex and, when activated for sufficient periods, have been implicated in nerve cell death and dysfunction (Heyes, 1992; Heyes, Brew et al., 1992; Heyes, Quearry, & Markey, 1989; Heyes, Saito et al., 1992; Saito, Markey, et al., 1992). On the other hand, kynurenic is an antagonist of NMDA receptors and could modulate the neurotoxic effects of QUIN as well as disrupt excitatory

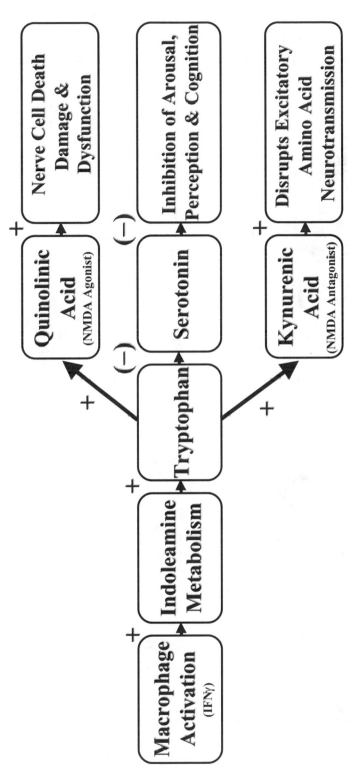

Figure 12.3. Immune activation has a variety of effects on cerebral neurotransmission. Bacterial, viral, fungal, and parasitic infections result in macrophage release of cytokines including those that activate indoleamine-2,3-dioxygenase (IDO). Increases in IDO activity accelerate the degradation of L-tryptophan to neuroreactive kynurenines, including the excitotoxin quinolinic acid (QUIN), and the antagonist of excitatory amino acid receptors, kynurenic acid (KYNA). QUIN and KYNA influence the activity of N-methyl-D-aspartate (NMDA) receptors. Degradation of L-tryptophan via this kynurenic pathway results in reduced serontonin levels. Consequences of this immune-to-brain pathway include neural damage and dysfunction, neurologic deficits and neurodegeneration, and inhibition of arousal, perception, and cognition.

amino acid transmission. Heyes and colleagues report that QUIN and kynurenic acid are mediators of neuronal dysfunction and nerve cell death in inflammatory diseases. A schematic diagram of the cerebral effects of cytokines is depicted in Figure 12.3.

It is apparent that many of the peripherally stimulated effects on the CNS result from activation of IL-1β in the brain (Quan, Sundar, & Weiss, 1994). That is, within hours after peripheral immune activation, expression of IL-1β transcripts is induced in the hippocampus, hypothalamus, and pituitary (Ban, Haour, & Lenstra, 1992; Laye, Parnet, Goujon, & Dantzer, 1994). Studies also show that IL-1 receptors are widely distributed throughout the brain and endocrine tissues (Cunningham & De Souza, 1993), with high densities observed in the hippocampal area and the choroid plexus (Takao, Tracy, Mitchell, & De Souza, 1990). Thus, it is not surprising that the behavioral and physiological effects can be mimicked by administration of IL-1β directly into the brain (Weiss et al., 1994), and that they can be attenuated by intracerebraventricular (i.c.v.) injection of the IL-1 receptor antagonist, IL-1ra (Bluthe, Dantzer, & Kelley, 1992).

Interestingly, circulating IL-1β does not cross the blood brain barrier (BBB) in humans. Rather, peripheral IL-1β somehow signals cytokine synthesis within the brain. Studies suggest that this process proceeds by humoral and neural pathways (see Dantzer, Konsman, Bluthe, & Kelley, 2000). The first studies carried out on the mechanisms by which peripheral immune stimuli signal the brain to induce fever, activate the HPA axis, and sickness behavior focused on primary and secondary signaling of proinflammatory cytokines in the circumventricular organs in the rodent. However, in the mid-1990s it was discovered that the subdiaphragmatic section of the vagus nerve attenuates the brain effects of systemic cytokines, suggesting cytokines are inducible in the brain. This observation shifted research attention away from the circumventricular organs to possible neural pathways. Since then, neuroanatomical pathways have been confirmed that reveal a fast route of communication from the immune system to the brain via the vagus nerves. This neural afferent pathway complements a humoral pathway that involves cytokines produced locally at the circumventricular organs and in the brain parenchyma (see reviews by Dantzer, Bluthe, Gheusi et al., 1998; Dantzer, Bluthe, Laye et al., 1998; Dantzer et al., 2000).

In summary, the biological pathways via which cytokines affect the CNS have been well characterized. The effects of cytokines in the brain involve changes in neurotransmission in regions (i.e., hippocampus, hypothalamus) with well-established links to learning and memory, emotion regulation, and the psychobiology of the stress response. It is tempting to speculate that man's sweeping elimination of natural predators and widespread application of medical interventions to eradicate infectious diseases (i.e., antibiotics, immunizations) may have created an opportunity for the expression of a wide range of individual differences in the activity of the cytokine network in the modern human population. The next sections detail our understanding of the links between immune activation and behavior, and cytokines and psychopathology.

CYTOKINE EFFECTS AT THE BEHAVIORAL SURFACE

The pioneering work of Robert Dantzer at the Neurobiologie Integrative, INSERUM, Bordeaux has defined the cutting edge of our knowledge regarding the behavioral effects of cytokines. Numerous animal-model studies show that IL-1β administration elicited anorexia (Hart, 1988; Moldawer, Andersson, Gelin, & Lundholm, 1988), increased sleep time (Opp, Orbal, & Kreuger, 1991), decreased social and nonsocial exploration (Sparado & Dunn, 1990), decreased sexual activity (Avitsur & Yirmiya, 1999), increased defensive withdrawal, and affected other behaviors characteristic of the nonspecific symptoms of sickness (Dantzer, 2001; Dantzer et al., 1993; Dunn, Antoon, & Chapman, 1991; Kent, Rodriguez, Kelley, & Dantzer, 1994; Kreuger, Walter, Dinarello, Wolff, & Chedid, 1984). At the behavioral level, some suggest that sickness behavior is the expression of a disruption in motivation and arousal that reorganizes the organism's priorities to cope with infectious pathogens (Aubert, 1999; Dantzer, 2001; Gahtan & Overmier, 2001).

Mild-to-moderate adverse effects of peripherally released cytokines such as IL-1β can be recognized in most individuals with an active systemic influenza (i.e., flu) infection. Tyrell and colleagues rigorously documented adverse effects of experimentally induced respiratory virus infection and cytokine administration on human psychomotor performance, mood, and memory (Smith et al., 1987; Smith, Tyrell, Coyle, & Higgins, 1988; Smith, Tyrell, Coyle, & Willman, 1987). Evidence of moderate-to-severe psychological effects of cytokines was first revealed in therapeutic clinical trials of interleukins and interferons as biological response modifiers. Many oncology patients treated with cytokines complained of headache, fever, anorexia, fatigue, and social withdrawal (Gutterman et al., 1982; Mannering & Deloria, 1986). Repeated prolonged exposure in oncology patients to cytokines resulted in increased irritability, short temper, agitation, and aggressiveness; extreme emotional liability, depression, and fearfulness; and severe cognitive changes including symptoms such as disorientation, paranoia, and suicidal ideation (e.g., Renault et al., 1987). Results from that study also showed that while these adverse effects were generally attenuated with the termination of the protocol, some participants remained emotionally vulnerable for weeks after the cessation. More recent studies show that oncology patients treated with cytokines (in this case interleukin-2 or interferon-alpha) have significantly higher depression and anxiety symptoms after only 3–5 days of therapy (Capuron, Bluthe, & Dantzer, 2001; Capuron, Ravaud, & Dantzer, 2000, 2001; Capuron, Ravaud, Gualde et al., 2001).

In summary, the experimental animal and clinical human studies provide strong support for the conclusion that cytokine production (or administration) is causally linked to the expression of atypical emotional, behavioral, and cognitive function. The severity of the symptoms clearly extends into the clinical range. The symptoms linked to cytokines include primarily those related to internalizing (such as cognitive processes, psychosis, anxiety, fearfulness, depression, thoughts about suicide) disorders. Generally, the effects of cytokines at the behavioral surface are consistent with our knowledge about the consequences cytokines have on the central nervous and neuroendocrine systems.

INTERNALIZING PROBLEM BEHAVIOR AND CYTOKINES

Very few published studies have been devoted to a comprehensive evaluation of the relationship between psychiatric disorder and cytokine regulation. Some studies report adult patients with severe depression, anxiety, and symptoms of stress-related psychiatric disorders have associated immune abnormalities (e.g., Kelly, Ganguli, & Rabin,

1987; Kronfol, Tandon, & Nair, 1990). The findings are not always consistent across studies, but the pattern largely supports the hypothesis of a close relationship between internalizing behavior problems and activation of the cytokine network (Connor & Leonard, 1998; Dantzer, Wollman, Vitkovic, & Yirmiya, 1999).

Depression. The rationale that cytokines play a role in the pathophysiology of major depression is based on assumptions that (1) depression is closely associated with stress and is often portrayed as an exaggerated response to stress, (2) depression is accompanied by atypical HPA axis activity, and (3) the cardinal manifestations of depression include changes in sleep, appetite, sex drive, social withdrawal, and cognitive slowing (Kronfol, 1999). There is evidence that cytokines are associated with, or influence, many of these individual symptoms (see Anderson et al., 1996; Herbert & Cohen, 1993a). For instance, in early studies Maes reported significant elevations of IL-1β and IL-6 in the plasma of depressed patients (Maes, Bosmans, Meltzer, Scharpe, & Suy, 1993; Maes et al., 1995). In the most recent studies, Owen, Eccleston, Ferrier, and Young (2001) report elevated levels of IL-1β in major depression and postviral depression. Musselman et al. (2001) report that cancer patients with depression had markedly higher plasma concentrations of IL-6 than healthy comparison subjects and cancer patients without depression. Berk, Wadee, Kuschke, and O'Neill-Kerr (1997) report that levels of c-reactive protein and IL-6 were significantly raised in a group with major depression. On the other hand, Haack and colleagues (1999) caution that the association between depressive symptoms and cytokines may be due in part to incomplete control of numerous potential confounding influences. In one of the largest studies to date (361 psychiatric patients, 64 health controls), they report that once age, body mass, gender, smoking habits, ongoing or recent infectious diseases, and medications are carefully taken into account, plasma levels of cytokines and cytokine receptors yield little, if any, evidence for immunopathology in major depression.

Very few studies have explored relationships between psychiatric symptoms or problem behavior and cytokine levels in youth. Birmaher et al. (1994) studied twenty adolescents with major depressive disorder, seventeen nondepressed subjects with conduct disorder, and seventeen healthy controls. Blood samples were drawn for total white blood cells, lymphocyte subsets, NK cell activity, and lymphocyte proliferation assays. Overall, there were no significant between-group differences, but the project did not measure cytokines. A preliminary study in our lab revealed that serum levels of cytokines were significantly correlated with behavior problems in clinic-referred youth, but not in nonreferred age-matched comparisons. In the study (M age $= 11.3$ years, range 8 to 17) we observed that individual differences in serum levels of IL-1 were positively correlated, r's (17) $= .59$ and $.55$, p's $< .05$, with self-reported anxiety/depression on the Youth Self-Report version of the Child Behavior Checklist (Achenbach, 1991a,b) and Children's Depression Inventory (Kovacs, 1983) in a clinic-referred group ($n = 20$) but not in a normally developing comparison ($n = 19$) group (Granger, Ikeda, & Block, 1997).

Anxiety Disorders. Depression is often accompanied by anxiety and other anxiety-related disorders, but in comparison to depression, data linking cytokines and anxiety disorders is scant. There is a growing body of evidence suggesting a role for autoimmune mechanisms in some specific cases of *obsessive compulsive disorder* (OCD; Garvey,

Giedd, & Swedo, 1998; Leonard et al., 1999; Swedo et al., 1998). Maes, Meltzer, and Bosmans (1994a) noted a positive association between IL-6 and the severity of compulsive symptoms. Mittleman et al. (1997) reported atypical cytokine levels in the cerebral spinal fluid in patients with childhood onset OCD. Studies do not consistently support a link between immune abnormalities and *panic disorders* (PD). Brambilla et al. (1992, 1994) reported plasma IL-1β was significantly higher in patients with PD than controls, before and after treatment with benzodiazepine. Studies by Rapaport and Stein (1994) and Weizman, Laor, Wiener, Wolmer, and Bessler (1999) failed to find that immune measures differentiated patients with PD from normal controls. Spivak et al. (1997) found circulating levels of IL-1β were significantly higher in patients with combat-related *Posttraumatic Stress Disorder* (PTSD), with IL-1β levels correlating with duration of PTSD, and severity of anxiety and depression. To our knowledge no studies have explored these relationships in children.

In summary, the findings to date suggest that cytokines cause rapid reorganization in several behavioral domains, the intensity of such effects ranges from mild to extreme, and that the duration of the effects can outlast the events that precipitated their release. The breadth, magnitude, and duration of the biobehavioral effects of cytokines underscore the plausibility that their dysregulation might alter the organization of human physiology and behavior in ways that affect microevolution and individual development. In particular, the adult and child literature highlights the possibility that variation in the expression of socioemotional, cognitive, and behavioral symptoms associated with depression and/or socially inhibited behaviors may be partially explained by differential sensitivities to the effects of exposure to naturally occurring ubiquitous immune stimuli (e.g., see Dantzer, 2001; Kronfol & Remick, 2000; Watson, Mednick, Huttunen, & Wang, 1999). However, the findings suggest that while cytokines are sufficient to cause psychiatric symptoms, they are not both *necessary and sufficient*; psychiatric symptoms occur in the absence of cytokine aberrations.

METHODS TO STUDY BEHAVIORAL EFFECTS OF CYTOKINES

Cytokines and their inhibitors can be measured in most biological fluids in the pg/ml (e.g., serum, plasma, urine, cerebrospinal fluid, and possibly saliva) range using immunosorbent (ELISA) and biological assays (Wadhwa & Thorpe, 1998). Reagents and materials for this purpose are now widely commercially available, and assays for these biomarkers are routine in most clinical and biomedical research laboratories. Under normal circumstances, the levels of many cytokines (particularly those responsible for the initiation and regulation of inflammation) are nondetectable using immunoassay methods. Many researchers thus depend on measuring cytokine mRNA transcripts using polymerase chain reaction (PCR) techniques. Kiecolt-Glaser and Glaser (1988), Vedhara, Fox, and Wang (1999), and Wadhwa and Thorpe (1998) present overviews of the measurement of the immune response with specific attention to cytokines.

There are several challenges to researchers studying cytokine-behavior relationships. As previously mentioned, under normal conditions, unless the immune system has been stimulated, the level of most cytokines is in the very low to undetectable range (Wadhwa & Thorpe, 1998). This creates considerable obstacles to evaluating correlates of individual differences as the range of scores is often restricted to present or absent.

Also, the variation in levels for the detectable scores can be considerable and is, in our experience, rarely normally distributed. To reveal the full range of individual differences, investigators are forced to study cytokine responses or production in reaction to an immune challenge. This is most often accomplished *in vitro* with lymphoid cells that have been isolated from the body and cultured. The ecological validity of such data has been questioned (Kiecolt-Glaser & Glaser, 1988).

On the other hand, a problem in studying the behavioral consequences of illness in whole organisms (especially in humans) is the difficulty of separating the effects of the infectious agent itself from the effects of the immune response to that agent. As noted above, our assumption is that some individuals generate more cytokines in response to immune challenge and/or that some individuals' nervous and/or endocrine system components are more sensitive to the effects of cytokines than others. Correspondingly, we are not particularly invested in the specifics of any particular pathogen or pathogenic process. Rather, we treat the pathogen as a stimulus, and are focused on characteristics of individuals that create exaggerated cytokine responses or sensitivities when exposed to any number of immune stimuli. To resolve this issue, in experimental paradigms it is common to employ a standard nonreplicating immune stimulus (e.g. lipopolysaccharide, LPS) as a proxy for systemic viral or bacterial infection (Tilders et al., 1994). LPS (also referred to as endotoxin) is the immunologically active component of gram-negative bacteria cell walls. LPS is derived from bacteria that are endemic to most mammalian species (*E. coli*, *Salmonella*), and vertebrates have specific LPS receptors on the surface of macrophages. Numerous animal studies show that LPS administration mimics the behavioral, neurochemical, and neuroendocrine response to cytokines (i.e., IL-1β) very closely (see Dunn, 1996). Use of substances like LPS also enables investigators to standardize exposure to the immune stimulus, a control that is not easy to implement in more ecologically valid contexts. In one of the few studies conducted with humans, Reichenberg et al. (2001) employed a double-blind cross-over design with twenty healthy male volunteers. Participants completed psychological questionnaires and neuropsychological tests one, three, and nine hours after intravenous injection of endotoxin (0.8 ng/kg, *Salmonella*). Reichenberg et al. (2001) observed that after endotoxin administration, the subjects showed a transient increase in anxiety and depressed mood, with decreased verbal and nonverbal memory. These changes were associated with increased levels of cytokine secretion (i.e., IL-1β, TNF-α, IL-6) released in response to endotoxin.

Interestingly, substances like endotoxin have been used as adjuvants in vaccine preparations (e.g., whole cell DPT vaccine). Adjuvants are added to stimulate the immune response sufficiently so that adequate antibody is produced to the particular antigen species included in the vaccine preparation. Investigators studying the effects of stress on immunity in adults have often taken advantage of immunizations as natural experiments (Bonneau, Sheridan, Feng, & Glaser, 1993; Kiecolt-Glaser, Glaser, Gravenstein, Malarkey, & Sheridan, 1996). Child immunizations offer a similar opportunity. In the United States, for instance, parents are encouraged to have their children immunized starting at three months of age and continuing on a regular basis through the preschool years. Studies of immunizations represent a natural experiment in which to explore individual differences in cytokine-behavior relationships (Morag, Yirmiya, Lerer, & Morag, 1998). Several studies predate the current rationale, but do show mild-to-moderate short-term behavioral effects of childhood immunizations (Cody, Baraff,

Cherry, Marcy & Manclark, 1981). The "side" effects include fever, irritability, lack of appetite, increased sleep, and parallel the "non-specific symptoms of sickness" induced by cytokines. Research on the efficacy of most childhood vaccines was conducted largely before cytokines were known as regulators of the neuro-endocrine-immune network. For instance, the whole cell version of the DPT vaccine contained endotoxin as an adjuvant. The vaccine was causally linked to adverse reactions and behavior disorders (e.g., Blumberg et al., 1993; Borg, 1958; Cody et al., 1981; Long, DeForest, Smith, Lazaro, & Wassilak, 1990). A government-mandated scientific panel called for studies of biobehavioral predictors of individual differences in the severity of adverse responses to vaccines, as well as the specific biological mechanisms responsible for vaccine-induced behavioral effects (Howson, Howe, & Fineberg, 1991). The use of the whole cell DTP vaccine was discontinued in the late 1990s.

CYTOKINES AFFECT DEVELOPMENTAL PLASTICITY OF THE BIOLOGICAL BASIS OF BEHAVIOR

It is clear that cytokines cause short-term behavioral changes, but is it possible that activation of the cytokine network could affect the long-term plasticity of biological systems underlying important behavioral, emotional, or cognitive capacities? Can cytokines change enduring aspects of our temperament or personality? The evidence of cytokine effects on cerebral and neuroendocrine systems underscores this may be biologically plausible. Yet, at first glance, this possibility seems to contradict our everyday experience. When adults have systemic viral or bacterial infections (e.g., influenza, *E. coli*) it is clear that the majority express "sickness behaviors," albeit to different degrees. But even those of us who become the most agitated, withdrawn, sleepy, and irritable when we are "sick" seemingly return to our "regular" selves soon after the infection subsides. Could there be periods in development when humans would be susceptible to longer-term or permanent effects? To adequately investigate this possibility, studies are needed that employ longitudinal designs and focus on the link between the activity of cytokines (and processes that influence their regulation), and the onset, changes, and continuities of atypical behavioral and biological function. Such studies have yet to be conducted with humans (to our knowledge). However, the evidence from animal studies is revealing.

Studies with rodents show conclusively that exposure to immune system products (i.e., cytokines) during early development permanently changes biological systems with well-known organizational influences on the brain and behavior. O'Grady and colleagues reported that immune activation during pre- and neonatal periods affects changes in the size of the adrenal glands, ovaries, and testes that persist into adulthood (O'Grady & Hall, 1990, 1991; O'Grady, Hall, & Goldstein, 1987). Shanks and colleagues (1995) showed that immune activation during a critical neonatal period of HPA axis development had profound effects on neuroendocrine (i.e., ACTH, corticosterone) responsiveness to environmental challenge during adulthood. Specifically, administration of endotoxin (0.05 mg/kg) on days 3 and 5 of life resulted in decreased glucocorticoid negative-feedback inhibition of ACTH synthesis, thereby potentiating HPA responsiveness to restraint stress. These studies are perhaps the first to reveal that exposure to immune products early in life can permanently alter neural systems, that is, HPA and hypothalamic-pituitary-gonadal (HPG) axes, governing the impact of maturational processes and environmental events on development. They suggest indirect effects on behavioral, emotional, and social processes via permanent changes induced in these biological systems.

This developmental phenomenon was first extended into the behavioral domain by Crnic and colleagues (Crnic, 1991; Segall & Crnic, 1990). Their studies reveal striking evidence that immune activation in neonates induced behavioral changes that persisted into adulthood. Neonatal mice administered Herpes Simplex Virus (HSV-1) or interferon became spontaneously hyperactive for life (Crnic & Pizer, 1988). Importantly, this radical reorganization of behavior was mediated by the impact of products of cellular immune activation, not necessarily viral pathogenesis, on the migration of granule cells from the cerebellum. Crnic's findings are groundbreaking in that they provide biological evidence of neuroanatomical changes induced by immune activation early in life that underly permanent behavioral change expressed later in life. Crnic (1991) postulated that individual differences in the development of atypical behavior may be caused by common immunological stimuli that have "uncommon effects" on the biological basis of behavior.

INDIVIDUAL AND DEVELOPMENTAL DIFFERENCES IN THE "UNCOMMON EFFECTS" OF COMMON IMMUNE STIMULI

We speculate that the specification of sources of individual differences in the uncommon effects of immune stimuli may hold considerable promise for extending our understanding of individual development and microevolution (Gottlieb, 1992). In a series of studies Granger and colleagues have employed a well-established model of genotype-environment interactions in relation to the major dimensions of atypical social development, internalizing and externalizing behavior problems. The model uses two lines of mice that have been selectively bred for differences in social interaction patterns for more than thirty generations and a control line of mice bred without selection for behavior. The advantages of the model include (a) demonstrated sensitive periods for early experiences that influence later social behavior (Cairns, Hood, & Midlam, 1985; Hood & Cairns, 1989), (b) line differences in the rate of development of aggressive behaviors (Cairns, Gariepy, & Hood, 1990; Hood & Cairns, 1988), and (c) line differences in immune responsiveness at the cellular level (Pettito et al., 1999; Pettito, Lysle, Gariepy, Clubb et al., 1994; Pettito, Lysle, Gariepy, & Lewis, 1992, 1994).

In the first study (Granger, Hood et al., 1997) to explore genetic-developmental differences in the biobehavioral effects of induced illness, adult males from two lines of mice selectively bred for high or low levels of aggressive behavior were injected with endotoxin (LPS: 0.25 mg/kg, 1.25 mg/kg or 2.5 mg/kg) or saline. Body temperature, weight, and locomotor activity were monitored before, injection, and eight and twenty-four hours after injection. Twenty-four hours after injection, social behaviors were assessed in a 10-min dyadic test, and spleens were collected. Males from the high-aggressive line had a lower threshold to endotoxin-induced effects on body temperature, weight loss, spleen weight, and corticosterone than males from the low-aggressive line. In the high-aggressive line only, social reactivity (startle response to mild social investigation) increased, and attack frequency and latency to attack decreased for endotoxin-treated compared to saline-treated mice. The interactions between selected line (genotype) and endotoxin treatment (environment) demonstrated that genetic-developmental differences in social and aggressive behavior may indicate the extent to which immune stimuli function as "biobehavioral" stressors.

In a second set of studies (Granger, Hood, & Banta, unpublished) male mice (45–50 days) from the high- and low-aggressive lines were administered endotoxin (1.25 mg/kg). Social behavior was assessed and serum harvested at 12 time points (0.5–24 hrs) post-injection. In contrast to low-aggressive line mice, high-aggressive line mice showed endotoxin-induced reduction in attack frequency and latency, more pronounced increases in behavioral immobility, socially reactive behaviors, and circulating levels of IL-1β. Endotoxin-related differences in levels of IL-1β, corticosterone, and behavior change were positively associated in the high-line only. A secondary experiment confirmed the basic findings at a five-fold lower dose (0.25 mg/kg). In a third experiment, high- and low-aggressive line mice were administered a standard dose of IL-1β (0.25–1.0 ug/ml). High-line mice showed an increase in circulating levels of IL-6 that was associated with higher levels of corticosterone, temperature loss, and behavioral immobility in observed social interactions.

Taken together with the findings of Pettito and associates with parallel lines of mice (Pettito et al., 1999; Pettito, Lysle, Gariepy, Clubb et al., 1994; Pettito et al., 1992; Pettito, Lysle, Gariepy, & Lewis, 1994), these data suggest that the observed pattern may in part be due to line differences in peripheral cytokine production. However, it cannot be ruled out at this time that there may be line-differential central nervous system or hypothalamic-pituitary-adrenal (HPA) axis sensitivity to the afferent signals of cytokines, other acute phase proteins, or endotoxin itself. The mechanisms responsible for the apparent linkage between these behavioral "traits," and immune function are yet to be determined. Pettito and colleagues (1999) raise two possibilities: that the association between selective line and immune function (in this case NK cell activation) may be due to a genetic linkage between subsets of genes involved in determining these complex traits, or that these results may represent a fortuitous association that occurred during selective breeding. There is some independent evidence supporting that the aggression-immunity link is not random. Experimental nonhuman primate studies (*Macaca Fascicularis*) revealed that changes in cellular immunity in response to the stress of repeated social reorganization are associated with individual differences in aggressive behavior (Cohen et al., 1997), and high-aggressive monkeys have higher lymphocyte counts than low-aggressive monkeys (Line et al., 1996). Also, among men ages 30–48 years ($n = 4,415$) there is a positive (curvilinear) relationship between individual differences in aggressive behavior and enumerative measures of B and T lymphocyte numbers (Granger, Booth, & Johnson, 2000).

In a third study, the expression of developmental differences in the biobehavioral consequences of immune activation in early life were investigated in the high- and low-aggressive mice (Granger, Hood, Ikeda, Reed, & Block, 1996). At age 5 or 6 days, male mice were administered saline or 0.05 mg/kg endotoxin. There was a transient endotoxin-induced reduction in the growth rate of the neonates from the high-aggressive line only. At adulthood, age 45–50 days, social behaviors were observed in a dyadic test. Hypothalmi and sera were harvested 20 minutes later. Rates of socially reactive behaviors to conspecific contact (i.e., kick, startle) were increased in the endotoxin-treated groups from both lines. For the high-aggressive line only, endotoxin treatment increased behavioral immobility, decreased attack frequency, and decreased levels of hypothalamic CRF. The effects of endotoxin exposure in early life on socially reactive behavior in later life were associated with endotoxin-induced individual differences in CRF levels in the high-aggressive but not low-aggressive line mice. These findings suggest that variation in the expression of socially inhibited behaviors in later life may be partially explained by differential sensitivities to the effects of exposure to immune stimuli in early life.

In mammalian species, early development is embedded in the social context of maternal caregiving (Hofer, 1994; Krasnegor & Bridges, 1990). Thus, the milieu of early social development may contribute to the effects of immune challenges on offspring (Hofer, 1994; Krasnegor & Bridges, 1990; Liu et al., 1997; Meaney, Aitken, Bhatnagar, Van Berkel, & Sapolsky, 1988). Two lines of evidence suggest that line-specific maternal responsiveness to endotoxin-treated pups may contribute to differences in early endotoxin exposure effects later in life. Shanks and colleagues (1995) reported anecdotal evidence of changes in mother-pup interactions that occur following endotoxin administration to neonatal rats. Also Gariepy, Nehrenberg, and Mills-Koonce (2000) have shown that dams from the high-aggressive line are naturally more active (more licking, handling of pups, more social contacts) in maternal caregiving than are dams from the low-aggressive line. The origins of individual differences in social behavior were examined in relation to early stress (immune challenge) and social milieu (maternal behavior) in the murine genetic-developmental model (Granger et al., 2001). Neonatal mice (5 or 6 days of age) from the selectively bred lines received a standard immune challenge (saline or 0.05 mg/kg LPS) and were reared by their line-specific biological dam or by a foster dam from a line bred without selection. As before, adult social behaviors were assessed in a dyadic test (45–50 days). Mice from the high-aggressive line show more developmental sensitivity to immune challenge than mice from the low-aggressive line, and line differences persist regardless of the early maternal environment. As adults, endotoxin-treated mice from the high-aggressive line have lower levels of aggressive behavior, longer latency to attack, and higher rates of socially reactive and inhibited behaviors compared to saline controls.

What are the implications of these findings for an integrative account of social development? The literature suggests two complementary models regarding the relation between selective breeding for social behavior and the developmental consequences of early immune challenge. One model posits a relationship stemming from an intrinsic difference in the sensitivity to immune stimuli associated with social behavioral predispositions (i.e., selective breeding for differences in social behavior). The second implies that the milieu of early social development may contribute to the effects of immune challenge on offspring. Based on the findings reported by Granger et al. (2001), we speculate that when intrinsic differences in immune responsiveness are extreme (as with individuals from the high- versus low-aggressive lines), maternal responsiveness to endotoxin-treated ("sick") pups may have little or no influence on social behavior outcomes later in life. The social environment's capacity to influence the developmental outcome under these conditions may be orders of magnitude less than the contribution made to the outcome by the intrinsic differences in immunologic reactivity (Granger et al., 2001). Alternatively, when intrinsic differences in immunologic reactivity are not as extreme (or within the "normal range" as depicted in Figure 12.2), the ontogenic process should be more open to the influence of social environmental processes.

Hood, Dreschel, and Granger (2003) examined the latter possibility. Neonatal mice (bred without selection for behavior or differences in immune reactivity) were fostered to dams that show differences in maternal behavior. Naturalistic observations of maternal behavior on postnatal days 2, 4, 5, 6, and 8 were conducted. On postnatal day 5, neonates were administered saline or 0.05 mg/kg endotoxin. As adults (day 45–50), fostered-reared subjects were observed in a dyadic test. At peak intensity of the transient illness induced by endotoxin (3 hrs post-injection), dams increase licking and decrease time off-nest for endotoxin but not saline-treated pups. Adult males that had been exposed to endotoxin early in life show changes in social behaviors that depend on the foster dam line and individual differences in maternal responsiveness among dams within lines. Taken together, the findings from this series of studies demonstrate that nonobvious but omnipresent features of the physical environment early in life, such as antigenic load, may interact with intrinsic differences in immunologic reactivity and the social environment to determine individual social developmental outcomes.

CONCLUDING COMMENTS AND FUTURE RESEARCH DIRECTIONS

Contemporary developmental theorists place behavioral adaptation in a pivotal position with respect to the bidirectional nature of environmental and biological influences on individual development. Cognitive-behavioral responsiveness to environmental events is thought to mediate or moderate the impact of such events on rapid (e.g., hormones, neurotransmitters) and slower (e.g., genetic activity) acting biological systems (Gottlieb, 1992). Subsequently, the effects of these biological systems manifest as adjustments in behavioral organization or responsiveness, or both. The functional and integrative integrity of the reciprocal influences among these systems is considered essential for optimal development. For instance, these processes enable individuals to continuously adapt to the ever-changing topography of social ecological landscapes, as well as appropriately engage the social context during life periods characterized by rapid developmental skills and abilities (e.g., infancy, toddlerhood, adolescence).

It seems reasonable that cytokines may affect developmental plasticity via their impact on these adaptive behavioral and cognitive processes. As noted above, there is unequivocal evidence that cytokines restrict the range of adaptive behaviors in several domains and may induce some maladaptive behavioral and psychological states. These cytokine-induced changes may potentiate the impact of environmental events on stress-responsive biological systems. For instance, cytokine effects may limit the behavioral surface's ability to effectively moderate the impact of environment challenge on HPA axis and sympathetic nervous system activation. Alternatively, cytokine-induced psychological states (maladaptive coping strategies or emotion regulation) may potentiate the responsiveness of environmentally sensitive biological systems. Still another possibility is that cytokine effects at the behavioral surface level restrict individual opportunities to engage contexts that nurture social, cognitive, or behavioral development. For instance, cytokine-induced social and defensive withdrawal or cognitive slowing would limit experiences in ways that would preclude vicarious or trial-and-error learning, parent-child interactions, or peer relationships.

In the field of child development, etiologic factors determining vulnerability to specific atypical developmental outcomes have for the most part consistently eluded detection. Even when the range of potential causal factors has been narrowed, it is clear that individual differences in the expression of their effects are the rule rather than the exception. Given this somewhat discouraging state of our knowledge, it is not surprising that developmental theorists commonly assume that atypical developmental outcomes represent the final common pathway of multiple independent and interacting factors. This perspective has proven useful for some purposes (i.e., identifying the range of prospective causal factors) but has not necessarily resulted in progress toward defining the nature of cause-and-effect. We forward an alternative perspective that a common set of biobehavioral processes may be responsible for causing subtle deviations in biological and behavioral plasticity. The effects of this "common initial pathway" may modify developmental processes impacting a range of atypical developmental outcomes. It follows that individual differences in the nature of these effects would be shaped by person factors (i.e., polygenic control of the immune response, central nervous system sensitivity to cytokines, critical periods of the development of the neuro-endocrine-immune network), environmental factors (i.e., frequency, duration, or timing of exposure to immunologic stimuli), as well as interactive effects.

A theoretical model representing the possible direct and indirect pathways between dysregulation of the cytokine network and developmental psychopathology is presented in Figure 12.4. At least five levels of analysis are relevant to understanding individual differences in the "uncommon effects" of common immune stimuli: (a) features of the physical environment or socioeconomic factors that increase risk or exposure to immune stimuli (e.g., population density, hygiene, water and food quality, heath care access or quality); (b) psychological factors that limit individuals' understanding or

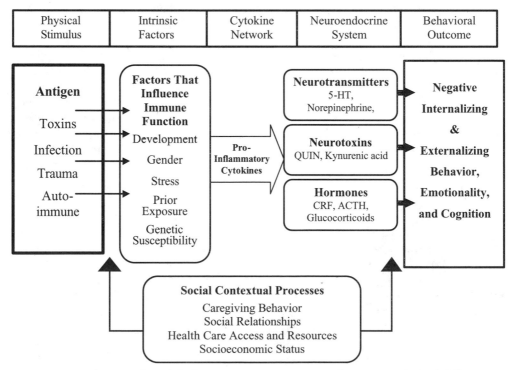

Figure 12.4. Theoretical model of interacting processes contributing to individual differences in the developmental effects of the activation of the cytokine network.

perceptions of susceptibility, severity of consequences, and risk or threat of exposure to antigens; (c) physiological predispositions or states that affect the synthesis of immune-derived molecules or that influence the sensitivity of target organs and tissues; (d) the capacity of the social environment to facilitate or disrupt recovery once a susceptible individual has been exposed; or (e) the competence of the individual at risk to elicit assistance and support from the social environment (Granger et al., 2001). Adopting this perspective leads to testable hypotheses at several levels of analysis regarding the mediation or moderation of a defined causal mechanism.

It is our expectation that the findings of studies that integrate this perspective and these psychoneuroimmunologic concepts into developmental science may engender strong inferences focused on explaining the nature of causation rather than describing phenomenan and their correlates. To adequately investigate this model, studies are needed that employ prospective longitudinal designs and focus on the link between the activity of cytokines and the onset, changes, and continuities of atypical behavioral and biological function in children. Studies focused to elaborate these uncommon effects in the context of childhood immunizations, early childhood infections or inflammatory diseases, and in special populations at high risk of exposure to immune stimuli early in life would seem an appropriate next step.

REFERENCES

Achenbach, T. M. (1991a). *Manual for the Youth Self-Report and 1991 profile*. Burlington: University of Vermont, Department of Psychiatry.

Achenbach, T. M. (1991b). *Manual for the Child Behavior Checklist/4-18 and 1991 profile*. Burlington: University of Vermont.

Adamson-Macedo, E. N. (2000). Neonatal psychoneuroimmunology: emergence, scope and perspectives. *Neuroendocrinol Lett, 21*(3), 175–186.

Ader, R. (1981). *Psychoneuroimmunology*. San Diego: Academic Press.

Ader, R. (1996). Historical perspectives on psychoneuroimmunology. In H. Friedman, T. W. Klein, & A. L. Friedman (Eds.), *Psychoneuroimmunology, stress and infection* (pp. 1–24). New York: CRC Press.

Ader, R. (2000). On the development of psychoneuroimmunology. *Eur J Pharmacol, 405*(1–3), 167–176.

Ader, R., Cohen, N., & Felten, D. (1995). Psychoneuroimmunology: interactions between the nervous system and the immune system. *Lancet, 345*(8942), 99–103.

Ader, R., Felten, D. L., & Cohen, D. J. (1991). *Psychoneuroimmunology*. San Diego: Academic Press.

Altman, F. (1997). Where is the "neuro" in psychoneuroimmunology? A commentary on increasing research on the "neuro" component of psychoneuroimmunology. *Brain Behav Immun, 11*(1), 1–8.

Anderson, J. A., Lentsch, A. B., Hadjiminas, D. J., Miller, F. N., Martin, A. W., Nakagawa, K., & Edwards, M. J. (1996). The role of cytokines, adhesion molecules, and chemokines in interleukin-2-induced lymphocytic infiltration in C57BL/6 mice. *J Clin Invest, 97*(8), 1952–1959.

Aubert, A. (1999). Sickness and behaviour in animals: a motivational perspective. *Neurosci Biobehav Rev, 23*(7), 1029–1036.

Avitsur, R., & Yirmiya, R. (1999). The immunobiology of sexual behavior: gender differences in the suppression of sexual activity during illness. *Pharmacol Biochem Behav, 64*, 787–796.

Ban, E. M., Haour, F. G., & Lenstra, R. (1992). Brain interleukin-1 gene expression induced by peripheral lipopolysaccharide administration. *Cytokine, 4*, 48–54.

Baraff, L. J., Cherry, J. D., Cody, C. L., Marcy, S. M., & Manclark, C. R. (1985). DTP vaccine reactions: effect of prior reactions on rate of subsequent reactions. *Dev Biol Stand, 61*, 423–428.

Benveniste, E. N. (1992a). Cytokines: Influence on glial cell gene expression and function. In J. E. Blalock (ed.), *Neuroimmunoendocrinology*, 2d ed. (pp. 106–153). New York: Karger.

Benveniste, E. N. (1992b). Inflammatory cytokines within the central nervous system: Sources, function and mechanism of action. *Cell Physiology, 32,* 1–16.

Berk, M., Wadee, A. A., Kuschke, R. H., & O'Neill-Kerr, A. (1997). Acute phase proteins in major depression. *J Psychosom Res, 43*(5), 529–534.

Berkenbosch, F., de Goeij, D. E., Rey, A. D., & Besedovsky, H. O. (1989). Neuroendocrine, sympathetic and metabolic responses induced by interleukin-1. *Neuroendocrinology, 50*(5), 570–576.

Berkenbosch, F., de Rijk, R., Del Rey, A., & Besedovsky, H. (1990). Neuroendocrinology of interleukin-1. *Adv Exp Med Biol, 274,* 303–314.

Berkenbosch, F., Van Dam, A.-M., DeRijk, R., & Schotanus, K. (1992). Role of the immune hormone interleukin-1 in brain adaptive responses to infection. In R. Kvetnansky, R. McCarty, & J. Axelrod (Eds.), *Stress: neuroendocrine and molecular approaches* (pp. 623–640). New York: Gordon and Breach Science.

Besedovsky, H. O., & del Rey, A. (1989). Mechanism of virus-induced stimulation of the hypothalamus-pituitary-adrenal axis. *J Steroid Biochem, 34*(1–6), 235–239.

Besedovsky, H., del Rey, A., Sorkin, E., Da Prada, M., Burri, R., & Honegger, C. (1983). The immune response evokes changes in brain noradrenergic neurons. *Science, 221*(4610), 564–566.

Birmaher, B., Rabin, B. S., Garcia, M. R., Jain, U., Whiteside, T. L., Williamson, D. E., al-Shabbout, M., Nelson, B. C., Dahl, R. E., & Ryan, N. D. (1994). Cellular immunity in depressed, conduct disorder, and normal adolescents: role of adverse life events. *J Am Acad Child Adolesc Psychiatry, 33*(5), 671–678.

Black, P. H. (1995). Psychoneuroimmunology: brain and immunity. *Scientific American Science and Medicine, 1,* 16–25.

Blalock, J. E. (1994). The immune system: our sixth sense. *The Immunologist, 2,* 8–15.

Blalock, J. E. (1997). The syntax of immune-neuroendocrine communication. *Immunology Today, 15,* 504–511.

Blumberg, D. A., Lewis, K., Mink, C. M., Christenson, P. D., Chatfield, P., & Cherry, J. D. (1993). Severe reactions associated with diphtheria-tetanus-pertussis vaccine: detailed study of children with seizures, hypotonic-hyporesponsive episodes, high fevers, and persistent crying. *Pediatrics, 91*(6), 1158–1165.

Blumberg, D. A., Morgan, C. A., Lewis, K., Leach, C., Holtzman, A., Levin, S. R., Baraff, L. J., & Cherry, J. D. (1988). An ongoing surveillance study of persistent crying and hypotonic-hyporesponsive episodes following routine DTP immunization: a preliminary report. *Tokai J Exp Clin Med, 13*(Suppl), 133–136.

Bluthe, R. M., Crestani, F., Kelley, K. W., & Dantzer, R. (1992). Mechanisms of the behavioral effects of interleukin 1. Role of prostaglandins and CRF. *Ann N Y Acad Sci, 650,* 268–275.

Bluthe, R. M., Dantzer, R., & Kelley, K. W. (1992). Effects of interleukin-1 receptor antagonist on the behavioral effects of lipopolysaccharide in rat. *Brain Res, 573*(2), 318–320.

Bonneau, R. H., Sheridan, J. F., Feng, N., & Glaser, R. (1993). Stress-induced modulation of the primary cellular immune response to herpes simplex virus infection is mediated by both adrenal-dependent and independent mechanisms. *J Neuroimmunol, 42*(2), 167–176.

Borg, J. M. (1958). Neurological complications of pertussis immunization. *British Medical Journal, 2,* 24.

Boyce, W. T., Chesney, M., Alkon, A., Tschann, J. M., Adams, S., Chesterman, B., Cohen, F., Folkman, S., & Ward, M. (1995). Psychobiologic reactivity to stress and childhood respiratory illness: results of two prospective studies. *Psychosomatic Medicine, 57,* 411–426.

Brambilla, F., Bellodi, L., Perna, G., Battaglia, M., Sciuto, G., Diaferia, G., Petraglia, F., Panerai, A., & Sacerdote, P. (1992). Psychoimmunoendocrine aspects of panic disorder. *Neuropsychobiology, 26*(1–2), 12–22.

Brambilla, F., Bellodi, L., Perna, G., Bertani, A., Panerai, A., & Sacerdote, P. (1994). Plasma interleukin-1 beta concentrations in panic disorder. *Psychiatry Res, 54*(2), 135–142.

Cairns, R. B., Gariepy, J. L., & Hood, K. E. (1990). Development, microevolution, and social behavior. *Psychol Rev, 97*(1), 49–65.

Cairns, B. D., Hood, K., & Midlam, J. (1985). On fighting mice: Is there a sensitive period for isolation effects? *Animal Behavior, 33,* 166–180.

Capuron, L., Bluthe, R. M., & Dantzer, R. (2001). Cytokines in clinical psychiatry. *Am J Psychiatry, 158*(7), 1163–1164.

Capuron, L., Ravaud, A., & Dantzer, R. (2000). Early depressive symptoms in cancer patients receiving interleukin 2 and/or interferon alfa-2b therapy. *J Clin Oncol, 18*(10), 2143–2151.

Capuron, L., Ravaud, A., & Dantzer, R. (2001). Timing and specificity of the cognitive changes induced by interleukin-2 and interferon-alpha treatments in cancer patients. *Psychosom Med, 63*(3), 376–386.

Capuron, L., Ravaud, A., Gualde, N., Bosmans, E., Dantzer, R., Maes, M., & Neveu, P. J. (2001). Association between immune activation and early depressive symptoms in cancer patients treated with interleukin-2-based therapy. *Psychoneuroendocrinology, 26*(8), 797–808.

Carr, D. J., Radulescu, R. T., DeCosta, B. R., Rice, K. C., & Blalock, J. E. (1992). Opioid modulation of immunoglobulin production by lymphocytes isolated from Peyer's patches and spleen. *Ann N Y Acad Sci, 650,* 125–127.

Chensue, S. W., Shmyre-Forsch, C., Otterness, I. G., & Kunkel, S. L. (1989). The beta form is the dominant interleukin-1 released by peritoneal macrophages. *Biochemical Biophysical Research Communications, 160,* 404–408.

Chuluyan, H. E., Saphier, D., Rohn, W. M., & Dunn, A. J. (1992). Noradrenergic innervation of the hypothalamus participates in adrenocortical responses to interleukin-1. *Neuroendocrinology, 56*(1), 106–111.

Cicchetti, D., & Lynch, M. (1995). Failures in the expectable environment and their impact on individual development: The case of child maltreatment. In D. Cicchetti & D. J. Cohen (Eds.), *Developmental psychopathology* (Vol 2. Risk, Disorder and Adaptation, pp. 32–71). New York: Wiley.

Clough, N. C., & Roth, J. A. (1998). *Understanding immunology.* St. Louis, Mo.: Mosby-Year Book.

Cody, C. L., Baraff, L. J., Cherry, J. D., Marcy, S. M., & Manclark, C. R. (1981). Nature and rates of adverse reactions associated with DTP and DT immunizations in infants and children. *Pediatrics, 68,* 650–659.

Coe, C. L. (1996). Developmental psychoneuroimmunology revisited. *Brain Behav Immun, 10*(3), 185–187.

Coe, C. K. (1999). Psychosocial factors and psychoneuroimmunology within a lifespan perspective. In D. P. Keating & C. Hertzman (Eds.), *Developmental health and the wealth of nations.* New York: Guilford Press.

Cohen, S., & Herbert, T. B. (1996). Health psychology: psychological factors and physical disease from the perspective of human psychoneuroimmunology. *Annu Rev Psychol, 47,* 113–142.

Cohen, S., Line, S., Manuck, S. B., Rabin, B. S., Heise, E., & Kaplan, J. R. (1997). Chronic stress, social status, and susceptibility to upper respiratory infections in nonhuman primates. *Psychosomatic Medicine, 59,* 213–221.

Connor, T. J., & Leonard, B. E. (1998). Depression, stress and immunological activation: the role of cytokines in depressive disorders. *Life Sciences, 62*(7), 583–606.

Cotman, C. W., Brinton, R. E., Glaburda, A., McEwen, B. S., & Schneider, D. M. (1987). *The neuro-immune-endocrine connection.* New York: Raven Press.

Crnic, L. S. (1991). Behavioral consequences of viral infection. In R. Ader, D. L. Felten, & N. Cohen (Eds.), *Psychoneuroimmunology* (2d ed., pp. 749–770). New York: Academic Press.

Crnic, L. S., & Pizer, L. I. (1988). Behavioral effects of neonatal herpes simplex type 1 infection of mice. *Neurotoxicol Teratol, 10*(4), 381–386.

Cunningham, E. T., & De Souza, E. B. (1993). Interleukin-1 receptors in the brain and endocrine tissues. *Immunology Today, 14,* 171–176.

Dantzer, R. (2001). Cytokine-induced sickness behavior: where do we stand? *Brain Behav Immun, 15*(1), 7–24.

Dantzer, R., Bluth, R.-M., & Goodall, G. (1993). Behavioral effects of cytokines: An insight into mechanisms of sickness behavior. *Methods in Neuroscience, 16,* 130–150.

Dantzer, R., Bluthe, R. M., Gheusi, G., Cremona, S., Laye, S., Parnet, P., & Kelley, K. W. (1998). Molecular basis of sickness behavior. *Ann N Y Acad Sci, 856,* 132–138.

Dantzer, R., Bluthe, R. M., Laye, S., Bret-Dibat, J. L., Parnet, P., & Kelley, K. W. (1998). Cytokines and sickness behavior. *Ann N Y Acad Sci, 840,* 586–590.

Dantzer, R., Konsman, J. P., Bluthe, R. M., & Kelley, K. W. (2000). Neural and humoral pathways of communication from the immune system to the brain: parallel or convergent? *Auton Neurosci, 85*(1–3), 60–65.

Hood, K. E., Dreschel, N. A., & Granger, D. A. (2003). Maternal behavior changes after immune challenge of neonates with developmental effects on adult social behavior. *Developmental Psychobiology, 42,* 17–34.

Howson, C. P., Howe, C. J., & Fineberg, H. V. (1991). *Adverse effects of pertussis and rubella vaccines: A report of the committee to review the adverse consequences of pertussis and rubells vaccines.* Unpublished manuscript. Washington, D.C: National Academy Press.

Janeway, C. A., Jr. (2001). How the immune system works to protect the host from infection: a personal view. *Proc Natl Acad Sci U S A, 98*(13), 7461–7468.

Kelly, R. H., Ganguli, R., & Rabin, B. S. (1987). Antibody to discrete areas of the brain in normal individuals and patients with schizophrenia. *Biological Psychiatry, 22,* 1488–1491.

Kemeny, M. E., & Gruenewald, T. L. (1999). Psychoneuroimmunology update. *Semin Gastrointest Dis, 10*(1), 20–29.

Kemeny, M. E., & Laudenslager, M. L. (1999). Introduction beyond stress: the role of individual difference factors in psychoneuroimmunology. *Brain Behav Immun, 13*(2), 73–75.

Kent, S., Rodriguez, F., Kelley, K. W., & Dantzer, R. (1994). Reduction in food and water intake induced by microinjection of interleukin-1 beta in the ventromedial hypothalamus of the rat. *Physiol Behav, 56*(5), 1031–1036.

Kiecolt-Glaser, J. K., & Glaser, R. (1988). Methodological issues in behavioral immunology research with humans. *Brain Behav Immun, 2*(1), 67–78.

Kiecolt-Glaser, J. K., & Glaser, R. (1989). Psychoneuroimmunology: past, present, and future. *Health Psychol, 8*(6), 677–682.

Kiecolt-Glaser, J. K., & Glaser, R. (1995). Psychoneuroimmunology and health consequences: data and shared mechanisms. *Psychosom Med, 57*(3), 269–274.

Kiecolt-Glaser, J. K., Glaser, R., Gravenstein, S., Malarkey, W. B., & Sheridan, J. (1996). Chronic stress alters the immune response to influenza virus vaccine in older adults. *Proc Natl Acad Sci U S A, 93*(7), 3043–3047.

Kluger, M. J. (1979). *Fever: Its biology, evolution, and function.* Princeton, N.J.: Princeton University Press.

Kopeloff, N., Kopeloff, L. M., & Raney, M. E. (1933). The nervous system and antibody production. *Psychiatry Quarterly, 7,* 84.

Kovacs, M. (1983). *The Children's Depression Inventory: A self-rated depression scale for school-aged youngsters.* Unpublished manuscript, University of Pittsburgh, School of Medicine.

Krasnegor, N. A., & Bridges, R. S. (1990). *Mammalian parenting: biochemical, neurological, and behavioral determinants.* New York: Oxford University Press.

Kreuger, J. M., Walter, J., Dinarello, C. A., Wolff, S. M., & Chedid, L. (1984). Sleep promoting effects of endogenous pyrogen (IL-1). *American Journal of Physiology, 246,* 9994–9999.

Kronfol, Z. (1999). Depression and immunity: The role of cytokines. In N. P. Plotnikoff, R. E. Faith, A. J., Murgo, & R. A. Good (Eds.), *Cytokines: Stress and immunit* (pp. 51–60), New York: CRC Press.

Kronfol, Z., Tandon, R., & Nair, M. (1990). Natural and lymphokine-activated killer cell activities in schizophrenia. *Biological Psychiatry, 27,* 41–179.

Kronfol, Z., & Remick, D. G. (2000). Cytokines and the brain: implications for clinical psychiatry. *Am J Psychiatry, 157*(5), 683–694.

Laye, S., Parnet, P., Goujon, E., & Dantzer, R. (1994). Peripheral administration of lipopolysaccharide induces the expression of cytokine transcripts in the brain and pituitary of mice. *Brain Res Mol Brain Res, 27*(1), 157–162.

Leonard, H. L., Swedo, S. E., Garvey, M., Beer, D., Perlmutter, S., Lougee, L., Karitani, M., & Dubbert, B. (1999). Postinfectious and other forms of obsessive-compulsive disorder. *Child and Adolescent Psychiatric Clinics of North America, 8*(3), 497–511.

Line, S., Kaplan, J. R., Heise, E., Hilliard, J. K., Cohen, S., & Rabin, B. S. (1996). Effects of social reorganization on cellular immunity in male cynomolgus monkeys. *American Journal of Primatology, 39,* 235–249.

Liu, D., Dioria, J., Tannenbaum, B., Caldji, C., Francis, D., Freedom, A., Sharma, S., Pearson, D., Plotsky, P. M., & Meaney, M. J. (1997). Maternal care, hippocampal, glucocorticoid receptors, and hypothalamic-pituitary-adrenal responses to stress. *Science, 277,* 1659–1662.

Long, S. A., DeForest, A., Smith, D. G., Lazaro, C., & Wassilak, S. G. F. (1990). Longitudinal study of adverse reactions following Diptheria-tetanus-pertusis vaccine in infancy. *Pediatrics, 85,* 294–302.

Maes, M., Bosmans, E., Meltzer, H. Y., Scharpe, S., & Suy, E. (1993). Interleukin-1 beta: a putative mediator of HPA axis hyperactivity in major depression? *American Journal of Psychiatry, 150,* 1189–1193.

Maes, M., Meltzer, H. Y., & Bosmans, E. (1994a). Psychoimmune investigation in obsessive-complusive disorder: Assays of plasma transferrin, IL-2 and IL-6 receptor, and IL-1β and IL-6 concentrations. *Neuropsychobiology, 30,* 57.

Maes, M., Meltzer, H. Y., & Bosmans, E. (1994b). Immune-inflammatory markers in schizophrenia: comparison to normal controls and effects of clozapine. *Acta Psychiatr Scand, 89*(5), 346–351.

Maes, M., Meltzer, H. Y., Bosmans, E., Bergmans, R., Vandoolaeghe, E., Ranjan, R., & Desnyder, R. (1995). Increased plasma concentrations of interleukin-6, soluble interleukin-6, soluble interleukin-2 and transferrin receptor in major depression. *J Affect Disord, 34*(4), 301–309.

Maier, S. F., & Watkins, L. R. (1998a). Bidirectional communication between the brain and the immune system: implications for behavior. *Animal Behaviour, 57,* 741–751.

Maier, S. F., & Watkins, L. R. (1998b). Cytokines for psychologists: implications of bidirectional immune-to-brain communication for understanding behavior, mood, and cognition. *Psychol Rev, 105*(1), 83–107.

Maier, S. F., Watkins, L. R., & Fleshner, M. (1994). Psychoneuroimmunology. The interface between behavior, brain, and immunity. *Am Psychol, 49*(12), 1004–1017.

Mannering, G. J., & Deloria, L. B. (1986). The pharmacology and toxicity of the interferones: An overview. *Annual Review of Pharmacology and Toxicology, 26,* 455–515.

Meaney, M. J., Aitken, D. H., Bhatnagar, S., Van Berkel, C., & Sapolsky, R. M. (1988). Postnatal handling attenuates neuroendocrine, anatomical, and cognitive impairments related to the aged hippocampus. *Science, 238,* 766–768.

Mittleman, B. B., Castellanos, F. S., Jacobsen, L. K., Rapoport, J. L., Swedo, S. E., & Shearer, G. M. (1997). Cerebrospinal fluid cytokines in pediatric neuropsychiatric disease. *Journal of Immunology, 159*(6), 2994–2999.

Moldawer, L. L., Andersson, C., Gelin, J., & Lundholm, K. G. (1988). Regulation of food intake and hepatic protein synthesis by recombinant-derived cytokines. *Am J Physiol, 254*(3 Pt 1), G450–456.

Morag, M., Yirmiya, R., Lerer, B., & Morag, A. (1998). Influence of socioeconomic status on behavioral, emotional and cognitive effects of rubella vaccination: a prospective, double blind study. *Psychoneuroendocrinology, 23*(4), 337–351.

Musselman, D. L., Miller, A. H., Porter, M. R., Manatunga, A., Gao, F., Penna, S., Pearce, B. D., Landry, J., Glover, S., McDaniel, J. S., & Nemeroff, C. B. (2001). Higher than normal plasma interleukin-6 concentrations in cancer patients with depression: preliminary findings. *Am J Psychiatry, 158*(8), 1252–1257.

O'Grady, M. P., & Hall, N. R. S. (1990). Postnatal exposure to Newcastles Disease virus alters endocrine development. *Teratology, 41,* 623–624.

O'Grady, M. P., & Hall, N. R. S. (1991). Long-term effects of neuroendocrine-immune interactions during early development. In R. Ader, D. L. Felten, & N. Cohen (Eds.), *Psychoneuroimmunology* 2d ed. (pp. 561–572).

O'Grady, M. P., Hall, N. R. S., & Goldstein, A. L. (1987). Developmental consequences of prenatal exposure to thymosin: long term changes in immune and endocrine parameters. *Society for Neuroscience, 13,* 1380.

Opp, M. R., Orbal, F., & Kreuger, J. M. (1991). Interleukin-1 alters rat sleep: Temporal and dose-related effects. *American Journal of Physiology, 260,* 52–58.

Owen, B. M., Eccleston, D., Ferrier, I. N., & Young, A. H. (2001). Raised levels of plasma interleukin-1 beta in major and postviral depression. *Acta Psychiatr Scand, 103*(3), 226–228.

Pettito, J. M., Gariepy, J., Gendreau, P. L., Rodriguiz, R., Lewis, M., & Lysle, D. T. (1999). Differences in NK cell function in mice bred for high and low aggression: Genetic linkage between complex behavior and immunological traits? *Brain, Behavior, and Immunity, 13,* 175–186.

Pettito, J. M., Lysle, D. T., Gariepy, J., Clubb, P. H., Cairns, B. D., & Lewis, M. (1994). Genetic differences in social behavior and cellular immune responsiveness: effects of social experience. *Brain, Behavior, and Immunity, 8,* 111–112.

Pettito, J. M., Lysle, D. T., Gariepy, J., & Lewis, M. (1992). The expression of genetic differences in social behavior in ICR mice correlates with differences in cellular immune responsiveness. *Clinical Neuropharmacology, 15,* 658–659.

Pettito, J. M., Lysle, D. T., Gariepy, J., & Lewis, M. (1994). Association of genetic differences in social behavior and cellular immune responsiveness. *Brain, Behavior, and Immunity, 8,* 111–112.

Quan, N., Sundar, S. K., & Weiss, J. M. (1994). Induction of interleukin-1 in various brain regions after peripheral and central injections of lipopolysaccharide. *J Neuroimmunol, 49*(1–2), 125–134.

Rapaport, M. H., & Stein, M. B. (1994). Serum cytokine and soluble interleukin-2 receptors in patients with panic disorder. *Anxiety, 1*(1), 22–25.

Reichenberg, A., Yirmiya, R., Schuld, A., Kraus, T., Haack, M., Morag, A., & Pollmacher, T. (2001). Cytokine-associated emotional and cognitive disturbances in humans. *Arch Gen Psychiatry, 58*(5), 445–452.

Renault, P. F., Hoofnagle, J. H., Parky, Y., Mullen, K. D., Peters, M., Jones, D., Rustigi, V., & Jones, F. A. (1987). Psychiatric complications of long-term interferon-alpha therapy. *Archives of Internal Medicine, 147,* 1577–1580.

Saito, K., Markey, S. P., et al. (1992). Effects of immune activation on quinolinic acid and neuroactive kynurenines in the mouse. *Neuroscience, 15,* 25–39.

Sameroff, A. J. (1983). Developmental systems: context and evolution. In W. Kessen (Ed.), *History, theory, and methods* (Vol. 1). In P. H. Mussen (Ed.), *Handbook of child psychology*. New York: Wiley.

Sapolsky, R., Rivier, C., Yamamoto, G., Plotsky, P., & Vale, W. (1987). Interleukin-1 stimulates the secretion of hypothalamic corticotropin- releasing factor. *Science, 238*(4826), 522–524.

Segall, M. A., & Crnic, L. S. (1990). An animal model for the behavioral effects of interferon. *Behav Neurosci, 104*(4), 612–618.

Shanks, N., Larocque, S., & Meaney, M. J. (1995). Neonatal endotoxin exposure alters the development of the hypothalamic-pituitary-adrenal axis: early illness and later responsivity to stress. *J Neurosci, 15*(1, Pt 1), 376–384.

Smith, A., Tyrell, D., Coyle, K., & Higgins, P. (1988). Effects of Interferon alpha on performance in man: A preliminary report. *Psychopharmacology, 96,* 414–416.

Smith, A. P., Tyrell, D. A., Al-Nakib, W., Coyle, K. B., Donovan, C. B., Higgins, P. G., & Willman, J. S. (1987). Effects of experimentally induced respiratory virus infection and illness on psychomotor performance. *Neuropsychobiology, 18,* 144–148.

Smith, E. (1992). Hormonal effects of cytokines. In J. E. Blalock (Ed.), *Neuroimmunoendocrinology* (pp. 154–169). New York: Krager.

Smith, R. W., Tyrell, D., Coyle, K., & Willman, J. S. (1987). Selective effects of minor illnesses on human performance. *British Journal of Psychology, 78,* 183–188.

Solomon, G. F. (1969). Emotions, stress, the central nervous system, and immunity. *Ann N Y Acad Sci, 164*(2), 335–343.

Solomon, G. F., Amkraut, A. A., & Kasper, P. (1974). Immunity, emotions and stress. With special reference to the mechanisms of stress effects on the immune system. *Ann Clin Res, 6*(6), 313–322.

Solomon, G. F., & Moos, R. H. (1965). Psychologic aspects of response to treatment in rheumatoid arthritis. *Gp, 32*(6), 113–119.

Sparado, F., & Dunn, A. J. (1990). Intracerebrovascular administration of interleukin-1 to mice alters investigation of stimulus in a novel environment. *Brain, Behavior, and Immunity, 4,* 308–322.

Spivak, B., Shohat, B., Mester, R., Avraham, S., Gil-Ad, I., Bleich, A., Valevski, A., & Weizman, A. (1997). Elevated levels of serum interleukin-1 beta in combat-related posttraumatic stress disorder. *Biol Psychiatry, 42*(5), 345–348.

Swedo, S. E., Leonard, H. L., Garvey, M., Mittleman, B. B., Allen, A. J., Perlmutter, S., Dow, S., Zamkoff, B. A., Dubbert, B. K., & Lougee, L. (1998). Pediatric autoimmune neuropsychiatric disorders associated with streptococcal infections: clinical description of the first 50 cases. *American Journal of Psychiatry, 155*(2), 264–271.

Takao, T., Tracy, D. E., Mitchell, W. M., & De Souza, E. B. (1990). Interleukin-1 receptors in the mouse brain-characterization and neuronal localization. *Endocrinology, 127,* 3070–3078.

Thomson, A. (1998). *The cytokine handbook*, 3rd ed. San Diego: Academic Press.

Tilders, F. J. H., DeRuk, R. H., VanDam, A.-M., Vincent, V. A. M., Schotanus, K., & Persoons, J. H. A. (1994). Activation of the hypothalamus-pituitary-adrenal axis by bacterial endotoxins: Routes and intermediate signals. *Psychoneuroendocrinology, 19,* 209–232.

Vedhara, K., Fox, J. D., & Wang, E. C. (1999). The measurement of stress-related immune dysfunction in psychoneuroimmunology. *Neurosci Biobehav Rev, 23*(5), 699–715.

Vilcek, J. (1998). The cytokines: An overview. In A. W. Thomson (Ed.), *The cytokine handbook* (pp. 1–20). San Diego: Academic Press.

Wadhwa, M., & Thorpe, R. (1998). Assays for cytokines. In A. W. Thomson (Ed.), *The cytokine handbook* (pp. 856–884). San Diego: Academic Press.

Watson, J. B., Mednick, S. A., Huttunen, M., & Wang, X. (1999). Prenatal teratogens and the development of adult mental illness. *Development and Psychopathology, 11,* 457–466.

Weiss, J. M., Quan, N., & Sundar, S. K. (1994). Widespread activation and consequences of interleukin-1 in the brain. *Annals of the New York Academy of Sciences, 741,* 338–357.

Weizman, R., Laor, N., Wiener, Z., Wolmer, L., & Bessler, H. (1999). Cytokine production in panic disorder patients. *Clin Neuropharmacol, 22*(2), 107–109.

Williams, J. M., Peterson, R. G., Shea, P. A., Schmedtje, J. F., Bauer, D. C., & Felten, D. L. (1981). Sympathetic innervation of murine thymus and spleen: evidence for a functional link between the nervous and immune systems. *Brain Res Bull, 6*(1), 83–94.

Woolski, B.M.R.N.J., Smith, E., Meyer, W. J., Fuller, G. M., & Blalock, J. E. (1985). Corticotrophin-releasing activity of monokines. *Science, 230,* 1035–1037.

THIRTEEN

The Hypothalamic–Pituitary–Adrenal System (HPA) and the Development of Aggressive, Antisocial, and Substance Abuse Disorders

Keith McBurnett, Jean King, and Angela Scarpa

It is often said that the only constant in life is change – in fact, responding to change might be considered the most fundamental aspect of life. As early as the 1930s, Selye used the term *stress* to refer to any condition (perceived or real) that threatens homeostasis (Selye, 1952, 1978), or in other words, signals the need for adaptive change. Responses to stress signals are believed to have developed as an alarm system for animals caught in a potentially dangerous situation, and as an activation system for animals faced with a competitive situation. These physiological responses to stress are coordinated by a rapidly responding sympathetic nervous system (SNS), and by a slower but longer-acting second stage involving the hypothalamus, the pituitary gland, and the outer cortex of the adrenal glands (collectively termed the hypothalamic–pituitary–adrenal axis, or HPA; Lopez, Akil, & Watson, 1999). Restorative biological processes (e.g., digestion, immune function, tissue building) are temporarily suppressed so that energy resources can be mobilized for activity (Sapolsky, Romero, & Munck, 2000). In the extreme, the stress response becomes a stereotypical set of behaviors and physiological reactions initially described by Cannon (1932) as the "fight or flight" response. Generally the physiological reaction returns to baseline levels soon after the offset of stress cues. If a stressful situation is prolonged or inescapable, the initial high state of physiological activation cannot be indefinitely sustained – eventually, exhaustion sets in. In some instances, the physiological substrates become unresponsive, and the behavioral result is depression or learned helplessness (Lopez et al., 1999).

Stressful conditions can be primarily physical or primarily psychological, and it is not uncommon for a given stressor to have both physical and psychological significance. As the role of stress in the etiology of mental health disorders becomes clearer (Bremner & Narayan, 1998; Holsboer, 2001; Lopez et al., 1999), researchers have been able to delineate key psychological components of the stress response. Limitations in an animal's ability to predict, control, and cope with change are reliably associated with exacerbation and prolongation of the stress response. If these mechanisms of psychological adaptation are sufficiently impeded, and the stress response is sufficiently intensified, then prolonged, or exhausted, psychopathology can result (Lopez et al., 1999). The same response that evolved to support adaptation to a stressor instead becomes maladaptive. Factors that promote maladaptive stress responses include environmental conditions (e.g., inescapable punishment), learning history and cognitive structures, and individual differences in the responsiveness of the SNS and HPA. Investigation of these factors has increased our understanding of how internalizing pathologies (anxiety, posttraumatic stress syndromes, depression) and psychosomatic illnesses develop and how they can be treated. However, the many ways in which these factors vary makes it very difficult to predict exactly *which* individuals will develop abnormalities in HPA and psychological functions, and exactly *what form* such abnormal outcomes may take. The term *multifinality* (Cicchetti & Richters, 1993; Cicchetti & Rogosch, 1996) has been applied to this type of developmental process whereby seemingly similar factors (e.g., undifferentiated stress) produce variable outcomes.

In contrast to internalizing disorders (anxiety and depression), which seem to have a basis in excessive or unsuccessful arousal, externalizing disorders seem to be linked both to excesses and to deficits in the optimal response to stressors. It has long been known that some chronically antisocial children and adults exhibit under-arousal or under-responsiveness in the rapidly responding stress system (the SNS; for reviews, see Lahey, Hart, Pliszka, Applegate, & McBurnett, 1993; McBurnett & Lahey, 1994). More recently, similar results have been found with the slower-responding system (the HPA) (McBurnett et al., 1991; McBurnett, Lahey, Rathouz, & Loeber, 2000; van Goozen et al., 1998). Not all antisocial individuals are under-responsive – in fact, many hostile, oppositional, or violent individuals seem over-aroused and highly reactive to perceived threats or confrontations. It is not a simple matter to determine just which antisocial individuals might exhibit unusually weak or unusually strong physiological reactions to a given type of stressor. In general, research has identified psychopathic, persistently aggressive, and undersocialized individuals as having muted physiological reactions. But such individuals represent a small fraction of the population of youth with behavior problems. Moreover, many children go through a transient developmental period in which they engage in antisocial behavior as teenagers and then improve to an extent by early adulthood (Aguilar, Sroufe, Egeland, & Carlson, 2000; Moffitt, 1993; Moffitt & Caspi, 2001). When researchers have tried to determine physiological correlates of antisocial youth, they sometimes have obtained null and even contradictory results (Banks & Dabbs, 1996; Kruesi, Schmidt, Donnelly, Euthymia, et al., 1989; Scarpa & Raine, 1997; Scerbo & Kolko, 1994; Schulz, Halperin, Newcorn, Sharma, & Gabriel, 1997; Targum, Clarkson, Magac-Harris, Marshall, & Skwerer, 1990). Reasons that may partially explain inconsistent findings are (a) the heterogeneity of antisocial and aggressive behavior, (b) the contextual moderation of the stress response, and (c) "noise" in the HPA output.

HETEROGENEITY OF CONDUCT DISORDER (CD) AND AGGRESSIVE BEHAVIOR

Previous reviews of the child literature on psychophysiology and antisocial behavior have been complicated by the fact that investigators have used different definitions and subtypes of conduct problems. The most consistent finding is that groups defined as psychopathic or as lacking significant anxiety, and groups defined as aggressive (rather than prone only to convert offending), tend to show lower arousal and responsiveness (Lahey et al., 1993; McBurnett & Lahey, 1994). In Table 13.1, the labels on the left side represent subtypes of antisocial samples that have shown underarousal of some type in psychophysiological studies.

identical stress stimuli, and thus any response differences can be attributed to subject characteristics. However, effects of the psychological context on responding can be extremely subtle. For example, in one psychophysiological study that compared adult male psychopaths to nonpsychopaths, it was found that despite otherwise tight control of the protocol, differences in the gender of the research assistants affected the results. Male psychopaths, compared to nonpsychopaths, responded differently when the research assistant was female. A possible theoretical explanation is that psychopathy is associated with a highly sensitive behavioral activation system, and the rewarding characteristics of the research assistant interacted with personality of the subjects.

In our studies of cohorts of clinic-referred children, we have assumed that samples of saliva gathered in the course of a clinic visit yield an index of "baseline" functioning of the HPA, as opposed to an index of HPA reactivity to a stress stimulus. This interpretation is somewhat arbitrary, as we have no way of determining whether the novelty of the clinic environment causes some children to secrete more cortisol than they otherwise might in their natural environment. If repeated samples of saliva are gathered (either during the same visit or at periodic returns to the clinic), any novelty effect associated with the first sample may be diminished. Moreover, the subjective meaning of a visit to a mental health clinic may differ according to nonrandom subject expectations, particularly if some children are normal volunteers and others are brought in because of problem behavior. Of course, the potential for variation in social context increases dramatically across labs and investigational protocols.

Not surprisingly, identifiable stressors (an approaching examination, the first weeks of a new school year, ets.) affect children's arousal and cortisol output (Davis, Donzella, Krueger, & Gunnar, 1999; Granger, Stansbury, & Henker, 1994; Gunnar, Tout, de Haan, Pierce, & Stansbury, 1997; Susman, Nottelmann, Dorn, Inoff-Germain, & Chrousos, 1988; Tennes & Kreye, 1985; Tennes, Kreye, Avitable, & Wells, 1986). Less noticeable are social influences such as subordinate status in a group, an unstable hierarchy of social status, and sustained social competition. These social conditions have been shown to stimulate the HPA in humans (Gunnar et al., 1997) and nonhuman primates (Sapolsky, 1982, 1989, 1990, 1992, 1995, 1996). It takes little stretch of imagination to hypothesize that adolescent subcultures that are continuously engaged in struggles for dominance (e.g., gangs, unstable criminal enterprises, etc.) may function to increase HPA arousal among antisocial youth whose physiological reactivity might otherwise be predicted to be low.

"NOISE" IN THE HPA AXIS

The HPA control of cortisol is affected by several factors that might be considered "noise" if we are primarily concerned with what kind of temperamental or antisocial features might be related to cortisol. These include multihierarchical regulation and adaptation, pulsatile release in response to homeostatic control, and diurnal variation.

Multihierarchical Regulation and Adaptation. (For references pertaining to this section, see Hadley, 2000; Nelson, 1995; Sapolsky et al., 2000; Schulkin, 1999.) There are three major levels of regulation of the HPA. In addition, limbic substrates of emotion and motivation feed into the top level of the HPA, and hence the system might also be termed the LHPA (limbic-hypothalamic-pituitary-adrenal axis). Cells in the hypothalamus release corticotrophic-releasing hormone (CRH), also referred to as corticotrophic-releasing factor (CRF). This travels to the anterior pituitary, which responds by releasing adrenocorticotrophic hormone (ACTH) into the general circulation. The cortices of the adrenal glands respond to elevated ACTH by releasing cortisol into general circulation. Cortisol has a number of actions which can be summarized as catabolic or activating: It tends to promote functions related to activity (protein catabolism, hepatic glycogenolysis and gluconeogenesis, increasing the sensitivity of arterioles to the action of norepinephrine) and to retard restorative and reparative functions.

Because cortisol is the "read-out" product of the HPA, its functional significance is related to higher levels of the system. A variety of factors such as anticipation of a stressful event, exposure to a pathogen, abnormal dietary intake, etc., can have an effect on baseline cortisol secretion. In addition, prolonged activation at any level of the HPA can result in adaptation (sensitization or desensitization) of feedback mechanisms, resulting in an abnormal relationship among outputs of different HPA levels (including hypo- or hyper-responsiveness). Abnormal cortisol levels may not themselves represent a sign of abundant or insufficient anxiety, but may instead reflect other hormones (e.g., CRH) that have a more direct or contributory role in modulating affect.

Pulsatile Response to Homeostatic Control. The different levels of the HPA control lower levels like a thermostat. A thermostat kicks on when the temperature goes below a preset threshold, and kicks off when the temperature exceeds that threshold. In a similar fashion, the HPA acts to release cortisol until the circulating levels rise, then to shut off release until the level of circulation falls off. Sampling blood or saliva at any one point in time is prone to catching the mean concentration level at the top or the bottom of its range. To offset this, it is recommended that multiple samples be gathered in order to aggregate a more precise estimate of average level.

Diurnal Variation. The classic diurnal rhythm of cortisol is to rise in the early morning hours to a peak level around the hour of awakening, then to steadily decline over the day before reaching a nadir around the hour of sleep (this pattern generally holds for group data but is not invariable across individuals). This makes intuitive sense, given cortisol's role in preparing the body for activity and in depressing restorative functions. The diurnal variation is so great that it can easily overshadow individual differences in cortisol levels. Hence, researchers have been advised to hold the time of collection constant across subjects. Although this is good advice for reducing extraneous variation, there are situations in which it is impractical. For example, Sapolsky and colleagues (Sapolsky et al., 2000) were only able to collect cortisol when subjects could be captured. Even so, they were able to find a relationship between social status and HPA function. Similarly, in studies conducted by McBurnett and colleagues (McBurnett, Lahey, Capasso, & Loeber, 1996; McBurnett et al., 1991; McBurnett et al., 1990), saliva sampling was "tacked on" to a clinical diagnostic evaluation scheduled for various times of the day. These studies, too, have been able to detect relationships between cortisol level and behavior. However, failing to control time of collection complicates the interpretation of findings. *If the time of collection does not systematically vary with the dependent variable*, the lack of control over diurnal variation does not invalidate any *significant* findings associating cortisol and the dependent variable. However, if no significant findings are obtained, it cannot be determined whether the additional "noise" (error variance) associated with time of collection obscured underlying behavior-hormone relationships, or whether such relationships simply did not exist. Attempts to statistically correct for diurnal variation may not fully partial out this variance. Thus, it is far preferable to hold collection times constant across subjects, as this affords both better control and more straightforward interpretation.

Because the top range of diurnal variation is observed in the morning hours, this may be the most opportune time at which to detect differences between groups hypothesized to have low cortisol and those with normal levels. The idea here is that the difference between normal cortisol secreters and hypo-secreters will be maximal at the peak level of secretion. On the other hand, reactivity paradigms may have the best chance of capturing individual differences in the afternoon hours. This is because as the normal diurnal curve falls off to a low level, there is more headroom for a large response to be reflected and less chance that the "law of initial values" (a ceiling effect or an inverse relationship between the magnitude of response to a stimulus and the pre-stimulus or baseline value; Fischer & Agnew, 1957; Wilder, 1957) will come into play and cushion the responses.

Control over many sources of variation in cortisol level may be achieved by collecting and aggregating repeated samples of cortisol. Increasing the number of cortisol samples results in more stable estimates of an individual's characteristic cortisol output (Pruessner et al., 1997). These returns quickly diminish with the number of repeated measures and become unsubstantial past five samples (Pruessner et al., 1997). McBurnnett et al. (2000) found that even one repeated sample separated from the original sample by an interval of one year substantially enhanced the relationship between persistent aggression and salivary cortisol concentration. The implication is that studies will have more power to detect cortisol-behavior relations if cortisol is collected between two and five times.

DEVELOPMENTAL MECHANISMS

Preclinical research, some of it going back decades, has provided much information about durable and plastic influences affecting behavior and the developing HPA.

Durable Genetic Effects. Investigators sometimes study animals that are bred for specific traits that occur across species and, in the extreme, resemble forms of human psychopathology. The HPA has been studied in rats predisposed to novelty-seeking (behavioral activation), harm avoidance (behavioral inhibition), and short latency to aggress (Benus, Bohus, Koolhaas, & van Oortmerssen, 1991; Benus, Bohus, Koolhass, & van Oortmerssen, 1989; de Kloet, Korte, Rots, & Kruk, 1996). Rats bred to respond to novel situations with behavioral activation (a) show similar strong behavioral activation to stimulant drugs, (b) have higher propensity to self-administer drugs, (c) have higher dopamine reactivity in the nucleus accumbens (a reward center) to stress and to drug, (d) have stronger corticosteroid response to stress, and (e) respond to glucocorticoids with greater levels of behavioral activation and mesolimbic dopamine release, compared to low responders to novelty (Piazza & Le Moal, 1997). Genetic influences on the HPA can be profound and can interact with early stress exposure (J. A. King, Mandansky, S. King, Fletcher, & Brewer, 2001). For example, the same early environmental stress can have directionall opposite effects on hormones, depending on genetic strain (King & Edwards,

1999). A recent study with a different species, however, found surprisingly consistent relationships between genetically determined cortisol reactivity and the establishment of dominance-subordinate roles. That study used the F2 generation of rainbow trout selectively bred for either high or low cortisol response to confinement. In forty-three out of forty-six novel pairings of high and low responders, the low-responding fish attained unequivocal dominance within three hours, even though pairs were carefully matched for physical size (Pottinger & Carrick, 2001).

Plasticity: The Adaptive Effects of Early "Stress Inoculation." The process of separating an infant rat from its mother and placing it in a different cage for a new minutes per day is described as "handling." In some strains of rats, daily handling for the first 1–3 weeks of life permanently increases sensitivity to glucocorticoids (GC, a collective term that includes cortisol and corticosterone), particularly in the hippocampus and forebrain. Greater sensitivity of feedback mechanisms to GC results in lower activity throughout the HPA, and in a more efficient and rapidly recovering response to stress throughout the lifespan (Frances et al., 1996; Levine & Lewis, 1958; Meaney, Aitken, Bodnoff, Iny, & Sapolsky, 1985; Meaney, Aitken, Bodnoff, Iny, Tatarewicz et al., 1985; Meany, Aitkin, Bodnoff, Ing, et al., 1995; Sapolsky, 1997). Two important features of this phenomenon are (a) it seems only to occur if mild stimulation is delivered during a "critical period," and (b) its effects on the developing HPA appear adaptive, as handled animals tend to have lower resting levels of CRF and corticosterone, and to quickly return to resting levels following termination of a stressor. The persistence of the handling effect can be seen even into the late stages of the lifespan, when age-related HPA hyperactivity, hippocampal cells loss, and memory deterioration is reduced in animals that were handled in infancy (Meaney, Aitken, Bhatnagar, & Sapolsky, 1991; Meaney, Aitken, van Berkel, Bhatnagar, & Sapolsky, 1988).

Plasticity: Prenatal Stress. On the other hand, severe prenatal stresses (delivered to mothers to a degree that affects placental hormones) are generally opposite those of handling. Prenatal stress of at least moderate severity *decreases* the number of hippocampal GR, decreases CRH in the paraventricular nucleus of the hypothalamus while increasing CRH in the central nucleus of the amygdala (one of the substrates of fear and anxiety), reduces endogenous opioid and GABA-ergic receptors, increases glucocorticoids (GC) in circulation, and ultimately leads to behavioral effects of attention deficits, hyperanxiety, and disturbed social behavior (Weinstock, 1997). Interestingly, the damaging effects of maternal stress on the fetus may be at least partially reversed by postnatal handling, suggesting that if such problem could be detected prior to the closing of the postnatal stress window, a clinical treatment could potentially be devised to mitigate the full impact of prenatal adversity.

Plasticity: Maternal Separation/Deviant Parenting. Brief separations of rat pups from their mothers activate the HPA in both offspring and parent, whereas reunion deactivates the response. An extended separation from mother, on the order of 8–24 hours in rats (Levine, 1994; Levine, Huchton, Wiener, & Rosenfeld, 1991), acutely elevates cortisol and appears to prime or sensitize the HPA to other stressors, as demonstrated by persistently exaggerated ACTH and cortisol responses to a variety of stressors. In nonhuman primates, incompetent parenting (such as peer-rearing rather than mother-rearing) results in lower levels of ACTH and cortisol, behavioral hyperactivity and increased instances of violence, and general dysregulation of brain neurochemistry and social behavior.

In humans, the acute effects of brief separation have been studied experimentally (Spangler & Grossman, 1993), and the effects of lengthier separation have been examined in naturally occurring situations. A recent review (Hennessy, 1997) concluded that the disruption of an affiliative relationship does not have uniform effects in all situations, and factors such as the quality of the preexisting attachment can moderate the response of the HPA (for an example of multifinality, see Cicchetti & Richters, 1993; Cicchetti & Rogosch, 1996). When human mothers briefly leave their children with babysitters who provide adequate but minimal response to child needs, moderate increases in cortisol have been reported (Gonzalez, Gunnar, & Levine, 1981; Larson, Gunnar, & Hertsgaard, 1991). When infant isolation or unresponsive parenting is prolonged, secure attachment cannot be achieved. The resulting abnormalities in affiliative capacity and in HPA function can be lifelong (Gunnar, Morison, Chisholm, & Schuder, 2001; Gunnar & Vazquez, 2001; Henry & Wang, 1998).

Abnormal attachment occurs across such diffferent syndromes as Separation Anxiety Disorder, autistic spectrum, and several personality disorders (e.g., dependent, schizoid personality, and antisocial). Little is known about how disrupted attachment develops in children who become psychopaths, and whether deviancies in parental behavior contribute to the development of psychopathy. A hallmark feature of psychopathy is the callous, unemotional objectification of other people, with diminished ability to form genuine attachments. Further investigation of individual differences in HPA response to separation from primary caretaker could potentially be an important means of understanding the roots and biological correlates of inability to attach.

Plasticity: Repeated Stress or Pharmacologic Stimulation. Experimental studies have demonstrated that long-lasting HPA sensitization can result from stressful stimuli or sustained drug exposure at different periods of development. Long-lasting sensitization is not uniformly observed across species and across experimental paradigms. When it does occur, the disruption of HPA feedback mechanisms results in failure to self-regulate or "suppress" endogenous production of GC following administration of an exogenous GC (e.g., dexamethasone). Other characteristics of stress-induced sensitization include increased self-administration of drugs, increased baseline HPA activity, and greater HPA responsiveness to new stressors (Deminiere et al., 1992; Haney, Maccari, Le Moal, Simon, & Piazza, 1995; Maccari et al., 1991).

Hypothetical Sources of Environmental Alteration of HPA in DBDs. Obviously, the effects of prolonged early stress cannot be examined experimentally in humans. However, we do know that children with DBDs have greater exposure to stressful conditions and poorer access to social buffers than children without such problems. Although we can only conclude that heightened exposure to stress is *correlated* with the development of DBDs, it is quite possible that causal mechanisms may account for some of these associations.

• Parents of DBD children are often in crisis (Loeber & Farrington, 2000; Loeber, Green, Lahey, Frick, & McBurnett, 2000). They have higher-than-average rates of police contacts, domestic violence, and substance abuse. They may be poor problem solvers, and often live in chaotic circumstances with frequent moves and job changes.

- Low socioeconomic status (SES) and multiple environmental stressors are more common in families of children with DBDs, especially CD, than in nonaffected families (Farrington, 1986). Children in lower SES environments are more likely to be exposed directly or vicariously to interpersonal violence.

- Mothers of children with DBDs have higher-than-average rates of depressive disorders (Nigg & Hinshaw, 1998). Prenatally, such problems in mothers may expose children to altered levels of stress hormones. Postnatally, maternal depression may reduce a mother's capacity of buffer her child's stress, as well as her capacity to provide a scaffold for her child to learn to self-regulate autonomic arousal.

- Children with DBDs (especially those with CD) are more likely to have been exposed to both illicit and legal drugs that affect the HPA, pre- and postnatally. Wakshlag et al. (1997) found that maternal smoking during pregnancy leads to increased incidence of CD in offspring, even when parental antisocial behavior and SES are controlled. Children with CD are more likely to live with parents who smoke, and thus to have lengthier exposure to the contents of second-hand smoke.

- Children with CD receive harsher physical punishment on a less consistent (hence more unpredictable) basis than other children (Patterson, Reid, & Dishion, 1992). The emotional tone of the family is likely to be hostile and pessimistic. This is partly because the child's deviant behavior leads to habitually coercive and conflictual parent-child interchanges (Hetherington & Martin, 1986).

- As children grow older and enter school, their attention and motivation deficits (and sometimes comorbid learning disabilities) make academic work more difficult than for the average unaffected student. They may internalize a negative self-worth, which becomes confirmed through low grades and disapproval from teachers.

- DBD children annoy others and break rules, incurring teacher punishment and peer rejection (Frick, 1998; Loeber & Farrington, 1998). Moreover, as adults' corrective statements and negative pronouncements go up, their rate of positive social interaction with children goes down (Barkley, 1998). Thus, not only does the behavior of children with CD elicit social stress, it also drives away the potential supports that might otherwise have buffered some of the effects of stress.

Knowing these correlates of DBDs, it is apparent that from the earliest point in development, the at-risk child may be exposed to more stress and fewer protective factors than is normal. It is plausible to hypothesize that such exposure increases the likelihood of permanently resetting HPA homeostasis, disrupting the normal adaptation to stress, and possibly contributing to the development of behavioral or emotional disorders.

EMPIRICAL STUDIES OF THE LOW CORTISOL–HIGH AGGRESSION LINK

This section discusses selected papers on the low cortisol–high aggression link. For the sake of focus, we omit papers that have not found this inverse relationship, but readers should be aware that there are several studies that have not found this pattern (see earlier discussion for citations of negative results and possible reasons for inconsistent findings).

through child physical abuse or exposure to community violence) may affect HPA-aggression relationships. In one study, salivary cortisol before and after a computerized provocation task was measured in nineteen clinic-referred children with disruptive behavior disorders (Scarpa, 1997; Scarpa & Kolko, 1996). The children were divided into reactors (i.e., those whose cortisol level increased after the computer provocation task) and nonreactors (i.e., those whose cortisol level remained the same or decreased after the task). Data on physical abuse history, cortisol reactivity, and staff reports of aggression were analyzed. The study found a statistical trend, suggesting that the highest rates of aggression were reported in children who had been abused and who meet the criteria for strong cortisol reaction.

Similar findings were obtained in a study of fifty-four university students who were selected from a screening sample based upon high and low scores on exposure to community violence (Scarpa, Fikretoglu, & K. A., 2000). Salivary cortisol was measured before and after a computerized stressor task. Results indicated that self-reported aggression was significantly associated with increased post-stressor cortisol. Follow-up analyses from this sample indicated that the significant cortisol-aggression link was found only in those who had been victims of violence, and not in subjects with no history of victimization (Scarpa, Bowser, Fikretoglu, Romero, & Wilson, 1999). Again, heightened HPA activity seemed related to increased risk for aggression only when coupled with a history of violent experiences.

On the other hand, King and colleagues (2001) compared young girls (ages 5–7) with documented abuse within the preceding two months to matched controls. The morning concentration of cortisol in saliva in the abused girls was less than half that of the nonabused girls. These findings do not contradict those reported by Scarpa, as there are obvious differences in the subjects' ages, the type and severity of traumatization, the use of baseline vs. reactivity paradigms, and in the intervening time between stress and cortisol measures. Moreover, the implication of Scarpa's work is that exposure to violence and aggression may interact in their influence on HPA activity.

A recent study addressed HPA function in relation to *type* of abuse and diurnal pattern (Cicchetti & Rogosch, 2001). Saliva samples were gathered at two different times of day from children attending a summer day camp. Children with a history of exposure to the widest variety of types of abuse (physical + sexual + neglect/emotional maltreatment) far exceeded children with fewer types of abuse (including those who had experienced physical but not sexual abuse and those who had experienced sexual but not physical abuse) in cortisol concentration both in the morning and in the afternoon. This difference was not accounted for by severity or developmental timing of abuse. Children who had experienced physical but not sexual abuse tended to show a restricted diurnal range, with lower cortisol in the morning and less of an afternoon decline in cortisol in the afternoon, compared to other groups.

ROLE OF HPA IN SUSCEPTIBILITY TO ADDICTION

There is considerable interest in how the HPA may be involved in the addictive process (King, Jones, Scheuer, Curtis, & Zarcone, 1990; Moss, Vanyukov, & Martin, 1995). Some studies suggest that activation of the HPA may be a mechanism that is involved in the development of addictive disorders. Pomerleau (Pomerleau, 1995; Pomerleau, Collins,

Shiffman, & Pomerleau, 1993; Pomerleau, Downey, Stelson, & Pomerleau, 1995) differentiated between the *exposure* model and the *sensitivity* model of addiction. The exposure model predicts that individuals who are initially sensitive to the aversive effects of nicotine may be discouraged from further use, but regardless of sensitivity, those individuals who continue to expose themselves to the drug will gradually develop dependence. The sensitivity model, on the other hand, assumes that (a) initial sensitivity to nicotine consists of *both* strongly aversive and strongly rewarding effects, and (b) repeated exposure rapidly induces physiological adaptation (tolerance) to the aversive effects, resulting in high-rate self-administration, and dependence. In this model, individual differences in susceptibility to addiction are related to the magnitude of physiological reactions (including that of the HPA axis) to a substance. In an unintended coincidence, sensitivity theory is also consistent with experimental findings that presentation of simultaneous cues for positive reinforcement and loss/punishment has a disinhibiting effect on antisocial individuals (Newman, 1987). Sensitivity theory is consistent with findings that high emotional reactivity is associated with higher rates and duration of drug use (Pandina, Johnson, & Labouvie, 1992), that neuroticism (strong reactivity to both positive and negative stimuli) is associated with risk for nicotine dependence (Gilbert, 1995; Gilbert & Gilbert, 1995), and that the highest risk for addiction is the cluster of "emotional/behavioral arousal, self-regulation difficulties, impulsivity, and hyperactivity/attention deficit disorder" (Glantz & Pickens, 1992). However, sensitivity theory is difficult to reconcile with other findings. Moss et al. (1995) selected high-risk boys on the basis of paternal psychoactive substance use disorder (PSUD) and found them to be hyporesponsive in anticipation of a stressful task. The association of paternal PSUD with low cortisol responsivity was entirely mediated by the boys' aggression and impulsivity, a finding more consistent with the chronic aggressive-low cortisol reactivity findings cited above. This points out the inadequacy of a single general theory to account for all varieties of substance abuse and antisocial behavior.

Glucocorticoid Response as a Mechanism of Reward. The classic neural substrate of reward is dopaminergic activity in the ventral tegmentum. New attention is being given to the participation of glucocorticoid receptors (GRs) in neural reward. GCs have relatively low affinity for GRs and tend not to bind to them unless HPA activation is sufficient to sharply raise the level of GC in circulation. GR occupation subsequently affects midbrain dopaminergic neurons. Careful programmatic research has demonstrated that GCs meet all of the conditions for a reward substrate (Piazza et al., 1993; Piazza & Le Moal, 1997). Animals will work to obtain exogenous infusion of corticosteroid, and will adjust their responding to maintain plasma levels in the upper physiological range (Weeks, 1962). The reward effect is dependent on physiological state and on corticosteroid "dose" (Piazza et al., 1996). GC secretion is increased by a variety of consummatory behaviors, natural reinforcers, and drugs of abuse (Caggiula et al., 1991). If human individual differences in GCs are a behaviorally important substrate of reward, or if state differences in HPA status moderate the response of midbrain reward centers and signals of available reinforcers, then these mechanisms would have profound explanatory value for understanding major DBD characteristics such as impulsivity, distractibility, inability to persevere on-task, proneness for risk-taking/thrill-seeking, and proneness to substance abuse.

FUTURE DIRECTIONS

There are many directions that future research can delve into the role of the HPA in the development of aggression, antisocial behavior, and substance abuse. For example:

- Knowing how cortisol levels vary as a function of bully and victim status would add to our understanding of the motivation and adverse effects of these social roles.

- Learning the time course of social outcomes and HPA activation would help clarify whether abnormal HPA activity is a contributor or a consequence of social successes and failures.

- Behavioral genetic decomposition of HPA activity into inherited and environmental components would help to determine how susceptible the HPA is to being reset by early environment. As discussed throughout this chapter, genetic influences on HPA function are modifiable by experience, but we do not know the extent to which this occurs in the natural course of development. Neither do we know much about gene-environment interaction questions, such as why some children exposed to deprivation or prolonged stress do not develop HPA abnormalities. Such understanding would have direct implications for prevention and childcare practices.

- By measuring the initial reactivity of children's HPA to a substance and then following them over several years, it would be possible to test the reactivity hypothesis (whether the intensity of the initial HPA response is a risk factor for progression to addiction). Longitudinal research is also needed to inform us of the outcomes of infants and children exposed to HPA-altering levels of stress.

- Studying the interaction of key personality variables (e.g., sensation-seeking) with cortisol reactivity to novel stimuli could provide a way to validate behavioral measures of personality traits (Davis et al., 1999; de Haan, Gunnar, Tout, Hart, & Stansbury, 1998; Rosenblitt, Soler, Johnson, & Quadagno, 2001; Wang et al., 1997). It could also lead to insights into how novelty is reinforcing to sensation-seekers.

- Although it is widely assumed that most of the population experiences the classic diurnal cycle of higher cortisol around awakening and lower cortisol around bedtime, this is simply a group average and many individuals do not show this pattern. It may be possible to link individual differences in the diurnal cortisol cycle (Boyce, Champoux, Suomi, & Gunnar, 1995) to such various behavioral patterns as sleep dysfunction (Born & Fehm, 1998), nocturnal behavioral activation (which seems to characterize at least some antisocial individuals), and poor academic or other cognitive performance at certain times of the day (Adam & Gunnar, 2001; Chapotot, Gronfier, Jouny, Muzet, & Brandenberger, 1998).

- The type of stressor that triggers cortisol release in a given individual is not well understood. The widely used stressor of simulated or actual public speaking is believed to probe for anxiety. However, in some research areas related to antisocial development, the more precise variable of interest is behavioral inhibition or harm avoidance. These variables are not perfectly correlated with social anxiety and may or may not be reflected by cortisol response to a social stressor.

- Studying the relationship between HPA function and other autonomic behaviors that are known to be related to psychopathy (SNS variables, startle reflex, etc.) could lead to the empirical derivation of a psychopathic endotype. Such an achievement would significantly help in validating and understanding the development of psychopathy and other antisocial patterns.

- New pharmacological therapies for abnormal HPA reactivity are under development. The hope is that medications that inhibit certain levels of the HPA (in particular, CRH release) will be proven to be safe and effective for managing internalizing disorders. But if research in this area continues, then medications that affect HPA function may eventually find applications in the treatment of some types of violent and temperamental behavior problems, or in the management or prevention of substance abuse and behavioral addictions (Frederick et al., 1998).

REFERENCES

Adam, E. K., & Gunnar, M. R. (2001). Relationship functioning and home and work demands predict individual differences in diurnal cortisol patterns in women. *Psychoneuroendocrinology, 26*(2), 189–208.

Aguilar, B., Sroufe, L. A., Egeland, B., & Carlson, E. (2000). Distinguishing the early-onset/persistent and adolescence-onset antisocial behavior types: From birth to 16 years. *Development and Psychopathology, 12*(2), 109–132.

Atkins, M. S., Osborne, M. L., Bennett, D. S., Hess, L. E., & Halperin, J. M. (2001). Children's competitive peer aggression during reward and punishment. *Aggressive Behavior, 27*(1), 1–13.

Banks, T., & Dabbs, J. M., Jr. (1996). Salivary testosterone and cortisol in a delinquent and violent urban subculture. *Journal of Social Psychology, 136*(1), 49–56.

Barkley, R. A. (1998). *Attention-deficit hyperactivity disorder: A handbook for diagnosis and treatment* (2d ed.). New York: Guilford Press.

Benus, R. F., Bohus, B., Koolhass, J. M., & van Oortmerssen, G. A. (1989). Behavioral strategies of aggressive and non-aggressive male mice in active avoidance. *Behavioral Processes, 20*, 1–12.

Benus, R. F., Bohus, B., Koolhaas, J. M., & van Oortmerssen, G. A. (1991). Heritable variation for aggression as a reflection of individual coping strategies. *Experientia, 47*, 1008–1019.

Born, J., & Fehm, H. L. (1998). Hypothalamus-pituitary-adrenal activity during human sleep: a coordinating role for the limbic hippocampal system. *Experimental and Clinical Endocrinology and Diabetes, 106*(3), 153–163.

Boyce, W. T., Champoux, M., Suomi, S. J., & Gunnar, M. R. (1995). Salivary cortisol in nursery-reared rhesus monkeys: Reactivity to peer interactions and altered circadian activity. *Developmental Psychobiology, 28*(5), 257–267.

Bremner, J. D., & Narayan, M. (1998). The effects of stress on memory and the hippocampus throughout the life cycle: implications for childhood development and aging. *Development and Psychopathology, 10*(4), 871–885.

Caggiula, A. R., Epstein, L. H., Antelman, S. M., Saylor, S. S., Perkins, S., Knopf, S., & Stiller, R. (1991). Conditioned tolerance to the anorectic and corticosterone-elevating effects of nicotine. *Pharmacology, Biochemistry and Behavior, 40*, 53–59.

Cannon, W. B. (1932). *The wisdom of the body*. New York: W. W. Norton.

Chapotot, F., Gronfier, C., Jouny, C., Muzet, A., & Brandenberger, G. (1998). Cortisol secretion is related to electroencephalographic alertness in human subjects during daytime wakefulness. *Journal of Clinical Endocrinology and Metabolism, 83*(12), 4263–4268.

Cicchetti, D., & Richters, J. E. (1993). Developmental considerations in the investigation of conduct disorder. *Development and Psychopathology, 5*(1–2), 331–344.

Cicchetti, D., & Rogosch, F. A. (1996). Equifinality and multifinality in developmental psychopathology. *Development and Psychopathology, 8*(4), 597–600.

Cicchetti, D., & Rogosch, F. A. (2001). Diverse patterns of neuroendocrine activity in maltreated children. *Development and Psychopathology, 13*(3), 677–693.

Davis, E. P., Donzella, B., Krueger, W. K., & Gunnar, M. R. (1999). The start of a new school year: individual differences in salivary cortisol response in relation to child temperament. *Developmental Psychobiology, 35*(3), 188–196.

de Haan, M., Gunnar, M. R., Tout, K., Hart, J., & Stansbury, K. (1998). Familiar and novel contexts yield different associations between cortisol and behavior among 2-year-old children. *Developmental Psychobiology, 33*(1), 93–101.

de Kloet, E. R., Korte, S. M., Rots, N. Y., & Kruk, M. R. (1996). Stress hormones, genotype, and brain organization: Implications for aggression. *Annals of the New York Academy of Sciences, 52*, 179–181.

Deminiere, J. M., Piazza, P. V., Guegan, G., Abrous, N., Maccari, S., Le Moal, M., & Simon, H. (1992). Increased locomotor response to novelty and propensity to intravenous self-administration in adult offspring of stressed mothers. *Brain Research, 586*, 135–139.

Farrington, D. P. (1986). The sociocultural context of child disorders. In H. C. Quay & J. S. Werry (Eds.), *Psychopathological disorders of childhood*, 3rd ed. (pp. 391–422). New York: Wiley.

Fischer, R., & Agnew, N. (1957). Addendum to a hierarchy of stressors. *Journal of Mental Science, 103*, 858–859.

Frances, D., Diorio, J., LaPlante, P., Weaver, S., Seckl, J. R., & Meany, M. J. (1996). The role of early environmental events in regulating neuroendocrine development. *Annals of the New York Academy of Sciences, 794*, 136–152.

Frederick, S. L., Reus, V. I., Ginsberg, D., Hall, S. M., Munoz, R. F., & Ellman, G. (1998). Cortisol and response to dexamethasone as predictors of withdrawal distress and abstinence success in smokers. *Biological Psychiatry, 43*(7), 525–530.

Frick, P. J. (1998). *Conduct disorders and severe antisocial behavior.* New York: Plenum.

Gilbert, D. G. (1995). *Smoking: Individual differences, psychopathology, and emotion.* Washington, D.C.: Taylor & Francis.

Gilbert, D. G., & Gilbert, B. O. (1995). Personality, psychopathology, and nicotine response as mediators of the genetics of smoking. *Behavior Genetics, 25*, 133–147.

Glantz, M. D., & Pickens, R. W. (1992). Vulnerability to drug abuse: Introduction and overview. In M. Glantz & R. Pickens (Eds.), *Vulnerability to drug abuse.* Washington, D.C.: American Psychological Association.

Goldstein, W. L. B. (2000). *The relationship among the symptoms associated with AD/HD subtypes and sociometric status among peers. (attention deficit hyperactivity disorder).* New York: Hofstra University.

Gonzalez, C. A., Gunnar, M. R., & Levine, S. (1981). Behavioral and hormonal responses to social disruption and infant stimuli in female rhesus monkeys. *Psychoneuroendocrinology, 6*(1), 53–64.

Granger, D., Stansbury, K., & Henker, B. (1994). Preschoolers' behavioral and neuroendocrine responses to social challenge. *Merrill-Palmer Quarterly, 40*(2), 190–211.

Gunnar, M. R., Morison, S. J., Chisholm, K., & Schuder, M. (2001). Salivary cortisol levels in children adopted from Romanian orphanages. *Development and Psychopathology, 13*(3), 611–628.

Gunnar, M. R., Tout, K., de Haan, M., Pierce, S., & Stansbury, K. (1997). Temperament, social competence, and adrenocortical activity in preschoolers. *Developmental Psychobiology, 31*(1), 65–85.

Gunnar, M. R., & Vazquez, D. M. (2001). Low cortisol and a flattening of expected daytime rhythm: Potential indices of risk in human development. *Development and Psychopathology, 13*(3), 515–538.

Hadley, M. E. (2000). *Endocrinology* (5th ed.). Upper Saddle River, N.J.: Prentice Hall.

Haney, M., Maccari, S., Le Moal, M., Simon, H., & Piazza, P. V. (1995). Social stress increases the acquisition of cocaine self-administration in male and female rats. *Brain Research, 698*, 46–52.

Hennessy, M. B. (1997). HPA responses to brief social separation. *Neuroscience and Biobehavioral Reviews, 21*(1), 11–29.

Henry, J. P., & Wang, S. (1998). Effects of early stress on adult affiliative behavior. *Psychoneuroendocrinology, 23*, 863–875.

Hetherington, E. M., & Martin, B. (1986). Family factors and psychopathology in children. In H. C. Quay & J. S. Werry (Eds.), *Psychopathological disorders of childhood*, 3rd ed. (pp. 332–390). New York: Wiley.

Hinshaw, S. P., Lahey, B. B., & Hart E. L. (1993). Issues of taxonomy and comorbidity in the development of conduct disorder. *Development and Psychopathology, 5*(1–2), 31–49.

Holsboer, F. (2001). Stress, hypercortisolism and corticosteroid receptors in depression: Implications for therapy. *Journal of Affective Disorders, 62*(1–2).

King, J. A., Abend, S., and Edwards, E. (2001). Genetic predisposition and the development of posttraumatic stress disorder in an animal model. *Biological Psychiatry, 50*(4), 231–237.

King, J. A., Barkley, R. A., & Barrett, S. (1998). Attention-deficit hyperactivity disorder and the stress response. *Biological Psychiatry, 44*(1), 72–74.

King, J. A., & Edwards, E. (1999). Early stress and genetic influences on hypothalamic-pituitary-adrenal axis functioning in adulthood. *Hormones and Behavior, 36*(2), 79–85.

King, R. J., Jones, J., Scheuer, J. W., Curtis, D., & Zarcone, V. P. (1990). Plasma cortisol correlates of impulsivity and suubstance abuse. *Personality and Individual Differences, 11*(3), 287–291.

King, J. A., Mandansky, D., King, S., Fletcher, K. E., and Brewer, J. (2001). Early sexual abuse and low cortisol. *Psychiatry and Clinical Neurosciences, 55*(1), 71–74.

Kruesi, M. J., Schmidt, M. E., Donnelly, M., Euthymia, D., et al. (1989). Urinary free cortisol output and disruptive behavior in children. *Journal of the American Academy of Child and Adolescent Psychiatry, 28*(3), 441–443.

Lahey, B. B., Applegate, B., Barkley, R. A., Garfinkel, B., McBurnett, K., Kerdyk, L., Greenhill, L., Hynd, G. W., Frick, P. J., Newcorn, J., Biederman, J., Ollendick, T., Hart, E. L., Perez, D., Waldman, I., & Shaffer, D. (1994). DSM-IV Field Trials for Oppositional Defiant Disorder and Conduct Disorder in children and adolescents. *American Journal of Psychiatry, 151*(8), 1163–1171.

Lahey, B. B., Applegate, B., McBurnett, K., Biederman, J., Greenhill, L., Hynd, G. W., Barkley, R. A., Newcorn, J., Jensen, P., Richters, J., Garfinkel, B., Kerdyk, L., Frick, P. J., Ollendick, T., Perez, D., Hart, E. L., Waldman, I., & Shaffer, D. (1994). DSM-IV Field Trials for Attention Deficit Hyperactivity Disorder in children and adolescents. *American Journal of Psychiatry, 151*(11), 1673–1685.

Lahey, B. B., Hart, E. L., Pliszka, S., Applegate, B., & McBurnett, K. (1993). Neurophysiological correlates of conduct disorder: A rationale and a review of research. *Journal of Clinical Child Psychology, 22*(2), 141–153.

Lahey, B. B., Loeber, R., Hart, E., Frick, P. J., Applegate, B., Zhang, Q., Green, S., & Russo, M. F. (1995). Four-year longitudinal study of conduct disorders in boys: Patterns and predictors of persistence. *Journal of Abnormal Psychology, 104*, 83–93.

Larson, M. C., Gunnar, M. R., & Hertsgaard, L. (1991). The effects of morning naps, car trips, and maternal separation on adrenocortical activity in human infants. *Child Development, 62*(2), 362–372.

Levine, S. (1994). The ontogeny of the HPA axis: The influence of maternal factors. *Annals of the New York Academy of Sciences, 746*, 275–288.

Levine, S., Huchton, S. D., Wiener, S. G., & Rosenfeld, P. (1991). Time course of the effect of maternal deprivation on the HPA axis in the infant rat. *Developmental Psychobiology* (24), 547–558.

Levine, S., & Lewis, G. W. (1958). The relative importance of experimenter contact in an effect produced by extrastimulation in infancy. *Journal of Comparative Physiological Psychology, 52*, 368–369.

Loeber, R., & Farrington, D. P. (Eds.). (1998). *Serious and violent juvenile offenders: Risk factors and successful interventions*. Thousand Oaks, Calif.: Sage Publication.

Loeber, R., & Farrington, D. P. (2000). Young children who commit crime: Epidemiology, developmental origins, risk factors, early interventions, and policy implications. *Development and Psychopathology, 12*(4), 737–762.

Loeber, R., Green, S. M., Lahey, B. B., Frick, P. J., & McBurnett, K. (2000). Findings on disruptive behavior disorders from the first decade of the Developmental Trends Study. *Clinical Child and Family Psychology Review, 3*(1), 37–60.

Lopez, J. F., Akil, H., & Watson, S. J. (1999). Neural circuits mediating stress. *Biological Psychiatry, 46*(11), 1461–1471.

Luecken, L. J. (1998). Childhood attachment and loss experiences affect adult cardiovascular and cortisol function. *Psychosomatic Medicine, 60*(6), 765–772.

Maccari, S., Piazza, P. V., Deminiere, J. M., Lemaire, V., Mormede, P., Simon, H., Angelucci, L., & Le Moal, M. (1991). Life events-induced decrease of type I corticosteroid receptors is associated with a decrease of corticosterone feedback and an increase of the vulnerability to amphetamine self-administration. *Brain Research, 547*, 7–12.

McBurnett, K. (1992). Psychobiological theories of personality and their application to child psychopathology. In B. B. Lahey & A. Kazdin (Eds.), *Advanced in child clinical psychology* (Vol. 14, pp. 107–164). New York: Plenum.

McBurnett, K., Kumar, A. M., Kumar, M., Perez, D., Lahey, B. B., & Shaw, J. A. (2000). Aggression, anxiety, and salivary cortisol in child psychiatry inpatients. *Biological Psychiatry (Supplement), 47* 150S–151S.

McBurnett, K., & Lahey, B. (1994). Psychophysiological and neuroendocrine correlates of conduct disorder and antisocial behavior in children and adolescents. In D. C. Fowles, P. Sutker, & S. Goodman (Eds.), *Progress in experimental personality and psychopathology research* (pp. 199–232). New York: Springer.

McBurnett, K., Lahey, B. B., Capasso, L., & Loeber, R. (1996). Aggressive symptoms and salivary cortisol in clinic-referred boys with Conduct Disorder. *Annals of the New York Academy of Sciences, 794* (Sept. 20: Understanding Aggressive Behavior in Children), 169–179.

McBurnett, K., Lahey, B. B., Frick, P. J., Hart, E. L., Christ, M. A. G., & Loeber, R. (1990). *Association of cortisol with peer nominations of popularity, aggression, and social inhibition in clinic-referred children.* Paper presented at the 24th annual meeting of the Association for the Advancement of Behavior Therapy, San Francisco.

McBurnett, K., Lahey, B. B., Frick, P. F., Risch, S. C., Loeber, R., Hart, E. L., Christ, M. A. G., & Hanson, K. S. (1991). Anxiety, inhibition, and conduct disorder in children: II. Relation to salivary cortisol. *Journal of the American Academy of Child and Adolescent Psychiatry, 30*, 192–196.

McBurnett, K., Lahey, B. B., Rathouz, P. J., & Loeber, R. (2000). Low salivary cortisol and persistent aggression in boys referred for disruptive behavior. *Archives of General Psychiatry, 57*(1), 38–43.

Meaney, M. J., Aitken, D. H., Bhatnagar, S., & Sapolsky, R. M. (1991). Postnatal handling attenuates certain neuroendocrine, anatomical, and cognitive dysfunctions associated with aging in female rats. *Neurobiol Aging, 12*(1), 31–38.

Meany, M. J., Aitken, D. H., Bodnoff, S. R., Ing, C. J., Tatarewicz, J. E., & Sapolsky, R. M. (1995). Early postnatal handling alters glucocorticoid postnatal handling in selected brain regions. *Behavioral Neuroscience, 99*, 765–770.

Meaney, M. J., Aitken, D. H., Bodnoff, S. R., Iny, L. J., & Sapolsky, R. M. (1985). The effects of postnatal handling on the development of the glucocorticoid receptor systems and stress recovery in the rat. *Progress in Neuropsychopharmacology and Biological Psychiatry, 9*(5–6), 731–734.

Meaney, M. J., Aitken, D. H., Bodnoff, S. R., Iny, L. J., Tatarewicz, J. E., & Sapolsky, R. M. (1985). Early postnatal handling alters glucocorticoid receptor concentrations in selected brain regions. *Behavioral Neuroscience, 99*(4), 765–770.

Meaney, M. J., Aitken, D. H., van Berkel, C., Bhatnagar, S., & Sapolsky, R. M. (1988). Effect of neonatal handling on age-related impairments associated with the hippocampus. *Science, 239* (4841 Pt 1), 766–768.

Moffitt, T. E. (1993). Adolescence-limited and life-course-persistent antisocial behavior: A developmental taxonomy. *Psychological Review, 100*, 674–701.

Moffitt, T. E., & Caspi, A. (2001). Childhood predictors differentiate life-course persistent and adolescence-limited antisocial pathways among males and females. *Development & Psychopathology, 13*(2), 355–375.

Moss, H. B., Vanyukov, M. M., & Martin, C. S. (1995). Salivary cortisol responses and the risk for substance abuse in prepubertal boys. *Biological Psychiatry, 38*, 547–555.

Nelson, R. J. (1995). *An introduction to behavioral endocrinology.* Sunderland, Mass.: Sinauer Associates.

Newman, J. P. (1987). Reaction to punishment in extraverts and psychopaths: Implications for the impulsive behavior of disinhibited individuals. *Journal of Research in Personality, 21*, 464–480.

Nigg, J. T., & Hinshaw, S. P. (1998). Parent personality traits and psychopathology associated with antisocial behaviors in childhood attention-deficit hyperactivity disorder. *Journal of Child Psychology and Psychiatry and Allied Disciplines, 39*(2), 145–159.

Pajer, K., Gardner, W., Rubin, R. T., Perel, J., & Neal, S. (2001). Decreased cortisol levels in adolescent girls with conduct disorder. *Archives of General Psychiatry, 58*(3), 297–302.

Pandina, R. J., Johnson, V., & Labouvie, E. W. (1992). Affectivity: A central mechanism in the development of drug dependence. In M. Glantz & R. Pickens (Eds.), *Vulnerability to drug abuse* (pp. 179–209). Washington, DC: American Psychological Association.

Patterson, G. R., Reid, J. B., & Dishion, T. J. (1992). *Antisocial boys*. Eugene, Ore.: Castalia Publishing.

Piazza, P. V., Deroche, V., Deminiere, J. M., Maccari, S., Le Moal, M., & Simon, H. (1993). Reinforcing properties of corticosterone demonstrated by intravenous self-administration: Possible biological basis of sensation-seeking. *Proceedings of the National Academy of Sciences, 90*, 11738–11742.

Piazza, P. V., & Le Moal, M. (1997). Glucocorticoids as a biological substrate of reward: Physiological and pathophysiological implications. *Brain Research Reviews, 25*, 359–372.

Piazza, P. V., Rouge-Pont, F., Deroche, V., Maccari, S., Simon, S., & Le Moal, M. (1996). Glucocorticoids have state dependent stimulant effects on the mesencephalic dopaminergic transmission. *Proceedings of the National Academy of Sciences, 93*, 8716–8720.

Pomerleau, O. F. (1995). Individual differences in sensitivity to nicotine: Implications for genetic research on nicotine dependence. *Behavior Genetics, 25*(2), 161–177.

Pomerleau, O. F., Collins, A. C., Shiffman, S., & Pomerleau, C. S. (1993). Why some people smoke and others do not: New perspectives. *Journal of Consulting and Clinical Psychology, 61* 723–731.

Pomerleau, O. F., Downey, K. K., Stelson, F. W., & Pomerleau, C. S. (1995). Cigarette smoking in adult patients diagnosed with attention deficit hyperactivity disorder. *Journal of Substance Abuse, 7*(3), 373–378.

Pottinger, T. G., & Carrick, T. R. (2001). Stress responsiveness affects dominant-subordinate relationships in rainbow trout. *Hormones and Behavior, 40*(3), 419–427.

Poulin, F., & Boivin, M. (2000). Reactive and proactive aggression: Evidence of a two-factor model. *Pschological Assessment, 12*(2), 115–122.

Pruessner, J. C., Gaab, J., Hellhammer, D. H., Lintz, D., Schommer, N., & Kirschbaum, C. (1997). Increasing correlations between personality traits and cortisol stress responses obtained by data aggregation. *Psychoneuroendocrinology, 22*(8), 615–625.

Rosenblitt, J. C., Soler, H., Johnson, S. E., & Quadagno, D. M. (2001). Sensation seeking and hormones in men and women: Exploring the link. *Homones and Behavior, 40*(3), 396–402.

Sapolsky, R. M. (1982). The endocrine stress-response and socail status in the wild baboon. *Hormones and Behavior, 16*(3), 279–292.

Sapolsky, R. M. (1989). Hypercortisolism among socially subordinate wild baboons originates at the CNS level. *Archives of General Psychiatry, 46*(11), 1047–1051.

Sapolsky, R. M. (1990). A. E. Bennett Award paper. Adrenocortical function, social rank, and personality among wild baboons. *Biological Psychiatry, 28*(10), 862–878.

Sapolsky, R. M. (1992). Cortisol concentrations and the social significance of rank instability among wild baboons. *Psychoneuroendocrinology, 17*(6), 701–709.

Sapolsky, R. M. (1995). Social subordinance as a marker of hypercortisolism. Some unexpected subtleties. *Annals of the New York Academy of Sciences, 771*, 626–639.

Sapolsky, R. M. (1996). Why stress is bad for your brain. *Science, 273*(5276), 749–750.

Sapolsky, R. M. (1997). The importance of a well-groomed child. *Science, 277*, 1620–1621.

Sapolsky, R. M., Romero, L. M., & Munck, A. U. (2000). How do glucocorticoids influence stress responses? Integrating permissive, suppressive, stimulatory, and preparative actions. *Endocrine Reviews, 21*(1), 55–89.

Scarpa, A. (1997). Aggression in physically abused children: The interactive role of emotion regulation. In A. Raine, P. A. Brennan, D. P. Farrington, & S. A. Mednick (Eds.), *Biosocial bases of violence* (pp. 341–343). New York: Plenum.

Scarpa, A., Bowser, F. M., Fikretoglu, D., Romero, N., & Wilson, J. W. (1999). Effects of community violence II: Interactions with psychophysiologica functioning. *Psychophysiology (Supplement), 36*, 102.

Scarpa, A., Fikretoglu, D., & K. A., L. (2000). Community violence exposure in a young adult sample: II. Psychophysiology and aggressive behavior. *Journal of Community Psychology, 28*, 417–425.

Scarpa, A., Friedman, B. H., Smalley, K. J., & Luscher, K. A. (1997). Physiological reactivity moderates stress-induced mood. *Psychophysiology (Supplement), 34*, 78.

Scarpa, A., & Kolko, D. J. (1996). Aggression in physically abused children. The role of distress proneness. *Annals of the New York Academy of Sciences, 794*, 405–407.

Scarpa, A., & Raine, A. (1997). Psychophysiology of anger and violent behavior. *Psychiatric Clinics of North America, 20*(2), 375–394.

Scerbo, A. S., & Kolko, D. J. (1994). Salivary testosterone and cortisol in disruptive children: relationship to aggressive, hyperactive, and internalizing behaviors. *Journal of the American Academy of Child and Adolescent Psychiatry, 33*(8), 1174–1184.

Scerbo, A. S., & Kolko, D. J. (1995). Child physical abuse and aggression: preliminary findings on the role of internalizing problem. *J Am Acad Child Adolesc Psychiatry, 34*(8), 1060–1066.

Schulkin, J. (1999). *The neuroendocrine regulation of behavior.* New York: Cambridge University Press.

Schulz, K. P., Halperin, J. M., Newcorn, J. H., Sharma, V., & Gabriel, S. (1997). Plasma cortisol and aggression in boys with ADHD. *Journal of the American Academy of Child and Adolescent Psychiatry, 36*(5), 605–609.

Selye, H. (1952). *The story of the adaptation syndrome.* Montreal: Acta.

Selye, H. (1978). *The stress of life.* (rev. ed). New York: McGraw-Hill.

Spangler, G., & Grossman, K. E. (1993). Biobehavioral organization in securely and insecurely attached infants. *Child Development, 64,* 1439–1450.

Suarez, E. C., Kuhn, C. M., Schanberg, S. M., Williams, R. B., Jr., & Zimmermann, E. A. (1998). Neuroendocrine, cardiovascular, and emotional responses of hostile men: the role of interpersonal challenge. *Psychosom Med, 60*(1), 78–88.

Susman, E. J., Nottelmann, E. D., Dorn, L. D., Inoff-Germain, G., & Chrousos, G. P. (1988). Physiological and behavioral aspects of stress in adolescence. *Advances in Experimental Medicine and Biology, 245,* 341–352.

Targum, S. D., Clarkson, L. L., Magac-Harris, K., Marshall, L. E., & Skwerer, R. G. (1990). Measurement of cortisol and lymphocyte subpopulations in depressed and conduct-disordered adolescents. *Journal of Affective Disorders, 18,* 91–96.

Tennes, K., & Kreye, M. (1985). Children's adrenocortical responses to classroom activities and tests in elementary school. *Psychosomatic Medicine, 47*(5), 451–460.

Tennes, K., Kreye, M., Avitable, N., & Wells, R. (1986). Behavioral correlates of excreted catecholamines and cortisol in second-grade children. *Journal of the American Academy of Child and Adolescent Psychiatry, 25*(6), 764–770.

van Goozen, S. H., Matthys, W., Cohen-Kettenis, P. T., Gispen-de Wied, C., Wiegant, V. M., & van Engeland, H. (1998). Salivary cortisol and cardiovascular activity during stress in oppositional-defiant disorder boys and normal controls. *Biological Psychiatry, 43*(7), 531–539.

Vanyukov, M. M., Moss, H. B., Plail, J. A., Blackson, T., Mezzich, A. C., & Tarter, R. E. (1993). Antisocial symptoms in preadolescent boys and in their parents: Associations with cortisol. *Psychiatry Research, 46,* 9–17.

Virkkunen, M. (1985). Urinary free cortisol secretion in habitually violent offenders. *Acta Psychiatrica Scandinavica, 72*(1), 40–44.

Wakschlag, L. S., Lahey, B. B., Loeber, R., Green, S. M., Gordon, R. A., & Leventhal, B. L. (1997). Maternal smoking during pregnancy and the risk of conduct disorder in boys. *Archives of General Psychiatry, 54*(7), 670–676.

Walker, J. L., Lahey, B. B., Russo, M., Frick, P. J., Christ, M. A. G., McBurnett, K., Loeber, R., Stouthamer-Loeber, M., & Green, S. (1991). Anxiety, inhibition, and conduct disorder in children: I. Relations to social impairment and sensation seeking. *Journal of the American Academy of Child and Adolescent Psychiatry, 30,* 187–191.

Wang, S., Mason, J., Charney, D., Yehuda, R., Riney, S., & Southwick, S. (1997). Relationships between hormonal profile and novelty seeking in combat-related posttraumatic stress disorder. *Biological Psychiatry, 41*(2), 145–151.

Weeks, J. R. (1962). Experimental morphine addiction: Method for automatic intravenous injections in unrestrained rats. *Science, 138,* 143–144.

Weinstock, M. (1997). Does prenatal stress impair coping and regulation of HPA axis? *Neuroscience and Biobehavioral Reviews, 21*(1), 1–10.

Wilder, J. (1957). The law of initial value in neurology and psychiatry. *Journal of Nervous and Mental Disease, 125,* 73–86.

Wilens, T. E., Biederman, J., Mick, E., Faraone, S. V., & Spencer, T. (1997). Attention Deficit Hyperactivity Disorder (ADHD) is associated with early onset substance use disorders. *Journal of Nervous and Mental Disease, 185*(8), 475–482.

FOURTEEN

Neuroendocrine Functioning in Maltreated Children

Dante Cicchetti

Cicchetti and Lynch (1995) asserted that child maltreatment may represent the greatest failure of the caregiving environment to provide many of the expectable experiences that are necessary to facilitate normal developmental processes. Maltreating parents also may be viewed as an aberration of the supportive, nurturant, sensitive, and protective adults that are expected by children in the evolutionary context of species-typical development (Belsky, 1984; Cicchetti & Lynch, 1995; Howes, Cicchetti, Toth, & Rogosch, 2000; Rogosch, Cicchetti, Shields, & Toth, 1995).

In contrast to what is anticipated in response to an average expectable environment, the ecological, social, biological, and psychological conditions that are associated with maltreatment set in motion a probabilistic path of epigenesis for maltreated children characterized by an increased likelihood of failure and disruption in the successful resolution of major stage-salient tasks of development, resulting in grave implications for functioning across the lifespan (Cicchetti, 1989; Cicchetti & Lynch, 1993; Egeland, 1997; Malinosky-Rummell & Hansen, 1993). These repeated developmental disruptions create a profile of relatively enduring vulnerability factors that increase the probability of the emergence of maladaptation and psychopathology as negative transactions between the child and the environment continue (Cicchetti & Lynch, 1993; Cicchetti & Rizley, 1981).

The notion that an average expectable environment is required for species-typical development suggests that competent outcomes in maltreated children should be highly improbable due to wide-ranging disturbances in the maltreatment ecology (Cicchetti & Lynch, 1993). Nonetheless, despite the fact that there is documented risk for maladaptation associated with maltreatment, the absence of a caregiving environment that provides opportunities for normal development does not necessarily condemn all maltreated children to negative developmental outcomes (Cicchetti & Rogosch, 1997; McGloin & Widom, 2001).

Although not all maltreated children exhibit maladaptive development and psychopathology, disturbances in their functioning are likely to emerge over the course of epigenesis. Specifically, maltreated children and adolescents have evidenced a wide

Work reported in this chapter was supported, in part, by grants from the William T. Grant Foundation, the Office of Child Abuse and Neglect, and the Spunk Fund.

range of disturbances and mental disorders, including clinical levels of internalizing and externalizing symptomatology, as well as higher rates of depression and anxiety disorders, conduct disorder and delinquency, and posttraumatic stress disorder (PTSD) (Cohen, Brown, & Smailes, 2001; De Bellis & Putnam, 1994; Famularo, Kinscherff, & Fenton, 1992; Pynoos, Steinberg, & Wraith, 1995; Shields & Cicchetti, 1998; Smith & Thornberry, 1995; Widom, 1989).

Until the past decade, scientific research conducted on the consequences of child maltreatment focused almost exclusively on psychological processes and outcomes (Cicchetti & Toth, 1995; Cicchetti & Toth, 2000; Trickett & McBride-Chang, 1995). These studies have revealed that child maltreatment exerts harmful effects on cognitive, social, emotional, representational, and linguistic development (Cicchetti, 1990; Cicchetti & Lynch, 1995), as well as disrupts the development of emotion regulation, secure attachment relationships, an autonomous sense of self, effective peer relations, and successful adaptation to school (Barnett, Ganiban, & Cicchetti, 1999; Bolger, Patterson, & Kupersmidt, 1998; Carlson, Cicchetti, Barnett, & Braunwald, 1989; Cicchetti, 1991; Shields, Cicchetti, & Ryan, 1994; Shonk & Cicchetti, 2001; Toth, Cicchetti, Macfie, & Emde, 1997).

During the past decade, research on the biological impact of child maltreatment has begun to receive more emphasis from researchers (De Bellis, 2001; De Bellis & Putnam, 1994). The examination of the neurobiological correlates and sequelae of child maltreatment holds great promise for enhancing the understanding of the mechanisms underlying maladaptive development in maltreated children.

A major impetus for the growing attention paid to the physiological impact of child maltreatment has been the empirical discoveries, theoretical influences, and technological advances in the study of brain-behavior relations (Cicchetti & Cannon, 1999; Nelson & Bloom, 1997). Previously, experience was not considered to be capable of exerting an impact on brain development. However, in present-day neuroscience, information in the brain is depicted as being represented and processed by distributed groups of neurons that maintain a functional interconnection based on experiential demands rather than by a strictly genetically predetermined scheme (Black & Greenough, 1992; Johnson, 1998). We now know that the mechanisms of neural plasticity cause the brain's anatomical differentiation to be dependent on stimulation from the environment (Cicchetti & Tucker, 1994; Greenough, Black, & Wallace, 1987).

Recognizing that mechanisms of neural plasticity are integral to the very anatomical structure of cortical tissue, and that they cause the formation of the brain to be an extended, malleable process, neuroscientists are presented with new avenues for understanding the vulnerability of the brain as a basis for the development of psychopathology (Cicchetti & Tucker, 1994). Environmental experience is now recognized to be critical to the differentiation of brain tissue itself (Cicchetti, 2002a). Nature's potential can be realized only as it is enabled by nurture.

Early stresses, either physiological or emotional, may condition young neural networks to produce cascading effects through later development, possibly constraining the child's flexibility to adapt to new challenging situations with new strategies rather than with old conceptual and behavioral prototypes. Thus, early psychological trauma may result not only in emotional sensitization (Cummings, Hennessy, Rabideau, & Cicchetti, 1994; Hennessy, Rabideau, Cicchetti, & Cummings, 1994; Maughan & Cicchetti, 2002), but also in pathological sensitization of neurophysiological reactivity (Pollak, Cicchetti, Klorman, & Brumaghim, 1997). Particularly in a temperamentally sensitive brain, less severe forms of psychological insult may create emotional sensitizations that ripple through the developmental process with effects that are neuropsychological more than neurophysiological, but that nonetheless compound themselves into relatively enduring forms of psychopathology.

Thus, children born with relatively normal brains may encounter a number of experiences (e.g., extreme poverty, community and domestic violence, physical abuse, sexual abuse, neglect, etc.) that can negatively impact upon developing brain structure, function, and organization and contribute to distorting these children's experiences of the world (De Bellis, 2001; Dodge, Pettit, & Bates, 1990; Pollak, Cicchetti, & Klorman, 1998; Rogosch, Cicchetti, & Aber, 1995). Children may be especially vulnerable to the effects of pathological experiences during periods of rapid creation or modification of neuronal connections (Black, Jones, Nelson, & Greenough, 1998). Pathological experience may become part of a vicious cycle, as the pathology induced in brain structure may distort the child's experience, with subsequent alterations in cognition or social interactions causing additional pathological experience and added brain pathology (Cicchetti & Tucker, 1994). Because experiential processes may continue to operate during psychopathological states, children who incorporate pathological experience may add neuropathological connections into their developing brains instead of functional connections (Black et al., 1998; Courchesne, Chisum, & Townsend, 1994).

Empirical evidence from rodent and primate models has demonstrated that the experience of traumatic events early in life can alter behavioral and neuroendocrine responsiveness, the morphological characteristics of the brain, and the activation of genes associated with negative behavioral and neurobiological outcomes (Sanchez, Ladd, & Plotsky, 2001). Furthermore, the results of animal studies reveal that early traumatic experience may impact upon the normative developmental processes that have been implicated in the etiology of mental disorders (Sanchez et al., 2001). In rodent and nonhuman primate investigations, early experiences of trauma have been shown to be associated with long-term alterations in coping, emotional and behavioral dysregulation, the responsiveness of the neuroendocrine system to stressful experiences, brain structure, neurochemistry, and gene expression (Cicchetti & Walker, 2001; Gunnar, Morison, Chisholm, & Schuder, 2001; Sanchez et al., 2001). In addition, research conducted with rodents has discovered that depriving rodent infants of adequate social and physical stimulation from their mothers influences the responsivity of the Limbic-Hypothalamic-Pituitary-Adrenal (LHPA) axis to stressors that occur later in life (Levine, 1994; Meaney et al., 1996; Plotsky & Meaney, 1993).

CHILD MALTREATMENT

The study of human child maltreatment also can be utilized to illustrate how traumatic social experiences can alter the activity of the hypothalamic–pituitary–adrenal (HPA) axis. Child abuse and neglect are stressful and threatening experiences that pose adaptational challenges, and the HPA axis is one of the physiological systems that has evolved in mammals to help focus and sustain cognitive, emotional, behavioral, and metabolic activity in response to conditions of threat (Lopez, Akil, & Watson, 1999; Vazquez, 1998). Basal activity of this neuroendocrine system follows a circadian rhythm such that the highest levels appear around the time of awakening and then decline to low

levels near the onset of sleep (Kirschbaum & Hellhammer, 1989). Basal levels of cortisol are essential to ensure normal brain growth and to support the metabolic activity
necessary to sustain general functioning (McEwen, 1998).

Stress reactions of the HPA system are regulated by multiple negative feedback
mechanisms that operate to maintain cortisol within the bounds set by the diurnal
cortisol rhythm. Negative feedback operates, in part, through cortisol receptors in the
hippocampus, hypothalamus, and pituitary (DeKloet, 1991). There tends to be a positive correlation between the number of receptors and the efficacy of negative feedback (Sapolsky, Krey, & McEwen, 1984). In animal models, early experiences have been
shown to affect receptor numbers, with normative levels of stress and challenge enhancing the number of receptors and adverse levels of stress and challenge decreasing
receptor numbers (Sanchez et al., 2001).

The capacity to elevate cortisol in response to acute trauma is necessary for survival.
Although brief elevations in glucocorticoids subsequent to acute stressors appear to improve the individual's ability to manage stressful experiences successfully, chronic hyperactivity of the HPA axis may bring about neuronal loss in the hippocampus, inhibit
the process of neurogenesis, slow down the development of myelination, eventuate in
abnormalities in synaptic pruning, and contribute to impairments in cognitive and affective functioning (Gould, Tanapat, McEwen, Flugge, & Fuchs, 1998; Sapolsky, 1992).
Moreover, hypocortisolism, or the elimination of glucocorticoids, also can cause damage to neurons (Gunnar & Vazquez, 2001; Heim, Ehlert, & Hellhammer, 2000). Thus,
some individuals who experience chronic stressors, such as ongoing physical abuse,
may manifest reduced adrenocortical secretion, decreased adrenocortical reactivity, or
enhanced negative feedback of the HPA axis (De Bellis, Keshavan, et al., 1999). Consequently, the avoidance of both chronic glucocorticoid hypersecretion and hyposecre-
tion is in the best interest of all individuals (Sapolsky, 1996).

Although the short- and long-term impact of child maltreatment on psychological outcomes has been the focus of considerable research (see, e.g., Cicchetti,
1994; Cicchetti & Carlson, 1989; Cicchetti & Manly, 2001; Cicchetti & Toth, 2000),
the psychobiological and neurobiological correlates and consequences of maltreatment have begun to be investigated relatively recently (see, e.g., Cicchetti & Tucker,
1994; De Bellis, 2001; De Bellis, Baum, et al., 1999; De Bellis, Keshavan, et al., 1999;
De Bellis & Putnam, 1994; Pollak et al., 1997). Examination of the neurobiological sequelae of abuse and neglect may enhance our understanding of the mechanisms supporting pathological development in maltreated children (Cicchetti & Tucker,
1994).

Instances of physical and sexual abuse can be viewed as potentially massive stressors. In animal research, threats of physical injury and pain have been demonstrated
to produce intense activation of physiological systems associated with fear and stress
(Kalin & Takahashi, 1990). Neglect by definition creates opportunities for unrelieved
fearfulness and discomfort, resulting in increased risk for accident, injury, and abusive
interactions that would also be expected to activate stress systems. One physiological
system that is likely to exhibit differences in functioning as a result of the stress associated with child maltreatment is the HPA system. The activity level of this system also
may be related to the psychological characteristics of maltreated children and may play
a role in the emergence of psychopathology among individuals with a history of child
maltreatment.

HPA Axis Functioning in Maltreated Children

A number of investigations have been conducted that indicate dysregulation of the HPA axis in maltreated children. To our knowledge, in the only study conducted with maltreated preschool children, Hart, Gunnar, and Cicchetti (1995) examined the relations between neuroendocrine activity and social competence. These investigators studied two groups of children for thirty-one days, either while they were attending a therapeutic preschool for abused and neglected children or while they were enrolled in a preschool serving economically disadvantaged nonmaltreating families. Daily saliva samples were collected from each child in the morning throughout the duration of the study. Each child's cortisol values over the days were used to compute measures of basal activity (median cortisol) and reactivity (ratio of quartile ranges). In addition, observations of social behavior, both within and outside the classroom, were collected in the hour prior to saliva sampling. At the conclusion of the study, teachers rated children's problems as well as competencies.

Hart and her colleagues (1995) found that median cortisol was not significantly correlated with social behavior measures. Cortisol reactivity was positively correlated with social competence and negatively correlated with shy/internalizing behavior. Moreover, maltreated children exhibited less cortisol reactivity than did comparison children. Consistent with prior findings in the literature (see Cicchetti & Toth, 1995, for a review), maltreated children also scored lower in social competence and higher in acting out/externalizing behaviors than did the comparison groups. Furthermore, maltreated preschool children failed to show elevations in cortisol on days of high versus low conflict in the classroom. Social competence also was found to correlate positively with cortisol levels on high-conflict days.

Taken together, the findings of this investigation suggest a reduction in cortisol reactivity in maltreated preschool children related to the impairment in social competence commonly noted among these children. The greater HPA reactivity found in the comparison group may be reflective of greater socioemotional health, at least when reactivity of the HPA system is examined within contexts that are familiar or typical for the child. Reduced activity of the HPA system may help to protect the maltreated child from some of the negative neural and immune consequences of high cortisol; however, the protection may have a socioemotional cost among children who would also exhibit decreases in competence and increases in fearful, anxious behavior. Future research will be needed to discover the processes relating competence to cortisol reactivity and the emergence and possible changes in these relations with development.

HPA dysregulation also has been found in children who have been sexually abused. Sexually abused girls have been shown to excrete significantly greater amounts of the dopamine (DA) metabolite, homovanillic acid (De Bellis, Lefter, Trickett, & Putnam, 1994). Furthermore, augmented mean morning serial plasma cortisol levels have been found in sexually abused girls, implicating altered glucocorticoid functioning in the HPA axis (Putnam, Trickett, Helmers, Susman, Dorn, & Everett, 1991). Moreover, the attenuated plasma adrenocorticotropin hormone (ACTH) response to the ovine corticotropin releasing hormone (CRH) stimulation test in sexually abused girls further suggests a dysregulatory disorder of the HPA axis, associated with hyporesponsiveness of the pituitary to exogenous CRH and normal overall cortisol secretion to CRH challenge (De Bellis et al., 1993). In addition, sexually abused children with posttraumatic stress disorder (PTSD) have been found to excrete significantly greater concentrations of baseline norepinephrine (NE) and DA in comparison to nonabused anxious and normal healthy comparison children (De Bellis, Baum, et al., 1999). Thus, it appears that the combination of sexual abuse experiences and PTSD is associated with enduring alterations of biological stress systems.

Two separate studies have revealed that maltreated school-age children with major depressive disorder (MDD) fail to display the expected diurnal decrease in cortisol secretion from morning to afternoon (Hart, Gunnar, & Cicchetti, 1996; Kaufman, 1991). Findings from another investigation revealed that when compared to depressed abused and normal comparison children, maltreated prepubertal depressed abused children who were living under conditions of chronic ongoing adversity exhibited an increased human CRH-induced ACTH response, but normal cortisol secretion. In contrast, depressed children with prior histories of abuse but now residing in a stable environment did not differ in their HPA functioning from the depressed abused or the normal comparison children (Kaufman et al., 1997).

To date, the investigations on HPA functioning in maltreated children have been characterized by an inconsistency in how the maltreatment variable has been operationalized. The maltreated children who have been participants in the aforementioned studies have been exposed to an array of traumatic experiences, including sexual abuse, with and without PTSD, physical abuse, with and without MDD, and neglect. Moreover, in many of the investigations on HPA functioning in maltreated children, the sample sizes have been small, thereby limiting the ability of the researchers to conduct a more fine-grained analysis of the maltreatment variables. In our laboratory, we recently have completed two large-scale studies that examined in greater detail aspects of child maltreatment and their relations to HPA axis functioning.

Study I: Diverse Patterns of Neuroendocrine Regulation in Maltreated Children

In the first study, Cicchetti and Rogosch (2001a) investigated cortisol regulation in a cohort of 175 school-aged maltreated and 209 nonmaltreated children from low-income socioeconomic status (SES) backgrounds. The research was carried out within the context of a research summer day camp program (see Cicchetti & Manly, 1990, for a description of the camp context).

The children did not know what to expect from the adults and children in the camp context. Moreover, children in the camp were unfamiliar with each other. Thus, the camp context constituted a social challenge for the children in attendance. An advantage of the naturalistic camp setting was that it permitted the collection of saliva from the children during uniform time periods. Saliva samples were obtained from the children at the same time in the morning (i.e., at 9:00 A.M., as soon as the children arrived at camp in a bus) and in the afternoon (i.e., at 4:00 P.M., shortly before they were bused home at the end of the day). The majority of the youngsters in this study were of minority racial-ethnic backgrounds (80%). Children on average were slightly over nine years of age and there were more boys ($N = 232$) than girls ($N = 152$) who participated.

Maltreatment subtypes, the severity of maltreatment incidents, the age of onset of maltreatment, and the developmental timing of the maltreatment experiences were obtained from coding the Child Protective Services (CPS) records for each maltreated child in the sample using the operational definitions provided in the Maltreatment Classification System (MCS), a measure developed in our laboratory and designed to delineate diverse features of child maltreatment that individual children had experienced (Barnett, Manly, & Cicchetti, 1993; Manly, Cicchetti, & Barnett, 1994; Manly, Kim, Rogosch, & Cicchetti, 2001). The MCS utilizes CPS records detailing investigations and findings regarding maltreatment occurrences in identified families. Instead of relying upon official DSS designations and case dispositions, the MCS is used to code all information available in a family's CPS case record, thereby yielding independent determinations of maltreatment experiences. Parents of the maltreated and nonmaltreated children gave their permission for research staff to check the CPS records at DSS and to examine the state registry for child abuse and neglect. Obtaining this permission from all parents ensures that there are no legally identified maltreated youngsters in the comparison group.

In terms of the operationalization of maltreatment subtypes, *sexual abuse* involves any attempted or actual sexual contact between a child and caregiver for purposes of the caregiver's sexual satisfaction or financial benefit. *Physical abuse* involves the infliction of physical injury on a child other than by accidental means (e.g., beating the child causing welts, bruises, broken bones, burns, choking). *Neglect* involves failure to provide for children's basic physical needs (i.e., for adequate food, clothing, shelter, medical treatment), lack of supervision (e.g., leaving child without adult supervision, leaving child in the care of dangerous caregivers), and/or moral-legal/educational neglect (e.g., exposing the child to criminal activity, failure to send a child to school). Finally, *emotional maltreatment* involves extreme thwarting of children's basic emotional needs for psychological safety and security, acceptance, and self-esteem, and age-appropriate autonomy (e.g., belittling and ridiculing the child, using fear and intimidation, suicidal and homicidal threats).

Cicchetti and Rogosch (2001a) found no group differences between maltreated and nonmaltreated children for average morning or average afternoon cortisol levels. Nonetheless, significant differences were obtained that were based on the subtypes of maltreatment that the children had experienced. Specifically, maltreated children who had been both physically and sexually abused, as well as neglected or emotionally maltreated, exhibited substantial elevations in morning cortisol levels; children who had cortisol levels that were greater than one standard deviation above the mean in both the morning and afternoon also were overrepresented in this multiple abuse group. The developmental timing of the occurrence of maltreatment did not account for these group differences, whereas the severity of sexual abuse was implicated. Both levels of average morning cortisol and of average afternoon cortisol were significantly correlated. Thus, the severity of sexual abuse appears to be a prominent contributor to the heightened cortisol levels exhibited by the subgroup of maltreated children who experienced physical and sexual abuse, as well as neglect or emotional maltreatment.

In contrast to the findings of the multiple abuse group, a subgroup of physically abused children evidenced a trend toward lower morning cortisol relative to nonmaltreated children. Additionally, the physically abused subgroup of children displayed a significantly smaller decrease in cortisol levels from morning to afternoon. This pattern suggests relatively less diurnal variation for the physically abused group of children, with trends toward relatively lower cortisol levels in the morning and significantly less decrease in cortisol over the day. Finally, no differences in patterns of cortisol regulation were obtained between the neglected and the emotionally maltreated groups of children and the comparison group.

The examination of HPA axis functioning in this investigation revealed that high levels of cortisol do not uniformly characterize the day-to-day functioning of maltreated children relative to nonmaltreated children. Rather, within the maltreatment groups, evidence for differential patterns of cortisol regulation was observed. Strikingly, the group of children who had experienced sexual and physical abuse, as well as neglect or emotional maltreatment, exhibited a high elevation in morning cortisol. Evidence also was obtained that a subgroup of this multiply abused group of children displayed high levels of cortisol in both the morning and afternoon. This sexually and physically abused group would appear to be closest to representing children who manifested hypercortisolism; however, the patterns of high morning and high afternoon cortisol found in the sexually and physically abused group were not characteristic of all children who had experienced maltreatment.

The group of children who had been physically but not sexually abused tended to exhibit a different pattern of cortisol regulation, one that was more akin to hypocortisolism. In the group of physically abused children, evidence of trends toward cortisol suppression and significantly less diurnal variation were found. Moreover, a subgroup of physically abused children with low cortisol also displayed a rise, rather than the expected decrease, in afternoon cortisol. Thus, once again there is evidence for atypical HPA regulation patterns in the physically abused children.

The pattern of cortisol suppression and less diurnal variation found in the group of physically abused children bears similarity to the link between the low levels of HPA activity and aggressiveness discovered by McBurnett, Lahey, Rathouz, and Loeber (2000). (See also McBurnett, King, & Scarpa, this volume.) Furthermore, the subgroup of physically abused children who exhibit low morning cortisol and rises in afternoon cortisol bear resemblance to the depressed physically abused or to the maltreated depressed children reported in the literature (Hart et al., 1996; Kaufman, 1991; Kaufman et al., 1997).

The absence of significant differences in patterns of cortisol regulation between the neglected and the emotionally maltreated group of children and the nonmaltreated comparison group must be considered within the context of the composition of the comparison sample. Because the comparison children did not differ from the maltreated children on any of the socioeconomic indicators, the nonmaltreated children comprise a very poor, high-risk minority group. In future research, it would be instructive to examine HPA axis functioning in maltreated and comparison groups of children from lower-risk backgrounds.

The divergent patterns of cortisol regulation for the varying subgroup configurations of maltreated children suggest that it is highly unlikely that the brains of all children are uniformly affected by the experience of maltreatment. Caution must be exercised before assertions that the early experience of child maltreatment results in permanent damage to the nervous system can be made (cf. Teicher, 2000). Not all maltreated children displayed HPA axis dysregulation. The group of children who experienced sexual and physical abuse, in combination with neglect or emotional maltreatment, exhibited patterns akin to hypercortisolism. These children's maltreatment also was characterized by high severity and occurred over multiple developmental periods.

It is quite conceivable that this group of children will be at extremely high risk for developing enduring neurobiological compromise. Similarly, the group of physically abused children, whose HPA axis functioning resembled hypocortisolism, also may be at enhanced risk for long-term negative neurobiological sequelae.

Even if the groups of maltreated children with HPA patterns of cortisol activation akin to hypercortisolism and hypocortisolism do manifest long-term neurobiological damage, these negative consequences may not prove to be irreversible. Because a significant portion of postnatal brain structuration and functioning occur through interactions of the child with the environment (Cicchetti & Tucker, 1994; Thompson & Nelson, 2001), changes in the internal and external environment may lead to improvements in the ability of the individual to grapple with developmental challenges. Thus, although historical factors canalize and constrain the adaptive process to some degree, neural plasticity may be possible throughout the life course as a result of adaptive neural and psychological self-organization (Cicchetti, 2002a). Cortical development and organization are not passive processes that depend solely upon genetic programming and environmental input. Rather, corticogenesis and organization are best conceived as processes of self-organization guided by self-regulatory mechanisms (Cicchetti & Tucker, 1994).

Study II: Child Maltreatment and Psychopathology: Their Impact on Neuroendocrine Functioning

In the second study, Cicchetti and Rogosch (2001b) examined the relations among child maltreatment, psychopathology, and neuroendocrine functioning. These investigators enlisted the participation of a large representative sample of maltreated and nonmaltreated children, with and without different forms of psychopathology. Because most studies that have investigated maltreatment and adrenocortical functioning either have controlled for gender, employed small samples sizes that precluded testing for gender effects, or utilized samples of only boys or girls, Cicchetti and Rogosch (2001b) chose to explore gender as a possible moderator of the links among maltreatment, psychopathology, and cortisol regulation.

The participants in this investigation included over 370 children (167 maltreated and 204 nonmaltreated), nine years of age on average, who attended a research summer camp program that was designed for maltreated and nonmaltreated disadvantaged children from low-SES backgrounds (Cicchetti & Manly, 1990). Saliva samples were obtained twice daily from the children. Upon their arrival at the camp site at 9:00 A.M. via bus, children provided a morning saliva sample. Shortly before being bused home at 4:00 P.M., children provided an afternoon saliva sample.

In the next to last day of the camp week, children completed the Children's Depression Inventory (CDI; Kovacs, 1985), a questionnaire widely used to assess depressive symptomatology in school-age children. At the conclusion of the camp week, which lasted thirty-five hours in duration, camp counselors, unaware of the maltreatment status of the various children in their group, completed the Teacher Report Form (TRF; Achenbach, 1991), a measure used to assess internalizing and externalizing symptomatology.

Consistent with Study I, maltreatment experiences were classified based on coding of the CPS records at DSS with the MCS. Parental permission to undertake CPS record

of morning cortisol than all of the other nonmaltreated groups (i.e., boys and girls with and without clinical levels of internalizing, externalizing, and comorbid psychopathology). Within the maltreatment group, maltreated girls with case-level externalizing problems had higher morning cortisol than did maltreated girls without externalizing problems. These differences were not observed among nonmaltreated girls. In addition, despite the absence of effects found for afternoon cortisol levels, the nonmaltreated boys who had clinical-level externalizing problems displayed the lowest average daily cortisol and were significantly lower than the maltreated girls without externalizing problems, the group that manifested the highest levels of average daily cortisol.

McBurnett and colleagues (McBurnett et al., 2000; McBurnett et al., this volume) have reported that lower levels of cortisol are associated with the early onset of aggressive conduct disorder. Furthermore, research also has demonstrated that youngsters with early onset conduct disorder evidence mild neuropsychological deficits, as well as more early family dysfunction, including child maltreatment (Aguilar, Sroufe, Egeland, & Carlson, 2002; Moffitt, 1993a, 1993b). Consequently, the apparently limited effects of maltreatment in relation to case-level externalizing problems and to cortisol secretion in Cicchetti and Rogosch's (2001b) investigation are surprising.

Although the small number of nonmaltreated children with clinical levels of comorbid internalizing and externalizing psychopathology precluded the inclusion of these youngsters in the statistical analyses, Cicchetti and Rogosch (2001b) examined the group of maltreated children and identified those who did not exhibit a decrease in cortisol levels across the day. These investigators discovered that maltreated children who had comorbid psychopathology were twice as likely to exhibit a lack of decrease or a rise from morning to afternoon cortisol levels than were maltreated children without clinical levels of comorbid problems.

In this investigation, Cicchetti and Rogosch (2001b) once again demonstrated that not all maltreated children display the same pattern of cortisol regulation. The finding that differential patterns of cortisol regulation were observed among the maltreated children provides additional evidence that the neurobiological functioning (and most probably, the neurobiological structures) of all maltreated children is not affected in the same way by the experience of maltreatment.

Future Directions

To date, the vast majority of the investigations that have examined HPA axis functioning in individuals who have been maltreated have focused on school-age or early adolescent children. In future research, it will be critical to undertake prospective longitudinal studies that are initiated as close in time to the initial maltreatment as possible and to assess HPA axis functioning repeatedly over time. Additionally, HPA axis regulation also should be investigated in children from families who are at high risk for maltreating their children (Cicchetti & Lynch, 1993; Cicchetti & Rizley, 1981). Because child maltreatment commonly occurs for the first time in the early years of life (Cicchetti & Toth, 2003), these high-risk for child maltreatment samples will largely be comprised of infants, toddlers, and preschoolers at the inception of the investigations.

Moreover, as most of the studies conducted on HPA axis functioning in maltreated children have either examined this physiological system in isolation or in relation to psychopathological outcomes, it is essential that future research incorporates both physiological and psychological measures into the assessments of adrenocortical regulation. Such work is important to carry out with maltreated children because, although there is a close correspondence between the biological and psychological consequences of stress, we have yet to produce enough information to be certain about the exact nature of the relations between these two domains of inquiry (Lopez, Akil, & Watson, 1999). If we can comprehend the neurobiology of stress through investigating which brain circuits are correlates of, or are altered by, the stress response, then this knowledge will provide important insights into the brain mechanisms that mediate the impact that stress exerts on mood, cognition, and behavior in both maltreated and nonmaltreated children.

Furthermore, it is essential for research on the effects of child maltreatment to adopt a multiple levels of analysis perspective (Cicchetti & Dawson, 2002). Multidisciplinary collaborations would enable scientists to develop a more comprehensive understanding of how maltreatment experiences at various points in the lifespan impact on the biological and psychological organization of traumatized individuals. Such research programs could include protocols for structural (MRI) and functional (fMRI) neuroimaging of the brain, potentiated startle to positive and negative emotional stimuli, EEG coherence and EEG hemispheric activation asymmetry, and brain event-related potentials (ERP) to positive and negative emotion stimuli. Additionally, each of the neurohormonal messengers involved in the HPA axis [i.e., adrenocorticotropin hormone (ACTH) and corticotropin releasing hormone (CRH)], as well as the other biological systems that play a role in the stress response (i.e., the autonomic, endocrinological, and immunological), also should be examined. A single measure is not sufficient to document the dynamic course of responsivity of the HPA axis. Finally, concurrent longitudinal assessments of developmentally salient tasks of adaptive functioning throughout the life course and across multiple contexts (e.g., affect regulation, attachment, self-development, peer relations, adaptation to school, friendships and dating relationships, identity development, and so on) and state of the art age-appropriate psychopathology assessments should be implemented. Prospective multiple levels of analysis investigations on large representative samples of maltreated and nonmaltreated children are necessary to more fully elucidate the mechanisms through which the adverse social experience of child maltreatment alters brain structure, function, and organization, as well as impairs basic psychological processes.

Animal studies have revealed that changes in the HPA axis mediate the longer term structural and functional changes in the brain that may arise due to stressful experiences (Meaney et al., 1996; Sanchez et al., 2001). One primary means through which hormones affect behavior is via their impact on gene expression (McEwen, 1994; Watson & Gametchu, 1999). Stress hormones have been shown to exert direct effects on the genes that control brain structure and function, including neuronal growth, neurotransmitter synthesis, receptor density and sensitivity, and neurotransmitter reuptake (McEwen, 1994; Watson & Gametchu, 1999). In recent years it has been demonstrated that chronic stress eventuates in a persistent inhibition of granule cell production and changes in the structure of the dentate gyrus, suggesting a mechanism whereby stress may alter hippocampal function (Gould & Tanapat, 1999). The identification of stress-sensitive neural processes may ultimately provide a basis for the formation of pharmacological and behavioral interventions to ameliorate the deleterious effects of early traumatic experiences (Kaufman, Plotsky, Nemeroff, & Charney, 2000; see also Post, Leverich, Weiss, Xing, Zhang, Li, & Smith, this volume).

Cicchetti and Rogosch's (2001a) findings of hypercortisolism in children who experience both sexual and physical abuse, as well as neglect and/or emotional maltreatment, suggest that this multiply abused group is at high risk for neurobiological and psychological dysfunction. Relatedly, adults who report having been physically or sexually abused in childhood and adult combat veterans with PTSD have been found to reveal a reduction in hippocampal volume during structural neuroimaging procedures (see Bremner & Vermetten, 2001, for a review). The hippocampus has neural connections with the prefrontal cortex and this latter structure may underlie some of the developmental sequelae related to child maltreatment (e.g., attentional anomalies, emotion dysregulation, and neuropsychological impairments in executive functions – see Cicchetti & Toth, 2000; Cicchetti & Tucker, 1994; Pollak, Cicchetti & Klorman, 1998; Pollak, Cicchetti, Klorman, & Brumaghim, 1997; Shields & Cicchetti, 1998).

In contrast to the studies of traumatized adults reported above, in an anatomical MRI study of maltreated children with PTSD, De Bellis and colleagues (De Bellis, Keshavan, et al., 1999) discovered that, although the experience of child maltreatment was associated with global adverse effects on brain development, including smaller intracranial and cerebral volumes and corpus callosum areas than nonmaltreated children from the low SES, there was no evidence for a reduction in hippocampal volume in maltreated children with PTSD. Moreover, in a recently published 2–3 year longitudinal follow-up study, De Bellis, Hall, Boring, Frustaci, and Moritz (2001) likewise did not find any structural changes in the hippocampus of maltreated children and young adolescents.

Attention to the process of development provides valuable information about some of the factors that contribute to moderating and mediating the link between maltreatment and its psychological and biological sequelae. Specifically, several investigative teams have recently discovered that there is an increase in cortisol release during the period of adolescence (Lupien, King, Meaney, & McEwen, 2001; Walker & Walder, this volume; Walker, Walder, & Reynolds, 2001). Relatedly, the hippocampus continues to undergo maturation beyond the period of adolescence (Spear, 2000, this volume). Thus, it is conceivable that there are maturational changes in the vulnerability of the HPA system. The absence of any signs of reduction in the hippocampal volume of maltreated children and young adolescents in the studies by De Bellis and colleagues (De Bellis, Keshavan, et al., 1999; De Bellis et al., 2001) may represent a true developmental difference between children and adolescents as compared to adults in the neurobiological sequelae of stress exposure.

In addition, because many of the maltreated children in the De Bellis et al. (De Bellis, Keshavan, et al., 1999; De Bellis et al., 2001) investigations not only had PTSD, but also had other psychopathological disorders (e.g., anxiety and depressive disorders), future anatomical neuroimaging studies need to enlist the participation of homogeneous groups of maltreated children, with and without psychopathology, as well as those with comorbid psychopathology. Such investigations will be essential in order to disentangle the effects of maltreatment on brain structure from those of other prenatal and postnatal environmental, as well as genetic, factors that contribute to the emergence of neurobiological dysfunction and that are causes or consequences of various psychopathological disorders. For example, several investigations that have utilized MRI have shown that there is a selective atrophy of the hippocampus in a number of mental disorders, as well as during aging in some individuals (McEwen, 2000). Clearly, it is critical to be cognizant of the fact that there are multiple converging pathways, some including the neural circuits that are activated by physical, psychological, and immunological stressors, others including the contributions of genetics, early experiences, and ongoing life events, that influence the neurobiological response to various stressors.

One way of minimizing the risk factors commonly associated with maltreatment (e.g., chronic poverty) would be to investigate maltreated children from middle- and upper-SES backgrounds. In theory, at least, investigations of these lower-risk maltreatment samples may enable researchers to obtain a clearer view of the impact of maltreatment on neurobiological development, thereby minimizing the need to tease apart the effects of other associated risk factors from those of child abuse and neglect, per se. For example, Cicchetti and Rogosch (2001a, 2001b) did not find any differences in HPA functioning between children who were neglected or emotionally maltreated and nonmaltreated comparison children from similar low-SES backgrounds. Although it is conceivable that more stressful methodologies such as reactivity paradigms or pharmacological challenge tests may prove to differentiate the neglected and emotionally maltreated children from nonmaltreated comparisons, investigations of neglected (e.g., lack of supervision) and emotionally maltreated children and nonmaltreated children from middle- or upper-SES backgrounds may reveal differences that are mitigated or eliminated by risk factors associated with membership in the lower SES.

A substantial research literature has demonstrated that not all persons who have been exposed to the same adverse experiences are uniformly affected (Luthar, Cicchetti, & Becker, 2000). For example, some maltreated children function well even though they have experienced the chronic stress of such caretaking casualty. As Cicchetti and Rogosch (2001a, 2001b) discovered, not all maltreated children appear to have the same pattern of HPA axis dysregulation. Not only did maltreated children with varying experiences exhibit different patterns of HPA regulation, but also some maltreated children appeared to manifest a normal HPA system.

To date, all of the research conducted in the area of resilience has focused on psychological factors as mediators, moderators, or developmental outcomes. In the future, it will be essential for researchers examining the pathways to resilient adaptation to incorporate biological assessments of these youngsters into their studies. Logical candidates to include in such investigations could involve assessments of neuroendocrine regulation, potentiated startle responses to positive and negative emotional stimuli, ERPs to positive and negative emotions, and structural and functional neuroimaging techniques. The latter two methods would help to ascertain whether the brains of resilient maltreated children differ structurally and/or functionally from those of nonresilient maltreated children.

Although we presently possess minimal knowledge about molecular genetics and child maltreatment, since social experiences have been demonstrated to affect gene expression and brain structure and function, and vice-versa, it is quite likely that maltreatment affects the expression of genes that impact brain structure and function as well as basic regulatory processes (Caspi et al., 2002; Cicchetti, in press). DNA microarrays can be utilized to index changes in the expression of genes that are essential for brain function (Greenberg, 2001). The implementation of such molecular genetic technologies into research on resilience may reveal the mechanisms responsible for inhibiting the expression of genes that are probabilistically associated with maladaptive outcomes and psychopathology in individuals who have been maltreated. Similarly, the incorporation of molecular genetic approaches may provide insights into the mechanisms that activate genes that may serve a protective function for maltreated persons.

Finally, as knowledge on the psychological and neurobiological sequelae of maltreatment, as well as their interrelation, continues to accrue, it will be important to implement preventive interventions with these children. Can the provision of developmentally sensitive interventions prevent, ameliorate, or even reverse, the adverse neurobiological and psychological consequences of the chronic stressor, child maltreatment? Is it possible for such preventive interventions to normalize brain structure, functioning, and organization only at particular developmental periods (i.e., are there sensitive periods during which such interventions will prove to be effective), or is neural plasticity operative across the life course (Cicchetti, 2002a)? Can interventions modify children's representations of caregiver and self and might such changes alter gene expression and brain organization? As our knowledge base matures, and if the answers to the aforementioned questions prove to be positive, then child maltreatment researchers will truly be able to provide maltreated children with an agenda of hope that can minimize or eradicate the adverse effects of their histories.

REFERENCES

Achenbach, T. M. (1991). *Manual for the Teacher's Report Form and 1991 Profile*. Burlington: University of Vermont, Department of Psychiatry.

Aguilar, B., Sroufe, L. A., Egeland, B., & Carlson, E. (2000). Distinguishing the early onset/persistent and adolescence-onset antisocial behavioral types: From birth to 16 years. *Development and Psychopathology, 12*, 109–132.

Barnett, D., Ganiban, J., & Cicchetti, D. (1999). Maltreatment, negative expressivity, and the development of Type D attachments from 12- to 24-months of age. *Monographs of the Society for Research in Child Development, 64*, 97–118.

Barnett, D., Manly, J. T., & Cicchetti, D. (1993). Defining child maltreatment: The interface between policy and research. In D. Cicchetti and S. L. Toth (Eds.), *Child abuse, child development, and social policy* (pp. 7–73). Norwood, NJ: Ablex Publishing.

Belsky, J. (1984). The determinants of parenting: A process model. *Child Development, 55*, 83–96.

Black, J. E., & Greenough, W. T. (1992). Induction of pattern in neural structure by experience: Implications for cognitive development. In M. Lamb, A. Brown, & B. Rogoff (Eds.), *Advances in developmental psychology* (Vol. 4, pp. 1–50). Hillsdale, NJ: Erlbaum.

Black, J. E., Jones, T. A., Nelson, C. A., & Greenough, W. T. (1998). Neuronal plasticity and the developing brain. In N. E. Alessi, J. T. Coyle, S. I. Harrison, & S. Eth (Eds.), *Handbook of child and adolescent psychiatry* (pp. 31–53). New York: Wiley.

Bolger, K. E., Patterson, C. J., & Kupersmidt, J. B. (1998). Peer relationships and self esteem among children who have been maltreated. *Child Development, 69*, 1171–1197.

Bremner, J. D., & Vermetten, E. (2001). Stress and development: Behavioral and biological consequences. *Development and Psychopathology, 13*, 473–490.

Carlson, V., Cicchetti, D., Barnett, D., & Braunwald, K. (1989). Disorganized/disoriented attachment relationships in maltreated infants. *Developmental Psychology, 25*, 525–531.

Caspi, A., M. Clay, J., Moffitt, T. E., Mill, J., Martin, J., Craig, I. W., Taylor, A., & Poulton, R. (2002). Role of genotype in the cycle of violence in maltreated children. *Science, 297*, 851–854.

Cicchetti, D. (1989). How research on child maltreatment has informed the study of child development: Perspectives from developmental psychopathology. In D. Cicchetti and V. Carlson (Eds.), *Child maltreatment: theory and research on the causes and consequences of child abuse and neglect* (pp. 377–431). New York: Cambridge University Press.

Cicchetti, D. (1990). The organization and coherence of socioemotional, cognitive, and representational development: Illustrations through a developmental psychopathology perspective on Down syndrome and child maltreatment. In R. Thompson (Ed.), *Nebraska Symposium on Motivation. Vol. 36. Socioemotional development* (pp. 259–366). Lincoln: University of Nebraska Press.

Cicchetti, D. (1991). Fractures in the crystal: Developmental psychopathology and the emergence of the self. *Developmental Review, 11,* 271–287.

Cicchetti, D. (Ed.) (1994). Special Issue: Advances and challenges in the study of the sequelae of child maltreatment. *Development and Psychopathology, 6*(1), 1–247.

Cicchetti, D. (2002a). How a child builds a brain: Insights from normality and psychopathology. In W. Hartup and R. Weinberg (Eds.) *Child Psychology in Retrospect and Prospect: Minnesota Symposia on Child Psychology, Volume 35* (pp. 23–71). Mahwah, N.J.: Erlbaum.

Cicchetti, D. (2002b). The impact of social experience on neurobiological systems: Illustration from a constructivist view of child maltreatment. *Cognitive Development, 17,* 1407–1428.

Cicchetti, D., & Cannon, T. D. (1999) Neurodevelopmental processes in the ontogenesis and epigenesis of psychopathology. *Development and Psychopathology, 11,* 375–393.

Cicchetti, D., & Carlson, V. (Eds.). (1989). *Child maltreatment: Theory and research on the causes and consequences of child abuse and neglect.* New York: Cambridge University Press.

Cicchetti, D., & Dawson, G. (2002). Multiple levels of analysis. *Development and Psychopathology, 14,* 417–420.

Cicchetti, D., & Lynch, M. (1993). Toward an ecological/transactional model of community violence and child maltreatment: Consequences for children's development. *Psychiatry, 56,* 96–118.

Cicchetti, D., & Lynch, M. (1995). Failures in the expectable environment and their impact on individual development: The case of child maltreatment. In D. Cicchetti & D. Cohen (Eds.), *Developmental psychopathology* (pp. 32–71). *Vol. 2 Risk, disorder, and adaptation.* New York: Wiley.

Cicchetti, D., & Manly, J. T. (1990). A personal perspective on conducting research with maltreating families: Problems and solutions. In G. Brody and I. Sigel (Eds.), *Methods of family research: Volume 2: Families at risk* (pp. 87–133). Hillsdale, N.J.: Erlbaum.

Cicchetti, D., & Manly, J. T. (Eds.) (2001). Operationalizing child maltreatment: Developmental proceses and outcomes. Special Issue: *Developmental and Psychopathology, 13* (4), 755–1048.

Cicchetti, D., & Rizley, R. (1981). Developmental perspectives on the etiology, intergenerational transmission and sequelae of child maltreatment. *New Directions for Child Development, 11,* 31–55.

Cicchetti, D., & Rogosch, F. A. (1997) The role of self-organization in the promotion of resilience in maltreated children. *Development and Psychopathology, 9,* 799–817.

Cicchetti, D., & Rogosch, F. A. (2001a). Diverse patterns of neuroendocrine activity in maltreated children. *Development and Psychopathology, 13,* 677–694.

Cicchetti, D., & Rogosch, F. A. (2001b). The impact of child maltreatment and psychopathology upon neuroendocrine functioning. *Development and Psychopathology, 13,* 783–804.

Cicchetti, D., & Toth, S. L. (1995). A developmental psychopathology perspective on child abuse and neglect. *Journal of the American Academy of Child and Adolescent Psychiatry, 34,* 541–565.

Cicchetti, D., & Toth, S. L. (2000). Developmental processes in maltreated children. In D. Hansen (Ed.), *Nebraska Symposium on Motivation, Vol. 46: Child Maltreatment* (pp. 85–160). Lincoln: University of Nebraska Press.

Cicchetti, D., & Toth, S. L. (2003). Child maltreatment: A research and policy agenda for the dawn of the Millennium. In R. P. Weissberg, L. H. Weiss, O. Reyes, and H. J. Walberg (Eds.), *Trends in the well-being of children and youth: Volume 2* (pp. 181–206). Washington, D.C.: CWLA Press.

Cicchetti, D., & Tucker, D. (1994). Development and self-regulatory structures of the mind. *Development and Psychopathology, 6,* 533–549.

Cicchetti, D., & Walker, E. F. (Eds.) (2001). Stress and development: biological and psychological consequences. Special Issue: *Development and Psychopathology, 13,* (3), 413–753.

Cohen, P., Brown, J., & Smailes, E. (2001). Child abuse and neglect and the development of mental disorders in the general population. *Development and Psychopathology, 13,* 981–1000.

Courchesne, E., Chisum, H., & Townsend, J. (1994). Neural activity-dependent brain charges in development: Implications for psychopathology. *Development and Psychopathology, 6,* 697–722.

McEwen, B. S. (1998). Protective and damaging effects of stress mediators. *Seminars in Medicine of the Beth Israel Deaconess Medical Center, 338,* 171–179.

McEwen, B. S. (2000). Effects of adverse environments for brain structure and function. *Biological Psychiatry, 48,* 721–731.

McGloin, J. M., & Widom, C. S. (2001). Resilience among abused and neglected children. *Development and Psychopathology, 13,* 1021–1038.

Meaney, M. J., Diorio, J., Francis, D., Widdowson, J., LaPlante, P., Caldji, C., Sharma, S., Seckl, J., & Plotsky, P. (1996). Early environmental regulation of forebrain glucocorticoid receptor gene expression: Implications for adrenocortical responses to stress. *Developmental Neuroscience, 18,* 49–72.

Moffitt, T. E. (1993a). Life course persistent and adolescence limited antisocial behavior: A developmental taxonomy. *Psychological Review, 100,* 674–701.

Moffitt, T. E. (1993b). The neuropsychology of conduct disorder. *Development and Psychopathology, 5,* 135–151.

Nelson, C. A., & Bloom, F. E. (1997). Child development and neuroscience. *Child Development, 68,* 970–987.

Plotsky, P. M., & Meaney, M. J. (1993). Early, postnatal experience alters hypothalamic corticotropin-releasing factor (CRF) mRNA, median eminence CRF content and stress-induced release in adult rats. *Molecular Brain Research, 18,* 195–200.

Pollak, S.D., Cicchetti, D., & Klorman, R. (1998). Stress, memory, and emotion: Developmental considerations from the study of child maltreatment. *Development and Psychopathology, 10,* 811–828.

Pollak, S. D., Cicchetti, D., Klorman, R., & Brumaghim, J. T. (1997). Cognitive brain event-related potentials and emotion processing in maltreated children. *Child Development, 68,* 773–787.

Post, R. M., Leverich, G. S., Weiss, S. R. B., Zhang, L., Xing, G., Li, H., & Smith, M. (this volume). Psychosocial stressors as predisposing factors to affective illness and PTSD: Potential neurobiological mechanisms and theoretical implications.

Putnam, F. W., Trickett, P. K., Helmers, K., Dorn, L., & Everett, B. (1991). Cortisol abnormalities in sexually abused girls. *Proceedings of the 144th Annual Meeting of the American Psychiatric Association, 107.*

Pynoos, R., Steinberg, A., & Wraith, R. (1995). A developmental model for childhood traumatic stress. In D. Cicchetti & D. Cohen (Eds.), *Developmental psychopathology: Risk, disorder, and adaptation* (pp. 72–95). New York: Wiley.

Rogosch, F. A., Cicchetti, D., & Aber, J. L. (1995). The role of child maltreatment in early deviations in cognitive and affective processing abilities and later peer relationship problems. *Development and Psychopathology, 7,* 591–609.

Rogosch, F., Cicchetti, D., Shields, A., & Toth, S. L. (1995). Parenting dysfunction in child maltreatment. In M. H. Bornstein (Ed.), *Handbook of parenting: Vol. 4* (pp. 127–159). Hillsdale, NJ: Erlbaum.

Sanchez, M. M., Ladd, C. O., & Plotsky, P. M. (2001). Early adverse experience as a developmental risk factor for later psychopathology: Evidence from rodent and primate models. *Development and Psychopathology, 13,* 419–450.

Sapolsky, R. M. (1992). *Stress, the aging brain, and the mechanisms of neuron death.* Cambridge, Mass.: MIT Press.

Sapolsky, R. M. (1996). Stress, glucocorticoids, and damage to the NS: The current state of confusion. *Stress, 1,* 1–19.

Sapolsky, R. M., Krey, L., & McEwen, B. (1984). Glucocorticoid-sensitive hippocampal neurons are involved in terminating the adrenal stress response. *Proceedings of the National Academy of Sciences of the United States, 81,* 6174–6177.

Shields, A. M., Cicchetti, D., & Ryan, R. M. (1994). The development of emotional and behavioral self regulation and social competence among maltreated school-age children. *Development and Psychopathology, 6,* 57–75.

Shields, A. M., & Cicchetti, D. (1998). Reactive aggression among maltreated children: The contributions of attention and emotion dysregulation. *Journal of Clinical Child Psychology, 27,* 381–395.

Shonk, S. M., & Cicchetti, D. (2001). Maltreatment, competency deficits, and risk for academic and behavioral maladjustment. *Developmental Psychology, 37,* 3–14.

Smith, C. A., & Thornberry, T. (1995). The relationship between child maltreatment and adolescent involvement in delinquency. *Criminology, 33,* 451–481.

Spear, L. P. (2000). The adolescent brain and age-related behavioral manifestations. *Neuroscience and Biobehavioral Reviews, 24,* 417–463.

Spear, L. P. (this volume). Neurodevelopment during adolescence.

Teicher, M. H. (2000). Wounds that time won't heal: The neurobiology of child abuse. *Cerebrum, 2,* 50–67.

Thompson, R. A., & Nelson, C. A. (2001). Developmental science and the media: Early brain development. *American Psychologist, 56,* 5–15.

Toth, S. L., Cicchetti, D., Macfie, J., & Emde, R. N. (1997). Representations of self and other in the narratives of neglected, physically abused, and sexually abused preschoolers. *Development and Psychopathology, 9,* 781–796.

Trickett, P., & McBride-Chang, C. (1995). The developmental impact of different types of child abuse and neglect. *Developmental Review, 15,* 311–337.

Vazquez, D. M. (1998). Stress and the developing limbic-hypothalamic-pituitary-adrenal axis. *Psychoneuroendocrinology, 23* 663–700.

Walker, E. F., & Walder, D. (this volume). Neurohormonal aspects of the development of psychotic disorders.

Walker, E. F., Walder, D., & Reynolds, F. (2001). Developmental changes in cortisol secretion in normal and at-risk youth. *Development and Psychopathology, 13,* 721–732.

Watson, C., & Gametchu, B. (1999). Membrane-initiated steroid actions and the proteins that mediate them. *Proceedings of the Society for Experimental Biology and Medicine, 220,* 9–19.

Widom, C. (1989). The cycle of violence. *Science, 244,* 160–166.

FIFTEEN

Toward Unraveling the Premorbid Neurodevelopmental Risk for Schizophrenia

Matcheri S. Keshavan

Over the past four decades several studies have attempted to investigate the potential premorbid indicators of risk for schizophrenia. These studies have involved either long-term follow-up investigation of mostly unselected at risk subjects, or follow-back studies, and have examined behavioral/physiological indicators of variable significance. The "first generation" prospective studies have revealed some important clues to putative markers of risk for schizophrenia such as attentional and neuromotor abnormalities. However, these studies have often been criticized for their expense and lack of statistical power. Over the past decade an impressive wealth of data suggest developmentally mediated neurobiological alterations preceding clinical manifestations of schizophrenia and the critical importance of adolescence for emergence of such alterations. In this chapter, we discuss the merits and disadvantages of approaches to ascertain premorbid risk for schizophrenic illness, and argue that at the dawn of the twenty-first century, it is time to launch a new generation of high risk studies in schizophrenia. To be successful, such studies need to: (a) use hypothesis-driven and established neurobehavioral and biological markers that are guided by the emerging neurodevelopmental models of schizophrenia; (b) use an "enhanced" high risk strategy which defines risk by the presence of both genetic risk and biobehavioral or psychopathological risk; (c) address issues of diagnostic reliability, specificity, and generalizability; (d) develop a prospective follow-up design through the critical risk period closer to illness onset such as adolescence; and (e) use coordinated multicenter studies which are likely to enhance statistical power in such studies.

The past several decades in schizophrenia can be characterized as manifesting a "shift to the left" in the emphasis on the different phases of the schizophrenic illness (Figure 15.1). Early studies of neurobiology of schizophrenic illness focused on cross-sectional studies of mostly chronic schizophrenic patients. The past two decades have seen an increasing emphasis on studies of *first episode* schizophrenia, a strategy which helps minimize the potential confounds of illness chronicity and treatment effects (Keshavan & Schooler, 1992). In recent years the focus has shifted to the *prodromal* phase of the schizophrenic illness because of the realization that early detection and

This work was supported in part by NIMH grants MH 01180, MH 43687, and MH 45156, and by a NARSAD grant.

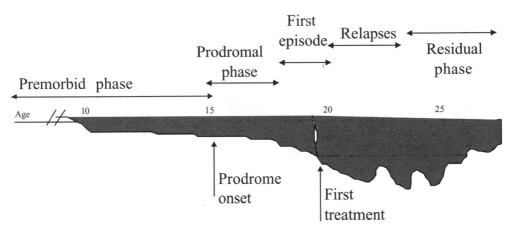

Figure 15.1. Natural course of schizophrenia showing the time frame for critical phases of the schizophrenic illness. The horizontal line represents the time dimension; the vertical dimension represents functional decline.

intervention in this phase may eventually improve outcome of this illness (McGlashan, 1998). The increasingly popular neurodevelopmental model of the schizophrenic illness has prompted interest in the *premorbid* phase of the schizophrenic illness with the renewed hope of identifying its potential precursors. Studies of the premorbid phase of the schizophrenic illness can potentially help us to identify vulnerability factors for schizophrenia, to examine the evolution of the early phase of the schizophrenic prodrome, to unravel the premorbid pathophysiology of this illness without the potential confounds of illness or treatment effects, and finally to facilitate early diagnosis and intervention efforts (Cornblatt & Obuchowski, 1997).

Over the past four decades several studies have examined premorbid risk factors for schizophrenia. While some important clues have emerged from these "high risk" studies as to the nature of risk factors for schizophrenia, several methodological difficulties have limited interpretation of such findings. The recent burgeoning of interest in the neurodevelopmental basis of schizophrenia as well as the accumulating knowledge on the neurobiological substrate of this illness have led to a renewed interest in unraveling the premorbid risk factors in schizophrenia. In particular, the advent of novel, noninvasive neuroimaging techniques allows investigation of in vivo neurobiological alterations in the individuals at risk of schizophrenia. The introduction of safe, effective treatments for psychotic illnesses as well as the possibility of therapeutic interventions in the prodromal phase (McGorry, 1998) make such efforts timely. In order for such studies to be fruitful, attention needs to be given to the following questions: (i) *who* are the most likely individuals that, when studied, will reveal useful insights about the nature of vulnerability to schizophrenia? (ii) *how* should such studies be designed, and what are the methodological issues that need to be addressed in these studies? (iii) *what* predictive/outcome factors, if studied, are likely to yield the best insights? and finally, (iv) *when*, that is, during which critical periods of development is it most fruitful to assess the risk factors? Focused, hypothesis-driven studies mindful of the above questions, and deploying the state of the art neurobiological tools of assessment, are likely to provide fresh impetus to this important, rather neglected field of research, and are reviewed here.

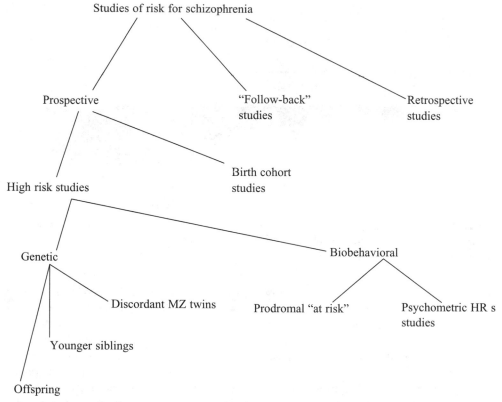

Figure 15.2. Approaches to examine premorbid risk in schizophrenia and other developmental neuropsychiatric disorders. HR = high risk; MZ = monozygotic.

WHO IS AT INCREASED RISK FOR SCHIZOPHRENIA?

Studies of the premorbid risk refer to the investigation of individuals who are considered more vulnerable to develop schizophrenia than are individuals in the general population. Several approaches have been used to assess premorbid risk (Figure 15.2). Studies of risk for schizophrenia can be retrospective or "follow-back" investigations (Walker et al., 1993) or prospective. Prospective studies could involve longitudinal investigation of large cohorts of unselected general populations (such as birth cohorts) or individuals selected for one or other index of high risk ("high risk" studies). High risk studies have utilized either neurobehavioral markers to identify the risk status, or genetic propensity. In this section we will outline the potential merits and disadvantages of these strategies, review the lessons learned from the early first generation high risk studies, and present a rationale for more focused "second generation" studies to examine premorbid risk.

Genetic High Risk Studies

This approach targets individuals at higher than normal genetic loading for schizophrenia. The benefits of this approach were first recognized by Pearson and Kley (1957).

Table 15.1. Ongoing "First Generation" Studies of High-Risk Offspring of Schizophrenic Parents

	Sample	Duration of follow-up	Outcome in the high risk group
New York Infant HR Study (Fish, 1992)	12 HR offspring/12 controls infancy	30 years	Scz – 8% Spectrum PD – 50%
Copenhagen HR Project (Parnas et al., 1993)	207 HR offspring/104 controls, mean age 15	30+ years	Psychosis – 20.8% Spectrum PD – 21.9%
Israel HR Study (Ingraham et al., 1995)	25 HR/25 controls, all raised in Kibbutz, age 8–14 years	27 years	Scz – 8% Aff – 24%
New York HR Project (Erlenmeyer-Kimling et al., 1995)	63 HR offspring/100 controls, 43 psychiatric controls	20+ years	Psychosis – 18.6% Spectrum PD – 18.1%
Finnish Adoptive Family Study (Tienari et al., 1994)	180 offspring of schizophrenic mothers adopted away; 200 offspring of mentally well mothers	20+ years	Scz – 5.2% Psychosis – 7.8%

Adapted from Cornblatt & Obuchowski, 1997

Offspring of schizophrenic parents represent an attractive high risk population for study since having one schizophrenic parent entails about 13 percent risk of developing the illness, and having two schizophrenic parents increases the risk to about 40 percent (Gottesman & Shields, 1982). Mednick and several other investigators initiated high risk studies in the early 1960s and 1970s, and some of these first generation studies have continued to date (Table 15.1). These studies typically involved follow-up of children of schizophrenic parents. Overall, these studies have supported the view that susceptibility to schizophrenia is mediated at least in part by hereditary factors, and have failed to identify any definitive environmental factors as contributing to the risk for this illness (Cornblatt & Obuchowski, 1997). These studies have also identified potential neurobehavioral markers of risk, such as attentional, eye movement, and neuromotor impairments, as will be discussed later.

The prospective high risk approaches are free from recall bias. Since subjects with a genetic propensity for a known disorder are studied, it is feasible to examine putative, disease-specific predictors. The main disadvantage of the earlier high risk studies, however, is the lack of statistical power, and the relatively modest cost effectiveness of the studies. Large samples of subjects will need to be studied, potentially limiting the number of feasible predictive variables. Another disadvantage is that the population, being chosen on the basis of family history, may be biased; if etiological heterogeneity exists, this may mean that the findings may be generalizable to only patients with familial schizophrenia. Finally, the low reproductive rates of schizophrenic patients make it hard to recruit adequate numbers of offspring. Despite these shortcomings, studies of high risk offspring have indicated that some individuals with genetic risk show evidence of increased liability to schizophrenia. However, the findings are highly variable across studies, and often lack specificity (see Gooding & Iacono, 1995; Cornblatt & Obuchowski, 1997, for reviews; and see Table 15.1).

The definition of the prodrome therefore needs to be stringent, and include both trait related (family history, personality traits) state related psychopathological criteria (sub-threshold positive and negative symptoms) and functional impairment (Keshavan & Cornblatt, 2000; Yung et al., 1998).

General Population Cohort Studies

Longitudinal studies of general population samples have been used to investigate developmental antecedents of schizophrenia. In Britain, two birth cohort studies have been published, the MRC National Survey of Health and Development of 1946 (Jones et al., 1994) and the National Child Development Study of 1958 (Done et al., 1994). Both of these studies, in which the participants have lived through most of the age of risk, showed that children destined to develop schizophrenia could be differentiated based on motor and cognitive dysfunction throughout childhood. David et al. (1997) showed a significant association between low IQ and later schizophrenia in a cohort study of male Swedish conscripts. Birth cohort studies can also reveal valuable information about potential etiological variables; the north Finland birth cohort (Rantakallio et al., 1997) revealed an association between central nervous system infections and later schizophrenia.

The main advantage with general population cohort studies is that they are an unbiased estimate of the at risk population; hence the findings, however limited, are generalizable and can be specifically applied to this illness (Table 15.2). However, large population samples are needed to yield a sufficient number of cases, and the number of predictive variables is often inadequate to address the specific questions. Further, birth cohort studies involve prolonged follow-up periods and are very expensive, leading to a delay of several decades before gaining predictive knowledge. However, prospective studies of young adult and adolescent cohorts (e.g. Davidson et al., 1999) may have an advantage of requiring a shorter follow-up. Finally, since large populations are involved, and most cohort studies have not begun with schizophrenia related research questions, the data collected at the outset is not fine-grained enough to ascertain neurodevelopmental antecedents of schizophrenia with any degree of specificity (Jones & Tarrant, 1999).

Follow-Back and Retrospective Studies

Follow-back studies examine precursors of adult onset psychopathology by examining medical or scholastic records of individuals with known outcome in adulthood. An innovative version of this strategy is the Archival-Observational Approach developed by Elaine Walker and colleagues (Walker & Lewine, 1990). These investigators collected old home movies from families of schizophrenic patients. Children who subsequently developed schizophrenia were distinguished by subtle but significant neuromotor abnormalities as compared to their unaffected siblings. These provocative findings support the view that dysmaturation of motor systems may occur in the future schizophrenic patient even in early childhood. The advantage of this approach is a relative freedom from recall bias (because of the archival source of information) that a representative sample of the schizophrenia population is obtained, and hence the findings are generalizable to this illness. However, the information available for such studies is severely limited and may or may not be related to pathophysiological questions of premorbid diathesis.

A distinction is often made between "follow-back" and retrospective studies; the former utilize archival sources of information that are relatively unbiased, and the latter studies are limited by the problems of recall bias. Retrospective studies rely on chart-review data, and other historical sources of information. The high prevalence of behavioral and cognitive difficulties in the general population can make them likely to be selectively attributed to the illness. Further, the information obtained in any retrospective analysis is likely to be too sketchy to allow examination of specific neurodevelopmental hypotheses.

Overall, it must be stated that all the above strategies seeking to elucidate premorbid neurodevelopmental risk factors have methodological limitations. Lack of statistical power, increased cost due to prolonged follow-up and the use of ill-established and "dated" predictive measures characterize high risk and birth cohort studies; the problems of recall bias and the inadequacy of retrospective information are limitations of retrospective studies. Studies of "super-high genetic risk" populations such as discordant MZ twins and children of two schizophrenic parents are limited by the fact that these are rare populations to find. Another way to enhance the power of high risk studies is to combine the genetic and psychobiological high risk strategies, rather than use either approach alone. Thus, one can select the subject initially for the presence of an affected relative, and then include only those who show one or other psychobiological markers, such as a personality deviation, SPEM impairment, attentional deviation, or ERP abnormality. In support of this approach are Moldin et al.'s (1991) observation that among offspring of schizophrenic parents, those with a deviant MMPI score had a higher risk of manifesting a schizophrenia outcome; and Cornblatt and Erlenmeyer-Kimling's (1989) observations of global attentional deviance being predictive of subsequent emergence of schizophrenia among the high risk offspring. Such an "enhanced high risk strategy" also suffers from the difficulty that findings from this design can not be generalized to all of schizophrenia because a narrowly defined population is studied. However, this approach is likely to have more statistical power to detect differences from controls, and can therefore be used to conduct the newer "second generation" high risk studies involving more expensive neurobiological studies (Table 15.2).

WHAT ARE THE METHODOLOGICAL ISSUES IN HIGH RISK RESEARCH?

Several studies of offspring of schizophrenics have been conducted worldwide over the last forty years. These studies have suggested several putative indicators of risk for schizophrenia (Table 15.3). However, "first generation" research of premorbid risk suffered from several methodological limitations that make it difficult to interpret many of the observations from these studies.

First, they were initiated at a time when explicit diagnostic criteria for diagnosis of psychiatric disorders had not yet been developed, and structured psychiatric diagnostic interviews were not used for obtaining reliable information for the diagnosis. Thus, many patients diagnosed as schizophrenic in these studies may not fulfill the current *DSM-IV* (*Diagnostic and Statistical Manual of Mental Disorders*, revised, 4th ed.) criteria for this illness. Diagnostic criteria are bound to change over time, but availability of

Table 15.3. Biobehavioral Predictors of Promise in "First Generation" High Risk Studies

- Neuromotor abnormalities in infancy and childhood (Fish et al., 1992)
- Schizotypy (Lenzenweger, 1994)
- Attentional deficits in childhood (Cornblatt & Keilp, 1994; Cornblatt et al., 1996)
- Working memory deficits in late childhood and adolescence (Erlenmeyer-Kimling, 1996)
- Eye movement dysfunction (Levy et al., 1994)
- Reduced or heightened electrodermal responsiveness (Cannon & Mednick, 1993)

comprehensive clinical information at baseline is critical to enable the researcher to apply future diagnostic schema to such information.

Second, several of these studies lacked a psychiatric control group, that is, offspring of parents with nonschizophrenic disorders, and thus failed to examine the issue of specificity. It is known that individuals at genetic risk for schizophrenia are at an increased risk for nonschizophrenic psychiatric disorder (Amminger et al., 1999). It is unclear whether this is due to a transmitted risk for a broad range of psychopathology, or whether nonschizophrenic psychopathology is a precursor, or a milder manifestation of schizophrenia. This question can best be addressed by having a psychiatric control group.

Third, previous studies have often suffered from difficulties in generalizability to schizophrenia. Children of schizophrenic patients are fewer and paternity may often be uncertain. For these reasons, in many studies, only children of female schizophrenic patients were included (Fish et al., 1992; Parnas et al., 1993; Tienari et al., 1994). Some studies excluded offspring because of lack of intact families (e.g., Erlenmeyer-Kimling et al., 1995). There are practical difficulties in conducting longitudinal studies of offspring from nonintact families. Recruiting nonrepresentative samples of high risk subjects could lead to loss of critical information on risk factors, leading to the problem of throwing the "baby out with the bathwater."

Thus, first generation studies have suffered from the problem of diagnostic reliability, specificity, and generalizability. Future studies need to address these limitations.

WHICH PREDICTIVE AND OUTCOME MEASURES SHOULD BE INVESTIGATED?

Our search for vulnerability markers has to begin by examining the possible trait-related alterations that characterize schizophrenia. A trait marker, to be useful in studies of familial vulnerability to schizophrenia, should (1) robustly distinguish the individuals with the illness from control populations; (2) be stable over time; (3) have greater prevalence in family members of identified schizophrenics than in the general population and be associated with psychotic spectrum disorder in family members; (4) be correlated with subsequent development of psychotic spectrum illness in high risk children and precede the development of clinical manifestations of psychotic spectrum disease; and (5) be relatively noninvasive and reliable (Garver, 1987).

Table 15.4. Putative
Neurobehavioral Markers of
Increased Risk for Schizophrenia

Psychometric Measures
Schizotypy
Psychosis proneness measures
Attentional measures
Working memory
Psychophysiological Measures
Eye movements
Electrodermal responsiveness
Evoked response potentials
Neurobiological Measures
Brain structural alterations (MRI)
Brain chemistry changes (MRS)

While none of the biobehavioral markers thus far examined in high risk studies fulfill all of these criteria, some are relatively more promising (Table 15.4); these include attentional impairment (Cornblatt & Obuchowski, 1997) and smooth pursuit eye movement abnormalities (Levy et al., 1994). The strongest evidence of impairment in relatives of schizophrenia patients appears to be in sustained attention, abstract thinking, and perceptual motor speed (Kremen et al., 1994). Among the various neuropsychological measures, the continuous performance test (CPT) appears to be consistently associated with liability to schizophrenia (Cornblatt & Keilp, 1994). A physiological measure that has received extensive attention is eye tracking abnormality (Levy et al., 1994), though most data are in adult relatives, and this measure has not been investigated as a predictor of schizophrenia risk in prospective studies (Cornblatt & Obuchowski, 1997). Cognitive evoked response potentials have also been proposed as measures of liability; prolonged latency and reduced amplitude of N100, p300, and p50 components have been observed among relatives (Friedman & Squires-Wheeler, 1994). Abnormal auditory event potentials (Schreiber et al., 1989) and electrodermal hypo- or hyperresponsiveness (Dykes et al., 1992; Hollister et al., 1994) have also been demonstrated, albeit less consistently.

The above measures are empirically derived, and only provide indirect clues as to what might be the neurobiological basis of these abnormalities. There is little evidence to suggest that neurochemical markers of dopaminergic or the serotonergic system predict increased risk for the development of schizophrenia (Csernansky & Newcomer, 1994). However, the advent of in vivo structural and physiological neuroimaging studies over the past two decades has raised the possibility that one may elucidate altered brain structure and function in the premorbid phase of schizophrenia. New in vivo approaches to examine the brain biology of abnormal neurodevelopment are beginning to be developed. Several studies, including our own (Keshavan et al., 1997; Lawrie et al., 1999; Schreiber et al., 1999), have shown evidence of structural brain abnormalities in young relatives of schizophrenic parents (Table 15.5). We have provided preliminary Magnetic Resonance Spectroscopy (MRS) data suggesting reductions in N-acetyl aspartate (NAA), an in vivo marker of neuronal integrity, in offspring at risk

Table 15.5. MRI Studies of Relatives at Familial Risk for Schizophrenia

Study	Subjects	Main Findings
Keshavan et al., 1997	11 adolescent offspring and 12 HC	Reduced AM, HCP, and increased third ventricles
Seidman et al., 1997	6 nonpsychotic siblings and 11 HC	Reduced AM, HCP, putamen, thalamus, and brain stem
Staal et al., 1998	32 healthy siblings 32 HC	Decreased thalamic volume
Sharma et al., 1998	31 schizophrenics, 57 relatives, and 39 HC	Larger left ventricles in "presumed" obligate carriers
Lawrie et al., 1999	100 relatives, 20 schizophrenics, and 30 HC	Bilateral HCP and thalamic volume reduction in relatives
Schreiber et al., 1999	15 adolescent offspring and 15 HC	Right AM and HCP volume reduction

HC: healthy controls; AM: amygdala; HCP: hippocampus

for schizophrenia (Keshavan et al., 1997). Using Blood Oxygenation Level Dependent (BOLD), and contrast Functional Magnetic Resonance Imaging (fMRI), it has now become possible to study regional brain activation during human development (Born et al., 1996); the development of neural networks as well as the changes in neural plasticity can thus be monitored noninvasively. It is also possible to conduct in vivo MRS studies prospectively from early in development (see Keshavan et al., 1997 for a review).

Choice of neurobiological and behavioral dependent parameters in schizophrenia high risk research has often been exploratory rather than hypothesis driven. The newer neurodevelopmental models allow formulation of predictors that are testable, and the newer in vivo imaging techniques make it feasible to examine several such hypotheses. The past two decades have witnessed a growing shift in viewing schizophrenia as a neurodevelopmental disorder. A detailed discussion of these models is beyond the scope of this chapter, and is detailed elsewhere (Keshavan & Hogarty, 1999). The timing of such a neurodevelopmental deviation has been a matter of debate, with both early (Murray & Lewis, 1987; Weinberger, 1987) and late models (Feinberg, 1982) being proposed. Briefly, the "early" model proposes a pre- or perinatal brain insult (viral, nutritional, autoimmune, or obstetric trauma) leading to a "fixed" developmental lesion (Weinberger, 1987); the "late" model, on the other hand, proposes an abnormality in postnatal developmental processes of dendritic pruning or myelination that occurs during late childhood and adolescence (Feinberg, 1982; Keshavan et al., 1994; Benes, 1995).

Several testable hypotheses can be generated from the early versus the late neurodevelopmental deviation models of schizophrenia which can potentially be tested in subjects at high risk for schizophrenia. For example, in *in vivo* anatomical studies, the "early" model would predict that subjects at high risk for schizophrenia have reduced cranial size (because growth in cranial size plateaus after the first two years of life), and reductions in both gray and white matter volumes (because of loss of both neurons and axons); on the other hand, the "late" neurodevelopmental models which do not invoke an early lesion predict a prominent reduction in gray matter (composed of synaptic neuropil which may decrease as a consequence of exaggerated dendritic pruning) without

(a) The hypothesis of exaggerated synaptic pruning in schizophrenia

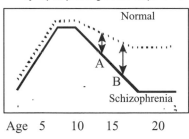

A = Baseline; B = Followup studies.

(b) The early developmental hypothesis of schizophrenia

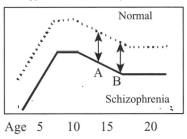

A = Baseline; B = Followup studies.

Figure 15.3. The "early" and "late" developmental models of schizophrenia.

changes in cranial size or white matter volume. A "late" neurodevelopmental model would predict that adolescent relatives at increased risk for schizophrenia may be more deviant from age matched controls than younger relatives. On the other hand, the "early" neurodevelopmental model would predict that high risk relatives would differ from age matched controls throughout childhood and adolescence (Figure 15.3). In designing future high risk studies, one should therefore consider putative neurobiological predictive variables demonstrated to have a significant association both with the schizophrenia diathesis as well as with brain maturation.

The choice of outcome measures in designing high risk studies also merits some fresh thinking. It should be kept in mind that developmental pathways can vary widely between individuals; one specific etiological factor can lead to diverse psychopathological outcomes (multi-finality) and several etiological variables and several developmental pathways can lead to a common clinical outcome (equi-finality). Thus, early high risk follow-up studies have suggested that offspring of schizophrenia patients have an increased risk not only for schizophrenia but also for a broader range of schizophrenia spectrum disorders (see Table 15.1). Additionally, the New York High Risk Project also showed that high risk subjects who eventually developed schizophrenia had an excess of nonpsychotic behavioral disturbances (Amminger et al., 1999). It is well known that a variety of nonpsychotic psychiatric difficulties may characterize the schizophrenia prodrome (Hafner, 1990). It may therefore be advantageous for follow up studies of high risk subjects to cast a broad range of outcome measures. This approach may be of advantage from a public health point of view, since such data may allow more than one outcome to be identified, as well as prevented (Jones & Tarrant, 1999).

WHEN, DURING DEVELOPMENT, IS IT MOST FRUITFUL TO ASCERTAIN PREMORBID RISK?

In designing studies of premorbid risk in schizophrenia, it is important to keep in mind the fact that certain periods during development may be particularly sensitive for the impact of adverse biological or environmental influences. Such "sensitive" periods include the fetal, neonatal, and early childhood periods as well as adolescence. Studies of adolescent individuals at risk for schizophrenia may be advantageous in designing studies of premorbid risk for schizophrenia for several reasons. First, the period of late

Table 15.6. Toward a Second Generation of High-Risk Studies

- An "enhanced" HR design may be more cost effective
- Multisite studies may be statistically more powerful
- Frontotemporal and subcortical structural and metabolic parameters may be the neurobiological markers worth pursuing
- Attention and executive functions may be the neurobehavioral markers of promise
- Need to consider a broad range of outcome measures of the schizophrenia diathesis
- Adolescence is a critical window of opportunity to study developmental risk for schizophrenia

postnatal development is unique as it involves an experience dependent reorganization of neural structures. Neurobiological phenomena that undergo major changes during such critical periods (e.g., delta sleep, membrane synthesis, and cortical gray matter structure) are also abnormal in schizophrenia, suggesting that an abnormality in the peri-adolescent brain maturational processes may underlie pathogenesis of schizophrenia (Keshavan & Hogarty, 1999; Feinberg, 1982). Second, adolescence represents an age period closer to the illness onset, since schizophrenia has its typical onset in adolescence; follow up of adolescent high risk subjects may therefore be cost-effective since a shorter duration of follow up may be needed to determine outcome. Third, there is evidence from genetic high risk studies (see review by Gooding & Iacono, 1995) suggesting that at least a subgroup of high risk subjects may become increasingly deviant with age during childhood and adolescence. Finally, recent data support the predictive ability of neurobehavioral indices in adolescence for schizophrenia related outcome. A recent "historical" prospective (or follow-back) study (Davidson et al., 1999) of healthy male young adult draftees to the Israeli draft board showed that schizophrenia could be predicted with a high specificity by deficits in social and intellectual functioning that were evident during adolescence. Neurobehavioral and neurobiological characterization of adolescent at risk subjects is therefore likely to be fruitful; however, it is important to ensure that the variables being examined have temporally stabilized, because of the enormous influence of age on several biological parameters of interest.

CONCLUSIONS

The "first generation" high risk studies have revealed noteworthy findings of impaired attentional and neurobehavioral abnormalities in individuals at genetic risk for schizophrenia. While these observations are consistent with the neurodevelopmental basis of schizophrenia, it is unlikely that such observations as yet have an established predictive value for schizophrenia at this time. However, these findings provide a good foundation for future studies; the goal of future high risk studies is to elucidate the premorbid neurobiological risk for schizophrenia and utilize such knowledge for early identification and intervention in this illness. The following caveats are worth keeping in mind while designing such studies (Table 15.6).

First, previous high risk studies are limited by their expense, as they involve prolonged follow-up periods with the likelihood of only a small proportion of the individuals developing the illness. Table 15.2 outlines the merits and disadvantages of the various approaches to studying premorbid developmental risk. It is proposed in this review that an "enhanced" high risk strategy that involves a genetically at risk population and the use of putative neurobehavioral/psychopathological markers of risk may increase the likelihood of identifying premorbid risk indicators in schizophrenia. Using a narrow approach of identifying only individuals with a genetic predisposition to schizophrenia is likely to limit generalizability of high risk studies to schizophrenia; an alternative is to define risk broadly, using both vulnerability indicators (family history, biological markers) as well as prodromal psychopathological indicators (e.g., "subthreshold" psychotic and negative symptoms; Yung et al., 1998). Such individuals are difficult to reliably identify and characterize, however. Carefully coordinated, multicenter studies of broadly defined high risk subjects are a valuable approach toward enhancing statistical power.

Second, the first generation high risk studies have often been explorative, at least in part, due to the lack of adequate theoretical models. During the past two decades, newer conceptualizations such as the neurodevelopmental models of schizophrenia have generated many testable predictions; the advent of noninvasive methodologies such as structural and functional neuroimaging allows testing of such predictions. Future high risk studies are therefore likely to be more hypothesis driven. The choice of predictive measures in future high risk studies should be driven by the emerging neurobiological hypotheses of schizophrenia. Among the promising predictive markers are neurobehavioral indices such as attentional impairment and neuroimaging measures reflecting the integrity of frontotemporal and subcortical brain structures. The follow-up studies should also include a broad range of outcome measures since previous studies have suggested that risk is increased not only for schizophrenia but a broader spectrum of schizophrenia related psychopathology. Issues of specificity and generalizability should also be carefully considered.

Third, the question of when it might be most fruitful to study premorbid risk for schizophrenia should also draw upon ongoing newer scientific research in schizophrenia. Over the past decade, adolescence has increasingly been viewed as a critical period of development during which the schizophrenia diathesis might unfold. Studies of adolescent high risk subjects also offer the advantage of proximity to the onset of schizophrenic illness and are therefore likely to be cost efficient.

Finally, while this review has focused on premorbid neurodevelopmental antecedents of schizophrenia, the approaches discussed herein are applicable to other neuropsychiatric developmental disorders as well. Bipolar disorder, which has been considered to have neurodevelopmental origins (Nasrallah & Tolbert, 1997), also has an onset in late adolescence or early adulthood; obsessive compulsive disorder has also been recently viewed as a neurodevelopmental disorder (Rosenberg & Keshavan, 1998).

The eventual aim of any investigative strategy in medicine is to help diagnosis and treatment monitoring for the benefit of the patient. The new generation of high risk studies can accomplish those goals. Recent advances in developmental neurobiology and neuroscience make it reasonable to expect a paradigm shift in research on schizophrenia. Studies of vulnerability as well as protective factors and studies of nature as well as nurture are needed. It is critical that such research is linked meaningfully to our efforts for early detection and intervention of this debilitating disorder. It is hoped that the third millennium will usher in a new generation of high risk research studies and move us closer to piecing together the puzzle of schizophrenia.

REFERENCES

Amminger, G. P., Pape, S., Rock, D., Roberts, S. A., Ott, S. L., Squires-Wheeler, E., Kestenbaum, C., & Erlenmeyer-Kimling, L. (1999). Relationship between childhood behavioral disturbance and later schizophrenia in the New York High-Risk Project. *American Journal of Psychiatry, 156,* 525–530.

Benes, F. M. (1995). A neurodevelopmental approach to the understanding of schizophrenia and other mental disorders. In D. Cicchetti & D. J. Cohen (Eds.), *Developmental psychopathology: Theory and methods* (pp. 227–253). New York: Wiley.

Born, P., Rostrup, E., Leth, H., Peitersen, B., & Lou, H. C. (1996). Changes of visually induced cortical activation patterns during development. *Lancet, 347,* 543–544.

Cannon, T. D., & Mednick, S. A. (1993). The schizophrenia high-risk project in Copenhagen: three decades of progress. *Acta Psychiatrica Scandinavica, Supplementum, 370,* 33–47.

Carter, J. W., Parnas, J., Cannon, T. D., Schulsinger, F., & Mednick, S. A. (1999). MMPI variables predictive of schizophrenia in the Copenhagen High-Risk Project: a 25-year follow-up. *Acta Psychiatrica Scandinavica, 99,* 432–440.

Chapman, L. J., Chapman, J. P., & Raulin, M. L. (1976). Scales for physical and social anhedonia. *Journal of Abnormal Psychology, 85,* 374–382.

Chapman, L. J., Chapman, J. P., & Raulin, M. (1978). Body-image aberration in schizophrenia. *Journal of Abnormal Psychology, 87,* 399–407.

Clark, V. P., Courchesne, E., & Grafe, M. (1992). In vivo myeloarchitecture analysis of human striate and extrastriate cortex using Magnetic Resonance Imaging. *Cerebral Cortex, 2,* 417–424.

Cornblatt, B. A., Dworkin, R. H., Wolf, L. E., & Erlenmeyer-Kimling, L. (1996). Markers, developmental processes, and schizophrenia. In M. F. Lenzenweger & J. J. Haugaard (Eds.), *Frontiers of developmental psychopathology* (pp. 125–147). New York: Oxford University Press.

Cornblatt, B., & Erlenmeyer-Kimling, L. (1985). Global attentional deviance as a marker of risk for schizophrenia: Specificity and predictive validity. *Journal of Abnormal Psychology, 94,* 470–486.

Cornblatt, B., & Erlenmeyer-Kimling. (1989). Attention and schizophrenia. *Schizophrenia Research, 2,* 58.

Cornblatt, B. A., & Keilp, J. G. (1994). Impaired attention, genetics, and the pathophysiology of schizophrenia. *Schizophrenia Bulletin, 20,* 31–46.

Cornblatt, B., & Obuchowski, M. (1997). Update of high risk research: 1987–1997. *International Review of Psychiatry, 9,* 437–447.

Csernansky, J. G., & Newcomer, J. W. (1994). Are there neurochemical indicators of vulnerability to schizophrenia? *Schizophrenia Bulletin, 20,* 89–102.

David, A. S., Malmberg, A., Brandt, L., Allebeck, P., & Lewis, G. (1997). IQ and risk for schizophrenia: a population-based cohort study. *Psychological Medicine, 27,* 1131–1323.

Davidson, M., Reichenberg, A., Rabinowitz, J., Weiser, M., Kaplan, Z., & Mark, M. (1999). Behavioral and intellectual markers for schizophrenia in apparently healthy male adolescents. *American Journal of Psychiatry, 156,* 1328–1335.

DeLisi, L. E., Goldin, L. R., Hamovit, J. R., Maxwell, M. E., Kurtz, D., & Gershon, E. S. (1986). A family study of the association of increased ventricular size with schizophrenia. *Archives of General Psychiatry, 43,* 148–153.

Done, D. J., Crow, T. J., Johnstone, E. C., & Sacker, A. (1994). Childhood antecedents of schizophrenia and affective illness: Social adjustments at ages 7 and 11. *British Medical Journal, 309,* 699–703.

Dykes, K. L., Mednick, S. A., Machon, R. A., Praestholm, J., & Parnas, J. (1992). Adult third ventricle width and infant behavioral arousal in groups at high and low risk for schizophrenia. *Schizophrenic Research, 7,* 13–18.

Erlenmeyer-Kimling, L., Squires-Wheeler, E., Hilldoff-Adamo, U. H., Bassett, A. S., Cornblatt, B. A., Kestenbaum, C. J., Rock, D., Roberts, S. A., & Gottesman, I. I. (1995). The New York High-Risk

Project. Psychoses and cluster A personality disorders in offspring of schizophrenic parents at 23 years of follow-up. *Archives of General Psychiatry, 52,* 857–865.

Feinberg, I. (1982). Schizophrenia and late maturational brain changes in man. *Psychopharmacology Bulletin, 18,* 29–31.

Fish, B., Marcus, J., Hans, S. L., Auerbach, J. G., & Perdue, S. (1992). Infants at risk for schizophrenia: Sequelae of a genetic neurointegrative defect: A review and replication analysis of pandysmaturation in the Jerusalem Infant Development Study. *Archives of General Psychiatry, 49,* 221–235.

Friedman, D., & Squires-Wheeler, E. (1994). Event-related potentials (ERPs) as indicators for risk for schizophrenia. *Schizophrenia Bulletin, 20*(1), 63–74.

Garver, D. L. (1987). Methodological issues facing the interpretation of high-risk studies: Biological heterogeneity (Review). *Schizophrenia Bulletin, 13,* 525–529.

Gooding, D. C., & Iacono, W. G. (1995). Schizophrenia through the lens of a developmental psychopathology perspective. In D. Cicchetti & D. J. Cohen (Eds.), *Developmental psychopathology: Risk, disorder, and adaptation* (pp. 535–580). New York: Wiley.

Gottesman, I. I., & Shields, J. (1982). *Schizophrenia: The epigenetic puzzle.* New York: Cambridge University Press.

Hafner, H. (1990). New perspectives in the epidemiology of schizophrenia. In H. Hafner & W. F. Gattaz (Eds.), *Search for the causes of schizophrenia* (pp. 408–431). Berlin: Springer-Verlag.

Hanson, D. R., Gottesman, I. I., & Heston, L. L. (1990). Long-range schizophrenia forecasting: many a slip twixt cup and lip. In J. Rolf, A. Masten, D. Cicchetti, K. Nuechterlein, & S. Weintraub (Eds.), *Risk and protective factors in the development of psychopathology.* New York: Cambridge University Press.

Hollister, J. M., Mednick, S. A., Brennan, P., & Cannon, T. D. (1994). Impaired autonomic nervous system-habituation in those at genetic risk for schizophrenia. *Archives of General Psychiatry, 51,* 552–558.

Holzman, P. S., Levy, D. L., & Proctor, L. R. (1976). Smooth pursuit eye movements, attention, and schizophrenia. *Archives of General Psychiatry, 33,* 1415–1420.

Ingraham, L. J., Kugelmass, S., Frenkel, E., Nathan, M., & Mirsky, A. F. (1995). Twenty-five year follow-up of the Israeli High-Risk Study: current and lifetime psychopathology. *Schizophrenia Bulletin, 21,* 183–192.

Jones, P., Rodgers, B., Murray, R., & Marmot, M. (1994). Child developmental risk factors for adult schizophrenia in the British 1946 birth cohort. *Lancet, 344,* 1398–1402.

Jones, P. B., & Tarrant, C. J. (1999). Specificity of developmental precursors to schizophrenia and affective disorders. *Schizophrenia Research, 39,* 121–125.

Josiassen, R. C., Shagass, C., Roemer, R. A., & Straumanis, J. J. (1985). Attention-related effects on somatosensory evoked potentials in college students at high risk for psychopathology. *Journal of Abnormal Psychiatry, 94,* 507–518.

Keshavan, M. S., Anderson, S., & Pettegrew, J. W. (1994). Is schizophrenia due to excessive synaptic pruning in the prefrontal cortex? *Journal of Psychiatric Research, 28,* 239–265.

Keshavan, M. S., & Cornblatt, B. (2000). Early pharmacotherapeutic intervention in the prodromal phase of schizophrenia: Is this a good idea? PRO/CON. *The Journal of Psychotic Disorders,* IV(2), 3.

Keshavan, M. S., & Hogarty, G. E. (1999). Brain maturational processes and delayed onset in schizophrenia. *Development and Psychopathology, 11,* 525–543.

Keshavan, M. S., Kapur, S., & Pettegrew, J. W. (1991). Magnetic resonance spectroscopy in psychiatry: Potential, pitfalls and promise. *American Journal of Psychiatry, 148,* 976–985.

Keshavan, M. S., Montrose, D. M., Pierri, J. N., Dick, E. L., Rosenberg, D., Talagala, L., & Sweeney, J. A. (1997). Magnetic resonance imaging and spectroscopy in offspring at risk for schizophrenia: Preliminary studies. *Progress in Neuro-Psychopharmacology and Biological Psychiatry, 21,* 1285–1295.

Keshavan, M. S., Pettegrew, J. W., Panchalingam, K., Kaplan, D., Brar, J., & Campbell, K. (1989). In vivo ^{31}P nuclear magnetic resonance (NMR) spectroscopy of the frontal lobe metabolism in neuroleptic naive first episode psychoses. *Schizophrenia Research, 2,* 122.

Keshavan, M. S., & Schooler, N. R. (1992). First-episode studies of schizophrenia: Criteria and characterization. *Schizophrenia Bulletin, 18,* 491–513.

SIXTEEN

Interactions of the Dopamine, Serotonin, and GABA Systems During Childhood and Adolescence

Influence of Stress on the Vulnerability for Psychopathology

Francine M. Benes

The past decade has been characterized by a significant change in the approach of psychologists and neuroscientists to the study of psychopathology (Cicchetti, 1993; Cicchetti & Cannon, 1999) and how we conceptualize the etiology of mental illness during childhood, adolescence, and adulthood (Benes, 1995). Among these disorders, schizophrenia and, more recently, bipolar disorder have received the most attention with recent postmortem studies having provided compelling evidence for a defect of GABAergic neurotransmission playing a role in its pathophysiology (for a review, see Benes & Berretta, 2001). For example, findings of a decreased density of interneurons (Benes, McSparren, Bird, SanGiovanni, & Vincent, 1991; Benes, Kwok, Vincent, & Todtenkopf, 1998), reduced GABA uptake (Simpson et al., 1989; Reynolds, Czudek, & Andrews, 1990), increased GABA receptor binding activity (Benes, Khan, Vincent, & Wickramasinghe, 1996; Benes, Vincent, Alsterberg, Bird, & SanGiovanni, 1992), decreased GABA terminals (Benes, Todtenkopf, Logiotatos, & Williams, 2000), and reduced expression of mRNA for GAD65 and GAD67 (Akbarian et al., 1995; Guidotti et al., 2000; Heckers et al., 2001; Volk, Austin, Pierri, Sampson, & Lewis, 2000) reported to date are consistent with the idea that there may be a decrease of GABAergic cells and/or activity in these disorders. Since the mechanism of action of antipsychotic medication involves blockade of both dopamine and serotonin receptors (Meltzer, 1994), a key question is how GABA cells interact with these monoaminergic systems in corticolimbic regions of schizophrenic brain. Thus far, studies of the dopamine (for a review, see Svensson, 2000) and serotonin (for a review, see Marek & Aghajanian, 1998) systems have failed to demonstrate consistent abnormalities that can be convincingly distinguished from neuroleptic effects. A recent report, however, has suggested that a subtle "mis-wiring" of the dopamine system with respect to pyramidal neurons and GABA cells may be present in the anterior cingulate cortex of subjects with schizophrenia (Benes, 2000). Such an abnormality could be present without there being any associated changes in the levels of biochemical and molecular markers for the dopamine system. If this latter hypothesis is correct, then it will be important to gain some insight into how aberrant connections between monoaminergic fibers and intrinsic cortical neurons may arise and how such changes may influence corticolimbic function.

The discovery that there are subtle alterations in the organization of the corticolimbic system in schizophrenia (Benes, Davidson, & Bird, 1986; Jakob & Beckmann,

1986; Kovelman & Scheibel, 1984) has resulted in the broadly held belief that this disorder is neurodevelopmental in nature (Benes, 1988; Weinberger, 1987). In addition, it seems likely that normal maturational changes in the corticolimbic system during late adolescence may act as a "trigger" for the onset of this illness in susceptible individuals (Benes, 1988, 1989; Keshavan & Hogarty, 1999). In order to understand further the implications of this hypothesis not only for schizophrenia, but also for other neuropsychiatric disorders that present during childhood and adolescence, the following discussion will examine the anatomic relationship of the monoaminergic systems to intrinsic cortical neurons, particularly GABAergic cells, and will consider how the development of these interactions could potentially go awry in relation to stress during the postnatal period.

INTERACTIONS OF DOPAMINE AND SEROTONIN FIBERS WITH CORTICAL NEURONS

It is now well established that the activity of cortical neurons is probably modulated by both the dopamine and serotonin systems. In rat medial prefrontal cortex, a homologue of the anterior cingulate cortex of human brain, serotoninergic fibers are abundantly present in both superficial and deep laminae (Lidov, Grzanna, & Molliver, 1980; Reader, 1981), while dopamine fibers are most densely distributed in layers V and VI (Emson & Koob, 1978; Lindvall & Bjorklund, 1978). Recent studies have demonstrated that both pyramidal (Goldman-Rakic, Leranth, Williams, Mons, & Geffard, 1989; Seguela, Watkins, & Descarries, 1988; Verney, Alvarez, Gerrard, & Berger, 1990), the principle projections cells of the cortex, and nonpyramidal (Verney et al., 1990; Benes, Vincent, & Molloy, 1993a) neurons, the local circuit cells that modulate their activity, both receive inputs from dopamine fibers. In some studies, each of these neuronal subtypes have both the D1 and D2 receptor binding activity (Benes, Vincent, & Molloy, 1993a; Vincent & Benes, 1995) and their respective messenger RNAs (Huntley, Morrison, Prikhozhan, & Sealfon, 1992) localized to their cell bodies. Rodent studies in which in situ hybridization has been used to localize mRNA for the two subtypes have demonstrated that projection cells of various laminae may express one or the other subtype (Gaspar, Bloch, & Le Moine, 1995), although the D2 receptor seemed to be principally associated with those in layer V. More recent work has demonstrated that mRNA for the D1 and D2 subtypes is also expressed by some but not all cortical GABAergic interneurons subtypes (Le Moine & Gaspar, 1998); the cells showing mRNA for both receptors were principally those containing parvalbumin, while those showing calbindin-immunoreactivity seemed to preferentially express the D1. Some immunocytochemical studies in primates have preferentially localized the D1 receptor to pyramidal neurons (Bergson, Mrzljak, Lidow, Goldman-Rakic, & Levenson, 1995; Smiley, Levey, Ciliax, & Goldman-Rakic, 1994), while others have found it in interneurons (Muly, Szigeti, & Goldman-Rakic, 1998); however, technical factors might account for this discrepancy. Using a very sensitive high resolution analysis of the distribution of D1 receptor binding activity, this receptor was found to be expressed by both projection cells and interneurons in rodent mPFC (Davidoff & Benes, 1998).

For the serotonin system, the activity of both pyramidal and nonpyramidal neurons can also be manipulated with either agonists or antagonists of its receptors (Gellman & Aghajanian, 1993; Sheldon & Aghajanian, 1990). While the $5HT_{2A}$ is expressed by both pyramidal cells (Jakab & Goldman-Rakic, 1998; Wu et al., 1998) and GABA neurons (Morilak & Ciaranello, 1993; Gellman & Aghajanian, 1993) in frontal cortices, the $5HT_{1A}$ subtype in hippocampus (Chalmers, Lopez, Vazquez, Akil, & Watson, 1994; Chalmers, Kwak, Mansour, Akil, & Watson, 1993) and the $5HT_{1C}$ subtype in pyriform cortex (Sheldon & Aghajanian, 1991) of rat brain may be preferentially expressed by pyramidal neurons. Thus, the pattern of expression for various receptor subtypes may vary from one region to another.

The above observations suggest that both projection cells and local circuit cells may be *potentially* influenced by the dopaminergic and serotonergic projections to mPFCx (Benes, Todtenkopf, & Taylor, 1997). It is noteworthy that a convergence of these fiber systems on to intrinsic cortical neurons could play an important role in the cortical stress response. Exposure to stress has not only been associated with changes in dopamine (Roth, Tam, Ida, Yang, & Deutch, 1988; Thierry, Tassin, Blanc, & Glowinski, 1976), but also serotonin (Chaouloff, 2000; Maines, Keck, Dugar, & Lakoski, 1998), particularly in key corticolimbic regions such as the hippocampus (Lopez, Chalmers, Vazquez, Akil, & Watson, 1993) and amygdala (Stutzmann, McEwen, & LeDoux, 1998), but has also been implicated in the regulation of pyramidal cells (Chalmers et al., 1993; Chalmers et al., 1994) and GABAergic interneurons (Corda & Biggio, 1986; Schwartz, Wess, Labarca, Skolnick, & Paul, 1987). Studies in which the learned helplessness model has been used to study stress have found a decrease of serotonergic function (Petty, Kramer, & Moeller, 1994). For schizophrenia and bipolar disorder, it seems likely that stress would contribute to the pathophysiology of these disorders by altering the modulation of monoaminergic inputs to GABAergic cells; the activity of these latter interneurons may also be influenced by exposure to stress, independent of its effect on monoaminergic activity.

To understand how the dopamine and serotonin systems may be interacting with intrinsic cortical neurons, it is important to know whether the respective fiber systems project to mutually exclusive neuronal subpopulations or whether perhaps there is a significant degree of overlap in the neurons receiving inputs from these two systems. In order to investigate this question, these two transmitter systems have been co-localized using a combination of single, double, and triple immunocytochemical approaches (Benes, Taylor, & Cunningham, 2000; Taylor & Benes, 1996).

When sections are processed simultaneously with antibodies against 5HT, TH, and glutamate decarboxylase (Benes & Berretta, 2001), two patterns of interaction have been observed. On the one hand, both serotonin and dopamine fibers are found in apposition with the same GABAergic interneuron, with approximately 25 percent of GABAergic cells showing a convergence of these two fiber systems. The second pattern observed with the triple localization involved appositions of serotonin, dopamine, and GABA fibers with pyramidal neurons. This so-called "trivergence" of these three types of fibers suggests that pyramidal neurons may not only receive traditional inhibitory inputs from GABAergic terminals, but also modulatory ones from the two monoaminergic systems. Taken together, it appears that the dopamine and serotonin systems may interact extensively with both pyramidal cells *and* interneurons (Figure 16.1). Although some of these interactions may be present at the level of the cell body, it is likely that the majority are occurring within the neuropil area where the dendritic branches of both cell types are localized.

EARLY ADOLESCENCE

LATE ADOLESCENCE

NORMAL

NORMAL

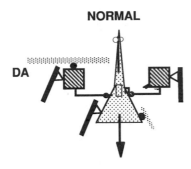
DA

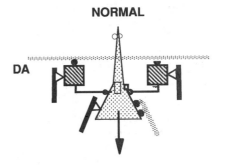
DA

PRE- AND POSTNATAL STRESS

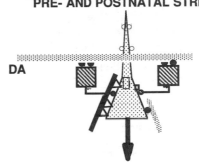
DA

 Inhibitory GABA Interneuron

Pyramidal Cell

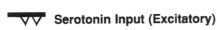 Dopamine Input (Inhibitory)

Serotonin Input (Excitatory)

Figure 16.1. A schematic diagram depicting a convergence of dopamine (DA) and serotonin (5HT) on pyramidal neurons and GABAergic interneurons in anterior cingulate cortex during early and late adolescence and in relation to pre- and postnatal stress. Early Adolescence: A pyramidal neuron is shown flanked by two inhibitory GABAergic interneurons. Both of these cells have already attained a mature pattern of connectivity with the pyramidal neurons. In addition, the 5HT inputs to the GABA cells (one per cell) and to the pyramidal neuron (two per cell) also have a distribution that is similar to that seen later during the adolescent period (right). Late Adolescence: The DA inputs to the GABA cell (one per cell) and to the pyramidal neuron (two per cell) have both increased to appropriate adult levels. The 5HT inputs to both cell types are similar to those seen during early adolescence. Pre- and Postnatal Stress: The GABA cells have an increased number of DA inputs; some may be relocated from the pyramidal neuron, while others may be produced by a sprouting of fibers. The 5HT inputs to the GABA cells have been decreased, but they have been relocated on to the pyramidal neuron. If DA fibers are inhibitory in nature, then this circuit predicts that the activity of the GABAergic cells may be significantly down-modulated. On the other hand, the activity of the pyramidal neuron would be markedly up-modulated as a result of (a) the decreased GABAergic activity influencing it, and (b) the increase of excitatory serotonergic inputs that once occupied termination sites on the GABA cells.

The responses associated with activation of the dopamine system are typically modulatory in nature and show a much longer duration than is typically observed with "classic" synaptic inputs (Bunney & Chiodo, 1984; Gulledge & Jaffe, 1998; Reader, Ferron, Descarries, & Jasper, 1979; Thierry, Mantz, Milla, & Glowinski, 1988), like those from GABAergic cells. In contrast, those responses associated with serotonergic inputs seem to exert a secondary influence on pyramidal neurons via GABAergic cells (Sheldon & Aghajanian, 1991). This arrangement may show some regional variation, as the action of serotonin in the medial prefrontal cortex appears to be a pre-synaptic one that is exerted on a subpopulation of glutamatergic terminals (Marek & Aghajanian, 1998). Further study is needed to identify the various ways in which dopamine and serotonin fibers may influence the activity of intrinsic cortical neurons.

POSTNATAL DEVELOPMENT OF MONOAMINERGIC FIBERS AND INTRINSIC CORTICAL NEURONS

It has long been suspected that the development of corticolimbic regions of human brain may continue well beyond birth (Benes, 1989; Benes, Turtle, Khan, & Farol, 1994; Flechsig, 1920; Yakovlev & Lecours, 1967). Recently, this idea has received increased attention with the growing realization that normal maturational changes probably play an important role in the appearance of various neuropsychiatric diseases at specific stages of postnatal life (Benes, 1988; Weinberger, 1987). Normal ontogenetic changes at critical stages of development could potentially act as "triggers" for the onset of various disorders at one or another stage of development. Many studies have demonstrated that there are significant changes in several key neurotransmitter systems at critical stages of the postnatal period (for comprehensive reviews, see Johnston, 1988; Parnavelas, Papadopoulos, & Cavanagh, 1988).

The Dopamine System

Dopaminergic projections to rat medial prefrontal cortex (mPFCx) have been found to increase progressively beyond the weanling stage until the early adult period (Kalsbeek, Voorn, Buijs, Pool, & Uylings, 1988; Verney, Berger, Adrien, Vigny, & Gay, 1982). During the first two postnatal weeks, the density of dopamine fibers in rat medial prefrontal cortex is quite low, but shows progressive increases into adulthood (Benes et al., 1993). A similar pattern of fiber staining occurs at all postnatal stages examined. Unlike the migration and differentiation of cortical neurons, the increase of dopamine fibers does not progress in a distinct "inside-out" manner (Benes, Vincent, Molloy, & Khan, 1996; Verney et al., 1982). The size of dopamine varicosities also doubles between the preweanling and adult periods.

Postnatal increases in the density of dopaminergic projections to rat mPFCx (Kalsbeek et al., 1988; Verney et al., 1982) are paralleled by an increase of D_2 receptor binding activity that begins prenatally (Bruinink, Lichtensteiner, & Schlumpf, 1983) and continues until the fourth postnatal week (Deskin, Seidler, Whitmore, & Slotkin, 1981). Interestingly, administration of 6-OH-dopamine prevents this latter increase of D_2 receptor binding (Deskin et al., 1981), an effect that is associated with dystrophic changes in the basal dendrites of pyramidal neurons (Kalsbeek et al., 1988). Lesions induced in the prefrontal cortex of adult monkeys using 6-OH-dopamine result in an impaired performance of the spatial delayed alternation task (Brozoski, Brown, Rosvold, & Goldman, 1979), and it seems likely that this functional deficit would be associated with changes in the D2 receptor on pyramidal neurons.

The GABA System

Gamma-aminobutyric acid (GABA) has long been considered the most important inhibitory neurotransmitter in the mammalian brain, and extensive neurochemical studies of its development in rodent brain suggest that its maturation continues well into the postnatal period (for a review, see Johnston, 1988). For example, GABA-accumulating cells show a progressive increase in numerical density until P11, the equivalent of childhood in rats (Chronwall & Wolff, 1980). In contrast, the concentration of GABA, the GABA-synthesizing enzyme GAD (Coyle & Enna, 1976), high affinity GABA receptor binding activity (Coyle & Enna, 1976; Palacios, Niehoff, & Kuhar, 1979), and the messenger [m]RNA that encodes this receptor protein (Gambarana, Pittman, & Siegel, 1990), all increase until the third postnatal week in rats. This latter interval marks the beginning of the postweanling period and is roughly equivalent to early adolescence, except that rodents have not as yet achieved reproductive capabilities.

At birth, the number of GABA cells in the cortex reaches a peak at approximately postnatal day 5, which is considered by some to be equivalent to the perinatal period in primates and humans. The number of these interneurons then diminishes until the start of the early adolescent period in rats (P20) when the cortical mantle has attained a maximum thickness (Vincent & Benes, 1995). This expansion of the cortex is synchronized with the increase in the relative amount of neuropil surrounding cell bodies and appears to be related to the presence of an increasing number of dendritic and axonal processes. At the same time, GABAergic cell bodies also show significant changes, such as a gradual increase in size and the appearance of prominent secondary and tertiary branches of their dendritic tree. Thus, the expansion of cortical neuropil probably involves, in part, an increase of both dendritic branches and terminals of GABAergic interneurons, and this process continues until the early postweanling period (P25) or early adolescence (Vincent, Khan, & Benes, 1995). This period also overlaps with the appearance of increased efficacy of GABAergic synaptic transmission (Luhmann & Prince, 1991). In rat cortex, the maturation of the GABA system continues for 3 postnatal weeks and appears to be complete by the equivalent of early adolescence.

Taking together the observations made in studies of the postnatal development of neurotransmitter systems, it appears that the full maturation of the GABA system is probably complete *before* the dopamine system has attained its full postnatal profile. Presumably, the dendritic tree of GABAergic interneurons may be lying in wait for the ingrowing dopamine fibers to target them for the formation of functional interactions.

The Development of Dopamine-GABA Interactions during Childhood and Adolescence

As previously reported using a double localization technique (Benes et al., 1996), both DA fibers and GABAergic cell bodies show a progressive increase in their interaction with one another between the preweanling period (equivalent to childhood) and the early stages of the postweanling period (equivalent to early adolescence). Moreover, an increasing number of DA fibers form contacts with GABAergic neurons as the postweanling period progresses, and this becomes most apparent at the beginning of the adult period (P60 in rats). When an *index of interaction* is computed by multiplying the percentage of GABA cell somata having apposed dopamine varicosities and the number of DA varicosities in contact with any given GABA-cell body, postweanling rats have an index that is 1.5 times higher than that seen in preweanling animals. By adulthood, this index increases 1.8 times with respect to postweanling rats and 2.5 times when compared to preweanling animals (Benes et al., 1993). Thus, the interaction of DA fibers with GABA cells increases dramatically during the periods equivalent to childhood and adolescence.

Taken together, the somata of GABAergic neurons probably act as a site with which sprouting dopaminergic fibers may form appositions. In this process, GABA cells may be a "passive" target for the formation of interactions; alternatively, they might exert an "active" neurotrophic influence on fiber sprouting and/or contact formation (Spoerri, 1988). Either way, it seems likely that dopaminergic fibers are capable of exerting an increasing modulatory influence on the activity of inhibitory interneurons during the equivalent of childhood and adolescence, particularly since DA receptors are localized on nonpyramidal cell bodies in rat mPFCx (Benes et al., 1993; Vincent & Benes, 1995). Moreover, both agonists and antagonists of DA can alter the postsynaptic potentials recorded in GABAergic interneurons in pyriform (Gellman & Aghajanian, 1993) and frontal (Zhou & Hablitz, 1999) cortices. Moreover, agonists of the D_2 receptor have been found to inhibit the release of $[^3H]$GABA (Retaux, Besson, & Penit-Soria, 1991; Tam & Roth, 1990) and dopamine itself can influence the firing of GABAergic neurons (Penit-Soria, Audinat, & Crepel, 1987). Thus, changes in the interaction of dopamine fibers with GABA cells during childhood and adolescence are probably associated with important functional consequences.

It has been postulated that a "mis-wiring" of dopamine fibers with GABA cells may be present in the anterior cingulate region of schizophrenics (Benes, Todtenkopf, & Taylor, 1997), although it is not clear whether such a change might have been present from birth or possibly have appeared *de novo* during adolescence as the disorder is becoming manifest. In a series of experiments that were designed to address this issue, rats were exposed to stress-simulating doses of corticosterone during the pre- and postnatal periods. Those rats exposed to corticosterone *both* pre- and postnatally showed an increase in the number of dopamine varicosities forming appositions with nonpyramidal cell bodies (Benes et al., 1997). In contrast, those rats exposed to glucocorticoid only during the postnatal period did not show this change. Direct effects of steroids on the expression of mRNA for TH (Iuvone & Dunn, 1986; Stone, Freedman, & Morgano, 1978; Stone & McCarty, 1983) could play a role in the induction of these changes during the postweanling and early adult periods. Interestingly, rats exposed prenatally to stress show persistently high levels of activity in the hypothalamo-pituitary axis (Takahashi & Kalin, 1991), as well as a potentiated response to stress during the pubertal period and later during adulthood (Fride, Dan, Feldon, Halvey, & Weinstock, 1986). Taken together, prenatal exposure to stress appears to enhance the subsequent response to stress later during adulthood. In a circuit where there is a pre-existing reduction of GABAergic activity (Figure 16.1), perhaps one related to obstetrical complications (Benes et al., 1997), the formation of superabundant connections between dopamine fibers and an impaired population of interneurons could lead to even further decreases of inhibitory modulation of pyramidal neurons generated by GABAergic cells and could even have a negative impact on the amount of serotonergic modulation being exerted (see discussion below). This latter scenario would likely be associated with a severe decompensation in the activity of the circuit shown in Figure 16.1 under stressful conditions.

The Influence of Serotonin Fibers on Dopamine Fiber Ingrowth

Recent evidence from studies of the anterior cingulate region of postmortem brain has suggested that the interaction of dopamine fibers with intrinsic cortical neurons may be abnormal where the distribution of dopamine fibers appears to be shifted from pyramidal cells to interneurons in layer II of schizophrenics (Benes et al., 1997). In the context of a possible "mis-wiring" of monoaminergic systems, it is important to emphasize that the dopamine fiber system in the anterior cingulate cortex (see above) is actively maturing during the adolescence. It is, therefore, appropriate to speculate as to whether perhaps neurotrophic mechanisms may potentially contribute to the plasticity of this system and the "mis-wiring" of these fibers thought to occur in schizophrenia. Likewise, it is important to consider whether serotonin fibers may also be impacting on the corticolimbic system, although, in this case, the postnatal maturation of this neuromodulatory system is probably completed during the equivalent of childhood (Lambe, Krimer, & Goldman-Rakic, 2000). Nevertheless, serotonin fibers have been found to promote the ingrowth of afferents originating in the thalamus during early cortical development (D'Amato et al., 1987). Thus, it is possible that serotonin fibers may be acting trophically to promote the ingrowth of dopamine fibers during adolescence and early adulthood. This possibility is particularly intriguing because a significant number of cortical neurons probably receive a convergence of these two monoaminergic systems (see above).

To assess the nature of this relationship, a series of experiments in which the 5HT projections from the nucleus raphe dorsalis (NRD) were lesioned during the neonatal period were recently undertaken (Taylor, Cunningham, & Benes, 1998). Contrary to the working hypothesis, dopamine fibers, rather than being decreased, appeared to be increased in the anterior cingulate cortex of rats having a marked reduction in the number of serotonin fibers. As discussed above, serotonergic fibers, like dopamine projections (see above), probably interact with both projection cells and interneurons (Benes et al., 2000; Morilak & Ciaranello, 1993; Sheldon & Aghajanian, 1990; Smiley & Goldman-Rakic, 1996; Taylor & Benes, 1996). Unlike the dopamine system, however, the serotonergic projections to the medial prefrontal cortex appear to be complete during the equivalent of childhood and show no further increases during adolescence (Lambe et al., 2000). Based on these various observations, it seems reasonable to conclude that changes in dopamine projections represent one of the most dynamic elements in the maturation of cortical circuitry during the postnatal period. Interestingly, lesioning of the ventral tegmental dopamine projections to the medial prefrontal cortex (anterior cingulate region) has been associated with a 30 percent decrease of basal dendritic branches of pyramidal neurons (Kalsbeek, de Bruin, Matthijssen, & Uylings, 1989), although serotonergic fibers were also reduced in this study. Thus, it is uncertain whether one or both of these monoaminergic systems contributed to the observed decrease in pyramidal cell dendrites.

Overall, the above studies were not consistent with the idea that 5HT may act trophically to facilitate the ingrowth of DA fibers during the late postweanling and early adult periods. Rather, it seems more likely that the opposite is the case, that is, the 5HT system seems to be exerting an inhibitory effect on the normal postnatal ingrowth of TH-IR fibers. One interpretation of these findings is that the 5HT and DA systems may be competing with one another for functional territory on the surface of intrinsic cortical neurons within rat mPFCx. An interaction of this type would tend to produce a reciprocal relationship between the two systems. An alternative possibility, however, is that the 5HT and DA systems mainly influence one another at the level of their respective brainstem nuclei, the dorsal raphe nucleus (NRD) and the ventral tegmental area (VTA), respectively. Accordingly, lesioning of the NRD may result in a stimulation of dopaminergic neurons within the VTA to sprout the distal portion of their fiber projections in various termination sites, such as the anterior cingulate cortex.

Physiological studies have yielded contradictory results regarding the manner in which the DA and 5HT systems may be influencing one another. On the one hand, some believe that 5HT can *increase* the release of DA in nucleus accumbens (Broderick & Phelix, 1997; Van Bockstaele, Cestari, & Pickel, 1994), corpus striatum (Broderick & Phelix, 1997; West & Galloway, 1996), and prefrontal cortex .(Gudelsky GA, 1996; Iyer & Bradberry, 1996). Conversely, some studies suggest that 5HT may actually decrease the release of DA, since exposure to selective 5HT receptor antagonists has been associated with an increase of extracellular DA concentrations (Howell et al., 1997; Pehek, 1996). The latter pattern is consistent with the idea that there may be a competitive interaction between these two monoaminergic systems. This idea is a particularly appealing one because the VTA receives a direct input from serotoninergic fibers (Van Bockstaele et al., 1994).

Behavioral Implications for the Normal and Abnormal Development of DA and 5HT Fibers

The anterior cingulate region plays a pivotal role in a corticolimbic network that mediates complex behaviors, such as motivation, selective attention, affective experience, and social interactions (Devinsky, Morrell, & Vogt, 1995). Accordingly, this region is also of central importance to the pathophysiology of schizophrenia and bipolar disorder because these same behaviors are typically found to be defective in both disorders (Benes, 1993b). Given the fact that there are abundant dopaminergic and serotonergic projections not only to the anterior cingulate region, but also to other corticolimbic regions, such as the amygdala, hippocampus, dorsolateral prefrontal cortex, frontal eye field 8, and inferior parietal lobe, it seems likely that alterations in the interaction of these two fiber systems with GABAergic interneurons could result in important changes in the functional output of this complex network. Normal developmental changes in this circuitry during adolescence are probably associated with more focused motivational responses, particularly ones that are associated with emotional reactions. On the other hand, the formation of abnormal connections between dopamine and serotonin fibers and intrinsic neurons within this system would be expected to result in *dysfunction*, appearing as poor motivation, inattention, inappropriate affect, and social withdrawal. In this latter setting, the administration of therapeutic agents, such as antipsychotic medications or even antidepressants, would tend to recalibrate the setpoint of this system back to normal as the functional interaction of dopamine and serotonin fibers with cortical neurons is corrected. For example, in schizophrenia, an excessive dopamine input to GABA cells would be blocked and would tend to reduce the inhibitory influence of this neuromodulator on dysfunctional GABA cells.

FUTURE DIRECTIONS

It is clear from the above direction that late postnatal changes in the convergence of dopamine and serotonin fibers onto GABAergic interneurons has the potential to help lay the groundwork for the formation of both normal and abnormal wiring patterns in the corticolimbic system of human brain. In those who carry the vulnerability for psychopathology, such changes may well contribute to the onset of mental illness during adolescence and adulthood. Our understanding of how these putative "mis-wirings" occur must rest on a solid neurobiological foundation, one in which the cellular and molecular mechanisms that control the plasticity of dopamine and serotonin fibers are better understood.

Future studies will consider the mechanisms that may be involved in the establishment of connnections between monoaminergic fibers and intrinsic cortical neurons. Toward this end, there are several proteins that comprise a family of trophic factors, such as nerve growth factor (NGF), brain derived neurotrophic factor (BDNF), and the neurotrophins NT-3 and NT4/5, that play a role in the differentiation, survival, and maintenance of central neurons (Caleo, Menna, Chierzi, Cenni, & Maffei, 2000). The effects of BDNF and NT-3 on long-term potentiation (LTP) in the hippocampus are mediated, at least in part, through specialized receptors, called Trk B and Trk C (Bramham, Southard, Sarvey, Herkenham, & Brady, 1996). This latter observation suggests that trophic changes at the molecular level contribute to the learning and memory associated with hippocampal function. During development of the cortex, GABAergic interneurons show a marked upregulation in the expression of the genes for BDNF, NT 4/5, and Trk B. It is noteworthy that these changes are believed to contribute to the intercellular signalling that occurs within nearby neurons, showing evidence of apoptosis (Wang, Sheen, & Macklis, 1998). In the nigrostriatal system, the expression of messenger ribonucleic acid (mRNA) for BDNF, NT-3, Trk B, and Trk C influences the differentiation of neurons; BDNF and Trk B also seem to work through a dopaminergic mechanism involving the D1 receptor (Jung & Bennett, 1996). Although BDNF and NT-3 are quite active during early development, they continue to play a role in the regulation of functions, such as long-term potentiation (LTP) during the adult period (Bramham et al., 1996; Castren et al., 1993). It will be important for future studies to focus attention on these various trophic factors and their associated receptors, so that we can learn more about the specific role that they may play not only in the differentiation of neurons, but also in the functional maintenance of mature synapses.

Relevant to the current discussion, it is also pertinent to consider what role trophic factors and/or their receptors might play in the competition of 5HT fibers with convergent DA inputs to GABA cells during the postnatal period. Under normal conditions, it seems reasonable to postulate that BNDF and/or its associated receptor Trk B, or possibly NT-3 and/or its receptor Trk C, might contribute to the establishment and/or maintenance of these monoaminergic connections with GABAergic interneurons. From the standpoint of normal development, it is possible that BDNF is synthesized and released by intrinsic cortical neurons and, once in the extracellular space, this trophin could help to promote the apposition of DA and 5HT fibers on their outer cell membrane. In other words, once released, trophic factors might be free to exert their action directly on dopaminergic fibers, particularly those that have the potential to sprout, when stimulated to do so by the appropriate molecular stimuli. In contrast, abnormal conditions may be associated with an inappropriate release of one or more trophic factors by intrinsic cortical neurons and this could theoretically provide the setting in which aberrant connection patterns emerge. An alternative possibility is that the elaboration of trophic factors by intrinsic neurons is relatively normal in some forms of psychopathology; however, the expression of their associated receptors (e.g., Trk B or Trk C) on extrinsic fiber systems like those from the ventral tegment dopamine neurons, might be abnormal. Either way, the net result could be the formation of increased numbers of appositions on one cell type (in this case, GABA cells), if it is releasing excessive amounts of trophic factor(s) and decreased contacts with another cell type, such as projections neurons, if these latter cells show a down-regulation of one or more trophic factor systems. If the dopamine fibers are subject to limitations in the amount of sprouting they can undergo, it may depend upon the amount of Trk B or Trk C receptors expressed by them. A second type of intrinsic neuron (e.g., a pyramidal cell) might show the opposite effect: a proportionate decrease in the number of DA fibers forming appositions.

It is clear from the above discussion that our understanding of the development of psychopathology will require sophisticated molecular approaches to analyze the expression of trophic factors and their receptors. Microscopic techniques, such as in situ hybridization and immunocytochemistry, that have a high degree of spatial resolution, will complement more encompassing approaches of gene expression profiling and proteomics. These latter technologies make it possible to examine 10–20,000 individual genes and proteins, respectively, and potentially offer an extraordinary view of the dynamics of cell regulation in the corticolimbic system. Such techniques are freeing neuroscientists from the constraints of studying one gene or protein at a time and are making it possible to study the complex cascades of changes that typically occur within corticolimbic neurons during normal and abnormal postnatal development.

CONCLUSIONS

The studies described above provide evidence in support of the idea that the dopamine and serotonin systems show a significant degree of convergence and plasticity in rat mPFCx, and the degree to which this occurs is probably similar for both pyramidal cells and GABAergic interneurons. Particularly noteworthy is the fact that the dopamine system may be capable of considerable plasticity at least until the start of the early adult period. If the dopamine system in human brain exhibits similar characteristics, the maturation of limbic cortex during adolescence and early adulthood may provide "a window of opportunity" for the induction of abnormal interactions of the monoaminergic systems with one another and with their intrinsic cortical targets. Indeed, some experimental evidence suggests that exposure to adrenal steroids during the postnatal period can result in an increase of dopamine interactions with interneurons in medial prefronal cortex of rats also exposed to these hormones prenatally (Benes, 1997). For GABAergic interneurons, complex changes in the regulation of GAD have been observed; however, these occur whether or not there has been exposure prenatally to adrenal steroid (Stone et al., 2001). Based on these studies, an important question to ask is whether pre- and/or postnatal stress might also result in an altered distribution of serotonergic projections in the anterior cingulate cortex, one that may be reciprocal in nature to that observed for the dopamine system (Figure 16.1). If this were the case, the model shown in Figure 16.1 would predict that the activity of GABAergic interneurons would be compromised by the presence of excessive dopaminergic inputs that are inhibitory in nature and diminished serotonergic inputs that are excitatory in nature. Since a combination of pre- and postnatal stress is believed to play a central role in the pathophysiology of some neuropsychiatric disorders (Benes, 1997; Walker & Diforio, 1997), it is plausible that changes in the way these two monoaminergic systems interact with one another might ultimately influence the activity of the individual cortical neurons upon which they both converge.

This model appears to have predictive validity in individuals with schizophrenia and/or bipolar disorder who have a higher expected occurrence of obstetrical complications. Such patients typically benefit from major tranquilizers that block dopamine receptors, as well as benzodiazepines that enhance the activity of the GABAA receptor. The model is also consistent with the fact that patients in the manic phase of bipolar disorder typically show an exacerbation of their symptoms with antidepressant medications. Since many of the latter drugs block the reuptake of serotonin, the model also predicts that the pyramidal neuron, if receiving an excessive excitatory input from this system, would show even more heightened activity. A weakness of this model is the fact that there have not as yet been systematic studies of the effects of pre- and postnatal stress on the relative numbers of dopamine *and* serotonin fibers on pyramidal cells versus GABA cells using a co-localization technique. Thus, some aspects of the model are purely inferential in nature. Accordingly, future studies should be directed at identifying further what effect stress might have on convergent dopaminergic and serotonergic fibers on target neurons of the cortex, how this interaction may be rendered influenced by exposure to pre- and postnatal stress, and how various psychotropic drugs may exert their action in relation to neuroplastic changes in these convergent monoaminergic fiber systems.

Overall, the work described above illustrates rather graphically that the study of abnormal conditions such as schizophrenia and bipolar disorder offer the potential to learn more about the structure and function of the human brain and how perturbations of its development during critical stages can result in dysfunction. Unlike Alzheimer's disease, where there is widespread degeneration of the corticolimbic system, these regions in individuals with schizophrenia and bipolar disorder do not show pronounced degrees of atrophy and neuronal cell death. Rather, in these latter disorders, there are subtle alterations in the pattern of connectivity between extrinsic and intrinsic neurons within complex circuits. By their very nature, the neuropsychiatric disorders provide a natural model system in which the wiring of the brain may be studied in order to understand how slight variations can result in profound disturbances of complex cognitive functions. In the years to come, it is reasonable to expect that our understanding of how the corticolimbic system is altered in schizophrenia and bipolar disorder will continue to expand, and there will be important new insights into how the corticolimbic system is functioning under both normal and abnormal conditions.

REFERENCES

Akbarian, S., Kim, J. J., Potkin, S. G., Hagman, J. O., Tafazzoli, A., Bunney, W. E., & Jones, E. G. (1995). Gene expression for glutamic acid decarboxylase is reduced without loss of neurons in prefrontal cortex of schizophrenics. *Archives of General Psychiatry, 52,* 258–278.

Benes, F. M. (1988). Post-mortem structural analyses of schizophrenic brain: study designs and the interpretation of data. *Psychiatric Developments, 6*(3), 213–226.

Benes, F. M. (1989). Myelination of cortical-hippocampal relays during late adolescence. *Schizophrenia Bulletin, 15*(4), 585–593.

Benes, F. M. (1993a). Neurobiological investigations in cingulate cortex of schizophrenic brain. *Schizophrenia Bulletin, 19*(3), 537–549.

Benes, F. M. (1993b). The relationship of cingulate cortex to schizophrenia. In B. A. Vogt & M. Gabriel (Eds.), *Neurobiology of cingulate cortex and limbic thalamus* (pp. 581–605). Boston: Birkhäuser.

Benes, F. M. (1995). A neurodevelopmental approach to the understanding of schizophrenia and other mental disorders. In D. Cicchetti & D. J. Cohen (Eds.), *Developmental psychopathology,* Volume 1: Theory and Methods (pp. 227–253). New York: Wiley.

Benes, F. M. (1997). The role of stress and dopamine-GABA interactions in the vulnerability for schizophrenia. *Journal of Psychiatric Research, 31*(2), 257–275.

Benes, F. M. (2000). Emerging principles of altered neural circuitry in schizophrenia. *Brain Research Reviews, 31*(2–3), 251–269.

Benes, F. M., & Berretta, S. (2001). GABAergic interneurons: Implications for understanding schizophrenia and bipolar disorder. *Neuropsychopharmacology.*

Benes, F. M., Davidson, B., & Bird, E. D. (1986). Quantitative cytoarchitectural studies of the cerebral cortex of schizophrenics. *Archives of General Psychiatry, 43,* 31–35.

Benes, F. M., Khan, Y., Vincent, S. L., & Wickramasinghe, R. (1996). Differences in the subregional and cellular distribution of GABAA receptor binding in the hippocampal formation of schizophrenic brain. *Synapse, 22*(4), 338–349.

Benes, F. M., Kwok, E. W., Vincent, S. L., & Todtenkopf, M. S. (1998). A reduction of nonpyramidal cells in sector CA2 of schizophrenics and manic depressives [see comments]. *Biological Psychiatry, 44*(2), 88–97.

Benes, F. M., McSparren, J., Bird, E. D., SanGiovanni, J. P., & Vincent, S. L. (1991). Deficits in small interneurons in prefrontal and cingulate cortices of schizophrenic and schizoaffective patients. *Archives of General Psychiatry, 48*(11), 996–1001.

Benes, F. M., Taylor, J. B., & Cunningham, M. C. (2000). Convergence and plasticity of monoaminergic systems in the medial prefrontal cortex during the postnatal period: implications for the development of psychopathology. *Cerebral Cortex, 10*(10), 1014–1027.

Benes, F. M., Todtenkopf, M. S., Logiotatos, P., & Williams, M. (2000). Glutamate decarboxylase(65)-immunoreactive terminals in cingulate and prefrontal cortices of schizophrenic and bipolar brain. *Journal of Chemistry and Neuroanatomy, 20*(3–4), 259–269.

Benes, F. M., Todtenkopf, M. S., & Taylor, J. B. (1997). Differential distribution of tyrosine hydroxylase fibers on small and large neurons in layer II of anterior cingulate cortex of schizophrenic brain. *Synapse, 25*(1), 80–92.

Benes, F. M., Turtle, M., Khan, Y., & Farol, P. (1994). Myelination of a key relay zone in the hippocampal formation occurs in the human brain during childhood, adolescence, and adulthood. *Archives of General Psychiatry, 51*(6), 477–484.

Benes, F. M., Vincent, S. L., Alsterberg, G., Bird, E. D., & SanGiovanni, J. P. (1992). Increased GABAA receptor binding in superficial layers of cingulate cortex in schizophrenics. *Journal of Neuroscience, 12*(3), 924–929.

Benes, F. M., Vincent, S. L., & Molloy, R. (1993a). Dopamine-immunoreactive axon varicosities form nonrandom contacts with GABA-immunoreactive neurons of rat medial prefrontal cortex. *Synapse, 15*(4), 285–295.

Benes, F. M., Vincent, S. L., Molloy, R., & Khan, Y. (1996). Increased interaction of dopamine-immunoreactive varicosities with GABA neurons of rat medial prefrontal cortex occurs during the postweanling period. *Synapse, 23*(4), 237–245.

Bergson, C., Mrzljak, L., Lidow, M. S., Goldman-Rakic, P. S., & Levenson, R. (1995). Characterization of subtype-specific antibodies to the human D5 dopamine receptor: studies in primate brain and transfected mammalian cells. *Proceedings of the National Academy of Science, 92*(8), 3468–3472.

Bramham, C. R., Southard, T., Sarvey, J. M., Herkenham, M., & Brady, L. S. (1996). Unilateral LTP triggers bilateral increases in hippocampal neurothrophin and *trk* receptor mRNA expression in behaving rats: evidence for inter-hemispheric communication. *Journal of Comparative Neurology, 368,* 371–382.

Broderick, P. A., & Phelix, C. F. (1997). I. Serotonin (5-HT) within dopamine reward circuits signals open-field behavior. II. Basis for 5-HT-DA interaction in cocaine dysfunctional behavior. *Neuroscience Biobehavioral Reviews, 21,* 227–260.

Brozoski, T., Brown, R. M., Rosvold, H. E., & Goldman, P. S. (1979). Cognitive deficit caused by depletion of dopamine in prefrontal cortex of rhesus monkey. *Science, 205,* 929–931.

Bruinink, A., Lichtensteiner, W., & Schlumpf, M. (1983). Pre- and postnatal ontogeny and characterization of dopaminergic D2, serotonergic S2, and spirodecanone binding sites in rat forebrain. *Journal of Neurochemistry, 40,* 1227–1237.

Bunney, B. S., & Chiodo, L. A. (1984). Mesocortical dopamine systems: further electrophysiological and pharmacological characteristics. In L. Descarries, T. A. Reader, & H. H. Jasper (Eds.), *Monoamine innervation of the cerebral cortex* (pp. 263–277). New York: Alan R. Liss.

Caleo, M., Menna, E., Chierzi, S., Cenni, M. C., & Maffei, L. (2000). Brain-derived neurotrophic factor is an anterograde survival factor in the rat visual system. *Current Biology, 10*(19), 1155–1161.

Castren, E., Pitkanen, M., Sirvio, J., Parsadanian, A., Lindholm, D., Thoenen, H., & Riekkinen, P. J. (1993). The induction of LTP increases BDNF and NGF messenger RNA but decreases NT-3 messenger RNA in the dentate gyrus. *Neuroreport, 4,* 895–898.

Chalmers, D. T., Kwak, S., Mansour, A., Akil, H., & Watson, S. (1993). Corticosteroids regulate brain hippocampal 5-HT1A receptor mRNA expression. *Journal of Neuroscience, 13,* 914–923.

Chalmers, D. T., Lopez, J. F., Vazquez, D. M., Akil, H., & Watson, S. J. (1994). Regulation of hippocampal 5-HT1A receptor gene expression by dexamethasone. *Neuropsychopharmacology, 10*(3), 215–222.

Chaouloff, F. (2000). Serotonin, stress and corticoids [In Process Citation]. *Journal of Psychopharmacology, 14*(2), 139–151.

Chronwall, B., & Wolff, J. R. (1980). Prenatal and postnatal development of GABA-accumulating cells in the occipital neocortex of rat. *Journal of Comparative Neurology, 190,* 187–208.

Cicchetti, D. (1993). Developmental pyschopathology: Reactions, reflections, projections. *Development and Psychopathology, 13,* 471–502.

Cicchetti, D., & Cannon, T. (1999). Neurodevelopmental processes in the ontogenesis and epigenesis of psychopathology. *Development and Psychopathology, 11,* 375–393.

Corda, M. G., & Biggio, G. (1986). Stress and GABAergic transmission: biochemical and behavioural studies. In G. Biggio & E. Costa (Eds.), *GABAergic transmission and anxiety* (pp. 121–135). New York: Raven Press.

Coyle, J. T., & Enna, S. (1976). Neurochemical aspects of the ontogenesis of GABAnergic neurons in the rat brain. *Brain Research, 111,* 119–133.

D'Amato, R. J., Blue, M., Largent, B., Lynch, D., Leobetter, D., Molliver, M., & Snyder, S. (1987). Ontogeny of the serotonergic projection of rat neocortex: Transient expression of a dense innervation of primary sensory areas. *Proceeding of the National Academy of Science, 84,* 4322–4326.

Davidoff, S. A., & Benes, F. M. (1998). High-resolution scatchard analysis shows D1 receptor binding on pyramidal and nonpyramidal neurons. *Synapse, 28*(1), 83–90.

Deskin, R., Seidler, F. J., Whitmore, W. L., & Slotkin, T. A. (1981). Development of noradrenergic and dopaminergic receptor systems depends on maturation of their presynaptic nerve terminals in the rat brain. *Journal of Neurochemistry, 36,* 1683–1690.

Devinsky, O., Morrell, M. J., & Vogt, B. A. (1995). Contributions of anterior cingulate cortex to behaviour. *Brain, 118*(Pt 1), 279–306.

Emson, P. C., & Koob, G. F. (1978). The origin and distribution of dopamine-containing afferents to rat frontal cortex. *Brain Research, 142*, 249–267.

Flechsig, P. (1920). Anatomie des menschlichen Gehirns und Ruckenmarks auf myelogenetischer Gundlange Leipzig, G. Thieme.

Fride, E., Dan, Y., Feldon, H., Halvey, G., & Weinstock, M. (1986). Effects of prenatal stress on vulnerability to stress in prepubertal and adult rats. *Physiology and Behavior, 37*, 681–687.

Gambarana, C., Pittman, R., & Siegel, R. E. (1990). Development expression of the GABA-A receptor g1 subunit mRNA in the rat brain. *Journal of Neurobiology, 21*(8), 1169–1179.

Gaspar, P., Bloch, B., & Le Moine, C. (1995). D1 and D2 receptor gene expression in the rat frontal cortex: cellular localization in different classes of efferent neurons. *European Journal of Neuroscience, 7*(5), 1050–1063.

Gellman, R. L., & Aghajanian, G. K. (1993). Pyramidal cells in piriform cortex receive a convergence of inputs from monoamine activated GABAergic interneurons. *Brain Research, 600*, 63–73.

Goldman-Rakic, P. S., Leranth, C., Williams, S. M., Mons, N., & Geffard, M. (1989). Dopamine synaptic complex with pyramidal neurons in primate cerebral cortex. *Proceedings of the National Academy of Science, 86*(22), 9015–9019.

Gudelsky GA, N. J. (1996). Carrier-mediated release of serotonin by 3,4methylenedioxymethamphetaine: implications for serotonin-dopamine interactions. *Journal of Neurochemistry, 66*, 243–249.

Guidotti, A., Auta, J., Davis, J. M., Gerevini, V. D., Dwivedi, Y., Grayson, D. R., Impagnatiello, F., Pandey, G., Pesold, C., Sharma, R., Uzunov, D., & Costa, E. (2000). Decrease in reelin and glutamic acid decarboxylase67 (GAD67) expression in schizophrenia and bipolar disorder: A postmortem brain study [In Process Citation]. *Archives of General Psychiatry, 57*(11), 1061–1069.

Gulledge, A. T., & Jaffe, D. B. (1998). Dopamine decreases the excitability of layer V pyramidal cells in the rat prefrontal cortex. *Journal of Neuroscience, 18*, 9139–9151.

Heckers, S., Stone, D. J., Walsh, J., Schick, J., Koul, P., & Benes, F. M. (2001). Decreased hippocampal expression of glutamic acid decarboxylase (GAD) 65 and 67 mRNA in bipolar disorder. *Archives of General Psychiatry.*

Howell, I. I., Czoty, P. W., & Burd, L. D. (1997). Pharmacological interactions between serotonin and dopamine on behavior in the squirrel monkey. *Psychopharmacology, 131*, 40–48.

Huntley, G. W., Morrison, J. H., Prikhozhan, A., & Sealfon, S. C. (1992). Localization of multiple dopamine receptor subtype mRNAs in human and monkey motor cortex and striatum. *Molecular Brain Research, 15*, 181–188.

Iuvone, P., & Dunn, A. (1986). Tyrosine hydroxylase activation in mesocortical 3,4-dihydroxyphenylethylamine neurons following footshock. *Journal of Neurochemistry, 47*, 837–844.

Iyer, R. N., & Bradberry, C. W. (1996). Serotonin-mediated increase in prefrontal cortex dopamine release: pharmacological characterization. *Journal of Pharmacology and Experimental Therapeutics, 277*, 40–47.

Jakab, R. L., & Goldman-Rakic, P. S. (1998). 5-Hydroxytryptamine2A serotonin receptors in the primate cerebral cortex: possible site of action of hallucinogenic and antipsychotic drugs in pyramidal cell apical dendrites. *Proceedings of the National Academy of Science, 95*(2), 735–740.

Jakob, H., & Beckmann, H. (1986). Prenatal developmental disturbances in the limbic allocortex in schizophrenics. *Journal of Neural Transmission, 65*, 303–326.

Johnston, M. V. (1988). Biochemistry of neurotransmitters in cortical development. In A. Peter & E. G. Jones (Eds.), *Cerebral Cortex*, Vol. 7: Development and Maturation of Cerebral Cortex (pp. 211–236). New York: Plenum.

Jung, A. B., & Bennett, J. P., Jr. (1996). Development of striatal dopaminergic function. III: Pre- and postnatal development of striatal and cortical mRNAs for the neurotrophin receptors trkBTK+ and trkC and their regulation by synaptic dopamine. *Brain Research: Developmental Brain Research, 94*(2), 133–143.

Kalsbeek, A., de Bruin, J. P., Matthijssen, M. A., & Uylings, H. B. (1989). Ontogeny of open field activity in rats after neonatal lesioning of the mesocortical dopaminergic projection. *Behavior and Brain Research, 32*(2), 115–127.

Kalsbeek, A., Voorn, P., Buijs, R. M., Pool, C. W., & Uylings, H. B. (1988). Development of the dopaminergic innervation in the prefrontal cortex of the rat. *Journal of Comparative Neurology, 269*(1), 58–72.

Keshavan, M. S., & Hogarty, G. E. (1999). Brain maturational processes and delayed onset in schizophrenia. *Development and Psychopathology, 11*, 524–543.

Kovelman, J. A., & Scheibel, A. B. (1984). A neurohistological correlate of schizophrenia. *Biological Psychiatry, 19*, 1601–1621.

Lambe, E. K., Krimer, L. S., & Goldman-Rakic, P. S. (2000). Differential postnatal development of catecholamine and serotonin inputs to identified neurons in prefrontal cortex of rhesus monkey. *Journal of Neuroscience, 20*(23), 8780–8787.

Le Moine, C., & Gaspar, P. (1998). Subpopulations of cortical GABAergic interneurons differ by their expression of D1 and D2 dopamine receptor subtypes. *Brain Research: Molecular Brain Research, 58*(1–2), 231–236.

Lidov, H. G. W., Grzanna, R., & Molliver, M. E. (1980). The serotonin innervation of the cerebral cortex in the rat – an immunocytochemical analysis. *Neuroscience, 5*, 207–227.

Lindvall, O., & Bjorklund, A. (1978). Anatomy of the dopaminergic neuron systems in the rat brain. In P. J. E. A. Roberts (Ed.), *Advances in biochemical psychopharmacology* (Vol. 19, pp. 1–23). New York: Raven Press.

Lopez, J., Chalmers, D., Vazquez, D., Akil, H., & Watson, S. (1993). Chronic unpredictable stress down-regulates serotonin 1A receptors in the hippocampus. *Society for Neuroscience Abstracts, 19*(1), 216.

Luhmann, H. J., & Prince, D. A. (1991). Postnatal maturation of the GABAergic system in rat neocortex. *Journal of Neurophysiology, 65*, 247–263.

Maines, L. W., Keck, B. J., Dugar, A., & Lakoski, J. M. (1998). Age-dependent loss of corticosterone modulation of central serotonin 5- HT1A receptor binding sites. *Journal of Neuroscience Research, 53*(1), 86–98.

Marek, G. J., & Aghajanian, G. K. (1998). The electrophysiology of prefrontal serotonin systems: therapeutic implications for psychosis. *Biological Psychiatry, 44*, 1118–1127.

Meltzer, H. Y. (1994). An overview of the mechanism of action of clozapine. J clin Psychiatry, 55 *Suppl B*, 47–52.

Morilak, D. A., & Ciaranello, R. D. (1993). Ontogeny of 5-hydroxytryptamine2 receptor immunoreactivity in the developing rat brain. *Neuroscience, 55*(3), 869–880.

Muly, E. C., 3rd, Szigeti, K., & Goldman-Rakic, P. S. (1998). D1 receptor in interneurons of macaque prefrontal cortex: distribution and subcellular localization. *Journal of Neuroscience, 18*(24), 10553–10565.

Palacios, J. M., Niehoff, D. L., & Kuhar, M. J. (1979). Ontogeny of GABA and benzodiazepine receptors: effects of Triton X-100, bromide and muscimol. *Brain Research, 179*, 390–395.

Parnavelas, J. G., Papadopoulos, G. C., & Cavanagh, M. E. (1988). Changes in neurotransmitters during development. In A. Peters & E. G. Jones (Eds.), *Cerebral Cortex*, Vol. 7: Development and Maturation of Cerebral Cortex (pp. 177–209). New York: Plenum.

Pehek, E. A. (1996). Local infusion of the serotonin antagonist ritanserin or ICS 205,930 increases in vivo dopamine release in the rat medial prefrontal cortex. *Synapse, 24*, 12–18.

Penit-Soria, J., Audinat, E., & Crepel, F. (1987). Excitation of rat prefrontal cortical neurons by dopamine: an in vitro electrophysiological study. *Brain Research, 425*, 363–374.

Petty, F., Kramer, G., & Moeller, M. (1994). Does learned helplessness induction by haloperidol involve serotonin mediation? *Pharmacology Biochemistry and Behavior, 48*(3), 671–676.

Reader, T. A. (1981). Distribution of catecholamines and serotonin in the rat cerebral cortex: Absolute levels and relative proportions. *Journal of Neural Transmission, 50*, 13–27.

Reader, T. A., Ferron, A., Descarries, L., & Jasper, H. H. (1979). Modulatory role for biogenic amines in the cerebral cortex: Microiontophoretic studies. *Brain Research, 160*, 217–229.

Retaux, S., Besson, M. J., & Penit-Soria, J. (1991). Opposing effects of dopamine D2 receptor stimulation on the spontaneous and the electrically evoked release of [3H]GABA on rat prefrontal cortex slices. *Neuroscience, 42*(1), 61–71.

Reynolds, G. P., Czudek, C., & Andrews, H. B. (1990). Deficit and hemispheric asymmetry of GABA uptake sites in the hippocampus in schizophrenia. *Biol Psychiatry, 27*(9), 1038–1044.

Roth, R. H., Tam, S. Y., Ida, Y., Yang, J. X., & Deutch, A. Y. (1988). Stress and the mesocorticolimbic dopamine systems. *Annals of the New York Academy of Sciences, 537,* 138–147.

Schuman, E. M. (1999). Neurotrophin regulation of synaptic transmission. *Current Opinion in Neurobiology, 9*(1), 105–109.

Schwartz, R., Wess, M., Labarca, R., Skolnick, P., & Paul, S. (1987). Acute stress enhances the activity of the GABA receptor-gated ion channel in brain. *Brain Research, 411,* 151–155.

Seguela, P., Watkins, K. C., & Descarries, L. (1988). Ultrastructural features of dopamine axon terminals in the anteromedial and suprarhinal cortex of rat. *Journal of Comparative Neurology, 289,* 11–22.

Sheldon, P. W., & Aghajanian, G. K. (1990). Serotonin (5-HT) induces IPSPs in pyramidal layer cells of rat piriform cortex: evidence for the involvement of a 5-HT2-activated interneuron. *Brain Research, 506,* 62–69.

Sheldon, P. W., & Aghajanian, G. K. (1991). Excitatory responses to serotonin (5-HT) in neurons of the rat piriform cortex: evidence for mediation by 5-HT1C receptors in pyramidal cells and 5-HT2 receptors in interneurons. *Synapse, 9,* 208–218.

Simpson, M. D. C., Slater, P., Deakin, J. F. W., Royston, M. C., & Skan, W. J. (1989). Reduced GABA uptake sites in the temporal lobe in schizophrenia. *Neuroscience Letters, 107,* 211–215.

Smiley, J. F., & Goldman-Rakic, P. S. (1996). Serotonergic axons in monkey prefrontal cerebral cortex synapse predominantly on interneurons as demonstrated by serial section electron microscopy. *Journal of Comparative Neurology, 367*(3), 431–443.

Smiley, J. F., Levey, A. I., Ciliax, B. J., & Goldman-Rakic, P. S. (1994). D1 dopamine receptor immunoreactivity in human and monkey cerebral cortex: Predominant and extrasynaptic localization in dendritic spines. *Proceedings of the National Academy of Science, 91,* 5720–5724.

Spoerri, P. E. (1988). Neurotrophic effects of GABA in cultures of embryonic chick brain and retina. *Synapse, 2,* 11–22.

Stone, D. J., Walsh, J. P., & Benes, F. M. (2001). Effects of pre- and postnatal stress on the rat GABA system. *Hippocampus, 11,* 492–507.

Stone, E., Freedman, L., & Morgano, L. (1978). Brain and adrenal tyrosine hydroxylase activity after chronic footshock stress. *Pharmacology Biochemistry and Behavior, 9,* 551–553.

Stone, E., & McCarty, R. (1983). Adaptation to stress: tyrosine hydroxylase activity and catecholamine release. *Neuroscience and Biobehavioral Reviews, 7,* 29–34.

Stutzmann, G. E., McEwen, B. S., & LeDoux, J. E. (1998). Serotonin modulation of sensory inputs to the lateral amygdala: dependency on corticosterone. *Journal of Neuroscience, 18*(22), 9529–9538.

Svensson, T. H. (2000). Dysfunctional brain dopamine systems induced by psychotomimetic NMDA-receptor antagonists and the effects of antipsychotic drugs. *Brain Research Reviews, 31,* 320–329.

Takahashi, L. K., & Kalin, N. H. (1991). Early developmental and temporal characteristics of stress-induced secretion of pituitary-adrenal hormones in prenatally stressed rat pups. *Brain Research, 558,* 75–78.

Tam, S., & Roth, R. (1990). Modulation of mesoprefrontal dopamine neurons by central benzodiazepine receptors. I. Pharmacological characterization. *Journal of Pharmacology and Experimental Therapeutics, 252,* 989–996.

Taylor, J., Cunningham, M. C., & Benes, F. M. (1998). Neonatal raphe lesions increase dopamine fibers in prefrontal cortex of adult rats. *Neuroreport, 9*(8), 1811–1815.

Taylor, J. B., & Benes, F. M. (1996). Colocalization of glutamate decarboxylase, tyrosine hydroxylase and serotonin immunoreactivity in rat medial prefrontal cortex. *Neuroscience-Net, 1,* 10001.

Thierry, A. M., Mantz, J., Milla, C., & Glowinski, J. (1988). Influence of the mesocortical/prefrontal dopamine neurons on their target cells. In P. W. Kalivas & C. B. Nemeroff (Eds.), *The mesocorticolimbic dopamine system,* Vol. 537 (pp. 101–111). New York: Ann. N.Y. Acad. Sci.

Thierry, A. M., Tassin, J. P., Blanc, G., & Glowinski, J. (1976). Selective activation of the mesocortical DA system by stress. *Nature, 263,* 242–244.

Van Bockstaele, E. J., Cestari, D. M., & Pickel, V. M. (1994). Synaptic structure and connectivity of serotonin terminals in the ventral tegmental area: potential sites for modulation of mesolimbic dopamine neurons. *Brain Research, 647*(2), 307–322.

Verney, C., Alvarez, C., Gerrard, M., & Berger, B. (1990). Ultrastructural double-labelling study of dopamine terminals and GABA-containing neurons in rat anteromedial cortex. *European Journal of Neuroscience, 2*, 960–972.

Verney, C., Berger, B., Adrien, J., Vigny, A., & Gay, M. (1982). Development of the dopaminergic innervation of the rat cerebral cortex. A light microscopic immunocytochemical study using anti-tyrosine hydroxylase antibodies. *Brain Research, 281*(1), 41–52.

Vincent, S. L., & Benes, F. M. (1995). Postnatal maturation of GABA-immunoreactive neurons of rat medial prefrontal cortex. *Journal of Comparative Neurology, 355*, 81–92.

Vincent, S. L., Khan, Y., & Benes, F. M. (1995). Cellular colocalization of dopamine D1 and D2 receptors in rat medial prefrontal cortex. *Synapse, 19*(2), 112–120.

Volk, D. W., Austin, M. C., Pierri, J. N., Sampson, A. R., & Lewis, D. A. (2000). Decreased glutamic acid decarboxylase67 messenger RNA expression in a subset of prefrontal cortical gamma-aminobutyric acid neurons in subjects with schizophrenia. *Archives of General Psychiatry, 57*(3), 237–245.

Walker, E., & Diforio, D. (1997). Schizophrenia: a neural diathesis-stress model. *Psychological Review, 104*, 667–685.

Wang, Y., Sheen, V. L., & Macklis, J. D. (1998). Cortical interneurons upregulate neurotrophins in vivo in response to targeted apoptotic degeneration of neighboring pyramidal neurons. *Experimental Neurology, 154*(2), 389–402.

Weinberger, D. R. (1987). Implications of normal brain development for the pathogenesis of schizophrenia. *Archives of General Psychiatry, 44*, 660–669.

West, A. R., & Galloway, M. P. (1996). Regulation of serotonin-facilitated dopamine release in vivo: the role of protein kinase A activating transduction mechanisms. *Synapse, 23*, 20–27.

Wu, C., Yoder, E. J., Shih, J., Chen, K., Dias, P., K., Shi, L., Ji, S. D., Wei, J., Conner, J. M., Kumar, S., Ellisman, M. H., & Singh, S. K. (1998). Development and characterization of monoclonal antibodies specific to serotonin 5-HT2A receptor. *Journal of Histochemistry and Cytochemistry, 46*, 811–824.

Yakovlev, P., & Lecours, A. (1967). The myelinogenetic cycles of regional maturation of the brain. In A. Minkowski (Ed.), *Regional development of the brain early in Life* (pp. 3–70). Oxford: Blackwell.

Zhou, F. M., & Hablitz, J. J. (1999). Dopamine modulation of membrane and synaptic properties of interneurons in rat cortex. *Journal of Neruophysiology, 81*, 967–976.

PART FOUR

The Neurodevelopmental Course of Illustrative High-Risk Conditions and Mental Disorders

SEVENTEEN

Neurobiology of Personality Disorders

Implications for a Neurodevelopmental Model

Larry J. Siever, Harold W. Koenigsberg, and Deidre Reynolds

The study of the neurobiology of personality disorders represents a unique opportunity to understand the interactions of genetics and environment with respect to the emergence of the persistent behavioral patterns and coping strategies that we label personality. In personality disorders such as schizotypal personality disorder or borderline personality disorder, temperamental vulnerabilities interacting with early and late environmental events may account for the constellation of behaviors that constitute the criteria for these disorders. In this chapter, the neurobiology of these two prototypic personality disorders will be reviewed in the context of the limited available evidence to examine how their underlying neurobiology unfolds in the context of the development of psychologic structures and behavior associated with personality.

The personality disorders constitute a level of pathology in between the persistent and chronic Axis I disorders, such as schizophrenia, and milder personality variations within the normal range. For this reason, they constitute an ideal set of disorders to evaluate individual differences and how individual differences in neurobiology translate into different patterns of psychopathology and behavioral traits. Genetic factors may "set" the initial susceptibility to these behavioral patterns that develop in the context of early intrauterine influences as well as early interactions with caretakers.

In order for a neurobiologic model to have heuristic value in generating new investigative approaches as well as contributing significantly to clinical work, the temperamental/behavioral traits to be studied need to be grounded in core psychobiologic domains such as affect regulation, cognitive organization, modulation of aggression, and anxiety (Siever & Davis, 1991). Individual differences in the regulation of each of these domains may provide the variability or biases that impact on later psychosexual development. Thus, personality disorder categories or inferential psychological structures are grounded in these fundamental dimensions which may have relatively specific neurobiologic correlates.

The neurobiologic approach is grounded in a dimensional rather than categorical model. All these dimensions may be altered in the major psychiatric syndromes or Axis I disorders as well: for example, mood regulation in the affective disorders, cognitive regulation in the schizophrenic disorders, impulse dysregulation in the impulse disorders, and anxiety in the anxiety disorders; Axis I disorders are marked by usually episodic emergence of symptoms that may cause considerable suffering for the patient. In contrast, the Axis II disorders are characterized by behavioral strategies which, although apparently maladaptive in adult functioning, attempt to compensate for the underlying temperamental vulnerabilities so that symptoms do not emerge or progress. Thus, the anxious individual may engage in avoidant or submissive behaviors to forestall the possibility of interpersonal rejection, thus minimizing the experience of anxiety symptoms, while unduly restricting their behavioral options. In contrast, the borderline patient marked by affective instability and impulsivity often acts impulsively and self-destructively in an attempt to alleviate the affective distress or imbalance following the feeling of abandonment or loss. These strategies may be ineffective so that, despite the borderline individual's attempt to relieve their distress with promiscuity, substance use, or binge eating, symptomatic depression may emerge. Analogously, the avoidant individual, unable to forestall experiences of potential intimacy, may experience overt symptoms of anxiety related to underlying conflicts about aggression or sexuality. However, the personality disorder itself is defined by these maladaptive strategies, rather than the symptomatic breakthroughs that are often inevitable in these personality disorders. We hypothesize that these behavioral strategies may be mediated by often unconscious assumptions and conflicts generated as the child with their specific vulnerabilities internalizes representation of themselves and the world around them (Greenspan, 1989). Their maladaptive strategies and often self-defeating schema of their world become understandable in the context of their underlying biologic vulnerabilities and specific environmental events that the developing child is struggling with (Schore, 1994).

Figure 17.1 presents a general model of personality development. Personality incorporates both mental or psychological components and characteristic behavioral patterns. The mental components include emotional state, impulses, cognitive organization, representations of self and others, and schemata for interpersonal interactions. They are mediated by experience and by neurobiological substrates. Behavioral strategies can be called upon to modulate mental state.

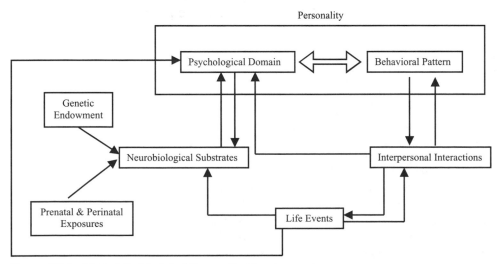

Figure 17.1. A Heuristic Model of Personality Development.

The neurobiologic substrates of personality disorder themselves do not remain static but are evolving in the course of the lifetime of the individual. They are grounded in the genetic makeup of each individual. Genetic differences themselves play an important role in personality development and it is likely that traits such as impulsivity or affective instability are prominent heritable components on the basis of studies of normal twins reared apart as well as monozygotic versus dizygotic twin studies that allow the disentanglement of genetic and environmental factors (Plomin & DeFries, 1981). Similarly, twin studies of personality disorders (Torgersen, 1984) also suggest the potential heritability for the impulsivity of the borderline or the eccentricity of the schizotypal individual. However, the role of neurobiology does not end at the genetic endowment of the individual. The expression of the genetic substrates is constantly being shaped by the environment in terms of specific gene expression by transcription factors that can be responsive to environmental stressors. Furthermore, environmental differences in the intrauterine environment, including variations in nutritional factors or the impact of viral infections, may also shape these neurobiologic substrates.

Human development is marked by a plasticity that is particularly great during the extended juvenile period. This delayed maturation allows environmental influences to have a particularly strong role in contrast to organisms with genetically preprogrammed or more simplistic influences of the surroundings, such as "imprinting." In infancy, the developing organism attempts to organize and regulate its internal state with the help of caretakers. In early infancy, sleeping may be punctuated by brief awakenings marked by hunger which is then alleviated by feeding by the mother. Thus, from very early on, the mother or other primary caretakers become centrally important in the development of adequate regulation of arousal, appetite, affect, and activity. The vulnerable infant who is prone to poorly modulated affective shifts or uncontrolled aggression may present a challenge for a mother who must help smooth out and reinforce appropriate regulation of these key cyclic biologic functions. Thus, from the very outset, these vulnerabilities translate themselves into an interpersonal context and are thus experienced and represented relationally.

Psychosocial influences in the family, school, and workplace will help shape personality development in a reciprocal interaction with the individual's evolving personality, for the individual is not a passive recipient of these forces, but indeed shapes and molds them by acting on their surroundings. While these experiences must, of course, be incorporated into the central nervous system, they presumably do so by means of potentiation of certain synaptic connections or by altering larger neural networks rather than resetting the more molar regulatory functions such as affective control or anxiety. However, massive trauma such as abuse and neglect can indeed, in principle, alter these psychobiologic regulatory domains and fundamentally shift these biologic vulnerabilities in the direction of severe psychopathology. Even relatively nontraumatic recurrent interactions that occur in the context of social learning may also be important in shifting, strengthening, or jeopardizing the regulation of anxiety, affect, action patterns, and cognition. These regulatory functions may also undergo a profound shift at the onset of adolescence with its accompanying hormonal changes and shifts in vulnerability patterns as well as resurgence of old injuries from past trauma. Finally, development does not end in adulthood. There is a considerable relearning and plasticity that may occur during the multiple phases of adult development, obviously a prerequisite for successful psychosocial intervention.

SCHIZOTYPAL PERSONALITY DISORDER

Schizotypal personality disorder (SPD) is the prototype of the schizophrenia spectrum. In the *DSM-IV* (*Diagnostic and Statistical Manual of Mental Disorders*, revised, 4th ed.), it is defined by the presence of five or more of the following features: (1) ideas of reference, (2) odd beliefs or magical thinking, (3) unusual perceptual experiences, (4) odd thinking and speech, (5) suspiciousness or paranoid ideation, (6) inappropriate or constricted affect, (7) odd, eccentric, or peculiar behavior, (8) lack of close friends, and (9) excessive social anxiety. Indeed, the criteria were formulated in part from characteristics identified in relatives of chronic schizophrenic individuals who had schizophrenia-related traits in the Danish Adoptive Studies (Kety et al., 1975, 1994). These adoption studies as well as family studies of schizophrenic individuals suggest that the milder, schizophrenia-related personality disorders may be more common phenotypic manifestations of underlying diatheses to schizophrenia than is chronic schizophrenia itself. Furthermore, it is likely that chronic schizophrenia represents the convergence of a number of interactive pathophysiologies involving cortical and subcortical brain structures. The study of schizotypal personality disordered individuals represents then a real opportunity to disentangle these various pathophysiologic processes.

An essential feature of schizotypal personality disorder, as well as other "odd cluster" personality disorders, is an underlying cognitive disorganization which appears to be grounded in altered brain circuitry. These brain abnormalities appear to be present quite early as part of an ongoing neurodevelopmental impairment. Deficits in information processing and cognitive function can interfere with effective social interaction as well as contribute to the cognitive/perceptional distortions in paranoia associated with this disorder.

Recent formulations of pathophysiology of schizophrenia suggest that it may be a neurodevelopmental disorder (Weinberger, 1987; Murray et al., 1992). Our studies of schizotypal personality disorder suggest the possibility that indeed schizotypal personality disorder is a more common manifestation of the neurodevelopemental susceptibilities that yield the schizophrenic disorders. Other pathophysiologic processes related to this neurodevelopmental impairment, including glutamatergic-dopaminergic imbalance, may drive this neurodevelopmental disorder toward or away from psychosis. Thus, studies examining schizotypal personality disorder patients in relation to appropriate normal controls, other personality disorder comparison groups, and schizophrenic patients may allow for a relative dissociation of these pathophysiologic processes.

Genetics

While the precise genetic locus of the susceptibility to schizophrenia has yet to be established, results of the large-scale linkage scale studies to date suggest some degree of heterogeneity in genetic underpinnings of schizophrenia, and an oligogenic model of several interactive genes remains a likely possibility. Large-scale family studies, such as the Roscommon County study, that have provided a basis for these linkage analyses, also suggests that the heritability for the schizophrenic disorders may be manifest in phenotypes ranging from chronic schizophrenia through schizotypal personality to some forms of schizoid and perhaps even avoidant personality disorder (Kendler et al., 1981). The Roscommon family study and other proceeding studies such as the Iowa non-500 (Tsuang et al., 1983) suggest that schizophrenia-related personality disorders are the most common schizophrenia-related diagnoses in the families of schizophrenic patients and both schizophrenic-related personality disorders and psychoses other than schizophrenia may be increased in prevalence in the families of schizophrenic patients, although not necessarily in the same individuals. These studies suggest that there may be familial genetic factors related to the "core" symptoms of the schizophrenia-related personality disorders, the social deficits and cognitive disorganization, and other genetic susceptibilities related to psychosis. Twin studies (Kendler et al., 1991) suggest independent heritability of factors related to the core social deficits and psychotic-like symptoms. Thus, genetic data are compatible with the model postulating some factors related to an underlying neurodevelopmental impairment with consequences for social and cognitive function and other genetic factors more related to susceptibility to psychosis.

Brain Structure

Neurodevelopmental abnormalities could alter brain structure to a degree that could be measurable by ventricle volume on CT scan or volume of brain regions of interest on magnetic resonance imaging (MRI). Indeed, several studies suggest that brain ventricular volume is increased in schizotypal personality disorder patients and schizophrenic patients (Siever et al., 1995). These studies have been confirmed by MRI studies (Buchsbaum, Yang, et al., 1997). Ventricular enlargement might be in part related to volume loss of cortical structures such as the temporal cortex. Indeed, reductions in volume of the temporal cortex, and, in particular, the superior temporal gyrus have constituted a hallmark finding in schizophrenic patients (McCarley et al., 1999). Two independent studies have now reported reduced temporal lobe volumes, including superior temporal gyrus in schizotypal individuals, as they have in schizophrenic patients (Downhill et al., 1997; Dickey et al., 1999). In contrast, frontal lobe volume appears to be normal in schizotypal personality disorder patients in contrast to reductions in schizophrenic patients (Kirrane et al., 2000; McCarley et al., 1999). Thalamic volume is also reduced, particularly in regions such as pulvinar which are linked to temporal cortex. But the medial dorsal nucleus which is linked to frontal cortex is not reduced. In contrast, schizophrenic patients show reductions in both pulvinar and medialdorsal nuclei and larger volume reductions in thalamus. Finally, striatal volumes, particularly putamen, are larger in schizophrenic patients compared to normal controls while the putamen is smaller in schizotypal personality disorder patients compared to controls. Even when schizotypal personality disorder patients that have never been medicated are compared to never-medicated chronic schizophrenic patients, the SPD patients showed reduced putamen size compared to the schizophrenic patients. These findings suggest that reductions in lateral structures, such as the temporal cortex, or medial temporal structures, such as the hippocampus, may be common throughout the schizophrenia spectrum disorders, but that schizotypal patients, in particular, may be better buffered in frontal regions which, in effect, may spare them the more severe executive deficits or social deficits of chronic schizophrenia. These differential volume reductions are evident in the corticothalamic relays as well, with thalamic nuclei projecting to lateral regions being reduced in schizotypal patients and those projecting to frontal cortex showing normal volumes. The relatively smaller putamen volumes in the schizotypal patients compared to both the normal controls and the schizophrenic patient volumes raise the possibility that reduced striatal tissue, possibly reflecting reductions in enervation by dopaminergic terminals or other afferents to this region, may reflect a better buffered striatal system, possibly with regard to dopaminergic activity.

Functional Imaging

Functional imaging studies suggest schizotypal personality disordered individuals have anomalous brain activation patterns, in some cases, with compensatory activation of regions that are not normally employed by control subjects in conjunction with task-induced activation. In an initial single photon emission computerized tomography (SPECT) study of patients with schizotypal personality disorder, schizotypal personality patients showed less activation of the precentral gyrus compared to controls and increased activation of the middle right frontal gyrus compared to controls, suggesting the possibility that they utilized these alternative regions to enable them to better perform the task. Greater activation of the middle frontal gyrus was correlated with better performance (Buchsbaum, Trestman, et al., 1997).

In flourode oxyglucose position emission tomography (FDG-PET), studies of schizophrenic patients, schizotypal patients, and normal controls, both schizophrenic and to a lesser degree schizotypal patients showed anomalous lateralization of activation of temporal structures during a verbal learning task. Both schizophrenic and schizotypal subjects did not activate Brodman area 46, the primary frontal area activated by normal controls, but schizotypal subjects showed activation of other frontal regions to a greater degree than either schizophrenic patients or normal controls, also consistent with compensatory activation of neighboring frontal regions. Finally, striatal activity was increased in schizotypal patients compared to controls subjects in the dopamine receptor–rich area of ventral putamen, suggesting reduced dopaminergic inhibitory tone. Other more dorsal striatal regions were less active in the schizotypal patients than the schizophrenic patients (Kirrane et al., 2000). The alternative activation patterns in frontal lobe is consistent with better buffered frontal cortical activity in schizotypal patients compared to schizophrenic patients, while the increased striatal activity is consistent with reduced dopaminergic activity in schizotypal patients compared to schizophrenic patients and control subjects, a possible protective factor against psychosis. This hypothesis is supported by the correlation between reduced activity and increased psychotic-like symptoms of SPD in ventral striatum.

Cognitive/Information Processing Capacity

Studies of schizotypal personality disorder patients identified in the clinic or among relatives of schizophrenic patients suggest similar but less severe attentional and cognitive impairment than in chronic schizophrenic patients. Abnormalities in smooth pursuit eye movements, backward masking, and sustained attention on a continuous performance task using more challenging stimulus presentations such as degraded stimuli or identical pairs have been demonstrated in schizotypal personality disorder patients just as they have in schizophrenic patients (Siever, Kalus, & Keefe, 1993). Abnormalities in executive function such as on the Stroop Color Word Interference Test and Wisconsin Card Sort have also been documented (Trestman et al., 1995; Siegel et al., 1996).

However, general intelligence seems to be spared in schizotypal patients, as does perceptual orientation (Trestman et al., 1995). Studies of more specific cognitive functions have documented impairment in visual spatial delayed response, partially mediated by dorsal lateral prefrontal cortex, and verbal learning, partially mediated by temporal and related lateral brain structures (Lees-Roitman et al., 2000; Bergman et al., 1998). Structural imaging studies suggest that these cognitive impairments are in part correlated with volumes of cortical structures implicated in their performance.

Initial data suggest that amphetamine, which enhances activity of two key neurotransmitter systems – the neuroadrenergic (neurotransmitter: norepinepherine) and dopaminergic (neurotransmitter: dopamine) – improves cognitive performance and visual spatial delayed response task (Kirrane et al., 2000), Continuous Performance Task, and a verbal learning task (Lees-Roitman et al., 1997).

Neurochemical Measures

Dopamine systems have been implicated in the psychotic symptoms of the schizophrenia spectrum. Studies of neuroleptic efficacy on psychotic symptoms associated with dopamine receptor occupancy, dopamine receptor number in postmortem samples, and direct studies of dopamine release following amphetamine suggest increased responses in schizophrenic patients associated with transient worsening of psychotic symptoms (Laruelle et al., 1996; Breier et al., 1997). Studies of cerebrospinal fluid (CSF) and plasma dopamine metabolites such as homovanillic acid (HVA) have been mixed but suggest increases associated with paranoid symptoms and decreases associated with negative anergic symptoms (Davis et al., 1991). The study of schizotypal personality disorder patients affords a better opportunity to disentangle the positive, psychotic-like symptoms from the negative or deficit-related symptoms. Increases in plasma HVA have been associated with psychotic symptoms in both schizotypal personality disorder patients and schizotypal relatives of schizophrenic patients, while decreases in plasma HVA have been associated with the negative symptoms of schizotypal personality disorder, particularly in schizotypal relatives of schizophrenic patients (Amin et al., 1997). Reductions in striatal volume and increases in ventral putamen metabolic activity are also consistent with hypothesis of reduced dopaminergic function in schizotypal patients. Initial results of studies of schizotypal personality disorder patients measuring dopamine release following amphetamine administration suggest normal release of dopamine in contrast to the increased release of dopamine following amphetamine in schizophrenic patients (Koenigsberg et al, 1999). Furthermore, the glycopyruvic stressor, 2-deoxyglucose, which results in increases in dopamine release measured by plasma HVA in schizophrenic patients that are greater than those observed in controls, results in HVA increases in schizotypal personality disorder patients which appear to be slightly lower than those of normal controls. These results are compatible with reduced dopaminergic activity in schizotypal patients (Amin et al., 1997). In studies of dopamine release measured by SPECT imaging following amphetamine, greater schizotypal symptoms were associated with lower dopamine release. Clearly, a range of dopaminergic activity exists in the schizophrenia-related disorder and differential activity of dopaminergic system in different brain region has been hypothesized (Davis et al., 1991; Weinberger et al, 1986). It appears that increased subcortical dopaminergic activity is associated with the psychosis-related symptoms of the schizophrenia spectrum, while reductions in dopaminergic activity in the frontal cortical regions may be implicated in the cognitive impairment of this disorder (consistent with its partial reversal by amphetamine in SPD patients). Patients with schizotypal personality disorder may be better buffered from subcortical increases in dopaminergic activity than patients susceptible to chronic schizophrenia; hence, they may display some of the social deficits and cognitive impairment without the serious psychotic symptoms.

A Neurodevelopmental Model of the Schizophrenia Spectrum Disorders

These findings are consistent with the model of the schizophrenia spectrum disorders implicating alterations in development of cortical structures and their relays to sub-cortical nuclei such as the mediodorsal nucleus of the thalamus and pulvinar. Lateral cortical structures such as the temporal or hippocampal cortex may be particularly vulnerable to such neurodevelomental aberrations, possibly in part because of their suscep-tibility to early environmental insults. Most studies suggest that genetic susceptibility factors interact with such environmental events to yield the phenotypic outcome of schizophrenia-related disorder. These observations are consistent with the reductions in temporal cortex found consistently in schizotypal personality disorder patients as well as schizophrenic patients, reductions that may even be comparable or greater in magnitude. However, other factors unrelated to the susceptibility to this neurodevelop-mental impairment may play a buffering role potentially protecting individuals with schizotypal personality disorder from the chronic psychosis and social and cognitive deterioration of schizophrenia. While there are probably a number of such factors, ge-netic factors relating to, for example, greater capacity or flexibility of frontal cortical structures perhaps associated with general intelligence may provide partial compensa-tion for the more serious social deficits and cognitive impairment of the schizophrenia spectrum. Better buffered subcortical dopaminergic activity, due to transient differences in dopaminergic activation potentials or in other neurotransmitter systems such as the glutaminergic system that may modulate the dopaminergic activity, may make it less likely that these cortical impairments translate into upregulation of dopaminergic ac-tivity subcortically, as they are hypothesized to do in chronic schizophrenia (Siever, Kalus, & Keefe, 1993).

A developmental model of schizotypal personality disorder will integrate what is known of the neurobiology of the disorder with the contribution of genetic suscep-tibility factors, environmental events, caregiver interactions, and other psychosocial influences. Figure 17.2 presents an approach to such a model.

Psychosocial Developmental Implications

A developmental trajectory of individuals with schizotypal personality disorder helps us to understand the social and cognitive difficulties of the schizophrenia spectrum in the absence of the deteriorating effects of chronic psychosis. Offspring of schizophrenic patients display an uneven neurologic maturation (Fish, 1987) resulting in develop-mental delays in motor coordination and social development. In this longitudinal study, many individuals with this kind of pandevelopmental dismaturation went on to develop schizotypal personality disorder. It is known that parent-infant interac-tions are very sensitive to children's psychomotor capability to integrate and respond

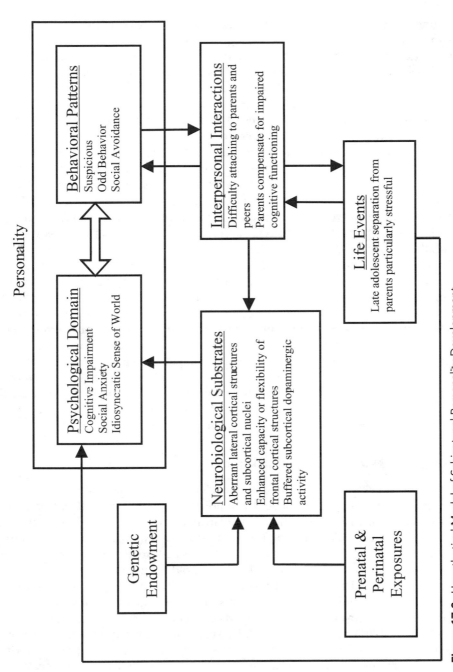

Figure 17.2. Hypothetical Model of Schizotypal Personality Development.

synchronously to verbal and nonverbal cues of the parents (Brazelton, 1978). Thus, these infants may have difficulty developing an attachment to parents and peers, and their experience becomes one of failed connections. As a result, such individuals often become isolated, preferring the familiarity of solitude to the uncomfortable challenge posed by any kind of interpersonal engagement, although they might ideally like to be able to feel connected to others. Their tendency to cognitive disorganization and distortion may result in eccentric or unusual ideas and distortions. The isolation they have chosen results in a lack of corrective feedback so that their sense of the world becomes more idiosyncratic. While most individuals destined to become schizotypal remain quietly eccentric, isolated, and cognitively challenged, those with a propensity for psychosis as well generally cannot withstand the stresses of separation from parents and caretakers, such as going away to school or a job. Often the parents have provided executive functions, compensating for areas of executive impairment in the pre-schizophrenic individual. The stress of separation may then trigger stress systems that result in unchecked dopaminergic overactivity and ultimately psychosis. Those less predisposed to psychosis such as the prototypic individual schizotypal personality disorder are able to develop self-contained, solitary, often eccentric lifestyles and are not so vulnerable to the stresses that might induce psychosis. This model, albeit simplified, is consistent with "high risk" studies of offspring of schizophrenic patients who show attentional and cognitive impairment on tasks such as the Continuous Performance Task at a relatively early age. Most of these individuals do not develop schizophrenia itself, but many end up having a diagnosis of schizotypal personality disorder or at least some degree of schizotypy. Thus, the schizotypal individual may be the more prototypic phenotype of the neurodevelopmental impairment of the spectrum, while other factors modulate this core "spectrum" vulnerability toward or away from the severe cognitive/social impairment and psychosis of chronic schizophrenia.

BORDERLINE PERSONALITY DISORDER

Borderline personality disorder (BPD) is characterized in the *DSM-IV* diagnostic system by the presence of five or more of the following features: (1) affective instability, (2) inappropriate intense anger, (3) impulsivity in at least two potentially self-damaging areas, (4) recurrent suicidal behavior, (5) unstable intense interpersonal relationships, (6) frantic efforts to avoid abandonment, (7) identity disturbance, (8) chronic feelings of emptiness, and (9) transient stress-related paranoid ideation or severe dissociative symptoms. Siever and Davis (1991) proposed that BPD entails the co-occurrence of two biologically determined personality traits, impulsive aggression and affective instability. Evidence from family studies supports this hypothesis. For example, Silverman and colleagues (1991) reported that the risk of either impulsive aggression or affective instability were greater in relatives of BPD probands than in those of probands with other personality disorders or schizophrenia, although both traits did not necessarily *co-occur* in the relatives of BPD probands as they did in the probands. While individuals with other personality disorders may experience dysregulation in either of these domains, the coincidence of affective instability and impaired impulse control thus appears to characterize BPD. Taken together, these two traits have a positive predictive value for diagnosing BPD of 75 percent when compared with other disorders of personality (Zanarini, et al., 1998). Biological studies of BPD, which will be discussed below, add additional support to this hypothesis by demonstrating neurobiological dysregulations associated with these traits. In a separate line of research relevant to a developmental model, investigators have turned attention to the relationship between childhood trauma and BPD (Perry and Herman, 1993). Studies of trauma survivors, in turn, have demonstrated lasting neurobiological changes consequent to trauma. These three lines of investigation converge to provide the basis for a neurodevelopmental model of BPD. We will first review each area separately and then consider their implications for a neurodevelopmental model of BPD.

Neurobiological Correlates of BPD

Impulsive Aggression

There is evidence that dysregulation in a number of neurotransmitter systems may play a role in impulsive aggression. The serotonin system has been the most extensively studied. Early studies of the serotonin (5-hydroxytraptamine, 5-HT) system relied on measurements of the levels of serotonin breakdown products in blood or cerebrospinal fluid (CSF). More recent studies have focused not only on the release of serotonin, but also on the sensitivity of a variety of specific types of receptors where the serotonin may act. Specific serotonin receptors that have been studied include the 5-HT$_{1A}$, 5-HT$_{1B}$, 5-HT$_{2A}$, and 5-HT$_{2C}$ receptors. These receptors have been examined using specific agents that stimulate them (agonists) or that block them (antagonists).

In 1976, Asberg and colleagues (Asberg et al., 1976) showed that CSF levels of the serotonin metabolite, 5-HIAA, were reduced in those depressed patients who had a history of suicide attempts, and to a greater degree if the attempts had been violent. Lower levels of CSF 5-HIAA have been reported in individuals who committed violent crimes or murder (Linnoila et al., 1983; Lindberg et al., 1984). While CSF studies provide an indirect measure of serotonin turnover, the reactivity of the serotonin system can be evaluated more directly by measuring prolactin release, which is under the control of serotonergic neurons at the level of the hypothalamus. Prolactin response to challenges with a variety of serotonergic agonists and releasing agents is reduced in personality disorder patients with impulsive aggression compared to normal controls and personality disorder patients without impulsive aggression. This has been demonstrated with the nonspecific serotonin releasing agent and reuptake inhibitor, fenfluramine (Coccaro et al., 1989), as well as with the 5-HT$_{1A}$ partial agonist, buspirone (Coccaro et al., 1990), the 5-HT$_{1A}$ selective agonist, ipsapirone (Moeller et al., 1998), and metachlorophenylpiperazine (m-CPP), which is a 5-HT$_{1A}$ and 5-HT$_{2C}$ agonist and a 5-HT$_{2A}$ antagonist (Coccaro, 1998). The neuroendocrine studies assay serotonin responsivity at the level of the hypothalmus. Recently, PET methodology has permitted a targeted examination of the serotonin systems in the frontal regions that are believed to control impulsive behavior. Siever et al. (1999) demonstrated blunted metabolic responses to d,l-fenfluramine in the orbital frontal, adjacent ventromedial, and cingulate cortex in patients with impulsive aggression compared with healthy controls.

Other neurotransmitters may also play a role in impulsive aggression. In a group of personality disordered patients, CSF levels of arginine vasopressin have been shown to positively correlate with life history of general aggression and aggression against persons (Coccaro et al., 1998). Some studies suggest that central norepinepherine (NE) may also be implicated in aggression. Siever and Trestman (1993) found that plasma

NE levels were correlated with impulsivity in male personality disordered patients. In a study using the growth hormone (GH) response to clonidine to assess the activity of central alpha-2 noradrenergic receptors, Coccaro et al. (1991) found an association between the magnitude of the GH response and self-reported irritability in personality disorder subjects and healthy controls. Other studies have found reduced levels of the norepinepherine metabolite, MHPG, in CSF or plasma in violent offenders (Virkkunen et al., 1987) and patients with a diagnosis of BPD (Coccaro, 1998), suggesting the possibility of reduced presynaptic noradrenergic activity and enhanced adrenergic receptor responsiveness associated with aggressive behavior.

Affective Instability

The cholinergic, noradrenergic, and GABAminergic systems may all play a role in affective instability. Several lines of evidence point to the involvement of cholinergic dysregulation. First, brain regions involved in emotion regulation such as the amygdala, hippocampus, and cingulate cortex have rich cholinergic enervation. REM sleep latency, which is under cholinergic control, is more variable among BPD patients than controls and more sensitive to the effect of cholinomimetic drugs. Cholinomimetics produce acute mood shifts to depression in patients with unipolar and bipolar depression (Janowsky & Overstreet, 1995). Among BPD patients, the cholinomimetic, physostigmine, has been shown to induce a mood shift to dysphoria that is of greater magnitude than among healthy control subjects (Steinberg et al., 1997). Moreover, the magnitude of the depressive response to physostigmine correlated with the degree of affective instability as indexed by the number of affective instability traits (i.e., affective instability per se, unstable relationships, identity disturbance, and chronic feelings of emptiness and boredom) in the borderline patients.

Noradrenergic systems may also contribute to affective instability, particularly by influencing reactivity to environmental stimuli. Personality disordered patients with high levels of irritability, verbal aggression, and risk taking, which may be associated with high engagement with the environment, have hyper-responsive noradrenergic systems (Steinberg et al., 1994). As described above, irritability in BPD patients and healthy controls correlates with growth hormone response to clonidine, a measure of reactivity of the alpha-2 receptor system.

GABA, a widely distributed neurotransmitter with inhibitory functions, could serve to damp down affective excursions, acting as an affect stabilizer. Decreased GABA activity could then contribute to affective instability. Lithium, valproate, and carbamezepine, mood stabilizers which have been reported to control affective instability in borderline patients, all increase GABAminergic transmission. On the level of intracellular signal transduction, these mood stabilizers also have been shown to affect G-protein, protein kinase C, MARCKS, and calcium activity (Ghaemi et al., 1999, Avissar & Schreiber, 1992). Thus, affective instability may be associated with disturbances in intracellular signaling mechanisms.

Genetic Factors

Family studies and candidate gene investigations both point to a role for inheritance in the development of BPD. While evidence for the familial transmission of BPD per se is mixed (Torgesen, 1994), there is stronger evidence that the BPD traits of affective instability and impulsivity run in families. Silverman et al. (1991) showed that each of these traits was more frequent in families of BPD patients than in families of those with other personality disorders or schizophrenia. In an analysis of 500 healthy monozygotic and dizygotic twin pairs raised together and apart, Coccaro and co-workers (1993) showed a heritability of 0.43 for the trait irritable impulsiveness. The genetic contribution was nonadditive (i.e., reflective of multiple genes contributing together to the phenotype, or of dominance). Their model also suggested that 54 percent of the variance was due to the influence of the nonshared environment. Interestingly, the contribution of shared environment was nonsignificant.

Specific mechanisms for the genetic transmission of borderline traits have not been established, but candidate gene studies suggest possible genetic contributions to the trait of impulsive aggression. Less data are available for the affective instability trait. Because impulsive aggression, whether self-directed or other directed, is associated with blunted serotonergic activity, attention has been focused on candidate genes which code for proteins involved in serotonergic neurotransmission. Studies of a nonfunctional polymorphism of the gene that codes for the serotonin $5-HT_{2A}$ receptor have found that the "1" allele of the gene is more strongly associated with self-mutilation in a group of personality disorder patients and with suicide attempts in males in that group than is the "2" allele of the gene (New et al., 1999a). A polymorphism involving two alleles ("G" and "C") that code for an amino acid in the gene for the $5-HT_{1B}$ receptor has also been studied in personality disorder patients. Among Caucasian patients, the "G" allele has been associated with a history of suicide attempts (New et al., 1999b). Two alleles ("U" and "L") of the tryptophan hydroxylase (TPH) gene have been studied. Although TPH is involved in serotonin synthesis, this polymorphism is not believed to be directly related to serotonin production. Nevertheless, it may be in linkage disequilibrium with components coding the regulatory region or with a neighboring gene. One study (New et al., 1998) reported an association between the LL genotype and impulsive aggression in a group of male Caucasian patients with personality disorders. Another study (Mann et al., 1997), examining Caucasian patients with a diagnosis of major depression, found an association between the "U" allele and suicidal acts.

The genetics of BPD has been difficult to elucidate, in part, because personality is likely to involve complex genetics (Burmeister, 1999), in which specific personality phenotypes may arise from the product of several genes acting together (epistasis), and particular personality phenotypes may be the common outcome of a number of different genotypes.

Environmental Influences

Twin studies indicate that nonshared environmental factors account for 54 percent of the variance in the occurrence of irritable impulsiveness (Coccaro et al., 1993). One such factor could be childhood trauma. Early abuse has been associated with various forms of psychopathology in adults, including BPD, but also with somatoform disorders, multiple personality disorder, and panic disorder (Teicher et al., 1994). Adult BPD patients report histories of physical or sexual abuse at rates ranging up to 81 percent (Herman et al., 1989). In female cohorts, physical abuse if present occurred in early childhood, while sexual abuse if present occurred in latency and adolescence (Zanarini et al., 1989). Community studies show that childhood sexual abuse was more often associated with the development of BPD in females (Jason et al., 1982; Paris et al., 1994); and physical abuse more often associated with the development of BPD in males (Herman et al., 1989; Paris et al., 1994). While childhood sexual abuse in BPD males was associated with the use of force and penetration by nonrelative strangers, trauma, loss, and problems with fathers were more important for male development of BPD (Paris et al., 1994).

Although such life experiences are clearly associated with the development of BPD, they are not uniquely associated with BPD (e.g., severe childhood trauma was found in 83 percent of adult patients with multiple personality disorder; Putnam et al., 1986). By the same token, most children who experience physical or sexual abuse do not go on to develop psychopathology. The data suggest, in fact, that only one in five have psychopathological outcomes (Paris, 1998). Childhood experiences other than sexual or physical abuse may play a role as well. Gudzer et al. (1991) report that borderline children, when compared with similarly impaired nonborderline children, had higher rates of parental neglect, parental criminality and substance abuse, and placements in foster homes, in addition to more sexual and physical abuse. Chronically disturbed caretakers and the presence of abuse were more significant than prolonged separation from caretakers and history of neglect respectively (Zanarini et al., 1989). In one study, borderline individuals retrospectively reported patterns of low care and overprotection by their caretakers, described as "affectionless control." There is some suggestion that duration may be more important than severity or frequency of physical abuse (Torgesen & Alnaes, 1992).

We are beginning to understand how life experience may be transduced into neurobiological changes. The brain continues to develop in response to experience throughout childhood and into adolescence. The prefrontal cortex, hippocampus, and amygdala are particularly plastic (Teicher et al., 1994). The prefrontal cortex, especially the orbitofrontal cortex, undergoes substantial growth during the first two years of life and some projections to the prefrontal cortex do not begin to myelinate until adolescence. Axonal and dendritic arborization and synaptogenesis are influenced by levels of sensory stimulation, by neurotransmitter release, and by stress hormones such as cortisol (Schore, 1994). Studies in rats and nonhuman primates have shown that chronic stress (psychosocial or restraint), which can elevate cortisol levels, or treatment with exogenous glucocorticoids causes atrophy or death of hippocampal neurons (Duman et al., 1997). Particularly relevant to BPD, in view of its association with blunted serotonergic activity, is the finding that exposure of rats to high levels of cortisol resulted in decreased binding at 5-HT_{1A} and 5-HT_{1B} receptors (Mendelson & McEwen, 1992).

In a study of 104 children and adolescents admitted to a psychiatric hospital, Teicher and colleagues (1994) report an association between history of physical or sexual abuse and electrophysiological abnormalities localized to the left frontotemporal and anterior regions. We would expect dysfunction in these areas to be implicated in the development of BPD since this region plays important roles both in the cognitive regulation of emotion and in impulse control. It has also been speculated that childhood trauma may lead to decreased interhemispheric communication and increased lateralization with greater right frontal function, leading to enhanced perception of emotion, or reactivity to negative affect (Teicher et al., 1994, Joseph, 1996). The hypothalamic–pituitary–adrenal (HPA) axis may be exquisitely sensitive to early childhood experiences and trauma (Figueroa & Silk, 1997) and alterations in CRF, ACTH, or cortisol may in turn influence neural development. Studies of posttraumatic stress disorder (PTSD) afford a valuable perspective, because of the high prevalence of childhood trauma in the histories of many of those who develop BPD and because PTSD per se is frequently associated with BPD. Characteristic neurobiological changes, such as decreased hippocampal volumes, increased glucocorticoid receptor sensitivity, and decreased cortisol release, have been identified in patients with PTSD (Yehuda, 1998). These findings are consistent with the possibility that similar changes could be induced in BPD as a result of childhood trauma.

In a study of twelve female BPD patients with impulsive self-damaging behavior and aggressiveness, Rinne and colleagues (2000) reported a blunted prolactin response to m-CPP in the subgroup with a history of sustained childhood physical and sexual trauma, compared to BPD patients without significant trauma and to controls. They also found that both trauma and nontrauma exposed BPD subgroups showed a similar blunted cortisol response to m-CPP, compared to controls. Since 5-HT_{1A} and 5-HT_{2C} receptors both play a role in prolactin release, while only 5-HT_{2C} receptors are required for cortisol release, the authors infer that sustained childhood trauma may downregulate 5-HT_{1A} receptors. Decreased 5-HT_{2C} receptor activity, on the other hand, appears present in the entire sample of impulsive aggressive borderline patients regardless of the presence of sustained childhood trauma. While the findings in this small sample require replication, they raise the possibility that reduced 5-HT_{2C} receptor activity may be a general feature in aggressive impulsive BPD patients, while exposure to sustained childhood trauma may add the additional complication of a decrease in 5-HT_{1A} receptor activity.

A Neurodevelopmental Model of BPD

A neurodevelopmental model of BPD should explain how the interaction between neurobiology and life experience over time culminates ultimately in the adult with borderline personality. While it is premature to propose such a model at present, we can draw upon the emerging data in the field to begin to sketch out the form such a model might take (see Figure 17.3).

The traits of impulsive aggression and affective instability, with their strong biological underpinnings, contribute to shaping the experience of the developing individual, but may themselves also be the consequences of powerful life experiences. The twin and family studies cited above indicate that children can be born with tendencies toward impulsive aggression and affective instability. Such traits will influence the nature of their early interactions with caregivers, which in turn will shape the developing child's preconceptions of social interactions and lead to the formation of particular internalized mental representations of others and the self. The infant who cries excessively, for example, may induce an irritable, impatient, or less empathic response in a caregiver. Over time the infant may not be able to develop the expectation that he will receive a positive or soothing interaction with a caregiver. In some cases, a consequence of trait aggression and affective instability may be the formation of extreme and unrealistic internalized representations of self and others, which set the stage for the disturbances in interpersonal relationships seen in the adult borderline patient. Conversely, life experience may shape neural development in such a way that impulsive aggression or affective instability are acquired. In some children, the proclivity toward impulsive aggression or affective instability is inherited. In others it may be instilled by negative

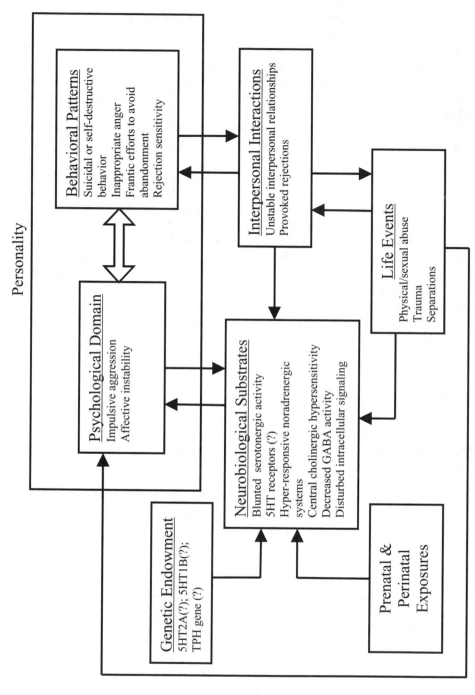

Figure 17.3. Hypothetical Model of Borderline Personality Development.

life experience. It is likely that those with a stronger inheritance of these trait predispositions require a smaller degree of adverse early life experience to develop BPD, while those with more robust impulse and affect control systems may not develop BPD unless they are exposed to extreme life experiences.

Children born with an impulsive aggressive or affectively unstable temperament may be more sensitive to frustration, pain, or discomfort, and may be less responsive to the efforts of the caregiver to soothe. This array of responses will evoke particular parental behaviors, partly co-determined by parental personality and temperament. Over time, on the basis of repeated patterns of interaction, the child develops mental representations of caregivers and other persons and of him or her self. In the context of high impulsive aggression, the self and others may come to be seen as unpredictable or dangerous. This can lead to distorted and maladaptive representations of the self and others. Affective instability could result in memories of quite similar interpersonal experiences being encoded with very different affective valences, depending upon the subject's affective state of the moment. This could lead to emotionally partitioned representations of the self or others, possibly contributing to the identity disturbances seen in BPD.

Animal studies and posttraumatic stress disorder research provide evidence that extreme early life experiences such as physical and sexual abuse can alter neural mechanisms. The effects of repeated or chronic abuse may be even more profound. One of the most clearly established neural sequella to intense or chronic stress is a loss of neurons in the hippocampus. The hippocampus is believed to play an important role in placing an emotional situation into a context based on prior emotional experiences (Ledoux, 1996). Thus, stress-related decreases in hippocampal volume might make it more difficult for the individual to draw upon emotional memories to assess and integrate current experience. Alterations in brain laterality might also alter the ability to process emotional information. Changes in cortisol levels and glucocorticoid receptor activity could influence the individual's ability to respond to stress. Impulsive aggression, a frequently seen component of adult PTSD, could develop in children exposed to trauma as well, possibly because of its effect in decreasing 5-HT_{1A} receptor activity. Neglect, untimely separations, and chronic stress may also affect the developing nervous system. In an animal model, Zhang and co-workers (1997) have shown that even brief maternal deprivation could lead to cell loss in the hippocampus. Serotonin, on the other hand, appears to promote the development of neurons in the cortex and hippocampus (Brezun & Daszuta, 1999; Gould, 1999). Individuals with robust serotonergic activity might have some protection from the deleterious effects of stress or separation. To the extent that individuals with impulsive aggression have downregulated serotonin systems, they may be more vulnerable to life's stressors. The effect of life experiences upon the developing brain is likely to depend heavily upon the biological maturity of the brain at the time of the experience. In the prefrontal cortex, for example, periods of substantial axonal and dendritic growth occur during the first two years of life. Schore (1994) has proposed that there is a critical period of synaptic growth involving the prefrontal limbic structures which occurs at the end of the first year of life and which is strongly affected by socioaffective interactions with the primary caregiver.

Thus, the neurodevelopment of BPD involves parallel and interacting developmental pathways of the individual's neural organization, on the one hand, and the social matrix in which the development takes place, on the other. Inborn temperamental traits evoke particular caregiver responses which, over time, both shape the individual's mental representations of the self and others and also directly influence neural development. Negative experiences such as abuse, neglect, and stress can alter the brain, giving rise to personality traits that in turn influence relationships first with caregivers and later with others in the individual life. In some individuals inheritance may play the greater role and in others, adverse life experience. Those whose genetic endowment predisposes to impulsive aggression or affective instability may develop BPD with less adverse early life exposures, while those with more robust impulse and affective systems may develop BPD only after more extreme early experiences.

DIRECTIONS FOR FURTHER RESEARCH

With the recent growth in knowledge of the ways in which neurobiology can contribute to personality, we are challenged with formulating a comprehensive model of personality development which integrates neurobiological processes with the psychosocial influences that shape personality. The models presented here are rudimentary at best and are offered as heuristics for further investigation. A research program to lay the groundwork for neurodevelopmental models of the personality disorders must address a number of areas. We need to identify those personality features that have biological underpinnings. At present, impulsive-aggression, affective instability, cognitive organization, reactive anxiety, novelty seeking, and reward dependence have been singled out as personality traits which have specific biological correlates. We do not know whether these traits are necessary and sufficient to account for the biology of the diverse personality disorders. Research focusing on the phenomenology of personality traits in tandem with family studies can be especially valuable here.

Despite important recent developments, additional research on the biological underpinnings of personality traits is called for. With respect to cognitive processing in SPD, we need to learn more about localized cortical and subcortical dopaminergic activity, and to better understand the role of noradrenergic systems and NMDA. In BPD, the role of serotonergic systems in impulsive-aggression has been established, but we have not yet identified the specific 5-HT receptors most strongly implicated and the possible role of other neurotransmitters such as norepinepherine and argenine vasopressin. We understand even less about the neurobiology of affective instability. In addition to identifying the neurotransmitter and intracellular communication systems that mediate affective experience, we need to learn more about the brain regions involved in affect modulation. Neuroimaging methods, particularly those with fast time resolution such as functional magnetic resonance imaging, offer the opportunity not only to learn which brain regions are involved in emotion regulation, but also to study differences in the time course of reactivity to emotional stimuli. We may thus be able to establish functional neuroanatomical correlates of affective instability and interpersonal sensitivity. The formulation of a neurodevelopmental model for the so-called cluster C personality disorders, avoidant, dependent, and obsessive-compulsive, will require greater knowledge of the neural systems involved in anxiety regulation.

Although we are beginning to learn about the genetics of impulsive-aggression, early findings have not always been replicable and the candidate gene strategies employed to date are limited by the availability of known genetic polymorphisms. Less is known about the genetics of affective instability and cognitive functioning. Family genetic studies with large sample sizes are needed to further this work. We need to study the effects of trauma, abuse, and neglect upon personality development and to extend this work to examine interactions between such life experiences and genetic endowment. Much of the research on early life experience and the development of personality disorders has been retrospective. Prospective studies of at-risk children which capture data on genetic endowment, prenatal and perinatal exposures, temperament, caregiver interactions, and life events will be needed to ultimately provide the necessary empirical grounding for neurodevelopmental models.

SUMMARY

Studies of two prototypical personality disorders, schizotypal and borderline, have increased our understanding both of the neurobiological underpinnings of these disorders and the reciprocal influence of neurobiology and environment on each other during the course of development. With this base, we can begin to consider heuristic models for the neurodevelopment of personality disorder. Biases in neuroregulatory systems may result from either a genetic susceptibility or the impact of physical or experiential (i.e., interpersonal) stressors during development. These biased systems, in turn, affect the nature of early social interactions that feed forward to form schemata for future interactions and to induce environmental consequences that may produce further neurobiological change.

An inherited vulnerability to impaired cognitive processing, perhaps augmented by exposure to physical insults to neuronal viability, sets the stage for the development of schizotypal personality disorder. There may be impaired information processing as well as diffuse neurodevelopmental anomalies that negatively influence the rhythms of early infant-caregiver interactions. Social interaction may thus become anxiety-laden for the individual, leading to the development of interpersonal coping strategies involving the distancing of self from others. This, in turn, may deprive the individual of the usual opportunities to correct initially idiosyncratic belief systems. In the presence of frontal and subcortical systems that buffer from outright psychosis, the individual is protected from schizophrenia, but may go on to develop schizotypal personality disorder.

In individuals with borderline personality disorder, the traits of impulsive aggression and affective instability co-occur. These traits may arise from either inheritance or such life experiences as early abuse or neglect, which can alter neuroregulatory systems. The traits of affective instability and impulsive aggression influence the interaction between infant and caregiver, which in turn may lead the developing individual to lay down representations of self and others that become maladaptive later in life. In addition, the child's temperament may elicit negative responses from caregivers that can generate high levels of stress, which can further alter developing neurobiological systems.

While such models must be regarded as highly tentative, they provide illustrations of how personality disorders may arise developmentally from a genetically predisposed neurobiology or environmentally induced alterations to developing brain systems, either of which in turn can influence key interpersonal interaction patterns, leading to the establishment of maladaptive social schemata or to further environmental experiences that may further affect neurobiological development.

REFERENCES

Amin, F., Siever, L.J., Silverman, J.M., et al. (1997). Plasma HVA in schizotypal personality disorder. In A.J. Friedhoff & F. Amin (Eds.), *Plasma homovanillic acid studies in schizophrenia, implications of presynaptic dopamine dysfunction* (pp. 133–149). Washington, D.C.: American Psychiatric Press Progress in Psychiatry Series.

Asberg, M., Traskman, L., & Thoren, P. (1976). 5-HIAA in the cerebrospinal fluid: A biochemical suicide predictor? *Archives of General Psychiatry, 33,* 1193–1197.

Avissar, S., & Schreiber, G. (1992). The involvement of guanine nucleotide binding proteins in the pathogenesis and treatment of affective disorders. *Biological Psychiatry, 31,* 435–459.

Bergman, A.J., Harvey, P.D., Lees-Roitman, S., Mohs, R.C., Marder, D., Silverman, J.M., & Siever, L.J. (1998). Verbal learning and memory in schizotypal personality disorder. *Schizophrenia Bulletin,* 24(4), 635–641.

Brazelton, T.B. (1978). The Brazelton Neonatal Behavior Assessment Scale: introduction. *Monogr Soc Res Child Dev,* 43 (5–6), 1–13.

Breier, A., Su, T.P., Saunders, R., et al. (1997). Schizophrenia is associated with elevated amphetamine induced synaptic dopamine concentrations: evidence from a novel positron emission tomography method. *Proc. Natl. Acad. Sci. USA, 94,* 2569–2574.

Brezun, J.M., & Daszulta, A. (1999). Depletion in serotonin decreases neurogenesis in the dentate gyrus and the subventricular zone of adult rats. *Neuroscience, 89,* 999–1002.

Buchsbaum, M.S., Trestman, R.L., Hazlett, E., Siegel, Jr., B.V., Schaefer, C.H., Luu-Hsia, C., Tang, C., Herrera, S., Solimando, A.C., Losonczy, M., Serby, M., Silverman, J., & Siever, L.J. (1997). Regional cerebral blood flow during the Wisconsin Card Sort Test in schizotypal personality disorder. *Schizophrenia Research, 27,* 21–28.

Buchsbaum, M.S., Yang, S., Hazlett, E., et al. (1997). Ventricular volume and asymmetry in schizotypal personality disorder and schizophrenia assessed with magnetic resonance imaging. *Schizophrenia Research, 27,* 45–53.

Burmeister, M. (1999). Basic concepts in the study of diseases with complex genetics. *Biological Psychiatry, 45,* 522–532.

Coccaro, E.F. (1998). Neurotransmitter function in personality disorders. In K.R. Silk (ed.), *Biology of Personality Disorders.* Washington, D.C.: American Psychiatric Press.

Coccaro, E.F., Bergeman, C.S., & McClearn, G.E. (1993). Heritability of irritable impulsiveness: A study of twins reared together and apart. *Psychiatry Research, 48,* 229–242.

Coccaro, E.F., Gabriel, S., & Siever, L.J. (1990). Buspirone challenge: Preliminary evidence for a role for 5HT1a receptors in impulsive aggressive behavior in humans. *Psychopharmacology Bulletin,* 26, 393–405.

Coccaro, E.F., Kavoussi, R.J., Hauger, R.L., Cooper, T.B., & Ferris, C.F. (1998). Cerebrospinal fluid vasopressin levels: correlates with aggression and serotonin function in personality-disordered subjects. *Arch Gen Psychiatry, 55,* 708–714.

Coccaro, E.F., Lawrence, T., Trestman, R., Gabriel, S., Klar, H.M., & Siever, L.J. (1991). Growth hormone responses to intravenous clonidine challenge correlates with behavioral irritability in psychiatric patients and healthy controls. *Psychiatry Research, 39,* 129–139.

Coccaro, E.F., Siever, L.J., Klar, H.M., et al. (1989). Serotonergic studies in affective and personality disorders: correlates with suicidal and impulsive aggressive behavior. *Archives of General Psychiatry, 46,* 587–599.

Davis, K.L., Kahn, R.S., Ko, G., & Davidson, M. (1991). Dopamine and schizophrenia: a reconceptualization. *American Journal of Psychiatry, 148,* 1474–1486.

Dickey, C.C., McCarley, R.W., Voglmaier, M.M., Niznikiewicz, M.A., Seidman, L.J., Hirayasu, Y.I., The, E.K., Van Rhoads, R., Jakab, M., Kikinis, R., Jolesz, F.A., & Shenton, M.E. (1999). Schizotypal personality disorder and the MRI abnormalities of temporal lobe gray matter. *Biological Psychiatry,* 45(11), 1393–1402.

Downhill, J.E., Buchsbaum, M.S., Hazlett, E.A., et al. (1997). Temporal lobe volume in schizotypal personality disorder and schizophrenia. *American Psychiatric Association Annual Meeting*, May 17–22, Abstract NR 172, Miami, Fla.

Duman, R.S., Heninger, G.R., & Nestler, E.J. (1997). A molecular and cellular theory of depression. *Arch Gen Psychiatry* 54, 597–606.

Figueroa, E., & Silk, K.R. (1997). Biological implications of childhood sexual abuse in borderline personality disorder. *Journal of Personality Disorders*, 11[1], 71–92.

Fish, B. (1987). Infant predictors of the longitudinal course of schizophrenic development. *Schizophrenia Bulletin*, 13, 395–409.

Ghaemi, S.N., Boiman, E.E., & Goodwin, F.K. (1999). Kindling and second messengers: An approach to the neurobiology of recurrence in bipolar disorder. *Biological Psychiatry*, 45, 137–144.

Gould, E. (1999). Serotonin and hippocampal neurogenesis. *Neuropsychopharmacology*, 21(2 suppl), 46S–51S.

Greenspan, S.I. (1989). *The development of the ego: Implications for personality theory, psychopathology, and the psychotherapeutic process.* Madison, Conn.: International Universities Press.

Gudzer, J., Paris, J., Zelkowitz, P., & Marchessault K. (1991). Risk factors for borderline pathology in children. *J. American Academy of Child and Adolescent Psychiatry*, 35(1), 26–33.

Gurvits, I.G., Koenigsberg, H.W., & Siever, L.J. (2000). Neurotransmitter dysfunction in borderline personality disorder. *The Psychiatric Clinics of North America*, 23, 27–40.

Herman, J.L., Perry, J.C., & van der Kolk, B.A. (1989). Childhood trauma in borderline personality disorder. *American Journal of Psychiatry*, 146, 490–495.

Janowsky, D.S., & Overstreet, D. (1995). The role of acetylcholine mechanisms in mood disorders. In F.E. Bloom & D.D. Kupfer (Eds.), *Psychopharmacology: The fourth generation of progress* (pp. 945–956). New York: Raven Press.

Jason, J., William, S.L., Burton, A., & Rochat, R. (1982). Epidemiological differences between sexual and physical abuse. *JAMA*, 247, 3344–3348.

Joseph, R. (ed.). (1996). *Neuropsychiatry, neuropsychology and clinical neuroscience, 2d Ed.* Philadelphia: Williams & Wilkins.

Kendler, K.S., Gruenberg, A.M., & Strauss, J.S. (1981). An independent analysis of the Copenhagen sample of the Danish adoption study of schizophrenia, II: the relationship between schizotypal personality disorder and schizophrenia. *Archive of General Psychiatry*, 38, 982–984.

Kendler, K.S., Ochs, A.L. Gorman, A.M., Hewitt, J.K., Ross, D.E., & Mirsky, A. (1991). The structure of schizotypy: a multitrait twin study. *Psychiatry Research*, 36, 19–36.

Kety, S.S., Rosenthal, D., & Wender, P.H. (1975). Mental illness in the biological and adoptive families of adopted individuals who have become schizophrenic: a preliminary report based on psychiatric interviews. In R. Fieve, D. Rosenthal, & H. Brill (Eds.), *Genetic research in psychiatry* (pp. 47–165). Baltimore: John Hopkins University Press.

Kety, S.S., Wender, P.H., Jacobsen, B., Ingraham, L.J., Jansson, L., Faber, B., & Kinney, D.K. (1994). Mental illness in the biological and adoptive relatives of schizophrenic adoptees. Replication of the Copenhagen Study in the rest of Denmark. *Archives of General Psychiatry*, 51(6), 442–455.

Kirrane, R., Mitropoulou, V., Nunn, M., New, A., Harvey, P., Schopick, F., Silverman, J., & Siever, L. (2000). Effects of amphetamine on visuospatial working memory performance in schizophrenia spectrum personality disorder. *Neuropsychopharmacology*, 22(1), 14–18.

Koenigsberg, H.W., Mitropoulou, V., Abi-Dargham, N., Nunn, M., Laruelle, M., & Siever, L.J. (1999). Subcortical dopaminergic activity in schizotypal personality disorder. *Annual Metting of the American Psychiatric Association*, NR212.

Laruelle, M., Abi-Dargham, A., van Dyck, C.H., Gil, R., D'Souza, C.D., Erdos, J., & McCance, E., et al. (1996). Single photon emission computerized tomography imaging of amphetamine-induced dopamine release in drug-free schizophrenic subjects. *Proc Natl Acad Sci USA*, 93(17), 9235–9240.

Ledoux, J. (1996). *The emotional brain.* New York: Simon & Schuster.

Lees-Roitman, S.E., Cornblatt, B.A., Bergman, A., Obuchowski, M., Mitropoulou, V., Keefe, R.S.E., Silverman, J.M., & Siever, L.J. (1997). Attentional functioning in Schizotypal Personality Disorder. *American Journal of Psychiatry*, 154, 655–660.

Lees-Roitman, S.E., Mitropoulou, V., Keefe, R.S.E., Silverman, J.M., Serby, M., Harvey, P.D., Reynolds, D.A., Mohs, R.C., & Siever, L.J. (2000). Visuospatial working memory in schizotypal personality disorder patients. *Schizophrenia Research*, 41, 447–455.

Lindberg, L., Asberg, M., Sunquist-Stensman, M., et al. (1984). 5-hydroxyindoleacetic acid levels in attempted suicides who have killed their children [letter]. *Lancet, 2*, 928.

Linnoila, M., Virkkunen, M., Scheinin, M., et al. (1983). Low cerebrospinal fluid 5-hydroxy-indoleacetic acid concentration differentiates impulsive from nonimpulsive violent behavior. *Life Science, 33*, 2609–2614.

Mann, J.J., Malone, K.M., Nielsen, D.A., Goldman D., Erdos, J., & Gelernter, J. (1997). Possible association of a polymorphism of the tryptophan hydroxylase gene with suicidal behavior in depressed patients. *American Journal of Psychiatry, 154*, 1451–1453.

McCarley, R.W., Wible, C.G., Frumin, M., Hirayasu, Y., Levitt, J.J., Fischer, I.A., & Shenton, M.E. (1999). MRI anatomy of schizophrenia. *Biological Psychiatry, 45*(9), 1099–1119.

Mendelson, S.D., & McEwen, B.S. (1992). Autoradiographic analyses of the effects of adrenalec-tomy and corticosterone on $5-HT_{1A}$ and $5HT_{1B}$ receptors in the dorsal hippocampus and cortex of the rat. *Neuroendocrinology, 55*, 444–450.

Moeller, F.G., Allen, T., Cherek, D.R., Dougherty, D.M., Lane, S., & Swann, A.C. (1998). Ipsapirone neuroendocrine challenge: relationship to aggression as measured in the human laboratory. *Psych. Res., 81*, 31–38.

Murray, R.M., O'Callaghan, E., Castle, D., & Lewis, S. (1992). A neurodevelopmental approach to the classification of schizophrenia. *Schizophrenia Bulletin, 18*, 319–333.

New, A.S., Gelernter, J., Mitropoulou, V., Koenigsberg, H.W., Siever, L.J. (1999b). Impulsive aggres-sion associated with HTR1B genotype in personality disorder. *Annual Meeting of the American Psychiatric Association*, NR388.

New, A.S., Gelernter, J., Mitropoulou, V., & Siever, L.J. (1999a). Serotonin related genotype and impulsive aggression. *Annual Meeting of the Society of Biological Psychiatry, 45*, Abstract #387.

New, A.S., Gelernter, J., Yovell, Y., Trestman, R.L., Nielsen, D.A., Silverman, J., Mitropoulou, V., & Siever, L.J. (1998). Tryptophan hydroxylase gene is associated with impulsive aggression: a preliminary study. *Am J Med Genet, 81*, 13–17.

Paris, J. (1998). Does childhood trauma cause personality disorders in adults? *Can J Psychiatry, 43*, 148–153.

Paris, J., Zweig-Frank, H., & Guzder, J. (1994). Risk factors for borderline personality in male outpatients. *Journal of Nervous and Mental Disease, 182*[7], 375–380.

Perry, J.C., & Herman, J.L. (1993). Trauma and defense in the etiology of borderline personality disorder. In J. Paris (Ed.), *Borderline Personality Disorder: etiology and treatment*. Washington, D.C.: American Psychiatric Press.

Plomin, R., & DeFries, J.C. (1981). Multivariate behavioral genetics and development: twin studies. *Prog Clin Biol Res, 69* Pt B, 25–33.

Putnam, F.W., Guroff, J.J., Silberman, E.K., Barban, L., & Post, R.M. (1986). The clinical phe-nomenology of multiple personality disorder: review of 100 recent cases. *Journal of Clinical Psychiatry, 47*(6), 285–293.

Rinne, T., Westenberg, H.G.M., den Boer, J.A., & van den Brink, W. (2000). Serotonergic blunting to meta-chlorophenylpiperazine (m-CPP) highly correlates with sustained childhood abuse in impulsive and autoaggressive female borderline patients. *Biol Psychiatry, 47*, 548–556.

Schore, A.N. (1994). *Affect regulation and the origin of the self: the neurobiology of emotional develop-ment*. Hillsdale, N.J.: Erlbaum.

Siegel, B.V., Trestman, R.L., O'Flaithbheartaigh, S., Mitropoulou, V., Amin, F., Kirrane, R., Silverman, J., Schmeidler, J., Keefe, R.S.E., & Siever, L.J. (1996). D-amphetamine challenge ef-fects on Wisconsin Card Sort Test performance in schizotypal personality disorder. *Schizophrenia Research, 20*, 29–32.

Siever, L.J., Buchsbaum, M.S., New, A.S., Speigel-Cohen, J., Wei, T., Hazlett, E.A., Sevin, M., Nunn, M., & Mitropoulou, V. (1999). d,l-fenfluramine response in impulsive personality dis-order assessed with [18F] flourodeoxyglucose positron emission tomography. *Neuropsychophar-macology, 20*, 413–423.

Siever, L.J., & Davis, K.L. (1991). A psychobiological perspective on the personality disorders. *American Journal of Psychiatry, 148*, 1647–1658.

Siever, L.J., Kalus, O.F., & Keefe, R.S. (1993). The boundaries of schizophrenia. *Psychiatry Clinics of North America, 16*, 217–244.

Siever, L.J., Rotter, M., Losonczy, M., et al. (1995). Lateral ventricular enlargement in schizotypal personality disorder. *Psychiatry Research*, 57, 109–118.

Siever, L.J., Rotter, M., Tresman, R.L., Coccaro, E.F., Losonczy, M., & Davis, K. (1993). Frontal lobe dysfunction and schizotypal personality disorder. *Proc. Amer. Psych. Assoc. Ann. Meeting*, NR502, 186.

Siever, L.J., & Tresman, R.L. (1993). The serotonin system and aggressive personality disorder. *International Clin. Psychopharmacology*, 8(suppl 2), 33–39.

Siever, L.J., Tresman, R.L., Siegel, B.V., Losonczy, M., Mitropoulou, V., Silverman, J., Keefe, R.S., Mohs, R., Buchsbaum, M.S., & Davis, K.L. (1995). Neuroimaging, neurobiological and neuropsychological abnormalities in SPD: implications for a model of the schizophrenia spectrum. *Schizophrenia Research*, 15 (1,2), 99.

Silverman, J.M., Pinkham, L., Horvath, T.B., Coccaro, E.F., Klar, H., Schear, S., Apter, S., Davidson, M., Mohs, R., & Siever, L.J. (1991). Affective and impulsive personality disorder traits in the relatives of patients with borderline personality disorder. *American Journal of Psychiatry*, 148[10], 1378–1385.

Steinberg, B.J., Tresman, R., Mitropoulou, V., et al. (1997). Depressive response to physostigmine challenge in borderline personality disorder patients. *Neuropsychopharmacology*, 17, 264–273.

Steinberg, B.J., Tresman, R., & Siever, L.J. (1994). The cholinergic and noradrenergic neurotransmitter systems and affective instability in borderline personality disorder. In K.R. Silk (Ed.), *Biological and neurobehavioral studies of Borderline Personality Disorder*. Washington, D.C.: American Psychiatric Press.

Teicher, M.H., Ito, Y., Glod, C.A., Schiffer, F., & Gelbard, H.A. (1994). Early abuse, limbic system dysfuncton, and borderline personality disorder. In K.R. Silk (Ed.), *Biological and neurobehavioral studies of Borderline Personality Disorder*. Washington, D.C.: American Psychiatric Press.

Torgersen, S. (1984). Genetics and nosologic aspects of schizotypal and borderline personality disorders: a twin study. *Archives of General Psychlatry*, 41, 546–554.

Torgersen, S. (1994). Genetics in borderline conditions, *Acta Psychiatr Scand*, suppl 379, 19–25.

Torgersen, S., & Alnaes, R. (1992). Differential perception of parental bonding in schizotypal and borderline personality disorder patients. *Comprehensive Psychiatry*, 33[1], 34–48.

Trestman, R.L., Keefe, R.S.E., Mitropoulou, V., Harvey, P.D., deVegvar, M.L., Lee-Roitman, S., Davidson, M., Aronson, A., Silverman, J., & Siever, L.J. (1995) Cognitive function and biological correlates of cognitive performance in schizotypal personality disorder. *Psychiatry Research*, 59, 127–136.

Tsuang, M.T., Bucher, K.D., & Fleming, J.A. (1983). A search for 'schizophrenia sectrum disorders.' An application of a muliple thershold model to blind family study data. *Br J Psychiatry*, 143, 572–577.

Virkkunen, M., Nuutila, A., Goodwin, F.K., & Linnoila, M. (1987). Cerebrospinal fluid monoamine metabolite levels in male arsonists. *Arch Gen Psychiatry*, 44, 241–247.

Weinberger, D.R. (1987). Implications of normal brain development for the pathogenesis of schizophrenia. *Archives of General Psychiatry*, 44, 660–669.

Weinberger, D.R., Berman, K.F., & Zec, R.F. (1986). Physiologic dysfunction of dorsolateral prefrontal cortex in schizophrenia. I. Regional cerebral blood flow evidence. *Archives of General Psychiatry*, 43, 114–124.

Yehuda, R. (1998). Neuroendocrinology of trauma and post-traumatic stress disorder. In R. Yehuda (Ed.), *Psychological trauma*. Washington, D.C.: American Psychiatric Press.

Zanarini, M.C., & Frankenburg, F.R. (1997). Pathways to the development of borderline personality disorder. *Journal of Personality Disorders*, 11[1], 93–104.

Zanarini, M.C., Frankenburg, F.R., & Dubo, E.D. (1998). Axis I comorbidity of borderline personality disorder. *American Journal of Psychiatry*, 155, 1733–1739.

Zanarini, M.C., Gunderson, J.G., & Marino, M.F. (1989). Childhood experiences of borderline patients. *Comprehensive Psychiatry*, 30[1], 18–25.

Zhang, L.X., Xing, G.Q., Levine, S., Post, R.M., & Smith, R.A. (1997). Maternal deprivation induces neuronal death. *Soc Neurosci Abstr*, 23, 1113.

EIGHTEEN

Genesis and Epigenesis of Psychopathology in Children with Depressed Mothers

Toward an Integrative Biopsychosocial Perspective

Sherryl H. Goodman

Even if scientists uncover a single, powerful determinant of behavior, whether it be a gene linked to a disorder, a toxic biological event that goes awry during fetal development, or an aspect of parental caregiving that interferes with the development of healthy relationships, it is now clear that not all individuals who share such risks will emerge with the same degree of mental health or disorder nor stay on the same, predicted developmental trajectory. In particular, little attention has been paid to the role of neurodevelopmental processes in enhancing or decreasing the opportunity for healthy development in individuals with environmental or genetic risks and vice versa. If we accept that neither environmental qualities nor genes or other biological mechanisms directly determine behavior or developmental course, then we are challenged to consider the potential explanatory power of the complexities of their possible interplay.

It is the purpose of this chapter to accept the challenge of such an integrative perspective for the understanding of risk for the development of psychopathology or other adverse outcomes in children with depressed mothers. Specifically, this chapter will examine current knowledge on outcomes and mechanisms of risk to children with depressed mothers from this perspective and propose future directions for such integrative research. An effort will be made to explore the influences on outcomes not only as a static event but also on alternative developmental pathways.

It needs to be stated at the outset that ideas about complex determinants of behavior are not new. Sameroff proposed systems theories of development in the 1970s and continues to evolve those ideas (Sameroff, 1975, 1995). Indeed, the field of developmental psychopathology emerged from the recognition of the benefits of considering multiple causal mechanisms, complex adaptational processes, and multidisciplinary perspectives (Cicchetti, 1989; Sroufe & Rutter, 1984). Moreover, proponents of ecological models remind us of the importance of considering not only parent and child characteristics and their interactions, but also the broader social context (Bronfenbrenner, 1992; Cicchetti & Lynch, 1993; Cicchetti & Toth, 1998). The challenge is to apply those models to a particular population at risk in such a way as to clarify existing findings and guide future research.

This chapter was written with financial support from an Emory University Research Committee Grant and National Institute of Mental Health, 1P50MH58922-01A1.

This chapter begins by briefly describing the reasons for concern about children with depressed mothers and the nature and extent of adverse outcomes in children and adolescents associated with depression in their mothers. The focus is on children whose mother, rather than father, has been depressed. They represent the majority of research that has been conducted. Although the depression in the mother may be considered the single risk factor for adverse outcomes in the children, in fact researchers have posited several potential etiological processes. These will be reviewed in turn, followed by a discussion of the alternative pathways to disorder and the particular adverse outcomes that are suggested by each. Next, a developmental psychopathology perspective is taken with an integrative model for understanding risk (Goodman & Gotlib, 1999). The model will be examined for its potential to provide insights for understanding causal mechanisms (etiological processes) and diverse pathways that might be pursued by children with depressed mothers.

Risk for depression and the other adverse outcomes unfolds over time and may emerge as disorder at different points across the lifespan. The integrative approach serves to direct attention to the interrelationships among the bio-psycho-social systems and how they may help to explain the associations between early developmental aberrations and later emerging signs of disorder. Since few of the studies of children with depressed mothers are longitudinal, these aspects of the model are speculative. Finally, implications for prevention and treatment are derived from the model and suggestions are made for further research.

NATURE AND EXTENT OF RISKS: ADVERSE OUTCOMES IN CHILDREN ASSOCIATED WITH MATERNAL DEPRESSION

Why Concerns About Children with Depressed Mothers?

Depression is the most common of psychiatric disorders. During the course of a lifetime, it is estimated that between 8 and 20 percent of the population will experience at least one clinically significant episode of depression (Kessler et al., 1994). Of those, approximately twice as many will be women rather than men (Frank, Carpenter, & Kupfer, 1988). A large-scale epidemiological survey of psychiatric disorders in adults found that 24 percent of women and 15 percent of men had experienced a diagnosable mood disorder in their lifetimes (Kessler et al., 1994). Depression rates are especially high among women of child-bearing ages (Blazer, Kessler, McGonagle, & Swartz, 1994; Weissman, 1984). Moreover, for many of these, the episode will not be their first or their last. Depression is a recurrent disorder. Over 80 percent of depressed patients have more than one depressive episode (Belsher & Costello, 1988). Over 50 percent relapse within two years of recovery (Keller & Shapiro, 1981). Thus, children are especially likely to be exposed to their mother's depression and, if so, to experience repeated exposures.

Researchers define clinically significant depression as either the set of symptoms, duration, and impairment by which an individual meets criteria for a Mood Disorder in the *Diagnostic and Statistical Manual of Mental Disorders* (*DSM-IV*; American Psychiatric Association, 1994) or individuals who score high on a self-report symptom rating scale of depression. The *DSM-IV* divides Mood Disorders into Depressive Disorders (sometimes referred to as Unipolar Depression) and Bipolar Disorders. Bipolar Disorder, which requires the presence of one or more Manic or Hypomanic Episodes, has less often been the focus of studies of maternal depression and will not be discussed in this chapter.

The *DSM-IV* further divides Depressive Disorders into Major Depression and Dysthymia. A diagnosis of Major Depression requires the occurrence of one or more episodes during which the individual exhibits, over a period of two weeks or more, depressed mood (in children or adolescents, this might be irritable mood) or a loss of interest or pleasure in almost all daily activities, along with a number of other symptoms of depression, including weight loss or gain, loss of appetite, sleep disturbance, psychomotor agitation or retardation, fatigue, feelings of guilt or worthlessness, and concentration difficulties. A diagnosis of Dysthymia requires a more chronic but less intense mood disturbance, with the individual having exhibited some symptoms of depression for most of a two-year period (one year in children and adolescents).

Other researchers forego the diagnostic system and study children whose mothers score above established cut-offs on self-report measures of depression symptoms. The most commonly used such measures are the Beck Depression Inventory (BDI; Beck, Steer, & Garbin, 1988; Beck, Ward, Mendelson, Mock & Erbaugh, 1961), or the revised BDI-II (Beck, Steer, & Brown, 1997), and the Centers for Epidemiological Studies–Depression Scale (CES-D; Radloff, 1977). High scores on these scales may not be specific to depression or may reveal more transient depression than would meet diagnostic criteria.

Thus, depression is common, especially among women of child-bearing and child-rearing ages, severe and impairing, and recurrent or persistent. It is not surprising that its presence in mothers has fueled concern for its potential to disrupt aspects of caretaking known to be critical for healthy child development. Knowledge of the heritability of depression adds further concern for the children of depressed parents. More recently, emerging knowledge of the neuroendocrinological correlates of depression during pregnancy has raised concern about possible adverse influences even on fetal development.

Adverse Child Outcomes Associated with Maternal Depression

Understanding that any risk factor will be differently associated with adverse outcomes depending on the developmental stage of the child at the time the risk factor occurs, this brief review will organize the findings by the broad age groupings of child development. That is, risk factors will have specific consequences depending on the time of exposure in relation to the particular developmental tasks of children, including the domains of cognitive, affective, social, and neurobiological development. Later, we will explain how this idea is not adequate to capture the complexity of either etiological or epigenetic models.

Because of concerns that development is rapidly occurring during infancy and early childhood when youngsters are most dependent on their parents, infants and toddlers of depressed mothers have most frequently been the subject of study (see reviews by Field, 1992; Gotlib & Goodman, 1999; Graham, Heim, Goodman, Miller, & Nemeroff, 1999). Infants of women with elevated symptom levels of depression, compared to those whose mothers score low, have been rated by observers as more drowsy or fussy, less relaxed or content, engaging in less toy exploration, less focused play (Abrams, Field, Scafidi, & Prodromidis, 1995). Their mothers rated them as crying more and more difficult to soothe (Zuckerman, Bauchner, Parker, & Cabral, 1990). Also, they have been found to have elevated levels of stress hormones (norepinephrine and cortisol), decreased vagal tone, and less left frontal EEG activation (greater relative right frontal EEG asymmetry) (Dawson, Hessl, & Frey, 1994; Field, Pickens, Fox, Nawrocki, & Gonzalez, 1995; Lundy et al., 1999). Similarly, observers rate infants of clinically diagnosed depressed mothers, compared to those with nondepressed mothers, as more tense, less happy, and as showing less tolerance for lab procedures, less distress during maternal separation, and having higher rates of insecure attachment (Campbell & Cohn, 1997; Cohn & Campbell, 1992; Teti, Gelfand, Messinger, & Isabella, 1995). Both groups have been found to score lower on the Bayley Scales of Infant Development or, for toddlers or preschool-aged children, on the McCarthy Scales of Children's Abilities (Field, Bendell-Estroff, Yando, et al., 1996; Hart et al., 1998; Hay, 1997; Murray, 1992; Whiffen & Gotlib, 1989). Between the ages of two and five, the children of clinically depressed mothers have been found to have more behavior problems than children of nondepressed mothers, including more dysregulated aggression (Radke-Yarrow, Nottelman, Martinez, & Fox, 1992). They also tend to suppress their emotions as a way of coping with stressful situations and show a pattern of more often disrupting their own activity when others were distressed, yet being less likely to express affect (Radke-Yarrow, Zahn-Waxler, Richardson, & Susman, 1994). They are more likely to attempt to appease a frustrated adult, but less likely to become physically aggressive across a variety of situations (Radke-Yarrow, 1998).

School-aged children with depressed mothers have been compared with controls on standardized measures of psychological functioning. As reviewed by Gotlib and Goodman (1999), researchers have reported higher rates of depression and other diagnosed psychiatric disorders, more internalizing and externalizing behavior problems, and more cognitive impairment in children with depressed mothers compared with well controls. They have also been found to have poorer peer relations and less adequate peer relations skills. On cognitive variables, children with depressed mothers have lower self-concepts, more negative cognitive style, are more self-critical and more likely to blame themselves for negative outcomes, and less likely to recall positive self-descriptive adjectives.

In sum, researchers have consistently found problems in development and the emergence of behavioral and emotional problems in children associated with maternal depression. These findings are supportive of hypotheses that the prevalence, impairment, chronicity or recurrence, heritability, and correlated stressors of depression are causal factors in these adverse outcomes. However, they fall short of explaining either mechanisms of causation or alternative pathways through development for children so exposed. The next section will discuss the etiological mechanisms that have been proposed.

ALTERNATIVE ETIOLOGICAL MECHANISMS AND THEIR IMPLICATIONS FOR EPIGENESIS

Genetic Influences

Genes might influence fetal development, be apparent, initially, in markers such as behavioral tendencies, negative affectivity, or stress reactivity, and, later, in precursors or early signs and ultimately in the full set of symptoms and duration required for a diagnosis of a depression disorder. Each of these possibilities will be discussed.

Heritability of Depression. Genetic influences have been posited to play an etiological role in the emergence of depression in children with depressed mothers, primarily in terms of the heritability of the depression disorder per se. Researchers have accumulated strong empirical support for the genetic transmission of depressive disorders in adults. The risk for an affective disorder in adult first-degree relatives of a patient with unipolar affective disorder is estimated at 20–25 percent compared with a general population risk of 7 percent (Nurnberger, Goldin, & Gershon, 1986; Tsuang & Faraone, 1990). Although not yet demonstrated, genetic influences are likely to be greater in children whose mothers have clinically significant levels of depression, in contrast to subclinical forms of depression. Recent twin studies revealed that additive genetic effects accounted for nearly 80 percent of the variance in narrowly defined major depression, whereas environmental factors were the predominant influence of milder forms of depression (Kendler et al., 1995; McGuffin & Katz, 1993; Plomin, 1990). Genetic influences are also likely to be greater in children whose mothers experienced postpartum depression compared to those whose mothers' first episode was later (O'Hara, 1986).

In contrast to the strong evidence for heritability of adult depression, heritability has not unequivocally been demonstrated for depressive disorders that first emerge in childhood or adolescence. Findings from studies of family history, or family aggregation, are consistent with a role for heritability. For example, risk of depression in children increases in a linear fashion with the number of affected relatives (Merikangas, Prusoff, & Weissman, 1988; Todd et al., 1993) and with the early onset of the mother's depression (i.e., before age 20; Weissman et al., 1987). Conversely, among children who become depressed, those with a depressed mother have an earlier onset (mean age of onset = 12.7) compared to those with nondepressed mothers (mean age of onset = 16.8 years; Weissman et al., 1987). Rates of affective disorder are even higher among adult relatives of depressed children than they are for depressed adolescents (Williamson et al., 1995) or depressed adults (Kovacs, Devlin, Pollock, Richards, & Mukerji, 1997), suggesting a greater role of heritability in depression that emerges in childhood than later. Among children of depressed parents, compared to children with parents with no depression, siblings have higher rates of aggregation for childhood onset anxiety disorders and for later emerging comorbid major depression and suicide attempts, suggesting that early emerging anxiety disorders may be the first indication of transmission of risk for depression from parent to child (Rende, Warner, Wickramarante, & Weissman, 1999).

Recent twin studies, although limited in that they studied genetic contribution to risk for depressive symptoms rather than for diagnosed depression, revealed that genetic influence is high, but only in particular circumstances. Genetic influence was found to vary considerably with three child characteristics. Heritability was more strongly associated with depressive symptoms than either shared or nonshared environmental influences among the subgroup of children with *fewer than* clinically significant levels of depression symptoms (Rende, Plomin, Reiss, & Hetherington, 1993), in older (7- to 12-year-old or 11- to 16-year old) rather than younger twins (4- to 6-year-old or 8- to 10-year old) (Harrington, Rutter, & Fombonne, 1996; Murray & Sines, 1996), and for girls rather than boys (Murray & Sines, 1996). Although these studies require replication using reliable diagnostic procedures, they are promising in revealing the specificity of the role of heritability in childhood- or adolescent-onset depression. Overall, it is important to remember that genes are probabilistic, not deterministic, in their influence.

Heritability of Other Disorders. Children with depressed mothers have also been diagnosed with disorders other than, or in addition to, depression, including externalizing behavior disorders. Heritability may play a role in the specificity of outcome. For example, depressed children or adolescents who had comorbid behavior disorders (e.g., attention deficit disorder, conduct disorder, and substance use-abuse disorders), compared to those with depression only, have been found to have first-degree relatives with higher rates of alcoholism, substance abuse, and antisocial personality disorders (Kovacs et al., 1997; Williamson et al., 1995). Thus, particular patterns of co-occurrence of disorders in the parents may influence whether the children inherit vulnerability to depression alone or with comorbid behavior disorders.

Heritability of Other Risks or Vulnerability to Depression. In addition to a direct role of heritability of depression per se, it is increasingly being recognized that genetics may contribute in less direct ways through heritability of traits or behavioral tendencies, which may predispose to depression, or of environmental risk factors, which increase the likelihood of depression. As reviewed by Loehlin (1992), several correlates of and possible vulnerability factors for depression are highly heritable, including the temperament dimension of sociability (Goldsmith, Buss, & Lemery, 1997; Plomin et al., 1993), behavioral inhibition and shyness (Cherny, Fulker, Corley, Plomin, & DeFries, 1994), low self-esteem (Loehlin & Nichols, 1976), neuroticism (Tellegen et al., 1988), subjective well-being (Lykken & Tellegen, 1996), and expression of negative emotion (Plomin et al., 1993). Although not yet tested, genetics may also account for variance in other psychological vulnerabilities such as social information processing deficit (Crick & Dodge, 1994). Among environmental variables that increase children's risk to depression, genetic mediation has been established for poor parenting quality, life stress, marital conflict, and divorce (Plomin, 1994). Thus, what is inherited may be a psychological or environmental vulnerability to depression rather than a biological risk for the disorder per se.

Implications of Heritability for Mechanisms of Epigenesis in Children with Depressed Mothers. Among a group of children born with high genetic risk for depression or other psychiatric disorders, or for psychological vulnerabilities to depressogenic traits or behavioral tendencies, multiple alternative developmental pathways are still possible. The concept of multifinality, referring to multiple pathways that may diverge from common origins, is essential for understanding the possible associations between genetic risk and outcomes (Cicchetti & Rogosch, 1996). Interactions and correlations among genes, cognitive, affective, interpersonal, and other biological systems help explain much of this variation and will be explored later in this chapter. Within genetic etiological mechanisms alone, nonetheless, it must be considered that genes may not only be expressed in infancy, may not be expressed uniformly throughout development, and may not be expressed at all until later in development. Mechanisms of gene activation and deactivation are just beginning to be understood and developmental variation of those mechanisms may explain alternative pathways. For example, as described by Cicchetti and Tucker (1994), genetic risk for depression could be expressed early in the development of anomalies in the brain structures that serve as receptors for neurotransmitters, predisposing the child to depression. Later gene activation and deactivation, as well as experience, may further modify those brain structures, ameliorating or exacerbating the risk. Thus multifinality, or multiple diverse pathways, can be expected even in association with heritability.

Innate Dysfunctional Neuroregulatory Mechanisms

Whether a manifestation of genetic risk or a function of *in utero* environmental hazards, some infants of depressed mothers may be born with dysfunctional neuroregulatory mechanisms. Infants with abnormal neuroendocrine functioning would be expected to show maladaptive stress reactivity, abnormal behavioral and affective functioning, and abnormal EEG patterns, each of which may represent trait markers for depression (Davidson & Fox, 1998; Gotlib, Ranganath, & Rosenfeld, 1998). There may be reasons to be particularly concerned about children who were exposed to high levels of cortisol prenatally in that such exposure could set off a cascade of neuroendocrine events, resulting in persistent changes that may mediate the development of major depression (Nemeroff, 1996).

Animal Models. In both rhesus monkeys and rats, stress during pregnancy (exposure to unpredictable and uncontrollable noise or light) has been associated with adverse outcomes. In Schneider and colleagues' studies of prenatally stressed rhesus monkeys, the infants had lower birth weight, poorer neuromotor maturation, delayed cognitive development, and showed less exploration of novel stimuli; as juveniles, they demonstrated abnormal social behavior and greater HPA activity at baseline and in response to stress, compared to monkeys who did not experience prenatal stress (Clarke & Schneider, 1993; Clarke, Wittwer, Abbott, & Schneider, 1994; Schneider, 1992). Offspring of prenatally stressed rats also have been found to have lower birth weight, vocalize less and explore less during isolation in a novel environment, and had suppressed immune function (Kay, Tarcic, Poltyrev, & Weinstock, 1998; Poltyrev, Keshet, Kay, & Weinstock, 1996; Williams, Hennessy, & Davis, 1998). The fetus's exposure to maternal stress hormones was hypothesized to be the causal agent in this set of abnormal outcomes.

Neonates Born to Mothers Depressed During Pregnancy. Behavioral observations of infants born to women depressed during pregnancy are consistent with the suggested innate dysfunctional neuroregulatory system. These infants show poorer performance on the Brazelton Neonatal Behavior Assessment Scale (see Field, 1992) and excessive crying and inconsolability (Zuckerman et al., 1990). Researchers have also found increased rates of premature births and lower birth weight associated with maternal depression (Copper et al., 1996).

Studies of the Fetal Environment. Researchers have examined how depression during pregnancy may contribute to adverse fetal environments, which, in turn, result in abnormal neuroregulatory mechanisms evident in the neonate. Three mechanisms have been considered as possible explanations of abnormal fetal development associated with depression during pregnancy. First, because the fetus's first transaction with the mother occurs at gestational days 13–14, when utero blood flow is established, the fetus might be affected by the neuroendocrine correlates of the mother's depression during most of fetal development. Studies of the neurobiology of pregnant, depressed women found higher urinary and plasma cortisol, norepinephrine, beta-endorphin, and corticotrophin releasing hormone (CRH) levels among women with elevated levels of depressed mood at 28 to 38 weeks of gestation (Field, 1998; Handley, Dunn, Waldron, & Baker, 1980; Smith et al., 1990). Most interest has focused on CRH, a major regulator of the stress response. In pregnant women, levels of the stress hormones gradually increase, the rate of increase determining the timing of labor and delivery. Increased CRH levels early in pregnancy predict early delivery (Wadhwa, Dunkel-Schetter, Chicz-DeMet, & Porto, 1996).

A critical question is whether these hormones cross the placenta to the fetus. Glover and colleagues (Gitau, Cameron, Fish, & Glover, 1998; Glover, Teixeira, Gitau, & Fisk, 1998) found that maternal levels of cortisol accounted for 50 percent of the variance in fetus's levels of cortisol at 20–36 weeks of pregnancy, supporting the notion that cortisol crosses the placenta. Correlations were not significant for the other hormones that researchers have found to be indicative of abnormal neuroendocrine functioning in depressed pregnant women.

A second possible explanation of abnormal fetal development associated with maternal depression is that the pregnancies are more medically complicated. For example, Glover et al. (1998; Teixeira, Fisk, & Glover, 1999) found reduced uterine blood flow associated with maternal trait anxiety in the third trimester of pregnancy in nonsmoking, healthy women, which, in turn, was directly associated with lower birth weight of the babies. Relatedly, Field (1992) found that fetuses of low-income, young, ethnic minority women with high self-reported symptom levels of depression during pregnancy had lower estimated weight and engaged in less movement compared to nondepressed, matched controls. Finally, Emory, Walker, and Cruz (1983) found that stress during pregnancy, itself a correlate of depression, was associated with higher heart rate, which, in uncomplicated pregnancies and deliveries, is associated with lower neonatal attention orientation and arousal.

The third possible explanation of abnormal fetal development associated with maternal depression is the less adequate prenatal care depressed women may obtain. Depressed pregnant women, compared to nondepressed women, report less healthy eating and sleeping patterns, and are more likely to smoke (Milberger, Beiderman, Faraone, Chen, & Jones, 1996). On the other hand, although there is some debate on the subject, antidepressant medications taken during pregnancy appear to not be associated with offsprings' neurocognitive development, especially once severity of depression is taken into account (Chambers, Johnson, Dick, Felix & Jones, 1996; Nulman et al., 1997; Pastuszak et al., 1993).

In sum, the fetuses of depressed women are exposed to higher levels of cortisol, experience less blood flow and more rapid heart rates, and, more generally, the consequences of less adequate prenatal care. As neonates, they tend to be smaller, are more likely to be born prematurely, and show poorer behavioral regulation. Thus, the atypical fetal environment of depressed women may increase infants' vulnerability.

Implications of Innate Dysfunctional Neuroregulatory Systems for Mechanisms of Epigenesis in Children of Depressed Mothers. The subset of children with depressed mothers who were born to women whose depression occurred during the pregnancy may be born with biological systems that predispose to depression. One possible developmental trajectory begins with the fetus being exposed to high levels of cortisol, reduced uterine blood flow, high heart rate, or inadequate nutrition. The trajectory continues with abnormal fetal development and then with the infant born with observable physical and psychological disadvantages, such as having low birth weight, being difficult to console, and having difficulty self-regulating.

Each of these steps in a hypothetical trajectory also can be considered risk factors for further adverse development in that they pose particular challenges for the developing child, including many that have implications for the emergence of depression. For example, fetal exposure to cortisol may result in persistent changes in corticotropin-releasing-factor (CRF)-containing neurons, the hypothalamic–pituitary–adrenal (HPA) axis, and the sympathetic nervous system, any of which may mediate the development of major depression (Nemeroff, 1996). In this and other ways, the offspring's biological system may be primed to react adversely to future adverse conditions. Others of the risks less directly predispose to depression, but impose additional challenges on the mother who, if depressed, may already find parenting a challenge. Examples of such parenting stressors are the infant being more difficult to console, less attentive, and less regulated. Later sections of this chapter will discuss possible modifiers of this proposed developmental course.

Depressed Mothers' Maladaptive Cognitions, Behaviors, and Affect

The most commonly posited single cause of adverse outcomes to children with depressed mothers is inadequate or detrimental parenting. Researchers have examined correlates of depression in mothers' cognitions, behaviors, and affect, typically derived from observations of mother-child interactions. Further, depressed mothers' inadequate parenting has been implicated in a broad set of interpersonal and social-cognitive consequences to the children. Note here that the assumption typically has been strictly that these psychosocial mechanisms have psychosocial consequences. Only recent and limited attention has been given to possible neuroendocrinological consequences of these psychosocial mechanisms, and these will be explored in a later section.

Goodman and Gotlib (1999) summarized the strong empirical evidence that depression in mothers is associated with their more negative cognitions (e.g., more negative parental efficacy beliefs), behaviors (e.g., less effective discipline), and affect (e.g., less positive and more sad, but also more irritable and angry affect). Children may be adversely affected by these maladaptive patterns as a function of social learning processes and through the parent being an inadequate social partner for the child's developmentally salient needs. Findings from several researchers demonstrate children's matching of their depressed mothers' sad and angry affect, low activity levels, inadequate relationship skills, and negative cognitions (e.g., low self-concept and negative cognitive style) (see Goodman & Gotlib, 1999). These findings support Bandura's (1986) social cognitive theory of how children of depressed mothers might be influenced, whether through modeling, direct instruction (e.g., reinforcement of the child's own negative views of the world), or performance outcomes (e.g., the child's experience of having been frequently criticized). However, these findings are not inconsistent with other explanations, including heritability of these affective, behavioral, or cognitive tendencies, as was discussed earlier; consequences of inadequate parenting of children's developmentally salient needs, as will be discussed next; or biobehavioral mechanisms that were set into play by adverse early parenting, as will be explored later in this section.

Depressed Mothers May Fail to Meet Children's Stage-Salient Needs. Given that children's parenting needs change over the course of development, etiological models of the depressed mother being an inadequate social partner for the child need to be specific to the developmental stage of the child at the time the mother is depressed. If, for example, depression were found to impair the aspects of parenting that are more critical for healthy development of infants than for adolescents, we would be able to limit our concern to children whose mothers are or were depressed during those developmental stages. In particular, concern is highest for the aspects of development that are both likely to be affected by inadequate parenting and are among those that have been hypothesized as risk factors for depression in children. For example, depressed mothers are more likely than well mothers to fail to provide the warm, contingently responsive environment necessary for the infant's development of healthy attachment and, subsequently, insecure attachment may be a risk factor for depression. However, as summarized in Table 18.1, researchers have shown that depression in mothers adversely affects essential aspects of parenting children throughout development, rather than being limited to a particular stage. Thus, regardless of when mothers become depressed, their children's needs may be inadequately met and essential aspects of development at risk for maladaptive outcomes.

Inadequate Early Parenting May Interfere with Healthy Development of Biobehavioral Mechanisms. Even children who did not experience adverse fetal environments, who are born with well-functioning neuroregulatory systems, may acquire dysfunctions via interaction with a depressed caregiver. It is now understood that important aspects of development of brain functions and neurobehavioral mechanisms are still developing after birth. Researchers are beginning to understand the extent to which the infant brain is sensitive to early life stress, with the major focus being on the frontal lobe, which plays a major role in the regulation of emotion (see Graham et al., 1999 for a review). Dawson et al. (1994) and Field (1992) have proposed that good quality parenting is required to support healthy brain development that continues into the first few years of postnatal life. Specifically, neurobiological development during early postnatal life may be adversely influenced by mothers being inadequately responsive, intrusive, or withdrawn, and by both expressing and eliciting an excess of negative emotion in interactions with the infants. Both Dawson and Field are accumulating evidence that such adverse early parenting is related to the reduced left frontal electrical brain activity that infants with depressed mothers demonstrate. Further, research is beginning to show that these neurobiological alterations are associated with a diminished capacity to experience joy and a heightened tendency to experience negative affect and, thus, may contribute to risk for developing depression and other emotional problems (e.g., Jones et al., 1997).

the mothers' dysphoric affect (Hops et al., 1987; Jaenicke et al., 1987; Radke-Yarrow, Belmont, Nottelmann, & Bottomly, 1990). Among children with depressed mothers, negative cognitions about the self (self-concept and negative self-schemata) predicted adjustment problems six months later (Hammen et al., 1988). How depressed mothers interpret and label their children's behavior (in ways that might make them angry or lead them to withdraw) may set in play a self-fulfilling prophecy in that children may develop negative expectations for themselves and others, which they then take with them into other contexts. Further support for this model comes from Joiner and Wagner (1995) who found, in children not selected for their mothers' depression, negative attributional style prospectively predicts increases in depressive symptoms in children.

In sum, regardless of the age at which children are first exposed to maternal depression, they are likely to be exposed to qualities of parenting that are inadequate to help the children meet their stage-salient needs. The children are likely to develop cognitive, affective, or interpersonal tendencies which, in turn, increase their vulnerability to the later development of depression. For children who are exposed at multiple points in development, these vulnerabilities would, at minimum, be cumulative and, possibly, interactive. An example of interactive influences is how children might be especially sensitive to later inadequate parenting having been primed by earlier mother-child relationship difficulties. More broadly, a negative cycle is likely to be set into place in that depressed mothers' parenting or general social skills deficits contribute to the development of atypical behavior or even symptoms in her child, which further taxes the mother and contributes to the mother's continuing to engage in inept parenting.

The Stressful Contexts of the Lives of Children with Depressed Mothers

In addition to the biological, genetic, and adverse parenting risks to children of depressed mothers, stressful life events associated with depression in adults, to which the children would also be directly and indirectly exposed, may also mediate the association between maternal depression and child psychopathology. Hammen (1997; 2002) delineates three different components of the stress to which children of depressed parents are exposed: the parent's depression itself, ongoing stressful conditions to which the child is exposed as a function of the parent's depression, and the child's own episodic and chronic stressors. The first component is similar to what was discussed in the previous section of this chapter.

Regarding the second and third components, Hammen et al. (1987) provided strong evidence for the higher levels of stress in families with depressed mothers compared not only to families with well parents but also to families with medically ill mothers. In particular, families with unipolar depressed mothers reported more stress in marital and social relationships, jobs, finances, and relations with children. The children concurred in that they reported more episodic and chronic stressors than did children with well mothers (Adrian & Hammen, 1990, reported in Hammen, 2002). Chronic strain predicted negativity of mother-child interactions beyond the contribution of depressive symptoms (Burge & Hammen, 1991). Hammen et al. (1987) found that both mothers' chronic stress and current depression (but not her lifetime history of depressive disorder) uniquely contributed to the prediction of children's diagnostic status and behavior problems. Similarly, Belle (1982) and Pound, Cox, Puckering, and Mills

(1985) reported that both maternal depression and stress associated with poverty were significant predictors of problems in children.

Moreover, the well-documented association, in adults, between depression and marital discord suggests that children with depressed mothers are likely to also be exposed to high levels of interparental conflict, parents' anger, and marital hostility (Gotlib & Beach, 1995). Marital discord, regardless of the presence of maternal depression, is known to be associated with poorer quality parent-child relationships (Erel & Berman, 1995). The quality of parent-child relationship is the purported mediator of the association between marital discord and child behavior problems. Marital discord may be more strongly associated with children's problems than is maternal depression (Emery, Weintraub, & Neale, 1982) or may mediate the association between maternal depression and children's psychological disturbance (Rutter & Quinton, 1984). Fendrich, Warner, and Weissman (1990) and Goodman et al. (1993) both found that marital discord exacerbates the negative effects of maternal depression on child functioning. Among school-aged children with depressed mothers, those whose parents were divorced were more likely to be rated by their teachers as undercontrolled and lower on ego resiliency (Goodman et al., 1993) and to have a conduct disorder (Fendrich et al., 1990). Thus, stress in general, and marital discord in particular, may be separate and important predictors of outcome in children with depressed mothers.

Implications of the Stressful Context of Depressed Mother's Lives for Mechanisms of Epigenesis in Children with Depressed Mothers. None of the studies of stress in families with depressed mothers has examined how the risks associated with stress might be differently associated with adverse outcomes depending on the developmental stage of the child at the time the stress occurs, nor how chronic or episodic stress might influence the developmental pathways for children with depressed mothers. One possibility is that the vulnerabilities in children that have been associated with having a depressed mother might compromise children's ability to cope with stressors (Compas et al., 2002). The children might be more inclined to have maladaptive neurobiological stress responses, have lower self-efficacy beliefs, generate less effective coping strategies, and perceive themselves as having fewer resources for coping with stress.

Summary: Alternative Etiological Mechanisms and Their Implications for Epigenesis

In sum, four mechanisms have been proposed to explain the association between maternal depression and adverse outcomes in children: genetic risks; innate dysfunctional neuroregulatory systems; exposure to mothers' negative or maladaptive cognitions, behaviors, and affect; and the stressful context of families with depressed mothers. Each of the mechanisms is supported by theory and, at least in part, by a network of empirical studies (see Goodman & Gotlib, 1999, for an evaluation of the relative strength of support for the mechanisms). Clearly much more work is needed, and ideas about future directions for research are provided in the closing section of this chapter.

More important, from the premise of this chapter, each of the proposed mechanisms is limited in that they offer only one particular perspective on how depressed mothers adversely affect their children. As has been reviewed here, most of the literature has taken the molecular approach of studying one particular aspect of the phenomenon. Although researchers typically acknowledge the role of other mechanisms, the single-mechanism approach misses the opportunities to test the complexities of how mechanisms may work together. Next, we argue that the additional explanatory power of a more integrative model offers advantages that outweigh the greater challenges to research design.

MULTIPLE INTERACTING CAUSES AND ALTERNATIVE DEVELOPMENTAL TRAJECTORIES

As much as the field has benefitted from studies of the individual hypothesized mechanisms, the concurrent consideration of multiple mechanisms within a causal model offers even greater potential. Several of the possibilities have already received significant attention. In this section, I will briefly describe examples of theories that highlight the interface of two or more mechanisms, that is, how causes might interact to produce unique outcomes. For each example, I will explore its implications for alternative developmental pathways that children of depressed mothers might follow, and point to research that has explored those possibilities as well as questions that have not yet been addressed. The ideas explored here extend from a developmental, integrative model for understanding mechanisms of transmission of risk for psychopathology in children of depressed mothers (Goodman & Gotlib, 1999), shown in Figure 18.1.

Moderators of Genetic Influence

Gene-Environment Correlation or Covariation. Researchers have begun to explore how genetic and environmental influences might work together. One possibility is that genetic vulnerability and environmental vulnerability (adverse parenting or stressors) might covary. Thus, over time, both genetics and environmental qualities will contribute to particular developmental trajectories. Behavior geneticists define three types of gene-environment (GE) correlations: passive, reactive, and active (Goldsmith, Gottesman, & Lemery, 1997; Plomin, DeFries, & Loehlin, 1977).

Passive GE correlations result from a child's genotype being correlated with the environment provided by parents and siblings, with that environment itself being associated with the heritable traits of the parents or siblings. Thus, depressed mothers' genes influence how they parent their children as well as increasing their children's genetic liability for depression. Rutter et al. (1997) persuasively argue for the necessity of research designed to distinguish between two alternative possibilities in passive GE correlations: first, that the association between parents' disorder and children's adverse outcomes is environmentally mediated, despite the genetic component in the parent's disorder; second, that an apparent environmental risk may actually reflect genetic mediation and is merely an epiphenomenon of the genetic liability (i.e., the supposed risk environment may have no direct risk impact on the children). Given the extent of the literature, there is little doubt that experiences increase individuals' vulnerability to depression. The remaining question is the extent to which that vulnerability is genetically or environmentally mediated. It will be important to distinguish the extent to which the environmental effects are shared or nonshared.

Reactive or evocative GE correlations result from others' reacting to a particular child based on some of the child's inherited characteristics. If what children inherit is

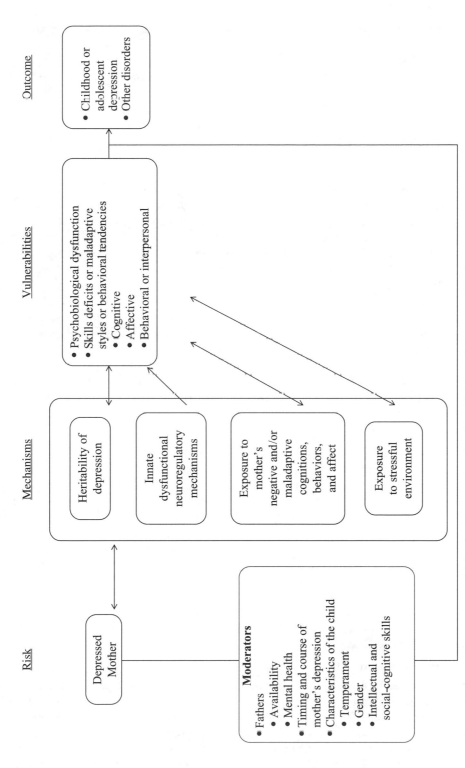

Figure 18.1. An Integrative Model for the Transmission of Risk to Children of Depressed Mothers.

a vulnerability to depression that is expressed in behavioral traits or tendencies, which are evident at birth, then those traits or tendencies may become part of evocative, gene-environment correlations. Children genetically liable to depression may evoke certain qualities in their environments. For example, the children, who might exhibit high levels of negative affect, may be rejected or neglected by peers. Or a depressed mother, herself sensitive to negative affect, may respond to her child's negative affect with intrusive involvement in order to prevent and reduce the child's distress. This maladaptive pattern may reinforce the child's vulnerability to depression by interfering with the child's developing capacity to self-regulate emotions. In these and similar ways, the environment becomes correlated with differences in genetic liabilities. These possibilities have received minimal attention from researchers.

Finally, an active GE correlation results from the child seeking an environment that facilitates further developing his or her inherited tendencies. Genetically vulnerable children may seek certain qualities in their environments. Or they may "experience" their environments differently than do children with well parents. For example, the children may engage the environment less actively or less positively. Or children may selectively attend to or be more sensitive to negative aspects of their environments. Thus over time, the expression of genetically influenced behavioral, cognitive, or affective traits or tendencies influences the environment as experienced by the individual, which feeds back to the traits or tendencies in ways that increase vulnerability to depression. Research with the longitudinal designs to test this aspect of a heritability model has not been reported. Particularly useful would be studies that take advantage of psychiatric or twin registries and test whether genetically vulnerable children are more susceptible than others to environmental stressors, and whether such associations vary at different points in development.

Gene-Environment Interactions – Stress-Diathesis Models. Infants come into the world with a set of genes which, if they include a genetic vulnerability to depression or to risk factors for depression, constitute a diathesis. The stress-diathesis model proposes that the diathesis will not be expressed unless the stress in the environment exceeds a certain threshold (Monroe & Simons, 1991). In this interactional perspective on stress-diathesis, the diathesis, in this case the genetic vulnerability to depression, is presumed not to change over the course of development. What might be expected to change is the context of the children's lives. Thus, particularly inept or pernicious qualities of parenting or stressful environments, when they exceed an unspecified threshold, will result in the expression of the depression vulnerability. Depression researchers might benefit from the stress-diathesis model developed by Walker et al. (1996), focusing on the moderating role of stress exposure and reactivity (i.e., biological stress responses) in the expression of the organic diathesis for schizophrenia.

Discontinuities in the Environment Relative to Genetic Vulnerability. Whether or not genetic vulnerability functions continuously in the child, the effects of genetic vulnerability are unfolding over time. Concurrently, the child is most likely experiencing discontinuities in the environment. Consider that depression is episodic and mothers will become depressed at different points in the child's development and be relatively nondepressed (although not necessarily parenting better) at other times. Researchers have not yet examined whether discontinuities in the environment might moderate continuities in the child.

Genetic Vulnerability Interacts with Other Biological Vulnerabilities. Genes may interact not only with environmental variables but also with other biological variables. One example of a possible interacting biological variable is the set of hormonal changes that occur at puberty. Thus, the higher genetic load for depression in girls than in boys (Murray & Sines, 1996) may interact with biological changes associated with puberty. Another possible interacting factor in such a model is gender-typical personality or behavioral styles (Nolen-Hoeksema & Girgus, 1994). These interactions may help explain the higher rates of depression observed in girls beginning in early adolescence (Angold & Rutter, 1992; Sheeber, Davis, & Hops, 2002).

Genetics might also influence biological functioning more directly. For example, Coccaro, Silverman, Klar, Horvath, and Siever (1994) found that a central 5-HT system abnormality was associated with an elevated morbid risk of impulsive personality disorder traits in the first-degree relatives of patients with personality disorder. This finding is consistent with the idea of genetic influences on set points for neurotransmitters, suggesting a specific mechanism by which genetics may influence heritability of depression.

Genes Interact with Other Genes. Although less often discussed, genes themselves are known to interact in ways that influence the likelihood of disorder. Even if a defect on a particular gene or set of genes were found to influence rates of depression, other genes might also be discovered to have converse, beneficial properties, thereby weakening the effect of the defective genes (Meehl, 1990). Goldsmith, Gottesman, and Lemery (1997) expand on this theme by hypothesizing that genetic liability consists of three components: specific genetic liability, general genetic liability, and genetic assets. Overall, they caution against speaking about genes for psychopathology. Rather, they suggest that "there may be *partially* genetically influenced *predispositions* for basic behavioral tendencies, that under certain experiential contexts, make the *probability* of developing psychopathology higher for individuals who possess greater than lesser degress of such behavioral tendencies" (p. 384).

Moderators of Other Biological Influences

Stress-Diathesis. The stress-diathesis model is relevant not only for genetic diatheses but also for other biological vulnerabilities. The proposed model suggests several possibilities for diatheses. Likely candidates are the psychobiological vulnerabilities that may be the result of a fetal abnormality associated with the mother's depression during pregnancy or of postnatal influences on still developing neuroregulatory systems. These include lowered vagal tone, abnormal stress response, and reduced left frontal activity. The children with depressed mothers who are born with inadequately functioning neuroregulatory systems, or those who acquire those vulnerabilities through inadequate early parenting, may have lower thresholds for stress-precipitated psychopathology.

An important distinction within stress-diathesis models is between an interactional model and a transactional one. As Sameroff (1995) explains, in an interactional model of stress-diathesis, the diathesis, or vulnerability, does not change. Only the particular

mothers' efficacy beliefs, arrangements for substitute care, support for fathers' and other relatives' healthy involvement with the child, and training in positive discipline.

It is also important to consider the needs of children whose mothers were depressed in the postpartum period and then recovered. Some researchers have found that preschool-aged children's cognitive deficits were unrelated to mothers' concurrent levels of depression but were significantly associated with maternal depression during the infant's first year (Cogill, Caplan, Alexandra, Roson, & Kumar, 1986; Sharp et al., 1995). Thus, it may be important to assess the child's prior exposure to the mother's depression even among mothers who are not currently depressed.

In contrast, children who are older when their mothers first become depressed may be better able to cope as a function of: (1) having acquired competencies through the successful development to this point, and (2) having the social-cognitive skills that allow them to express their fears, more accurately perceive situations, to reason about the consequences of their mother's depression, and generate alternative solutions. On the other hand, they may feel guilty or responsible for the mother's sad moods, blaming themselves when she has re-occurrences, and worrying about the likelihood of developing depression themselves, or experiencing other adverse consequences. For early adolescents, the mother's depression may add another set of stressors at a time when multiple life changes already place them at risk for problems in adjustment (Petersen, 1988). The depressed mother may be so distressed by confrontations with a challenging teen that she withdraws further and fails to provide the monitoring so essential to teen development (Dishion & McMahon, 1998). It is even possible that a genetic vulnerability only gets expressed at this time of accumulated stressors. Opportunities for preventive and therapeutic intervention include: helping youths to establish and build on supports outside of the home (Gladstone & Beardslee, 2002), teaching adaptive coping strategies (Compas et al., 2002), and assessing and challenging dysfunctional cognitions (Garber & Martin, 2002).

Finally, the proposed model suggests a set of considerations for intervention that stretch the traditional boundaries for practitioners. That is, the ideal targets of early intervention might include the proposed mechanisms themselves and the vulnerabilities in the child that are associated with the mechanisms. With regard to the four proposed mechanisms, work with the first component, heritability, might include genetic counseling so that parents are aware of the risks from personal and family histories of depression. The second mechanism, innate neuroregulatory dysfunctions, might be minimized if depressed pregnant women are treated for their depression, their stress is reduced, and their prenatal care improved. Children might be less adversely affected by their mothers' depression if mothers are quickly and effectively treated for their depression in a way that minimizes the child's exposure to the depressed mother's negative or maladaptive cognitions, behaviors, and affect, the third mechanism. There is some evidence for significant prevention of deficits in children's functioning as a result of interventions into the parent-child relationship (Cicchetti, Rogosch, & Toth, 2000; Cicchetti, Toth, & Rogosch, 1999; Gladstone & Beardslee, 2002; Lyons-Ruth, Connell, Grunebaum, & Botein, 1990). Finally, the fourth mechanism, exposure to stressful environments, would be targeted by interventions for depressed women that treat the distressed marriage (Beach, Fincham, & Katz, 1998; Whisman & Uebelacker, 1999) and work to minimize the consequences of other stressors, including those associated with poverty. Each of these implications for intervention must be considered in light of

Silberg and Rutter's (2002) caveat that some of the seemingly environmentally mediated risks are actually associated with genetic mediation and would not be effective targets of intervention. This is by no means to suggest that qualities that have high genetic loading cannot be altered by experience (Meehl, 1972). Rather, some of the evidence for environmentally mediated risks may be misleading. Nonetheless, the many influences on gene expression offer challenging opportunities to intervene.

Interventions into the proposed vulnerabilities would include enhancing children's developing competencies such as affective regulation, peer relationships, school achievement, and so forth. Children with depressed mothers might be helped to develop accurate understandings and coping efficacy beliefs about the mother's depression. Early interventions into the mother-child relationship might include parent coaching to enhance the parent's support and gradual intervention into the children's risk-increasing behavioral tendencies, which have been noted, such as negative affectivity, dysfunctional neuroregulatory tendencies, and challenges to the development of a secure attachment organization. Each of the proposed ideas for intervention might not only benefit an individual child and family but also serve as experiments to further test the value of the proposed model (Dickey, 1996).

FUTURE RESEARCH DIRECTIONS

Earlier in this chapter, it was argued that four mechanisms offer strong promise for explaining the transmission of risk for depression from parent to child: genetics, dysfunctional neuroregulatory mechanisms, adverse parenting, and exposure to stressful environments. Research has been accumulating to document the differences between children with depressed parents and others on each of these mechanisms (Goodman & Gotlib, 1999). On the other hand, little research has examined the mediational role specified by the mechanisms, that is, the functional or causal roles of the mechanisms. In particular, few studies have used either statistical models (Baron & Kenny, 1986; Holmbeck, 1997) or experimental manipulations to test whether the mechanisms *explain* the association between maternal depression and the vulnerabilities in the children or, ultimately, the emergence of depression or other disorders in the children. Even fewer have moved beyond the interactionist/modifier variable model in ANOVA or regression designs, both of which assume that the critical influences are separable rather than interdependent.

Even more daunting steps need to be taken to design studies that test aspects of the proposed integrative model (Goodman & Gotlib, 1999). For example, longitudinal studies could be used to explore transactional patterns such as how a depressed mother might respond to her child's tendency to display negative affect by intrusive involvement, which, in turn, interferes with the child's development of emotion regulation abilities. Research designs using multilevel modeling might reveal the levels of contextual variables that are necessary for affective, behavioral, or cognitive tendencies or predispositions to be expressed, resulting in depression vulnerability. Other advances will come from behavior or molecular genetically informed designs, such as testing whether children with high heritability for depression are more susceptible than others to adverse parenting or high levels of stressors.

Finally, more developmental consideration is needed in regard to research on etiological mechanisms. Important questions remain as to what aspects of inadequate parenting, stress, and so forth children are most vulnerable to at different times in their lives. Some understanding is emerging with regard to how children at different ages are differently vulnerable to depression (Cicchetti & Toth, 1998). Overall, an integrative, biopsychosocial model that takes a developmental psychopathology perspective offers tremendous promise for understanding the genesis and epigenesis of psychopathology in children with depressed mothers. Such work is essential to guide the development of empirically based interventions to prevent the now well established adverse outcomes in these children.

REFERENCES

Abrams, S.M., Field T., Scafidi, F., & Prodromidis, M. (1995). Newborns of depressed mothers. *Infant Mental Health Journal, 16,* 233–239.

American Psychiatric Association. (1994). *Diagnostic and statistical manual of mental disorders, 4th edition.* Washington, D.C.: American Psychiatric Association.

Angold, A., & Rutter, M. (1992). Effects of age and pubertal status on depression in a large clinical sample. *Development and Psychopathology, 4,* 5–28.

Bandura, A. (1986). *Social foundations of thought and action: A social cognitive theory.* Englewood Cliffs, N.J.: Prentice-Hall.

Baron, R.M., & Kenny, D.A. (1986). The moderator-mediator variable distinction in social psychological research: Conceptual, strategic, and statistical considerations. *Journal of Personality and Social Psychology, 51,* 1173–1182.

Beach, S.R., Fincham, F.D, & Katz, J. (1998). Marital therapy in the treatment of depression: Toward a third generation of therapy and research. *Clinical Psychology Review, 18,* 635–661.

Beck, A.T., Steer, R.A., & Brown, G.K. (1997). *Beck Depression Inventory, 2d edition.* San Antonio, Tex., The Psychological Corporation.

Beck, A.T., Steer, R.A., & Garbin, M.G. (1988). Psychometric properties of the Beck Depression Inventory. Twenty-five years of evaluation. *Clinical Psychology Review, 8,* 77–100.

Beck, A.T., Ward, C.H., Mendelson, M., Mock, J.E., & Erbaugh, J. (1961). An inventory for measuring depression. *Archives of General Psychiatry, 4,* 561–571.

Beiderman, J., Rosenbaum, J.F., Hirshfeld, D.R., Faraone, S.V., Bolduc, E.A., Gersten, M., Meminger, S.R., Kagan, J., Snidman, N., & Reznick, S. (1990). Psychiatric correlates of behavioral inhibition in young children of parents with and without psychiatric disorders. *Archives of General Psychiatry, 47,* 21–26.

Belle, D. (1982). *Lives in stress.* Beverly Hills: Sage Publications.

Belsher, G., & Costello, C.G. (1988). Relapse after recovery from unipolar depression: A critical review. *Psychological Bulletin, 104,* 84–96.

Belsky, J., Hsieh, K-H, & Crnic, K. (1998). Mothering, fathering, and infant negativity as antecedents of boys' externalizing problems and inhibition at age 3 years: Differential susceptibility to rearing experience? *Development and Psychopathology, 10,* 301–319.

Bettes, B.A. (1988). Maternal depression and motherese: Temporal and intonational features. *Child Development, 59,* 1089–1096.

Blazer, D., Kessler, R., McGonagle, K., & Swartz, M. (1994). The prevalence and distribution of major depression in a national community sample: The National Comorbidity Survey. *American Journal of Psychiatry, 151,* 979–986.

Breznitz, Z., & Friedman, S.L. (1988). Toddlers' concentration: Does maternal depression make a difference? *Journal of Child Psychology and Psychiatry, 29,* 267–279.

Bronfenbrenner, U. (1992). Ecological systems theory. In R. Vasta (Ed.), *Six theories of child development: Revised formulations and current issues* (pp. 187–249). London: Jessica Kingsley Publishers.

Bugental, D.B., Blue, J., Cortez, V., Fleck, K., & Rodriguez, A. (1992). Influences of witnessed affect on information processing in children. *Child Development, 63,* 774–786.

Burge, D., & Hammen, C. (1991). Maternal communication: A predictor of children's outcomes at follow-up in a high risk sample. *Journal of Abnormal Psychology, 100,* 174–180.

Campbell, S.B., & Cohn, J.F. (1997). The timing and chronicity of postpartum depression: Implications for infant development. In P. Murray (Ed.), *Postpartum depression and child development* (pp. 165–197). New York: Guilford Press.

Chambers, C.D., Johnson, K.A., Dick, L.M., Felix, R.J., & Jones, K.L. (1996). Birth outcomes in pregnant women taking fluoxetine. *New England Journal of Medicine, 335*, 1010–1015.

Cherny, S.S., Fulker D.W., Corley R.P., Plomin R., & DeFries J.C. (1994). Continuity and change in infant shyness from 14 to 20 months. *Behavior Genetics, 24*, 365–379.

Cicchetti, D. (1989) (Ed). *The emergence of a discipline: Rochester Symposium on Developmental Psychopathology, Vol. 1.* Hillsdale, N.J.: Erlbaum.

Cicchetti, D., & Lynch, M. (1993). Toward an ecological/transactional model of community violence and child maltreatment: Consequences for children's development. *Psychiatry, 56*, 96–118.

Cicchetti, D., & Rogosch, F. (1996). Equifinality and multifinality in developmental psychopathology. *Development and Psychopathology, 8*, 597–600.

Cicchetti, D., Rogosch, F.A., & Toth, S.L. (2000). The efficacy of toddler-parent psychotherapy for fostering cognitive development in offspring of depressed mothers. *Journal of Abnormal Child Psychology, 28*, 135–148.

Cicchetti, D., & Schneider-Rosen, K. (1984). Toward a transactional model of childhood depression. *New Directions for Child Development. No. 26*, 5–27.

Cicchetti, D., & Schneider-Rosen, K. (1986). An organizational approach to childhood depression. In M. Rutter, C. Izard, & P. Read (Eds.), *Depression in young people: Clinical and developmental perspectives* (pp. 71–134). New York: Guilford Press.

Cicchetti, D., & Toth, S.L. (1998). The development of depression in children and adolescents. *American Psychologist, 53*, 221–241.

Cicchetti, D., Toth, S.L., & Rogosch, F.A. (1999). Toddler-parent psychotherapy as a preventive intervention to alter attachment organization in offspring of depressed mothers. *Attachment and Human Development, 1*, 34–66.

Cicchetti, D., & Tucker, D. (1994). Development and self-regulatory structures of the mind. *Development and Psychopathology, 6*, 533–549.

Clarke, A.S., & Schneider, M.L. (1993). Prenatal stress has long-term effects on behavioral responses to stress in juvenile rhesus monkeys. *Developmental Psychobiology, 26*, 296–304.

Clarke, A.S., Wittwer, D.J., Abbott, D.H., & Schneider, M.L. (1994). Long-term effects of prenatal stress on HPA axis activity in juvenile rhesus monkeys. *Developmental Psychobiology, 27*, 256–269.

Coccaro, E.F., Silverman, J.M., Klar, H.M., Horvath, T.B., & Siever, L.J. (1994). Familial correlates of reduced central serotonergic system function in patients with personality disorders. *Archives of General Psychiatry, 51*, 318–324.

Cogill, S.R., Caplan, H.L., Alexandra, H., Robson, K.M., & Kumar, R. (1986). Impact of maternal depression on cognitive development of young children. *British Medical Journal, 292*, 1165–1167.

Cohn, J., & Campbell, S. (1992). Influence of maternal depression on infant affect regulation. In D. Cicchetti & S. Toth (Eds.), *Developmental perspectives on depression, Vol. 4* (pp. 103–130). Rochester, N.Y.: University of Rochester Press.

Cohn, J., & Tronick, E.J. (1983). Three-month-old infants' reaction to simulated maternal depression. *Child Development, 54*, 185–190.

Compas, B.E., Langrock, A.M., Keller, G., Merchant, M.J., & Copeland, M.E. (2002). Children coping with parental depression: Processes of adaptation to family stress. In S. Goodman & I. Gotlib (Eds.), *Children of depressed parents: Alternative pathways to risk for psychopathology.* Washington, D.C.: American Psychological Association Press.

Copper, R.L., Goldenberg, R.L., Das, A., Elder, N., Swain, M., Norman, G., Ramsey, R., Cotroneo, P., Collins, B.A., Johnson, F., Jones, P., & Meier, A.M. (1996). The preterm prediction study: maternal stress is associated with spontaneous preterm birth at less than thirty-five weeks' gestation. *American Journal of Obstetrics and Gynecology, 175*, 1286–1292.

Crick, N.R., & Dodge, K.A. (1994). A review and reformulation of social information-processing mechanisms in children's social adjustment. *Psychological Bulletin, 115*, 74–101.

Cummings, E.M., & Cicchetti, D. (1990). Toward a transactional model of relations between attachment and depression. In M.T. Greenberg, D. Cicchetti, & E.M. Cummings (Eds.), *Attachment in the preschool years: Theory, research, and intervention. The John D. and Catherine T. MacArthur Foundation series on mental health and development* (pp. 339–372). Chicago: University of Chicago Press.

Cummings, E.M., & Davies, P.T. (1994). Maternal depression and child development. *Journal of Child Psychology and Psychiatry, 35,* 73–112.

Davidson, R.J. & Fox, N.A. (1988). Cerebral asymmetry and emotion: Development and individual differences. In D.L. Molfese & S.J. Segalowitz (Eds.), *Brain lateralization in children: Developmental implications* (pp. 191–206). New York: Guilford Press.

Dawson, G., Frey, K., Panagiotides, H., Osterling, J., & Hessl, D. (1997). Infants of depressed mothers exhibit atypical frontal brain activity: A replication and extension of previous findings. *Journal of Child Psychology & Psychiatry & Allied Disciplines, 38,* 179–186.

Dawson, G., Hessl, D., & Frey, K. (1994). Social influences on early developing biological and behavioral systems related to risk for affective disorder. *Development and Psychopathology, 6,* 759–779.

Deater-Deckard, K., & Dodge, K.A. (1997). Spare the rod, spoil the authors: Emerging themes in research on parenting and child development. *Psychological Inquiry, 8,* 230–235.

Dickey, M.H. (1996). Methods for single-case experiments in family therapy. In D.H. Sprenkle & S.M. Moon (Eds.), *Research methods in family therapy* (pp. 264–285). New York: Guilford Press.

Dishion, T.J., & McMahon, R.J. (1998). Parental monitoring and the prevention of child and adolescent problem behavior: A conceptual and empirical formulation. *Clinical Child and Family Psychology Review, 1,* 61–75.

Emery, R., Weintraub, S., & Neale, J.M. (1982). Effects of marital discord on the children of schizophrenic, affectively disordered, and normal parents. *Journal of Abnormal Child Psychology, 10,* 215–228.

Emory, E., Walker, E., & Cruz, A. (1983). Fetal heart rate: II. Behavioral correlates. *Psychophysiology, 19,* 680–686.

Erel, O., & Berman, B. (1995). Interrelatedness of marital relations and parent-child relations: A meta-analytic review. *Psychological Bulletin, 118,* 108–132.

Fendrich, M., Warner, V., & Weissman, M.M. (1990). Family risk factors, parental depression, and psychopathology in offspring. *Developmental Psychology, 26,* 40–50.

Field, T. (1984). Early interactions between infants and their postpartum depressed mothers. *Infant Behavior and Development, 7,* 517–522.

Field, T. (1992). Infants of depressed mothers. *Development and Psychopathology, 4,* 9–66.

Field, T. (1994). The effects of mother's physical and emotional unavailability on emotion regulation. In N.A. Fox (Ed.). *The development of emotion regulation: Biological and behavioral considerations. Monographs of the Society for Research in Child Development, 59,* 208–227.

Field, T.M. (1998). Depressed mothers and their newborns. Paper presented at the 11th Biennial Conference on Infant Studies, Atlanta, GA, April 2–5.

Field, T., Bendell-Estroff, D., Yando, R., Del Valle, C., Malphurs, J., & Hart, S. (1996). "Depressed" mothers' perceptions of infant vulnerability are related to later development. *Child Psychiatry and Human Development, 27,* 43–53.

Field, T., Healy, B., Goldstein, S., & Guthertz, M. (1990). Behavior state matching and synchrony in mother-infant interactions of nondepressed versus depressed dyads. *Developmental Psychology, 26,* 7–14.

Field, T., Healy, J.B., Goldstein, S. Perry, S., Bendell, D.J., Schanberg, S., Zimmerman, E.A., & Kuhn, C. (1988). Infants of depressed mothers show "depressed" behavior even with non-depressed adults. *Child Development, 59,* 1569–1579.

Field, T., Pickens, J., Fox, N.A., Nawrocki, T., & Gonzalez, J. (1995). Vagal tone in infants of depressed mothers. *Development and Psychopathology, 7,* 227–231.

Field, T., Sandberg, D., Garcia, R., Vega-Lahr, N., Goldstein, S., & Guy, L. (1985). Prenatal problems, postpartum depression, and early mother-infant interactions. *Developmental Psychology, 12,* 1152–1156.

Fleming, A., Ruble, D., Flett, G., & Shaul, D. (1988). Postpartum adjustment in first-time mothers: Relations between mood, maternal attitudes, and mother-infant interactions. *Developmental Psychology, 24,* 71–81.

Forehand, R., Lautenschlager, G.J., Faust, J., & Graziano, W.G. (1986). Parent perceptions and parent-child interactions in clinic-referred children: A preliminary investigation of the effects of maternal depressive moods. *Behavior Research and Therapy, 24,* 73–75.

Fox, N.A. (1994). Dynamic cerebral processes underlying emotion regulation. In N.A. Fox (Ed.), The development of emotion regulation: Biological and behavioral considerations. *Monographs of the Society for Research in Child Development, 59* (2–3, Serial No. 240) (pp. 152–166).

Fox, N.A., & Calkins, S.D. (1993). Multiple-measure approaches to the study of infant emotion. In M. Lewis, J.M. Haviland, et al. (Eds.), *Handbook of emotions.* (pp. 167–184). New York: Guilford Press.

Frank, E., Carpenter, L.L., & Kupfer, D.J. (1988). Sex differences in recurrent depression: Are there any that are significant? *American Journal of Psychiatry, 145,* 41–45.

Garber, J. & Martin, N.C. (2002). Negative cognitions in offspring of depressed parents: Mechanisms of risk. In S. Goodman & I. Gotlib (Eds.), *Children of depressed parents: alternative pathways to risk for psychopathology.* Washington, D.C.: American Psychological Association Press.

Gianino, A., & Tronick, E. (1985). The mutual regulation model: The infant's self and interactive regulation and coping and defensive capacities. In T. Field, P. McCabe, & N. Schneiderman (Eds.), *Stress and coping* (pp. 47–68). Hillsdale, N.J.: Erlbaum.

Gitau, R., Cameron, A., Fisk, N.M., & Glover, V. (1998). Fetal exposure to maternal cortisol. *Lancet, 352,* 707–708.

Gladstone, T.R.G., & Beardslee, W.R. (2002). Treatment, intervention and prevention with children of depressed parents: A developmental perspective. In S.H. Goodman & I.H. Gotlib (Eds.), *Children of depressed parents: Alternative pathways to risk for psychopathology.* Washington, D.C.: American Psychological Association Press.

Glover, V., Teixeira, J., Gitau, R., & Fisk, N. (1998). Links between antenatal maternal anxiety and the fetus. Paper presented at the 11th Biennial Conference on Infant Studies, Atlanta, GA, April 2–5.

Goldsmith, H.H., Buss, K.A., & Lemery, K.S. (1997). Toddler and childhood temperament: expanded content, stronger genetic evidence, new evidence for the importance of environment. *Developmental Psychology, 33,* 891–905.

Goldsmith, H.H., Gottesman, I.I., & Lemery, K.S. (1997). Epigenetic approaches to developmental psychopathology. *Development and Psychopathology, 9,* 365–387.

Goldsmith, D.F., & Rogoff, B. (1997). Mothers' and toddlers' coordinated joint focus of attention: Variations with maternal dysphoric symptoms. *Developmental Psychology, 33,* 113–119.

Goodman, S.H., Adamson, L.B., Riniti, J., & Cole, S. (1994). Mothers' expressed attitudes: Associations with maternal depression and children's self-esteem and psychopathology. *Journal of the American Academy of Child and Adolescent Psychiatry, 33,* 1265–1274.

Goodman, S.H., Brogan, D., Lynch, M.E., & Fielding, B. (1993). Social and emotional competence in children of depressed mothers. *Child Development, 64,* 516–531.

Goodman, S.H. & Gotlib, I.H. (1999). Risk for psychopathology in the children of depressed parents: A developmental approach to the understanding of mechanisms. *Psychological Review, 106,* 458–490.

Gotlib, I.H., & Beach, S.R.H. (1995). A marital/family discord model of depression: Implications for therapeutic intervention. In N.S. Jacobson & A.S. Gurman (Eds.), *Clinical handbook of couple therapy* (pp. 411–436). New York: Guilford Press.

Gotlib, I.H., & Goodman, S.H. (1999). Children of parents with depression. In W.K. Silverman & T.H. Ollendick (Eds.), *Developmental issues in the clinical treatment of children and adolescents* (pp. 415–432). Boston: Allyn & Bacon.

Gotlib, I.H., Ranganath, C., & Rosenfeld, J.P. (1998). Frontal EEG alpha asymmetry, depression, and cognitive functioning. *Cognition and Emotion, 12,* 449–478.

Graham, Y.P., Heim, C., Goodman, S.H., Miller, A.H., & Nemeroff, C.B. (1999). The effects of neonatal stress on brain development: Implications for psychopathology. *Development and Psychopathology, 11,* 545–565.

Hammen, C. (1997). Children of depressed parents: The stress context. In S.A. Wolchik & I.N. Sandler (Eds.), *Handbook of children's coping: Linking theory and intervention. Issues in clinical child psychology* (pp. 131–157). New York: Plenum.

Hammen, C. (2002). The context of stress in families of children with depressed parents. In S.H. Goodman & I.H. Gotlib (Eds.), *Children of depressed parents: Mechanisms of risk and implications for treatment*, Washington, D.C.: American Psychological Association Press.

Hammen, C., Adrian, C., & Hiroto, D. (1988). A longitudinal test of the attributional vulnerability model in children at risk for depression. *British Journal of Clinical Psychology, 27*, 37–46.

Hammen, C., Burge, D., & Stansbury, K. (1990). Relationship of mother and child variables to child outcomes in a high risk sample: A causal modeling analysis. *Developmental Psychology, 26*, 24–30.

Hammen, C., Gordon, D., Burge, D., Adrian, C., Jaenicke, C., & Hiroto, D. (1987). Maternal affective disorders, illness, and stress: Risk for children's psychopathology. *American Journal of Psychiatry, 144*, 736–741.

Handley, S.L., Dunn, T.L., Waldron, G., & Baker, J.M. (1980). Tryptophan, cortisol and puerperal mood. *British Journal of Psychiatry, 136*, 498–508.

Harrington, R., Rutter, M., & Fombonne, E. (1996). Developmental pathways in depression: Multiple meanings, antecedents, and endpoints. *Development and Psychopathology, 8*, 601–616.

Hart, S., Jones, N.A., Field, T., & Lundy, B. (1999). One-year-old infants of intrusive and withdrawn depressed mothers. *Child Psychiatry and Human Development, 30*, 111–120.

Hay, D.F. (1997). Postpartum depression and cognitive development. In L. Murray & P.J. Cooper (Eds.), *Postpartum depression and child development* (pp. 85–110). New York: Guilford Press.

Holmbeck, G.N. (1997). Toward terminological, conceptual, and statistical clarity in the study of mediators and moderators: examples from the child-clinical and pediatric psychology literatures. *Journal of Consulting and Clinical Psychology, 65*, 599–610.

Hops, H., Biglan, A., Sherman, L., Arthur, J., Friedman, L., & Osteen, V. (1987). Home observations of family interactions of depressed women. *Journal of Consulting and Clinical Psychology, 55*, 341–346.

Jaenicke, C., Hammen, C., Zupan, B., Hiroto, D., Gordon, D., Adrian, C., & Burge, D. (1987). Cognitive vulnerability in children at risk for depression. *Journal of Abnormal Child Psychology, 15*, 559–572.

Joiner, T.E., & Wagner, K.D. (1995). Attributional style and depression in children and adolescents: A meta-analytic review. *Clinical Psychology Review, 15*, 777–798.

Jones, N., Field, T., Davalos, M. & Pickens, J. (1997). Brain electrical activity stability in infants/children of depressed mothers. *Child Psychiatry and Human Development, 28*, 326–339.

Kagan, J. (1994). On the nature of emotion. In N. Fox (Ed.), *The development of emotion regulation: Biological and behavioral considerations*. Monographs of the Society for Research in Child Development, 59 (Nos. 2–3), pp. 7–24.

Kagan, J., Arcus, D., & Snidman, N. (1993). The idea of temperament: Where do we go from here? In R. Plomin, G.E. McClearn, et al., (Eds.), *Nature, nurture and psychology* (pp. 197–210). Washington, DC: American Psychological Association.

Kagan, J., & Snidman, N. (1991). Temperamental factors in human development. *American Psychologist, 46*, 856–862.

Kay, G., Tarcic, N., Poltyrev, T., & Weinstock, M. (1998). Prenatal stress depresses immune function in rats. *Physiology and Behavior, 63*, 397–402.

Keller, M.B., & Shapiro, R.W. (1981). Major depressive disorder: Initial results from a one-year prospective naturalistic follow-up study. *Journal of Nervous and Mental Disorders, 169*, 761–768.

Kendler, K.S., Kessler, R.C., Walters, E.E., MacLean, C.J., Sham, P.C., Neale, M.C., Heath, A.C., & Eaves, L.J. (1995). Stressful life events, genetic liability and onset of an episode of major depression in women. *American Journal of Psychiatry, 152*, 833–842.

Kessler, R., McGonagle, K., Zhao, S., Nelson, C., Hughes, M., Eshleman, S., Wittchen, H.-U., & Kendler, K. (1994). Lifetime and 12-month prevalence of DSM-III-R psychiatric disorders in the United States: Results from the National Comorbidity Study. *Archives of General Psychiatry, 51*, 8–19.

Kochanska, G., Kuczynski, L., & Maguire, M. (1989). Patterns of mutual influence between well and depressed mothers and their 5-year-old children. Paper presented at the Society for Research in Child Development, April 27–30. Kansas City, Missouri.

Kochanska, G., Kuczynski, L., Radke-Yarrow, M., & Welsh, J.D. (1987). Resolutions of control episodes between well and affectively ill mothers and their young children. *Journal of Abnormal Child Psychology, 15*, 441–456.

Kovacs, M., Devlin, B., Pollock, M., Richards, C., & Mukerji, P. (1997). A controlled family history study of childhood-onset depressive disorder. *Archives of General Psychiatry, 54,* 613–623.

Livingood, A.B., Daen, P., & Smith, B.D. (1983). The depressed mother as a source of stimulation for her infant. *Journal of Clinical Psychology, 39,* 369–375.

Loehlin, J.C. (1992). *Genes and environment in personality development.* Beverly Hills: Sage Publications.

Loehlin, J.C., & Nichols, R.C. (1976). *Heredity, environment, and personality.* Austin: University of Texas Press.

Lundy, B.L, Jones, N.A., Field, T., Nearing, G., Davalos, M., Pietro, P.A., Schanberg, S., & Kuhn, C. (1999). Prenatal depression effects on neonates. *Infant Behavior and Development, 22,* 119–129.

Lykken, D., & Tellegen, A. (1996). Happiness is a stochastic phenomenon. *Psychological Science, 7,* 186–189.

Lyons-Ruth, K., Connell, D., Grunebaum, H., & Botein, S. (1990). Infants at social risk: Maternal depression and family support services as mediators of infant development and security of attachment. *Child Development, 61,* 85–98.

McGuffin, P., & Katz, R. (1993). Genes, adversity, and depression. In R. Plomin & G.E. Mc-Clearn (Eds.), *Nature and nurture and psychology* (pp. 217–230). Washington, D.C.: American Psychological Association.

Meehl, P.E. (1972). Specific genetic etiology, psychodynamics, and therapeutic nihilism. *International Journal of Mental Health, 1,* 10–27.

Meehl, P.E. (1990). Toward an integrated theory of schizotaxia, schizotypy, and schizophrenia. *Journal of Personality Disorders, 4,* 1–99.

Merikangas, K.R., Prusoff, B.A., & Weissman, M.M. (1988). Parental concordance for affective disorders: Psychopathology in offspring. *Journal of Affective Disorders, 15,* 279–290.

Milberger, S., Beiderman, J., Faraone, S.V., Chen, L., & Jones, J. (1996). Is maternal smoking during pregnancy a risk factor for attention deficit hyperactivity disorder in children? *American Journal of Psychiatry, 153,* 1138–1142.

Monroe, S.M., & Simons, A.D. (1991). Diathesis-stress theories in the context of life-stress research: Implications for depressive disorders. *Psychological Bulletin, 110,* 406–425.

Murray, K.T., & Sines, J.O. (1996). Parsing the genetic and nongenetic variance in children's depressive behavior. *Journal of Affective Disorders, 36,* 23–34.

Murray, L. (1992). The impact of postnatal depression on infant development. *Journal of Child Psychology and Psychiatry, 33,* 543–561.

Nemeroff, C. (1996). The corticotropin-releasing factor hypothesis of depression: New findings and new directions. *Molecular Psychiatry, 1,* 336–342.

Nolen-Hoeksema, S., & Girgus, J.S. (1994). The emergence of gender differences in depression during adolescence. *Psychological Bulletin, 115,* 424–443.

Nulman, I., Rovet, J., Stewart, D.E., Wolpin, J., Gardner, H.A., Theis, J.G., Kulin, N., & Koren, G. (1997). Neurodevelopment of children exposed in utero to antidepressant drugs. *New England Journal of Medicine, 336,* 258–262.

Nurnberger, J., Goldin, L.R., & Gershon, E.S. (1986). Genetics of psychiatric disorders. In G. Winokur & P. Clayton (Eds.), *The medical basis of psychiatry* (pp. 486–521). Philadelphia: WB Saunders.

O'Hara, M.W. (1986). Social support, life events, and depression during pregnancy and the post partum. *Archives of General Psychiatry, 43,* 569–573.

Pasamanick, B., & Knobloch, H. (1966). Retrospective studies on the epidemiology of reproductive casualty: Old and new. *Merrill-Palmer Quarterly, 12,* 7–26.

Pastuszak, A., Schick-Boschetto, B., Zuber, C., Feldkamp, M., Pinelli, M., et al. (1993). Pregnancy outcome following first-trimester exposure to fluoxetine (Prozac). *Journal of the American Medical Association, 269,* 2246–2248.

Patterson, G.R. (1982). *Coercive family process.* Eugene, Ore.: Castalia.

Petersen, A.C. (1988). Adolescent development. *Annual Review of Psychology, 39,* 583–607.

Plomin R. (1990). The role of inheritance in behavior. *Science, 248,* 183–188.

Plomin, R. (1994). *Genetics and experience: The interplay between nature and nurture.* Thousand Oaks, Calif.: Sage Publications.

Plomin, R., DeFries, J.C., & Loehlin, J.C. (1977). Genotype-environment interaction and correlation in the analysis of human behavior. *Psychological Bulletin, 84,* 309–322.

Plomin, R., Emde, R.N., Braungart, J.M., Campos, J., Corley, R., Fulker, D.W., Kagan, J., Reznick, J.S., Robinson, J., Zahn-Waxler, C., et al. (1993). Genetic change and continuity from fourteen to twenty months: The MacArthur Longitudinal Twin Study. *Child Development, 64,* 1354–1376.

Poltyrev, T., Keshet, G.I., Kay, G., & Weinstock, M. (1996). Role of experimental conditions in determining differences in exploratory behavior of prenatally stressed rats. *Developmental Psychobiology, 29,* 453–462.

Pound, A., Cox, A., Puckering, C., & Mills, M. (1985). The impact of maternal depression on young children. In J.E. Stevenson (Ed.), *Recent research in developmental psychopathology* (pp. 3–10). Oxford: Pergamon Press.

Radke-Yarrow, M. (1998). *Children of depressed mothers: From early childhood to maturity.* New York: Cambridge University Press.

Radke-Yarrow, M., Belmont, B., Nottelmann, E., & Bottomly, L. (1990). Young children's self-conceptions: Origins in the natural discourse of depressed and normal mothers and their children. In D. Cicchetti & M. Beeghly (Eds.), *The self in transition: Infancy to childhood* (pp. 345–361). Chicago: University of Chicago Press.

Radke-Yarrow, M., Cummings, E.M., Kuczynski, L., & Chapman, M. (1985). Patterns of attachment in two- and three-year-olds in normal families and families with parental depression. *Child Development, 56,* 884–893.

Radke-Yarrow, M., Nottelmann, E., Martinez, P., & Fox, M.B. (1992). Young children of affectively ill parents: A longitudinal study of psychosocial development. *Journal of the American Academy of Child & Adolescent Psychiatry, 31,* 68–77.

Radke-Yarrow, M., Zahn-Waxler, C., Richardson, D.T., & Susman, A. (1994). Caring behavior in children of clinically depressed and well mothers. *Child Development, 65,* 1405–1414.

Radloff, L.S. (1977). The CES-D scale: A self-report depression scale for research in the general population. *Applied Psychological Measurement, 1,* 385–401.

Rende, R.D., Plomin, R., Reiss, D., & Hetherington, E.M. (1993). Genetic and environmental influences on depressive symptomatology in adolescence: Individual differences and extreme scores. *Journal of Child Psychology and Psychiatry, 34,* 1387–1398.

Rende, R., Warner, V., Wickramarante, P., & Weissman, M.M. (1999). Sibling aggregation for psychiatric disorders in offspring at high and low risk for depression: 10-year follow up. *Psychological Medicine, 29,* 1291–1298.

Rubin, K.H., & Lollis, S.P. (1988). Origins and consequences of social withdrawal. In J. Belsky, T. Nezworski, et al. (Eds.), *Clinical implications of attachment. Child psychology* (pp. 219–252). Hillsdale, N.J.: Erlbaum.

Rutter, M., Dunn, J., Plomin, R., Simonoff, E., Pickles, A., Maughan, B., Ormel, J., Meyer, J., & Eaves, L. (1997). Integrating nature and nurture: Implications of person-environment correlations and interactions for developmental psychopathology. *Development and Psychopathology, 9,* 335–364.

Rutter, M., & Quinton, P. (1984). Parental psychiatric disorder: Effects on children. *Psychological Medicine, 14,* 853–880.

Sameroff, A.J. (1975). Transactional models in early social relations. *Human Development, 18,* 65–79.

Sameroff, A.J. (1995). General systems theories and developmental psychopathology. In D. Cicchetti & D.J. Cohen (Eds.) (1995). *Developmental psychopathology, Vol. 1: Theory and methods* (pp. 659–695). New York: Wiley.

Scarr, S., & Deater-Deckard, K. (1997). Family effects on individual differences in development. In S.S. Luthar, J.A. Burack, et al. (Eds.). *Developmental psychopathology: Perspectives on adjustment, risk, and disorder* (pp. 115–136). New York: Cambridge University Press.

Schaughency, E.A., & Lahey, B.B. (1985). Mothers' and fathers' perceptions of child deviance: Roles of child behavior, parental depression, and marital satisfaction. *Journal of Consulting and Clinical Psychology, 53,* 718–723.

Schneider, M.L. (1992). Prenatal stress exposure alters postnatal behavioral expressions under conditions of novelty challenge in rhesus monkey infants. *Developmental Psychobiology, 25,* 529–540.

Sharp, D., Hay, D.F., Pawlby, S., Schmucker, G., Allen, H., & Humar, R. (1995). The impact of postnatal depression on boys' intellectual development. *Journal of Child Psychology and Psychiatry and Allied Disciplines, 36,* 1315–1336.

Sheeber, L., Davis, B., & Hops, H. (2002). Gender specific vulnerability to depression in children of depressed mothers. In S.H. Goodman & I.H. Gotlib (Eds.), *Children of depressed parents: Alternative pathways to risk for psychopathology*, Washington, D.C.: American Psychological Association Press.

Silberg, J., & Rutter, M. (2002). Nature-nurture interplay in the risks associated with parental depression. In S.H. Goodman & I.H. Gotlib (Eds.), *Children of depressed parents: Mechanisms of risk and implications for treatment*, Washington, D.C.: American Psychological Association Press.

Singer, J.M., & Fagen, J.W. (1992). Negative affect, emotional expression, and forgetting in young infants. *Developmental Psychology, 28,* 43–57.

Smith, R., Cubis, J., Brinsmead, M., Lewin, T., Singh, B., Owens, P., Eng-Cheng, C., Hall, C., Adler, R., Lovelock, M., Hurt, D., Rowley, M., & Nolan M. (1990). Mood changes, obstetric experience and alterations in plasma cortisol, beta-endorphin and corticotrophin releasing hormone during pregnancy and the puerperium. *Journal of Psychosomatic Research, 34,* 53–69.

Snyder, J. (1991). Discipline as a mediator of the impact of maternal stress and mood on child conduct problems. *Development and Psychopathology, 3,* 263–276.

Sroufe, L.A., & Rutter, M. (1984). The domain of developmental psychopathology. *Child Development, 55,* 17–29.

Suomi, S.J. (1995). Influence of attachment theory on ethological studies of biobehavioral development in nonhuman primates. In S. Goldberg, R. Muir, et al. (Eds.), *Attachment theory: Social, developmental, and clinical perspectives* (pp. 185–201). Hillsdale, N.J.: Analytic Press.

Teixeira J.M., Fisk, N.M., & Glover, V. (1999). Association between maternal anxiety in pregnancy and increased uterine artery resistance index: cohort based study. *British Medical Journal, 318,* 153–157.

Tellegen, A., Lykken, D.T., Bouchard, T.J., Jr., Wilcox, K.J., Segal, N.L., & Rich, S. (1988). Personality similarity in twins reared apart and together. *Journal of Personality and Social Psychology, 54,* 1031–1039.

Teti, D.M., & Gelfand, D.M. (1991). Behavioral competence among mothers of infants in the first year: The mediational role of maternal self-efficacy. *Child Development, 62,* 918–929.

Teti, D.M., & Gelfand, D.M. (1997). Maternal cognitions as mediators of child outcomes in the context of postpartum depression. In L. Murray & P.J. Cooper, (Eds.), *Postpartum depression and child development* (pp. 136–164). New York: Guilford Press.

Teti, D.M., Gelfand, D.M., Messinger, D.S., & Isabella, R. (1995). Maternal depression and the quality of early attachment: An examination of infants, preschoolers, and their mothers. *Developmental Psychology, 31,* 364–376.

Todd, R.D., Neuman, R., Geller, B., Fox, L.W., & Hickok, J. (1993). Genetic studies of affective disorders: Should we be starting with childhood onset probands? *Journal of the American Academy of Child and Adolescent Psychiatry, 32,* 1164–1171.

Tronick, E.Z., & Gianino, A.F. (1986). The transmission of maternal disturbance to the infant. In E.Z. Tronick & T. Field (Eds.), *Maternal depression and infant disturbance* (pp. 5–12). San Francisco: Jossey-Bass.

Tsuang, M.T., & Faraone, S.V. (1990). *The genetics of mood disorders.* Baltimore: Johns Hopkins University Press.

Wadhwa, P.D., Dunkel-Schetter, C., Chicz-DeMet, A., & Porto, M. (1996). Prenatal psychosocial factors and the neuroendocrine axis in human pregnancy. *Psychosomatic Medicine, 58,* 432–446.

Walker, E., Neumann, C.C., Baum, K., Davis, D.M., DiForio, D., & Bergman, A. (1996). The developmental pathways to schizophrenia: Potential moderated effects of stress. *Development and Psychopathology, 8,* 647–666.

Webster-Stratton, C., & Hammond, M. (1988). Maternal depression and its relationship to life stress, perceptions of child behavior problems, parenting behaviors, and child conduct problems. *Journal of Abnormal Child Psychology, 16,* 299–315.

Weissman, M.M. (1984). The epidemiology of depression: An update on sex differences in rats. *Journal of Affective Disorders, 7,* 179–188.

Weissman, M.M., Bland, R.C., Canino, G.J., Faravelli, C., Greenwald, S., Hwu, H.G., Joyce, P.R., Karam, E.G., Lee, C.K., Lellouch, J., Lepine, J.P., Newman, S.C., Rubio-Stipec, M., Wells, J.E., Wickramaratne, P.J., Wittchen, H., & Yeh, E.K. (1996). Cross-national epidemiology of major depression and bipolar disorder. *Journal of the American Medical Association, 276,* 24–31.

Weissman, M.M., Gammon, G.D., John, K., Merikangas, K.R., Warner, V., Prusoff, B., & Sholom-skas, D. (1987). Children of depressed parents: Increased psychopathology and early onset of major depression. *Archives of General Psychiatry, 44,* 847–853.

Whiffen, V.E., & Gottlib, I.M. (1989). Infants of postpartum depressed mothers: Temperament and cognitive status. *Journal of Abnormal Psychology, 98,* 274–279.

Whisman, M.A., & Uebelacker, L.A. (1999). Integrating couple therapy with individual therapies and antidepressant medications in the treatment of depression. *Clinical Psychology-Science and Practice, 6,* 415–429.

Williams, M.T., Hennessy, M.B., & Davis, H.N. (1998). Stress during pregnancy alters rat offspring morphology and ultrasonic vocalizations. *Physiology and Behavior, 63,* 337–343.

Williamson, D.E., Ryan, N.D., Birmaher, B., Dahl, R.E., et al. (1995). A case-control family history study of depression in adolescents. *Journal of the American Academy of Child and Adolescent Psychiatry, 34,* 1596–1607.

Zahn-Waxler, C., Denham, S., Iannotti, R.J., & Cummings, E.M. (1992). Peer relations in children with a depressed caregiver. In R.D. Parke, G.W. Ladd, et al. (Eds.), *Family-peer relationships: Modes of linkage* (pp. 317–344). Hillsdale, N.J.: Erlbaum.

Zahn-Waxler, C., Iannotti, R.J., Cummings, E.M., & Denham, S. (1990). Antecedents of problem behaviors in children of depressed mothers. *Development and Psychopathology, 2,* 271–291.

Zuckerman, B.S., Bauchner, H., Parker, S., & Cabral, H. (1990). Maternal depressive symptoms during pregnancy and newborn irritability. *Developmental and Behavioral Pediatrics, 11,* 190–194.

NINETEEN

The Neurobiology of Child and Adolescent Depression

Current Knowledge and Future Directions

Joan Kaufman and Dennis Charney

Not much is known about neurodevelopmental factors involved in the pathophysiology of child and adolescent depression. Neuroendocrine and sleep EEG research paradigms have been used in the majority of published studies examining the neurobiological correlates of early-onset depression. Although these procedures have their merits, the "window to the brain" afforded by these methods is extremely limited. Emerging neuroimaging technologies will provide a unique opportunity to investigate the brain mechanisms underlying child and adolescent depression. To date, however, the application of these techniques in the study of early-onset depression is in its infancy.

The existence of major depressive disorder (MDD) in children and adolescents was controversial until relatively recently, and the diagnosis of MDD was not included in any child psychiatric text prior to the late 1970s (Puig-Antich & Gittleman, 1982). Research over the past two decades, however, has clearly demonstrated that children are capable of experiencing episodes of depression which meet standard *DSM-IV* (*Diagnostic and Statistical Manual of Mental Disorders*, 4th ed.) criteria for MDD (Birmaher et al., 1996c; Ryan et al., 1987). In addition, MDD in children and adolescents is common, recurrent, and associated with significant morbidity and mortality (Birmaher et al., 1996c). Epidemiological studies estimate that the prevalence of depression is 2 percent in children (Kashani et al., 1983) and 5–8 percent in adolescents (Lewinsohn, Clarke, Seeley & Rohde, 1994). Early-onset episodes of depression are associated with significant and persistent functional impairment (Puig-Antich et al., 1993), and within five years of the onset of MDD, 70 percent of clinically referred depressed children and adolescents will experience a recurrence (Kovacs et al., 1984; Rao et al., 1995). In addition, longitudinal follow-up studies estimate that as many as 5–10 percent of depressed adolescents will complete suicide within fifteen years of their initial episode of MDD (Rao, Weissman, Martin, & Hammond, 1993; Weissman et al., 1999).

Despite similarities in the clinical picture and longitudinal course of MDD in children, adolescents, and adults, there are notable differences in the neurobiological

The preparation of this manuscript was supported by the Connecticut and Massachusetts Mental Illness Research Clinical Center (MIRECC) which is funded by a grant from the U.S. Department of Veterans Affairs (Director: Bruce J. Rounsaville, M.D.).

correlates and treatment response of depressed patients in these different age cohorts that warrant careful consideration. Most notably, depressed children and adolescents do not show evidence of hypercortisolemia as is frequently reported in adults (Kaufman & Ryan, 1999; Ryan & Dahl, 1993), and depressed children and adolescents fail to respond to tricyclic antidepressants (Hazell, O'Connell, Heathcote, Robertson, & Henry, 1995; Keller et al., in press).

These and other findings reviewed in this chapter make it unclear whether or not child-, adolescent-, and adult-onset depression are the same or distinct disorders. In this chapter we review extant data on the neurobiological correlates and treatment response of depressed children and adolescents, and highlight differences in research findings across the lifecycle. Alternate explanations to account for the discrepancies are delineated, and clinical and preclinical studies that provide support for these alternate explanations are discussed. Directions for future research are outlined, with emphasis placed on the role of utilizing neuroimaging approaches. The application of these techniques, and the cross fertilization of clinical and basic research strategies will help to elucidate the neurodevelopmental processes involved in the pathophysiology of child and adolescent depression (Cicchetti & Cannon, 1999), and help to determine if child-, adolescent-, and adult-onset depression are one and the same disorder.

The data reviewed in this chapter are very consistent with the principles of developmental psychopathology emphasized throughout this text (Cicchetti & Rogosch, 1996). For example, the field of developmental psychopathology emphasizes the mutual interplay between normality and psychopathology. This concept is highlighted in the discussion of the constraints in our knowledge about the pathophysiology of early-onset affective disorders which is due to the limits in our understandings of the typical development of the neural substrates underlying the affective and cognitive processes that are disturbed in depressed children. The concept *equifinality* is delineated repeatedly as well, since there are multiple pathways to the etiology of child and adolescent depression. Multifinality is also stressed, as there are a range of outcomes associated with early-onset affective disorders (e.g., sustained recovery, recurrence, new onset bipolar disorder). Preliminary data suggest that the neurobiology of depression in children and adolescents with different etiological pathways and developmental trajectories is distinct. A central theme reiterated throughout this chapter is the concept of heterogeneity, with careful attention to the pathways to early onset affective disorders, and the outcomes of depressed children, recommended in attempting to uncover relevant subtypes of child- and adolescent-onset mood disorders, and the underlying pathophysiology associated with each.

NEUROBIOLOGICAL CORRELATES AND TREATMENT RESPONSE OF DEPRESSION ACROSS THE LIFECYCLE

Although there are significant differences in the neurobiological correlates and treatment response of depression in children, adolescents, and adults, there are also a few similarities. In this chapter, the similarities are discussed first, followed by a discussion of the discrepancies in research findings across the lifecycle. In some of the research where inconsistencies have been reported, children and adolescents differ from one another, and only one cohort is similar to adults, with the group similar

Table 19.1. HPA Axis Measures

Measure	Children		Adolescents		Adults	
	Finding	Replicability	Finding	Replicability	Finding	Replicability
DST (% Non-suppression)	50–70%	++	40–60%	++	50–70%	++
24-hour Basal Cortisol	Normal	++	Normal	++	Elevated	++
Nighttime Cortisol	Elevated	+/−	Elevated	+/−	Elevated	++
ACTH post-CRH	Normal	+	Normal	+	Blunted	++

Replicability Code:
+/− = Inconsistent findings reported
+ = One controlled study
++ = Replicated finding

to adults changing depending on the parameter under investigation. In other studies, children and adolescents are similar to each other, but both differ from adults. (For a more detailed review of the literature, readers are referred to Kaufman et al., 2001.)

Similar Findings Reported across the Lifecycle

Dexamethasone Suppression Test. The Dexamethasone Suppression Test (DST) has been more extensively studied in children and adolescents than any other psychobiological parameter. Dexamethasone is a synthetic substance like cortisol that has been used to investigate the integrity of feedback mechanisms in the Hypothalamic–Pituitary–Adrenal (HPA) axis. Administration of dexamethasone normally causes the HPA axis to shut down and cortisol levels to decrease markedly. DST nonsuppression suggests that the normal feedback mechanisms in place to shut off the HPA axis are deficient. Approximately 50–70 percent of adults with depression are considered DST nonsuppressors, and have elevated cortisol secretion after dexamethasone administration.

As reviewed by Dahl et al. (1992), there have been twenty-nine studies that conducted the DST in depressed children and adolescents. The results of these studies are summarized in Table 19.1. Half the studies were conducted with preadolescents, and the majority (79%) utilized inpatient samples. Approximately half of the published reports included twenty or more depressed children or adolescents, and a comparable number of controls. Averaging across studies, rates of nonsuppression were somewhat higher among children than adolescents, and about twice as high in subjects from inpatient settings than subjects from outpatient settings. An estimated 50–70 percent of depressed children and 40–60 percent of depressed adolescents were reported to be DST nonsuppressors. The rates of DST nonsuppression reported in these studies are more or less comparable to the rates reported in adult samples (APA, 1987; Carroll, 1982). Also consistent with the studies conducted in adults, higher rates of nonsuppression were reported in children and adolescents with endogenous symptoms

Table 19.2. Double-Blind Placebo-Controlled Clinical Trials

	Children		Adolescents		Adults	
	Finding	Replicability	Finding	Replicability	Finding	Replicability
SSRI Medications Fluoxetine	Effective	+	Effective	+	Effective	++
Paroxetine	–	–	Effective	+	Effective	++
TCA Medications Imipramine	Ineffective	++	Ineffective	++	Effective	++
Amitriptyline	Ineffective	+	Ineffective	++	Effective	++
Nortriptyline	Ineffective	+	Ineffective	+	Effective	++
Desipramine	–	–	Ineffective	++	Effective	++

Replicability Code:
+   = One controlled study
++ = Replicated finding

(Robbins, Alessi, Yanchyshyn, & Colfer, 1983), psychotic features (Freeman, Poznanski, Grossman, Buchsbaum, & Banegas, 1985), and a prior history of MDD (Klee & Garfinkel, 1984). In the one study that assayed dexamethasone levels (Birmaher et al., 1992), as expected, plasma dexamethasone levels correlated negatively with plasma cortisol levels. MDD and normal control subjects, however, did not differ in rates of dexamethasone metabolism.

Treatment with Selective Serotonin Reuptake Inhibitors. As mentioned in the introduction, tricyclic antidepressants (TCAs), which include the older antidepressant medications like imipramine, are no more effective than placebo in the treatment of child and adolescent depression (Keller et al., 2001). In contrast, selective serotonin reuptake inhibitors (SSRIs) preliminarily appear effective in this age cohort. Emslie and colleagues (1997) conducted a randomized, double-blind, placebo-controlled eight-week clinical trial of fluoxetine (e.g., Prozac) in ninety-six child and adolescent outpatients with nonpsychotic MDD. At the end of the study, using the intent to treat sample, significantly more patients who received fluoxetine were rated "much" or "very much" improved on the Clinical Global Impression Scale (56% versus 33%). After week five of treatment, there were also significant differences between the two groups on depression symptom severity ratings. The significant differences in depression severity ratings were maintained for each subsequent assessment point, with the gap between the two groups maximal at the conclusion of the study. In addition, equivalent response rates were found for patients twelve and younger ($N = 48$) and those thirteen and above ($N = 48$). These results are consistent with the findings of Keller and colleagues (2001) demonstrating efficacy of the SSRI paroxetine over placebo in the treatment of adolescent depression. (See Table 19.2 for a summary of double-blind pediatric placebo-controlled clinical trials.) As will be discussed further later in this chapter, there are differences in the mechanism of action of SSRI and TCA medications which may provide valuable insights into the underlying neurobiology of early onset depression (Guidotti & Costa, 1998).

Table 19.3. EEG Sleep Parameters

Measure	Children		Adolescents		Adults	
	Finding	Replicability	Finding	Replicability	Finding	Replicability
REM Latency	Normal	+/−	Decreased	++	Decreased	++
REM Density	Normal	++	Increased	+/−	Increased	++
Delta Sleep	Normal	++	Normal	++	Decreased	++

Replicability Code:
+/− = Inconsistent findings published
+ = One controlled study
++ = Replicated finding

Research Suggesting Children and Adolescents Differ from One Another

EEG Sleep. EEG sleep studies utilize electrodes to monitor changes in brain waves to assess various aspects of sleep architecture. EEG changes associated with MDD in adults are among the best-replicated findings in biological psychiatry (Reynolds, Gillen, & Kupfer, 1987). The most consistently reported sleep alterations include prolonged sleep latency, sleep continuity disturbances, reduced time until first rapid eye movement (REM) period, increased REM density, and decreased delta (Stage 3 and Stage 4) sleep. Alterations in EEG sleep measures consistent with findings reported in adults are more common in depressed adolescents than in depressed children, and more frequent in inpatient versus outpatient cohorts. As reviewed elsewhere (Kaufman & Ryan, 1999; Ryan & Dahl, 1993), six of the eight EEG sleep studies conducted with adolescents reported reduced REM latency, and four of the eight studies reported REM density differences (see Table 19.3). Of the studies conducted with children, only one reported REM latency differences and no other EEG sleep findings (Emslie, Rush, Weinberg, Rintelmann & Roffwarg, 1990). The remaining three studies conducted with this age group failed to detect differences between depressed and control children on any of the EEG sleep summary measures, despite inclusion of inpatients, ample sample size in two studies, and excellent methodology in all three studies (Dahl et al., 1991a; Puig-Antich et al., 1982; Young, Knowles, MacLean, Boag & McConville, 1982). As summarized in Table 19.3, no studies with children or adolescents have detected delta (Stage 3 and 4) sleep differences between depressed and control subjects.

Growth Hormone Probes. In contrast to the EEG sleep findings reviewed above, Growth Hormone (GH) probe studies with children have produced quite robust results similar to those reported in depressed adults, and predominantly negative results in studies with adolescents. Most studies with adolescents, however, had very small sample sizes, making conclusions in this area tentative. The results of studies examining GH probes in depressed children and adolescents are summarized in Table 19.4. When compared to normal controls, depressed children have been reported to have blunted GH response to clonidine (Jensen & Garfinkel, 1990; Meyer et al., 1991); insulin induced hypoglycemia (Meyer et al., 1991; Puig-Antich et al., 1984; Ryan et al., 1994); L-Dopa (Jensen & Garfinkel, 1990); and GH releasing hormone (Ryan et al., 1994).

Table 19.4. GH Response to Several Neuroendocrine Probes

Probe	Children		Adolescents		Adults	
	Finding	Replicability	Finding	Replicability	Finding	Replicability
Clonidine	Blunted	++	Normal	+	Blunted	++
ITT	Blunted	++	–	–	Blunted	++
L-Dopa	Blunted	++	Normal	+	Blunted	++
GHRH	Blunted	++	–	–	Blunted	+/−
Dextroamphetamine	–	–	Normal	+	Blunted	+
Desipramine	–	–	Blunted	+	Blunted	++

Replicability Code:
+/− = Inconsistent findings published
+   = One controlled study
++ = Replicated finding

In comparison, no overall group differences were found between depressed and control adolescents in GH secretion after administration of clonidine (Jensen & Garfinkel, 1990), L-Dopa (Jensen & Garfinkel, 1990), or Dextroamphetamine (Waterman et al., 1991). One study did report blunted GH secretion in adolescents after Desmethylimipramine administration; however, findings were restricted to depressed adolescents with suicide ideation and plan (Ryan et al., 1988).

Children and Adolescents Similar to Each Other – Both Differ from Adults

Basal Cortisol. Approximately one-half of depressed adults show evidence of cortisol hypersecretion (Schildkraut, Green, & Mooney, 1989). As stated above, classic cortisol hypersecretion as frequently reported in depressed adults is rare in depressed children and adolescents (see Table 19.1). To the extent that dysregulation of basal cortisol is found in subjects in this age range, it appears more subtle, and is manifest as alterations in the normal diurnal pattern of cortisol secretion. Rather than have increased twenty-four-hour cortisol secretion, depressed youngsters are more likely to only have elevated cortisol output close to the period of sleep onset, a time when the HPA axis is normally quiescent. Two studies examining cortisol secretion in depressed children failed to detect differences between depressed and normal control children on any of the summary measures of twenty-four-hour plasma cortisol samples, and hypercortisolemia was reported in less than 10 percent of the subjects (Birmaher et al., 1992; Puig-Antich et al., 1989a). In two other combined investigations of depressed children and adolescents that did not collect twenty-four-hour specimens, nighttime cortisol was reportedly increased in the depressed subjects (Goodyer et al., 1996; Kutcher et al., 1991). One other report similarly found increased cortisol secretion after sleep onset in depressed inpatient/suicidal adolescents, but no overall difference in twenty-four-hour mean cortisol secretion (Dahl et al., 1991b). This finding was not observed in another large study with predominantly outpatient adolescents (Dahl et al., 1989). Studies with adults with unipolar depression report a correlation between age and cortisol hypersecretion (Asnis et al., 1981; Halbreich, Asnis, Zumoff, Nathan & Shindledecker, 1984).

This may account for the observed differences in rates of hypercortisolemia in child, adolescent, and adult cohorts, but as discussed later, other factors may also contribute.

Corticotropin Releasing Hormone. The cortisol secretion abnormalities observed in depressed adults have been hypothesized to be due to alterations in endogenous Corticotropin Releasing Hormone (CRH) secretion (Gold et al., 1986; Plotsky, Owens, & Nemeroff, 1998). Consequently, several investigators have administered CRH to depressed patients. Adults with MDD have repeatedly been found to have elevated baseline cortisol and blunted ACTH secretion after CRH infusion (see Birmaher et al., 1996a for a review). In contrast, as summarized in Table 19.1, when CRH was administered to a cohort of thirty-four children with MDD and twenty-two normal controls, there were no overall group differences on any of the basal or post-CRH cortisol or ACTH measures (Birmaher et al., 1996a). Likewise, when CRH was administered to a group of twenty-one MDD and twenty normal control adolescents, no group differences were found on any measures (Dorn et al., 1996). Despite adequate sample size, these studies failed to replicate the pattern of results observed in adult depressed samples.

Serotonin Probes. Most studies using serotonergic probes in children (e.g., depressed and aggressive children) report findings that are opposite most studies conducted with adults. After administration of serotonin precursors and serotonin direct and indirect agonists, depressed adults have been reported to have blunted prolactin secretion, with post-challenge prolactin levels found to correlate negatively with dimensional measures of depression, aggression, and/or suicidality (Maes & Meltzer, 1995). In contrast, most studies conducted with either depressed or aggressive children report augmented prolactin secretion after serotonergic presynaptic probes in both diagnostic groups (e.g., fenfluramine, L-5-HTP), and a positive correlation between prolactin levels and dimensional clinical scales (Birmaher et al., 1997; Kaufman et al., 1998b; Pine et al., 1997; Ryan et al., 1992). In depressed adults, postsynaptic $5HT_{1B}$ serotonergic receptors have been hypothesized to be intact, given the absence of differences in prolactin secretion after m-Chlorophenylpiperazine (mCPP) administration (Anand et al., 1994). This finding in adults is likewise contradicted by a recent report of a small cohort of depressed adolescents who were found to have an augmented prolactin response after administration of the serotonergic postsynaptic probe mCPP (Ghaziuddin, King, Zaccagnini, & Weidmer-Mikhail, 1997). As one study with older adolescents did find depressed adolescents secreted significantly less prolactin after clorimpramine administration than age matched controls (Sallee et al., 1998), more work is needed to understand developmental influences on serotonergic indices. While children, adolescents, and adults all show evidence of serotonergic system dysregulation, the nature of these alterations appear to vary across the lifecycle. Available research studies conducted in depressed children and adolescents are summarized in Table 19.5.

Tricyclic Antidepressant Medications. Unlike in adults, tricyclic antidepressants (TCAs) do not appear effective for the treatment of depression in children and adolescents (Birmaher, Ryan, Williamson, Brent, & Kaufman, 1996b; Keller et al., in press). As indicated in Table 19.2, a number of placebo-controlled clinical trials in depressed children and adolescents failed to demonstrate efficacy of several different TCA medications, including imipramine, amitriptyline, desipramine, and nortriptyline.

Table 19.5. Prolactin Secretion After Serotonergic Probes

Probe	Children		Adolescents		Adults	
	Finding	Replicability	Finding	Replicability	Finding	Replicability
L-5HTP	Augmented	++	–	–	Blunted	++
MCPP	–	–	Augmented	+	Normal	+
Clomipramine	–	–	Blunted	+	Blunted	++

Replicability Code:
+ = One controlled study
++ = Replicated finding

Conclusions from the early TCA studies were limited due to small sample size (Martin, Kaufman, & Charney, 2000); however, a recent multi-site double-blind, placebo-controlled trial of 275 depressed outpatients 12–19 years of age randomized to paroxetine, imipramine, or placebo provides conclusive evidence regarding the inefficacy of TCA medications in this age cohort (Keller et al., 2001). Patients randomized to imipramine received comparable ratings as patients receiving placebo on all of the clinical outcome measures. In contrast, as mentioned earlier, paroxetine proved superior to placebo on measures of affect, global improvement, and remission of depressive symptoms. Given the accumulating negative evidence against the efficacy of TCAs in this age cohort, the increased reporting of adverse side effects with these medications, and the potential for lethality with overdose, TCA medications appear to be of questionable utility in the treatment of depression in children and adolescents.

Summary

Although there are some similarities in the neurobiological correlates and treatment response of depressed children, adolescents, and adults, the differences far outnumber the similarities. Both children and adolescents differ from depressed adults on measures of basal cortisol secretion, ACTH stimulation post-CRH infusion, response to several serotonergic probes, and efficacy of TCA medications. Given the consistent inconsistencies in research findings across the lifecycle, it seems reasonable to pose the question, "Are child-, adolescent-, and adult-onset depression one and the same disorder?"

REASONS FOR DISCREPANCIES IN RESEARCH FINDINGS ACROSS THE LIFECYCLE

There are many precedents in medicine in which earlier- and later-onset forms of disease represent illnesses with distinct neurobiological mechanisms, despite similarity in clinical picture (Childs & Scriver, 1986). A classic example is the comparison of juvenile to adult onset diabetes (Geller & Luby, 1997). While child-onset depression may be distinct from adult-onset depression, there are alternate plausible explanations for the discrepant findings in child, adolescent, and adult studies. The differences in the neurobiological correlates and treatment response of depressed patients across the lifecycle may be due to: (1) developmental factors; (2) stage of illness factors (e.g., number of episodes, total duration of illness); or (3) heterogeneity in clinical outcome (e.g., recurrent unipolar course vs. new onset bipolar disorder). These alternate explanations are discussed further in the remainder of this section.

Developmental Factors

Many of the neurobiological systems implicated in the pathophysiology of adult depression are not fully developed until adulthood. While the expression of serotonin, norepinephrine, and dopamine receptors occur very early in life and are highly synchronized across the cortex (Lidow & Rakic, 1992), the development of monoaminergic storage capacity and synthetic processes is more variable (Goldman-Rakic & Brown, 1982). Serotonin content and synthetic activity matures relatively early (Goldman-Rakic & Brown, 1982), with the adult pattern of serotonergic innervation to the prefrontal cortex achieved by approximately six months in primates (Kye, Woo & Lewis, 1996), or roughly five to six years in humans. In contrast, the development of norepinephrine and dopamine content and synthetic activity continues through puberty, with dopamine innervation to the prefrontal cortex not finalized until early adulthood (Rosenberg & Lewis, 1995).

The neuronal circuits that mediate the performance of various cognitive tasks have also been found to change and become more refined with development. For example, when the functioning of the dorsolateral prefrontal cortex was experimentally temporarily interrupted through the use of reversible cyrogenic inhibition (e.g., cooling), no notable changes in a delayed response performance memory task were reported in primates 18 months or younger, mild deficits (8%) were noted in monkeys 19–31 months of age, and significant (22%) deficits were noted in postpubertal monkeys 34–36 months of age (Alexander & Goldman, 1978). These findings suggest that the dorsolateral prefrontal cortex is central in mediating the performance of delayed response memory tasks in mature, but not young, non-human primates (Alexander & Goldman, 1978). Consistent with this pre-clinical work, recent developmental neuroimaging studies examining cortical activity during memory tasks report greater and more diffuse activation in the prefrontal region in children relative to adults (Casey, Giedd, & Thomas, 2000). At younger ages, connections from a wider range of prefrontal brain regions are utilized in the performance of delayed memory tasks. With development, there appears to be refinement of the circuits that mediate memory performance, and increased specialization of the dorsolateral prefrontal cortex for the performance of this type of cognitive task.

Interestingly, deficits in the performance of delayed memory tasks have been repeatedly reported in adult depressed cohorts, especially among older patients with recurrent episodes of illness (Sweeney, Strojwas, Mann, & Thase, 1998). Adults with depression have also been found to have reduced structure and function in the dorsolateral prefronal cortex in neuroimaging studies (Drevets, Gadde, & Krishnan, 1999). In contrast, depressed children do not appear to have difficulties in the performance of delayed memory tasks. While there is a need for more work in this area, preliminary data suggest that deficits in visual-spatial reasoning are more prominent than memory deficits in youngsters with depression (Frost, Moffitt, & McGee, 1989; McClure, Rogeness, & Thompson, 1997; McGee, Anderson, Williams, & Silva, 1986). Neuroimaging studies have yet to examine the structure and function of the dorsolateral prefrontal cortex in pediatric depressed cohorts. Studies that assess oculomotor basal ganglia-thalamocortical circuits that mediate the performance of visual-spatial reasoning tasks, as opposed to dorsolateral and other prefrontal cortical circuits utilized in delayed memory paradigms, may be more fruitful in neuroimaging studies of early onset depression (Alexander, DeLong, & Strick, 1986). If there are true differences in neuropsychological correlates of depression in juvenile and adult samples, and the differences reflect true differences in affected underlying neuronal pathways, the examination of both types of tasks in functional neuroimaging studies in children, adolescents, and adults could provide valuable insights into potential developmental changes in the neural circuits that mediate depression across the lifecycle.

Stage of Illness Factors

Based on findings from preclinical studies, it has been hypothesized that the biological correlates and treatment response of patients with recurrent episodes of depression may differ from patients with a single episode of MDD (Post, 1992). Through kindling mechanisms, and stress-induced neurotoxicity and alterations in neurotrophic factors, recurrent episodes of depression may enhance neurobiologic alterations associated with depression (for further discussion of these mechanisms, see the following authors: Duman & Charney, 1999; Kupfer, 1991; Post, 1992). In accordance with these assertions, hippocampal volume reductions are significantly more common in adult depressed patients with recurrent episodes of disorder than patients with single episodes of MDD, with degree of hippocampal atrophy found to correlate significantly with lifetime duration of depressive illness (Sheline, Wang, Gado, Csernansky, & Vannier, 1996). Given the demonstrated importance of stage of illness on hippocampal volume measures, it is not surprising that the one study that examined hippocampal volume in children and adolescents with Posttraumatic Stress Disorder ($N = 43$), about half of whom met criteria for comorbid MDD, failed to find evidence of hippocampal atrophy (De Bellis et al., 1999). Developmental factors are likely also relevant, however, as preclinical studies have found age dependent changes in sensitivity to NMDA receptor blockade neurotoxicity in corticolimbic regions, with cell death minimal or absent in childhood, and reaching peak in early adulthood (Farber et al., 1995).

As most children and adolescents who participated in the studies reviewed in this chapter only had one episode of depression, differences from adult studies may be attributable to differences in the proportion of patients with recurrent episodes of disorder included in the investigations. Consistent with this hypothesis, adults with recurrent depression are more likely to have EEG sleep alterations than adults experiencing a first episode of depression (Thase et al., 1995). There is also some evidence to suggest that HPA axis alterations may be more likely in depressed children with recurrent illness than in depressed children experiencing their first episode (Klee & Garfinkel, 1984). In addition, when post-hoc analyses were conducted in one study comparing prolactin values after serotonergic challenge in depressed children with and without a prior history of MDD, similar to findings in adults, children with recurrent depression secreted significantly less prolactin than children with single episodes of disorder (Birmaher et al., 1997). Therefore, differences in the neurobiological correlates of depression across the lifecycle may reflect course of illness factors – and not fundamental differences in the pathophysiology of the disorder. Careful classification of patients by stage of illness (e.g., first episode vs. recurrent), and repeat longitudinal neurobiological assessments after a recurrence will help to resolve this question.

Heterogeneity in Clinical Outcome

Given the protracted period of risk for the development of affective disorders, studies with child and adolescent probands have a high likelihood of including subjects who will change their group status over time. For example, although not reported in all studies (Weissman et al., 1999), several studies have reported that as many 20–40 percent of children and adolescents with depression experience a manic episode within five years of their initial episode of MDD (Rao et al., 1996; Strober, Lampert, Schmidt, & Morrell, 1993). In one longitudinal follow-up study of depressed adolescents who completed a comprehensive psychobiological protocol during their index episode of depression (Rao et al., 1996), differences between depressed and normal control subjects on measures of basal cortisol secretion were only evident after removal of subjects who switched to Bipolar Disorder. Utilization of the longitudinal clinical course data was essential in "cleaning" the Time 1 biological data.

Children and adolescents who serve as "normal" controls in studies of the neurobiological correlates of early onset depression may also switch group status over time. In the longitudinal study referenced above, 23 percent of the "normal" controls had an episode of MDD during the seven-year interval follow-up (Rao et al., 1996). These subjects likewise differed from "true normal controls" on several of the Time 1 psychobiological measures. For example, controls who developed depression over the follow-up interval had significantly higher REM density and a trend toward reduced REM latency when compared to controls with no disorder at follow-up. In high-risk studies, youngsters at risk for MDD have also been found to have biological alterations similar to depressed children prior to the onset of any affective disorder. Like depressed children, when compared to low-risk normal controls, high-risk children have been found to have augmented prolactin secretion after L-5-HTP administration and blunted growth hormone secretion after GHRH administration (Birmaher et al., 2000). Given the protracted period of risk for the onset of depression, studies that failed to utilize normal controls at low familial risk for affective disorder may have obscured group differences in neurobiological studies with child and adolescent probands. These findings highlight the need for careful characterization of normal controls, and the importance of longitudinal follow-up data to "clean" Time 1 psychobiological measures.

Summary

As discussed in this section, differences in the neurobiological correlates and treatment response of depressed patients across the lifecycle may be due to: (1) developmental factors; (2) stage of illness factors (e.g., number of episodes, total duration of illness); or (3) heterogeneity in clinical outcome (e.g., recurrent unipolar course vs. new onset bipolar disorder). There is compelling evidence to support each of these possibilities. Unfortunately, available data preclude definitive conclusions regarding the merits of these alternate hypotheses. Further systematic research will be required to determine if child-, adolescent-, and adult-onset depression are one and the same disorder.

DIRECTIONS FOR FUTURE RESEARCH

The pattern of findings observed in the neruobiological correlates and treatment re-sponse of depressed children, adolescents, and adults is not entirely consistent nor easily understood (e.g., DST nonsuppression, normal basal cortisol secretion, normal ACTH post-CRH infusion). The incorporation of neuroimaging measures in neurobio-logical studies of early-onset affective disorders will allow for more direct examinations of similarities, differences, and potential developmental changes in the neural circuits implicated in the pathophysiology of depression across the lifecycle. As stated previ-ously, most studies of the neurobiological correlates of early-onset depression have uti-lized neuroendocrine paradigms. Although these methods have their merits, especially for the study of the Hypothalamic–Pituitary–Adrenal axis stress system, the "window to the brain" afforded by these methods is extremely limited. To determine if child-, adolescent-, and adult-onset depression are one and the same disorder, we recommend: (1) utilizing the same neuroimaging paradigms in child, adolescent, and adult depressed cohorts; (2) carefully characterizing subjects' stage of illness; and (3) conducting longi-tudinal clinical and repeat neurobiological assessments of patients of different ages at various stages of illness.

Important foci for future research in early-onset affective disorders are discussed in the remainder of this section. The first two sections discuss research methods that have not been applied, or only little applied to the study of early-onset affective disorders (e.g., neuroimaging, genetics). The next two parts discuss factors affecting heterogeneity in depressed cohorts (e.g., family history of psychiatric illness, life events, and traumatic experiences), and the last section discusses gender influences on depression.

Central Measures of Brain Function

As stated in the introduction, the development of new, noninvasive imaging techniques afford a unique opportunity to investigate the brain mechanisms underlying child- and adolescent-onset depression. The methods typically considered "noninvasive" include structural and functional Magnetic Resonance Imaging (MRI), Magnetic Resonance Spectroscopy (MRS), and Diffusion Tensor Imaging (DTI), as these methods do not require the injection of radioactive tracers and have no known adverse side effects. The application of these procedures in children and adolescents with unipolar depression is in its infancy, however, with only a few published reports and abstracts of imaging studies produced to date.

Structural MRI studies are easily accomplished in pediatric populations (Rosenberg et al., 1997), and permit the identification of neuroanatomical variations associated with early onset MDD. Steingard and colleagues (Steingard et al., 1996) conducted the only published report of structural MRI in children and adolescents with depressive disorders (e.g., major depression and dysthymia). Children with depressive disorders were found to have reduced frontal lobe/cerebral volume ratios and increased lateral ventrical/cerebral volume ratios when compared to psychiatric control subjects. The finding of reduced frontal lobe volume is consistent with results of studies conducted with adults, but lateral ventrical enlargement has not typically been reported in non-delusional mid-life depression (Drevets et al., 1999). These findings need to be replicated and future studies extended to include normal control comparison subjects and the examination of more refined subregions of the frontal lobes. In particular, given repli-cated MRI and Positron Emission Tomography (PET) studies showing reduced structure and function in the dorsolateral (Brodamanns area 9) region of the prefronal cortex, this region needs to be examined in child and adolescent cohorts.

In depressed adults, in the subgenual prefrontal cortex (e.g., Brodmanns area 24), an area ventral to the genu of the corpus callosum and sometimes referred to as the anterior cingulate, gray matter volume reductions as high as 40 percent have also been reported (Drevets et al., 1997). Preliminary yet to be published structural MRI work under way at Washington University in adolescent twins with adolescent or earlier onset MDD suggest subgenual prefrontal cortex/anterior cingulate volume is similarly reduced in early-onset depression (Botteron, Raichle, Heath, & Todd, 1999). In addition, the volume reduction appears to represent a "scar" marker, as it is observed in identical twins with a history of MDD, but not present in co-twins without a history of affec-tive illness. In adults, increased blood flow in the subgenual cingulate (Broadmanns area 25) has also been reported in normal controls during experimentally induced transient sadness and in depressed patients during episodes of illness (Mayberg et al., 1997).

Depressed adults have also been reported to have reductions in amygdala volume (Sheline, Gado, & Price, 1998). Preliminary results from the ongoing twin study cited above suggest that adolescent twins with adolescent or earlier onset MDD similarly have reduced amygdala volume (Botteron et al., 1999). Interestingly, the volume reduction in this region appears to represent a potential putative "risk" marker, and was observed in identical twins with a history of MDD, *and* in co-twins without a history of affective illness. Longitudinal follow-up of this cohort will be very informative in determining the predictive significance of this marker over time.

Hippocampal volume assessments have not been obtained in children and ado-lescents with primary affective disorders. As mentioned previously, no hippocampal volume reductions were reported in a study of children and adolescents with PTSD, half who had comorbid MDD (De Bellis et al., 1999). Reduction in hippocampal vol-ume has been reported in several (Bremner et al., 2000; Shah et al., 1998; Sheline et al., 1996; Mervaala et al., 2000), but not all studies of adults with depression (Axelson et al., 1993; Hauser et al., 1989; Vakili et al., 2000). In two of the positive studies, degree of hippocampal atrophy was found to correlate with total duration of illness (Bremner et al., 2000; Sheline et al., 1996). This raises questions as to whether these changes rep-resent primary disturbances associated with the onset of disorder, or secondary brain changes related to recurrence and extended glucocorticoid exposure. There may be some structural abnormalities associated with depression in adults which represent pri-mary disturbances and are evident across the lifecycle (e.g., frontal lobe; amygdala), and others (e.g., hippocampal atrophy) which are only evident later in development or secondary to biological alterations (e.g., excess cortisol) associated with persistence and recurrence of disorder. More research is needed in this area.

Preclinical studies have shown that the dorsolateral prefrontal cortex, the cingulate, and other subcortical structures including the hippocampus are functionally linked. The subgenual cingulate projects directly to the dorsolateral prefrontal cortex, and there are many bidirectional indirect pathways between these structures through sev-eral different limbic and paralimbic nodes including the hippocampus, posterior cin-gulate, and anterior insula. The importance of these regions in mediating mood and attention and emotional homeostasis has been implicated in multiple neuroimaging studies with depressed (Baxter et al., 1989; Bench et al., 1992; Mayberg et al., 1999) and normal control (George et al., 1995; Lane, Reiman, Ahern, Schwartz, & Davidson, 1997; Mayberg et al., 1999) adults. The relevance of these neural circuits in child- and adolescent-onset depression has yet to be established and will require utilization of functional neuroimaging techniques.

Functional MRI (fMRI) studies permit the identification of the different regions in the brain that are utilized in processing different types of information or solving various types of problems. There is one ongoing investigation of functional MRI in depressed children and adolescents. Consistent with the structural MRI findings reported above (Botteron et al., 1999), preliminary reports from this study suggest depressed adolescents have reduced amygdala activation when processing fearful and neutral faces compared to adolescents with anxiety disorders and normal controls (Thomas et al., 2001). Therefore, both structural and functional abnormalities have been reported in the amygdala in association with early-onset MDD.

In addition to structural and functional MRI methodology, Magnetic Resonance Spectroscopy (MRS) is another noninvasive imaging technique that warrants further application in studies of child and adolescent depression. MRS allows for the direct monitoring of brain neurochemistry, and can be used to quantify steady-state metabolic levels of neurotransmitters such as glutamate-amino acid butyric acid (GABA), and compounds involved in membrane phospholipid metabolism. In a recent abstract, Steingard and colleagues (Steingard & Renshaw, 1996) reported that depressed adolescents had a trend toward reduced N-acetyl-L-aspartate (NAA) to creatine and phosphocreatine (CR) ratios in the orbitofronal cortex when compared to normal controls (Brodmanns area 47). As NAA is thought to arise largely from neurons, the preliminary data reported by Steingard and colleagues suggest the possibility that abnormal development of the orbitofrontal cortex may be associated with early-onset depression. In studies with adults, abnormalities of the orbitofrontal cortex appear to be linked to serotonergic processes. Adults with depression have been found to have reduced serotonergic receptor binding in the orbitofronal cortex (Biver et al., 1997), and recovered depressed adult patients that experience a relapse in symptoms after experimentally induced depletion of tryptophan, the amino acid that is the precursor to serotonin, show decreased metabolism in this region as well (Bremner et al., 1997). In addition, in a recent postmortem study of adult depressed patients (Rajkowska et al., 1999), cortical thickness was found to be significantly reduced in the rostral orbitofrontal cortex (Brodmanns areas 10 and 47). The reduced cortical volume was associated with a reduction in the size of the largest class of neurons located in supragranular layers, and an increase in density of small neurons found in this area. Consistent with the data discussed above, primate studies have found that the neurons in this region are targets of serotonergic input. The overall smaller neuronal size in this cortical region was attributed to neuronal shrinkage or a developmental deficiency, rather than neuronal loss by the authors of the study. If neuronal loss had occurred, density of large neurons would have been decreased without associated increases in the density of small neurons (Rajkowska et al., 1999). Additional MRS studies examining phospholipid metabolism, structural MRI studies, and postmortem studies in child and adolescent depression will help to determine the potential relevance of the orbitofrontal cortex in the pathophysiology of early-onset depression.

The use of MRS technology to examine GABA is also of interest in the study of child and adolescent depression given: emerging conceptualizations of the role of GABA in mood disorders (Petty, 1995); a report documenting reduced plasma GABA in a subset of depressed children and adolescents (Prosser et al., 1997); a recent MRS study demonstrating reduced cortical GABA in depressed adults (Sanacora et al., 1999); and new insights into the unique mechanism of action of SSRI medications (Guidotti & Costa, 1998). While both TCA and SSRI medications enhance serotonergic transmission and reduce glutamate N-methyl-D-aspartate (NMDA) glutamate receptor function (Kilts, 1994), amelioration of depressive symptoms with SSRI treatment is uniquely correlated with increases in the neurosteroid 3-alpha, 5-alpha, tetrahydroprogesterone (ALLO). ALLO binds with high affinity to GABA receptors, and potently facilitates GABA transmission at these sites (Gambarana, Ghiglieri, & Graziella de Montis, 1995). In contrast, Imipramine and other TCA agents that are ineffective in child- and adolescent-onset depression do not promote changes in brain ALLO or GABA transmission. The use of MRS methodology to study glutamate in early-onset depression is warranted as well, as preclinical studies with glutamatergic agents produce animals with the two most prominent characteristics of patients with early-onset depression: animals with learned helplessness which is nonresponsive to TCA treatments (Petty, McChesney, & Kramer, 1985), and animals who display "depression-like" behaviors in the absence of hypercortisolemia (Biagini et al., 1993).

Diffusion Tensor Imaging (DTI) is another noninvasive neuroimaging methodology that permits the evaluation of the integrity of white matter tracts – axonal pathways (Pierpaoli, Jezzard, Basser, Barnett, & Di Chiro, 1996). The use of DTI may be of special interest in studies designed to investigate the neurobiology of affective disorders in children with a history of significant trauma. Preclinical research examining the effects of early stress in *mature* animals, and clinical studies of *adults* with Postraumatic Stress Disorder, suggest that stress early in life is associated with changes in the Hypothalamic–Pituitary–Adrenal (HPA) axis, central Corticotropin Releasing Hormone (CRH) system, and the hippocampus, a brain structure vulnerable to the neurotoxic effects of stress-induced elevations in circulating glucocorticoids (e.g., cortisol) and amino acids (e.g., glutamate).

Emerging evidence in human and nonhuman primates suggests that the neurobiological changes associated with early stress may vary at different developmental periods. HPA axis changes are not especially robust in juvenile samples, and contradictory findings have been reported (Kaufman & Charney, 1999). In addition, early stress may not be associated with the same pattern of brain changes in adult and juvenile samples. To the best of our knowledge, there is only one published structural MRI study in *prepubescent* nonhuman primates subjected to early stress, and the one previously cited published structural MRI study in maltreated children and adolescents with PTSD (De Bellis et al., 1999; Sanchez, Hearn, Do, Rilling, & Herndon, 1998). Neither study reported hippocampal atrophy. Both studies, however, reported reductions in the medial and caudal portions of the midbody of the corpus callosum.

The corpus callosum contains the majority of inter-hemispheric axonal projections in the brain. The medial and caudal portions of the midbody of the corpus callosum contains inter-hemispheric projections from the auditory cortices, posterior cingulate, retrospenial cortex, insula, and somatosensory and visual cortices to a lesser extent. It also includes connections from the inferior parietal lobe to the contralateral inferior

for such signaling molecules, and have been proposed to play a central role in a variety of forms of synaptic plasticity. Consistent with this hypothesis: neurotrophins have been found to be present in sites of CNS development and adult plasticity; neurotrophin expression and secretion is activity dependent; and neurotrophins have been found to regulate aspects of neuronal function that change activity in neural circuits, including synaptic function, membrane excitability, neuronal morphology, and neuronal connectivity (McAllister et al., 1999). Recent studies have also demonstrated that antidepressant medications promote the expression of the neurotrophin brain-derived neurotrophic factor (BDNF) in certain populations of neurons in the hippocampus and cerebral cortex (Duman, Heninger, & Nestler, 1997). The importance of these changes is highlighted by the discovery that stress can decrease the expression of BDNF and lead to atrophy in these same stress-vulnerable hippocampal neurons. These findings lead to a molecular and cellular hypothesis of depression that posits stress-induced vulnerability to depression is mediated by intracellular mechanisms that decrease neurotrophic factors necessary for the survival and optimal function of particular neurons in key circuits implicated in the pathophysiology of depression (Duman et al., 1997). Genes encoding and regulating neurotrophic factors may be important candidates to study in future genetic investigations of affective disorders in children, adolescents, and adults.

The research potentials afforded by the Human Genome and Brain Molecular Anatomy projects, as well as some of the emerging technologies discussed in the next section, are profound. As recently discussed by Watson and Akil (1999), there will be many challenges in defining the genes involved in depression and other psychiatric disorders, elucidating their functions, and understanding their interactions with developmental and environmental factors. Through collaborations among geneticists, neurobiologists, and clinicians, however, much progress in understanding the pathophysiology of these disorders is possible.

Life Events and Early Childhood Trauma

While genetic and environmental factors have traditionally been conceptualized as independent contributors to the etiology of depression, twin studies have highlighted the interdependence of these factors. Specifically, twin studies with adult and adolescent probands suggest genetic factors influence: (1) risk of exposure to traumatic events; and (2) sensitivity to the negative impact of environmental stressors (Kendler, 1998; Kendler et al., 1995; Silberg et al., 1999). In accordance with these data, several studies have demonstrated that depressed children and adolescents are significantly more likely than controls to have experienced adverse life events in the year preceding the onset of their depression (Goodyer, Herbert, Tamplin, Secher, & Pearson, 1997; Williamson et al., 1998). Nevertheless, not all depressed children and adolescents have a history of significant life stressors.

There are preliminary data to suggest that children and adolescents who develop depression independent of a history of adversity may differ significantly on a number of parameters than those who develop depression in the context of such experiences. For example, depressed abused and depressed nonabused children have been found to differ on a number of neurobiological indices. Specifically, consistent with preclinical studies examining the impact of early adverse rearing conditions on serotonergic function (Kraemer, 1992), depressed abused children have been found to secrete significantly more prolactin after L-5-HTP administration than depressed nonabused children (Kaufman et al., 1998b). In addition, while HPA axis alterations are rare in nontraumatized depressed children, they have been reported in several studies of depressed abused children (Hart, Gunner, & Cicchetti, 1996; Kaufman, 1991; Kaufman et al., 1997).

In addition to differing on numerous neurobiological parameters, depressed abused and depressed nonabused children have also been found to have different patterns of psychiatric disorders among their first-degree relatives (Kaufman et al., 1998a). When compared to controls, both depressed abused and depressed nonabused children have significantly elevated rates of depression in their first-degree relatives, with more than 50 percent of the first-degree relatives of both depressed cohorts having a lifetime history of MDD. The relatives of the depressed abused children, however, also have elevated rates of alcoholism and antisocial personality disorder. In fact, 77 percent of the depressed abused children had relatives with Depressive Spectrum Disorders. In contrast, 62 percent of the depressed nonabused children met Winokur's (1982) criteria for Familial Pure Depressive Disorder subtype. The relatives of the nonabused depressed children were also significantly more likely to meet criteria for non-PTSD anxiety disorders. This finding is also of significant interest, as Weissman and colleagues (1984) found offspring of depressed patients with comorbid anxiety (e.g., Panic) disorders to be two times more likely to develop child onset depression than offspring of depressed patients without anxiety disorders. While both depressed abused and depressed nonabused children have high familial loading of depression, the pattern of psychiatric illness in the relatives of these two groups of children suggest a different underlying vulnerability to depression in the two cohorts. These studies highlight the need for further systematic examination of familial/genetic and experiential factors in studies of the neurobiological correlates and treatment of early-onset depression.

Preclinical studies will help to identify the mechanisms by which experiential factors (e.g., stress) confer vulnerability to depression, and examine genetic factors that effect sensitivity to these experiences. For example, chronic stress has been found to decrease $5HT_{1A}$ receptor number and binding in the hippocampus, and produce changes in mineralocorticoid and glucocorticoid receptor ratios in this same region (Lopez, Chalmers, Little, & Watson, 1998). Examination of this sort of animal model of depression in mice strains with high versus low behavioral responses to stress will allow for an examination of differences in the expression of genes due to inherent differences between the high stress and low stress breeds, and differences resulting from the stress and nonstress experimental conditions. Candidate genes of interest to examine mRNAs for would include corticotropin releasing hormone, glucocorticoid receptors, 5HT receptors, and other genes known to be involved in the stress response (Watson & Akil, 1999).

Evolving methodologies, such as gene chips and complimentary DNA (cDNA) clones derived from the expressed sequence tag (EST) data base developed as part of the Human Genome Project, will allow for the simultaneous study of thousands of genes or mRNAs involved in the complex genetics of depression and other brain disorders (Watson & Akil, 1999). Currently, in conducting the stress reactivity experiment described above, 5–10 genes could be examined. The evolving technologies of gene chips that contain 10,000 or more oligonucleiotides of 10 to 20 nuceotides per chip can be used to scan thousands of genes simultaneously. ESTs are fragments of DNA sequences several hundred nucleotides in length that represent sequences that are complementary to stretches of the genome which encode mRNA and are eventually translated into proteins. The EST/cDNA arrays similarly allow for the simultaneous examination of thousands of potentially relevant genes. These evolving technologies when used in animal studies with various developmental manipulations will provide very powerful tools for unraveling the genetic and developmental factors that influence the pathophysiology of child and adolescent depression, and the interaction of environmental factors.

Gender Influences on Depression

Among pre-adolescents, MDD occurs at approximately the same rate in boys and girls. With the onset of adolescence, the gender ratio of depression shifts to 2:1. Paralleling the gender distribution of depression observed in adult cohorts, female adolescents are approximately two times more likely to develop depression than male adolescents (Angold, Costello, & Worthman, 1998; Birmaher et al., 1996c). Although the shift in gender distribution of depression that occurs in adolescence appears to be linked to changes in pubertal status, more research is needed to understand the mechanisms responsible for this shift, and the overall 2–3-fold increased rate of depression that occurs in adolescence.

Oxytocin is one neurohormone hypothesized to influence the shift in the gender distribution of depression that occurs with the onset of puberty (Cyranowski, Frank, Young, & Shear, 2000), but currently there are no data examining this. The relationship between sex steroid levels and depressed mood has been examined in several investigations of normal adolescents, but no studies of depressed teenagers. In nonclinical samples of adolescents, low testosterone has been associated with higher ratings of sad affect in boys (Susman et al., 1987). Interestingly, in depressed men with low basal testosterone secretion, testosterone replacement therapy in an open clinical trial was found to be an effective augmentation treatment for SSRI refractory MDD (Seidman & Rabkin, 1998). Within normal samples of girls, the rapid increase of estradiol that corresponds with puberty onset has also been associated with higher ratings of depression (Warren & Brooks-Gunn, 1989). Investigations with adult women have not consistently reported abnormal circulating levels of estrogen in association with Premenstrual Mood Syndrome (PMS); however, several studies suggest a role of gonadal steroids in precipitating symptoms of PMS (Rubinow, Schmidt, & Roca, 1998).

Little data exist on PMS in adolescence. Studies with normal adolescents suggest that close to 90 percent of female adolescents experience at least one PMS symptom of moderate or greater severity (Cleckner-Smith, Doughty, & Grossman, 1998; Fisher, Trieller, & Napolitano, 1989). In normal adolescents, physical PMS symptoms are associated with greater ratings of emotional distress (Freeman, Rickels, & Sondheimer, 1993), and in a study of normal health and development, it was estimated that up to 14 percent of female adolescents met diagnostic criteria for PMS (Raja et al., 1992).

PMS has not been systematically evaluated in most clinical or neurobiological research studies with depressed adolescents. The role of sex steroids in the pathophysiology of early-onset affective disorders warrants further investigation given the data reviewed in this section, and preclinical studies which suggest a role for sex steroids in mediating serotonergic functioning and stress reactivity. Both testosterone and estrogen influence multiple parameters of serotonergic tone (Rubinow et al., 1998; Simon, Cologer-Clifford, Lu, McKenna, & Hu, 1998). Sex steroids also effect gene expression of hypothalamic CRH and hipppocampal and hypothalamic glucocorticoid receptor mRNA levels (Patchev & Almeida, 1998). Consequently, it has been suggested that better understanding of gender differences in neuroendocrine response to stress will enhance understanding of the development of disorders like depression which have a higher prevalence in women (Jezova, Jurankova, Mosnarova, Kriska, & Skultetyova, 1996). Focused preclinical work in this area will help to refine hypotheses on the role of sex steroids in the pathophysiology of early-onset depression, and attainment of sex steroid measures in clinical studies may help to delineate gender influences on the pathophysiology of depression.

Summary

This section reviewed a range of research strategies to be used to unravel the neurodevelopmental factors and processes that promote the development of depression in children and adolescents. A key theme reiterated throughout the section is the concept of heterogeneity – heterogeneity in pathways to the etiology of depression, and heterogeneity in the outcome of children with depression. If the onset of depressive symptoms appears independent of any life stressors, within the context of a history of child maltreatment, or in association with the onset of the menstrual cycle, the underlying pathophysiology is apt to be different. Likewise, the neurobiology of depression in children with single episodes of disorder, a recurrent course of illness, or a switch to bipolar disorder preliminarily appears to be distinct. Familial loading for psychopathology and depressive subtypes are also important factors to consider in future studies. The utilization of neuroimaging and genetic research approaches with carefully characterized samples will help to unravel the neuroanatomical structures and circuits implicated in the etiology of early-onset MDD. This work must proceed, however, in close association with normal developmental studies, as the neural circuits that mediate the control of affect at different developmental stages is poorly understood. The longitudinal follow-up of high risk and clinical populations will also help to identify primary disturbances associated with the onset of disorder, and secondary alterations associated with recurrence and/or persistence of depressive symptomatology.

The mechanisms responsible for the development of depression may change with age. While those who study adult depression have developed cogent theories of potential mechanisms responsible for the etiology of depression, like those of Nemeroff and colleagues which focuses on alterations in the stress hormone CRH (Heim, Owens, Plotsky, & Nemeroff, 1997), the application of these theories is apt to be limited in early-onset affective illness. Given the relative absence of HPA axis and hippocampal volume changes in juvenile depressed samples, and emerging data focusing on other structures such as the amygdala in nontraumatized populations, and the corpus callosum in those with a history of significant early adversity, alternate theories are required to explain the pathophysiology of early-onset mood disorders. The research will require an iterative process, and will benefit greatly from a strong cross-fertilization between developmental, basic, and clinical research approaches.

CONCLUSION

Depression in children and adolescents is common, recurrent, and associated with significant morbidity and mortality. Over the past fifteen years we have learned that we cannot extrapolate down from what we know about depression in adults. There are many differences in the neurobiological correlates and treatment response of depressed children, adolescents, and adults. Systematic longitudinal research that carefully accounts for developmental, stage of illness, familial, and experiential factors is required to understand the pathophysiology of depression across the lifecycle. The application of multidisciplinary research approaches will help to elucidate the neurodevelopmental processes involved in the pathophysiology of child and adolescent depression, and help to determine if child-, adolescent-, and adult-onset depression are one and the same disorder.

REFERENCES

Alexander, G. E., DeLong, M. R., & Strick, P. L. (1986). Parallel organization of functionally segregated circuits linking basal ganglia and cortex. *Annu Rev Neurosci, 9,* 357–381.

Alexander, G. E., & Goldman, P. S. (1978). Functional development of the dorsolateral prefrontal cortex: an analysis utlizing reversible cryogenic depression. *Brain Res, 143*(2), 233–249.

Anand, A., Charney, D. S., Delgado, P. L., McDougle, C. J., Heninger, G. R., & Price, L. H. (1994). Neuroendocrine and behavioral responses to intravenous m-chlorophenylpiperazine (mCPP) in depressed patients and healthy comparison subjects [see comments]. *Am J Psychiatry, 151*(11), 1626–1630.

Angold, A., Costello, E. J., & Worthman, C. M. (1998). Puberty and depression: the roles of age, pubertal status and pubertal timing. *Psychol Med, 28*(1), 51–61.

Angst, J., & Merikangas, K. (1997). The depressive spectrum: diagnostic classification and course. *J Affect Disord, 45*(1–2), 31–39; discussion 39–40.

APA. (1987). The dexamethasone suppression test: an overview of its current status in psychiatry. The APA Task Force on Laboratory Tests in Psychiatry. *Am J Psychiatry, 144*(10), 1253–1262.

Asnis, G. M., Sachar, E. J., Halbreich, U., Nathan, R. S., Novacenko, H., & Ostrow, L. C. (1981). Cortisol secretion in relation to age in major depression. *Psychosom Med, 43*(3), 235–242.

Axelson, D. A., Doraiswamy, P. M., McDonald, W. M., Boyko, O. B., Tupler, L. A., Patterson, L. J., Nemeroff, C. B., Ellinwood, Jr., E. H., & Krishnan, K. R. (1993). Hypercortisolemia and hippocampal changes in depression. *Psychiatry Res, 47,* 163–173.

Baxter, L. R., Schwartz, J. M., Phelps, M. E., Mazziotta, J. C., Guze, B. M., Selin, C. E., Gerner, R., & Sumida, R. (1989). Reduction of prefrontal cortex glucose metabolism common to three types of depression. *Arch Gen Psychiatry, 46,* 243–250.

Bench, C., Friston, K., Brown, R., Scott, L., Frackowiak, R., & Dolan, R. (1992). The anatomy of meloncholia-focal abnormalities of cerebral blood flow in major depression. *Psychological Medicine, 22,* 607–615.

Biagini, G., Pich, E. M., Carani, C., Marrama, P., Gustafsson, J. A., Fuxe, K., & Agnati, L. F. (1993). Indole-pyruvic acid, a tryptophan ketoanalogue, antagonizes the endocrine but not the behavioral effects of repeated stress in a model of depression. *Biol Psychiatry, 33*(10), 712–719.

Birmaher, B., Dahl, R. E., Perel, J., Williamson, D. E., Nelson, B., Stull, S., Kaufman, J., Waterman, G. S., Rao, U., Nguyen, N., Puig-Antich, J., & Ryan, N. D. (1996a). Corticotropin-releasing hormone challenge in prepubertal major depression. *Biol Psychiatry, 39*(4), 267–277.

Birmaher, B., Dahl, R. E., Williamson, D. E., Perel, J. M., Brent, D. A., Axelson, D. A., Kaufman, J., Dorn, L. D., Stull, S., & Ryan, N. D. (2000). Growth hormone secretion in children and adolescents at high risk for major depressive disorder. *Arch Gen Psychiatry, 57,* 867–872.

Birmaher, B., Kaufman, J., Brent, D. A., Dahl, R. E., Perel, J. M., al-Shabbout, M., Nelson, B., Stull, S., Rao, U., Waterman, G. S., Williamson, D. E., & Ryan, N. D. (1997). Neuroendocrine response to 5-hydroxy-L-tryptophan in prepubertal children at high risk of major depressive disorder. *Arch Gen Psychiatry, 54*(12), 1113–1119.

Birmaher, B., Ryan, N. D., Dahl, R., Rabinovich, H., Ambrosini, P., Williamson, D. E., Novacenko, H., Nelson, B., Lo, E. S., & Puig-Antich, J. (1992). Dexamethasone suppression test in children with major depressive disorder [published erratum appears in *J Am Acad Child Adolesc Psychiatry* 1992 May 31(3):561]. *J Am Acad Child Adolesc Psychiatry, 31*(2), 291–297.

Birmaher, B., Ryan, N. D., Williamson, D. E., Brent, D. A., & Kaufman, J. (1996b). Childhood and adolescent depression: a review of the past 10 years. Part II. *J Am Acad Child Adolesc Psychiatry, 35*(12), 1575–1583.

Birmaher, B., Ryan, N. D., Williamson, D. E., Brent, D. A., Kaufman, J., Dahl, R. E., Perel, J., & Nelson, B. (1996c). Childhood and adolescent depression: a review of the past 10 years. Part I. *J Am Acad Child Adolesc Psychiatry, 35*(11), 1427–1439.

Biver, F., Wikler, D., Lotstra, F., Damhaut, P., Goldman, S., & Mendlewicz, J. (1997). Serotonin 5-HT2 receptor imaging in major depression: focal changes in orbito-insular cortex. *Br J Psychiatry, 171*, 444–448.

Botteron, K. N., Raichle, M. E., Heath, A. C., & Todd, R. D. (1999). *Twin study of prefrontal brain morphometry in adolescent onset depression.* Paper presented at the Child Depression Consortium, Pittsburgh.

Bremner, J. D., Innis, R. B., Salomon, R. M., Staib, L. H., Ng, C. K., Miller, H. L., Bronen, R. A., Krystal, J. H., Duncan, J., Rich, D., Price, L. H., Malison, R., Dey, H., Soufer, R., & Charney, D. S. (1997). Positron emission tomography measurement of cerebral metabolic correlates of tryptophan depletion-induced depressive relapse. *Arch Gen Psychiatry, 54*(4), 364–374.

Bremner, J. D., Narayan, M., Anderson, E. R., Staib, L. H., Miller, H. L., & Charney, D. S. (2000). Hippocampal volume reduction in major depression. *Am J Psychiatry, 157*(1), 115–118.

Carroll, B. J. (1982). The dexamethasone suppression test for melancholia. *Br J Psychiatry, 140*, 292–304.

Casey, B. J., Giedd, J. N., & Thomas, K. M. (2000). Structural and functional brain development and its relation to cognitive development. *Biol Psychol, 54*(1–3), 241–257.

Childs, B., & Scriver, C. R. (1986). Age at onset and causes of disease. *Perspect Biol Med, 29*(3 Pt 1), 437–460.

Cicchetti, D., & Cannon, T. D. (1999). Neurodevelopmental processes in the ontogenesis and epigenesis of psychopathology [editorial]. *Dev Psychopathol, 11*(3), 375–393.

Cicchetti, D., & Rogosch, F. A. (1996). Equifinality and mutlifinality in developmental psychopathology. *Development and Psychopathology, 8*, 597–600.

Cleckner-Smith, C. S., Doughty, A. S., & Grossman, J. A. (1998). Premenstrual symptoms. Prevalence and severity in an adolescent sample. *J Adolesc Health, 22*(5), 403–408.

Collier, D. A., Stober, G., Li, T., Heils, A., Catalano, M., Di Bella, D., Arranz, M. J., Murray, R. M., Vallada, H. P., Bengel, D., Muller, C. R., Roberts, G. W., Smeraldi, E., Kirov, G., Sham, P., & Lesch, K. P. (1996). A novel functional polymorphism within the promoter of the serotonin transporter gene: possible role in susceptibility to affective disorders [see comments]. *Mol Psychiatry, 1*(6), 453–460.

Cyranowski, J. M., Frank, E., Young, E., & Shear, M. K. (2000). Adolescent onset of the gender difference in lifetime rates of major depression: a theoretical model. *Arch Gen Psychiatry, 57*(1), 21–27.

Dahl, R., Puig-Antich, J., Ryan, N., Nelson, B., Novacenko, H., Twomey, J., Williamson, D., Goetz, R., & Ambrosini, P. J. (1989). Cortisol secretion in adolescents with major depressive disorder. *Acta Psychiatr Scand, 80*(1), 18–26.

Dahl, R. E., Kaufman, J., Ryan, N. D., Perel, J., al-Shabbout, M., Birmaher, B., Nelson, B., & Puig-Antich, J. (1992). The dexamethasone suppression test in children and adolescents: a review and a controlled study [published erratum appears in *Biol Psychiatry* 1993 Jan 1;33(1):64–9]. *Biol Psychiatry, 32*(2), 109–126.

Dahl, R. E., Ryan, N. D., Birmaher, B., al-Shabbout, M., Williamson, D. E., Neidig, M., Nelson, B., & Puig-Antich, J. (1991a). Electroencephalographic sleep measures in prepubertal depression. *Psychiatry Res, 38*(2), 201–214.

Dahl, R. E., Ryan, N. D., Puig-Antich, J., Nguyen, N. A., al-Shabbout, M., Meyer, V. A., & Perel, J. (1991b). 24-hour cortisol measures in adolescents with major depression: a controlled study. *Biol Psychiatry, 30*(1), 25–36.

De Bellis, M. D., Keshavan, M. S., Clark, D. B., Casey, B. J., Giedd, J. N., Boring, A. M., Frustaci, K., & Ryan, N. D. (1999). Developmental traumatology. Part II: Brain development. *Biol Psychiatry, 45*(10), 1271–1284.

Dorn, L. D., Burgess, E. S., Susman, E. J., von Eye, A., DeBellis, M. D., Gold, P. W., & Chrousos, G. P. (1996). Response to oCRH in depressed and nondepressed adolescents: does gender make a difference? *J Am Acad Child Adolesc Psychiatry, 35*(6), 764–773.

Drevets, W. C. (1998). Functional neuroimaging studies of depression: the anatomy of melancholia. *Annu Rev Med, 49*, 341–361.

Drevets, W., Gadde, K., & Krishnan, K. (1999). Neuroimaging studies of mood. In D. Charney, E. Nestler, & B. S. Bunney (Eds.), *Neurobiology of mental illness* (pp. 394–418). New York: Oxford University Press.

Drevets, W. C., Price, J. L., Simpson, J. R., Jr., Todd, R. D., Reich, T., Vannier, M., & Raichle, M. E. (1997). Subgenual prefrontal cortex abnormalities in mood disorders. *Nature, 386*(6627), 824–827.

Duman, R. S., & Charney, D. S. (1999). Cell atrophy and loss in major depression [editorial; comment]. *Biol Psychiatry, 45*(9), 1083–1084.

Duman, R. S., Heninger, G. R., & Nestler, E. J. (1997). A molecular and cellular theory of depression [see comments]. *Arch Gen Psychiatry, 54*(7), 597–606.

Emslie, G. J., Rush, A. J., Weinberg, W. A., Kowatch, R. A., Hughes, C. W., Carmody, T., & Rintelmann, J. (1997). A double-blind, randomized, placebo-controlled trial of fluoxetine in children and adolescents with depression. *Arch Gen Psychiatry, 54*, 1031–1037.

Emslie, G. J., Rush, A. J., Weinberg, W. A., Rintelmann, J. W., & Roffwarg, H. P. (1990). Children with major depression show reduced rapid eye movement latencies. *Arch Gen Psychiatry, 47*(2), 119–124.

Farber, N. B., Wozniak, D. F., Price, M. T., Labruyere, J., Huss, J., St. Peter, H., & Olney, J. W. (1995). Age-specific neurotoxicity in the rat associated with NMDA receptor blockade: potential relevance to schizophrenia? *Biol Psychiatry, 38*(12), 788–796.

Fisher, M., Trieller, K., & Napolitano, B. (1989). Premenstrual symptoms in adolescents. *J Adolesc Health Care, 10*(5), 369–375.

Freeman, E. W., Rickels, K., & Sondheimer, S. J. (1993). Premenstrual symptoms and dysmenorrhea in relation to emotional distress factors in adolescents. *J Psychosom Obstet Gynaecol, 14*(1), 41–50.

Freeman, L. N., Poznanski, E. O., Grossman, J. A., Buchsbaum, Y. Y., & Banegas, M. E. (1985). Psychotic and depressed children: a new entity. *J Am Acad Child Psychiatry, 24*(1), 95–102.

Frisch, A., Postilnick, D., Rockah, R., Michaelovsky, E., Postilnick, S., Birman, E., Laor, N., Rauchverger, B., Kreinin, A., Poyurovsky, M., Schneidman, M., Modai, I., & Weizman, R. (1999). Association of unipolar major depressive disorder with genes of the serotonergic and dopaminergic pathways. *Mol Psychiatry, 4*(4), 389–392.

Frost, L. A., Moffitt, T. E., & McGee, R. (1989). Neuropsychological correlates of psychopathology in an unselected cohort of young adolescents. *J Abnorm Psychol, 98*(3), 307–313.

Gambarana, C., Ghiglieri, O., & Graziella de Montis, M. (1995). Desensitization of the D1 dopamine receptors in rats reproduces a model of escape deficit reverted by imipramine, fluoxetine and clomipramine. *Prog Neuropsychopharmacol Biol Psychiatry, 19*(5), 741–755.

Geller, B., & Luby, J. (1997). Child and adolescent bipolar disorder: a review of the past 10 years. *J Am Acad Child Adolesc Psychiatry, 36*(9), 1168–1176.

George, M., Ketter, T., Parekh, P., Horwitz, B., Herscovitch, P., & Post, R. (1995). Brain activity during transient sadness and happiness in healthy women. *Am J Psychiatry, 152*, 341–351.

Ghaziuddin, N., King, C., Zaccagnini, J., & Weidmer-Mikhail, M. (1997). *Responses to serotonergic prob (mCPP) in depressed and control adolescents*. Paper presented at the Society for Biological Psychiatry Annual Convention and Scientific Program, San Diego.

Gold, P. W., Calabrese, J. R., Kling, M. A., Avgerinos, P., Khan, I., Gallucci, W. T., Tomai, T. P., & Chrousos, G. P. (1986). Abnormal ACTH and cortisol responses to ovine corticotropin releasing factor in patients with primary affective disorder. *Prog Neuropsychopharmacol Biol Psychiatry, 10*(1), 57–65.

Goldman-Rakic, P. S., & Brown, R. M. (1982). Postnatal development of monoamine content and synthesis in the cerebral cortex of rhesus monkeys. *Brain Res, 256*(3), 339–349.

Goodyer, I. M., Herbert, J., Altham, P. M., Pearson, J., Secher, S. M., & Shiers, H. M. (1996). Adrenal secretion during major depression in 8- to 16-year-olds, I. Altered diurnal rhythms in salivary cortisol and dehydroepiandrosterone (DHEA) at presentation. *Psychol Med, 26*(2), 245–256.

Goodyer, I. M., Herbert, J., Tamplin, A., Secher, S. M., & Pearson, J. (1997). Short-term outcome of major depression: II. Life events, family dysfunction, and friendship difficulties as predictors of persistent disorder. *J Am Acad Child Adolesc Psychiatry, 36*(4), 474–480.

Guidotti, A., & Costa, E. (1998). Can the antidysphoric and anxiolytic profiles of selective serotonin reuptake inhibitors be related to their ability to increase brain 3 alpha, 5 alpha-tetrahydroprogesterone (allopregnanolone) availability? *Biol Psychiatry, 44*(9), 865–873.

Halbreich, U., Asnis, G. M., Zumoff, B., Nathan, R. S., & Shindledecker, R. (1984). Effect of age and sex on cortisol secretion in depressives and normals. *Psychiatry Res, 13*(3), 221–229.

Harrington, R., Rutter, M., Weissman, M., Fudge, H., Groothues, C., Bredenkamp, D., Pickles, A., Rende, R., & Wickramaratne, P. (1997). Psychiatric disorders in the relatives of depressed probands. I. Comparison of prepubertal, adolescent and early adult onset cases. *J Affect Disord, 42*(1), 9–22.

Hart, J., Gunner, M., & Cicchetti, D. (1996). Altered neuroendocrine activity in maltreated children related to symptoms of depression. *Develop and Psychopathology, 8,* 201–214.

Hauser, P., Altshuler, L. L., Berrettini, W., Dauphinais, I. D., Gelernter, J., & Post, R. M. (1989). Temporal lobe measurement in primary affective disorder by magnetic resonance imaging. *J Neuropsychiatry Clin Neurosci, 1,* 128–134.

Hazell, P., O'Connell, D., Heathcote, D., Robertson, J., & Henry, D. (1995). Efficacy of tricyclic drugs in treating child and adolescent depression: a meta-analysis. *Bmj, 310*(6984), 897–901.

Heim, C., Owens, M. J., Plotsky, P. M., & Nemeroff, C. B. (1997). The role of early adverse life events in the etiology of depression and posttraumatic stress disorder. Focus on corticotropin-releasing factor. *Ann N Y Acad Sci, 821,* 194–207.

Hyman, S. E. (1999). Introduction to the complex genetics of mental disorders [editorial]. *Biol Psychiatry, 45*(5), 518–521.

Jensen, J. B., & Garfinkel, B. D. (1990). Growth hormone dysregulation in children with major depressive disorder [see comments]. *J Am Acad Child Adolesc Psychiatry, 29*(2), 295–301.

Jezova, D., Jurankova, E., Mosnarova, A., Kriska, M., & Skultetyova, I. (1996). Neuroendocrine response during stress with relation to gender differences. *Acta Neurobiol Exp (Warsz), 56*(3), 779–785.

Kashani, J. H., McGee, R. O., Clarkson, S. E., Anderson, J. C., Walton, L. A., Williams, S., Silva, P. A., Robins, A. J., Cytryn, L., & McKnew, D. H. (1983). Depression in a sample of 9-year-old children: prevalence and associated characteristics. *Arch Gen Psychiatry, 40*(11), 1217–1223.

Kaufman, J. (1991). Depressive disorders in maltreated children. *J Am Acad Child Adolesc Psychiatry, 30*(2), 257–265.

Kaufman, J., Birmaher, B., Brent, D., Dahl, R., Bridge, J., & Ryan, N. D. (1998a). Psychopathology in the relatives of depressed-abused children. *Child Abuse Negl, 22*(3), 171–181.

Kaufman, J., Birmaher, B., Perel, J., Dahl, R. E., Moreci, P., Nelson, B., Wells, W., & Ryan, N. D. (1997). The corticotropin-releasing hormone challenge in depressed abused, depressed nonabused, and normal control children. *Biol Psychiatry, 42*(8), 669–679.

Kaufman, J., Birmaher, B., Perel, J., Dahl, R. E., Stull, S., Brent, D., Trubnick, L., al-Shabbout, M., & Ryan, N. D. (1998b). Serotonergic functioning in depressed abused children: clinical and familial correlates. *Biol Psychiatry, 44*(10), 973–981.

Kaufman, J., & Charney, D. S. (1999). Neurobiological correlates of child abuse [editorial; comment]. *Biol Psychiatry, 45*(10), 1235–1236.

Kaufman, J., Martin, A., King, R., & Charney, D. (2001). Are child-, adolescent-, and adult-onset depression one and the same disorder? *Biological Psychiatry, 49,* 1012–1033.

Kaufman, J., & Ryan, N. (1999). The neurobiology of child and adolescent depression. In D. Charney, E. Nestler, & B. Bunny (Eds.), *The neurobiological foundation of mental illness.* New York: Oxford University Press.

Keller, M. B., Ryan, N., Birmaher, B., Klein, R., Papathoedorou, G., Strober, M., Wagner, K. D., Winters, N., Emslie, G., Weller, E., Carlson, G., Clarke, G., Geller, B., Gergel, I., Kutcher, S.,

McCafferty, J. P., & Fristad, M. (2001) Multi-center trial of paroxetine and imipramine in the treatment of adolescent depression. *JAMA*.

Keller, M. B., Ryan, N. D., Strober, M., Klein, R. G., Kutcher, S. P., Birmaher, B., Hagino, O. R., Koplewicz, H., Carlson, G. A., Clarke, G. N., Emslie, G. J., Feinberg, D., Geller, B., Kusumakar, V., Papatheodorou, G., Sack, W. H., Sweeney, M., Wagner, K. D., Weller, E. B., Winters, N. C., Oakes, R., & McCafferty, J. P. (2001). Efficacy of paroxetine in the treatment of adolescent major depression: a randomized, controlled trial. *J Am Acad Child Adolesc Psychiatry, 40*, 762–772.

Kendler, K. S. (1998). Anna-Monika-Prize paper. Major depression and the environment: a psychiatric genetic perspective. *Pharmacopsychiatry, 31*(1), 5–9.

Kendler, K. S., Kessler, R. C., Walters, E. E., MacLean, C., Neale, M. C., Heath, A. C., & Eaves, L. J. (1995). Stressful life events, genetic liability, and onset of an episode of major depression in women. *Am J Psychiatry, 152*(6), 833–842.

Kilts, C. D. (1994). Recent pharmacologic advances in antidepressant therapy. *Am J Med, 97*(6A), 3S–12S.

Klee, S. H., & Garfinkel, B. D. (1984). Identification of depression in children and adolescents: the role of the dexamethasone suppression test. *J Am Acad Child Psychiatry, 23*(4), 410–415.

Kovacs, M., Devlin, B., Pollock, M., Richards, C., & Mukerji, P. (1997). A controlled family history study of childhood-onset depressive disorder. *Arch Gen Psychiatry, 54*(7), 613–623.

Kovacs, M., Feinberg, T. L., Crouse-Novak, M., Paulauskas, S. L., Pollock, M., & Finkelstein, R. (1984). Depressive disorders in childhood. II. A longitudinal study of the risk for a subsequent major depression. *Arch Gen Psychiatry, 41*(7), 643–649.

Kraemer, G. (1992). A psychobiological theory of attachment. *Behavioral and Brain Sciences, 15*, 493–541.

Kunugi, H., Ishida, S., Kato, T., Tatsumi, M., Sakai, T., Hattori, M., Hirose, T., & Nanko, S. (1999). A functional polymorphism in the promoter region of monoamine oxidase-A gene and mood disorders. *Mol Psychiatry, 4*(4), 393–395.

Kupfer, D. J. (1991). Long-term treatment of depression. *J Clin Psychiatry, 52 Suppl*, 28–34.

Kupfer, D. J., Frank, E., Carpenter, L. L., & Neiswanger, K. (1989). Family history in recurrent depression. *J Affect Disord, 17*(2), 113–119.

Kutcher, S., Malkin, D., Silverberg, J., Marton, P., Williamson, P., Malkin, A., Szalai, J., & Katic, M. (1991). Nocturnal cortisol, thyroid stimulating hormone, and growth hormone secretory profiles in depressed adolescents [see comments]. *J Am Acad Child Adolesc Psychiatry, 30*(3), 407–414.

Kye, C. H., Woo, T. U., & Lewis, D. A. (1996). Postnatal development of monoamine contact and synthesis in the cerebral cortex of rhesus monkeys (abstract). *Neuroscience, 22*, 905.

Lane, R., Reiman, E., Ahern, G., Schwartz, G., & Davidson, R. (1997). Neuroanatomical correlates of happiness, sadness, and disgust. *Am J Psychiatry, 154*, 926–933.

Leboyer, M., Bellivier, F., Nosten-Bertrand, M., Jouvent, R., Pauls, D., & Mallet, J. (1998). Psychiatric genetics: search for phenotypes. *Trends Neurosci, 21*(3), 102–105.

Lepore, F., Ptito, M., & Jasper, H. H. (1986). *Neurology and neurobiology* (Vol. 17). New York: Alan R. Liss.

Lewinsohn, P. M., Clarke, G. N., Seeley, J. R., & Rohde, P. (1994). Major depression in community adolescents: age at onset, episode duration, and time to recurrence [see comments]. *J Am Acad Child Adolesc Psychiatry, 33*(6), 809–818.

Lidow, M. S., & Rakic, P. (1992). Scheduling of monoaminergic neurotransmitter receptor expression in the primate neocortex during postnatal development. *Cereb Cortex, 2*(5), 401–416.

Lopez, J. F., Chalmers, D. T., Little, K. Y., & Watson, S. J. (1998). A.E. Bennett Research Award. Regulation of serotonin1A, glucocorticoid, and mineralocorticoid receptor in rat and human hippocampus: implications for the neurobiology of depression. *Biol Psychiatry, 43*(8), 547–573.

Maes, M., & Meltzer, H. (1995). The serotonin hypothesis of major depression. In F. Bloom & D. Kupfer (Eds.), *Psychopharmacology: the fourth generation of progress* (pp. 933–944). New York: Raven Press.

Martin, A., Kaufman, J., & Charney, D. (2000). Pharmacotherapy of early-onset depression. Update and new directions. *Child Adolesc Psychiatr Clin N Am, 9*(1), 135–157.

Mayberg, H. S., Brannan, S. K., Mahurin, R. K., Jerabek, P. A., Brickman, J. S., Tekell, J. L., Silva, J. A., McGinnis, S., Glass, T. G., Martin, C. C., & Fox, P. T. (1997). Cingulate function in depression: a potential predictor of treatment response [see comments]. *Neuroreport, 8*(4), 1057–1061.

Mayberg, H. S., Liotti, M., Brannan, S. K., McGinnis, S., Mahurin, R. K., Jerabek, P. A., Silva, J. A., Tekell, J. L., Martin, C. C., Lancaster, J. L., & Fox, P. T. (1999). Reciprocal limbic-cortical function and negative mood: converging PET findings in depression and normal sadness. *Am J Psychiatry, 156*(5), 675–682.

McAllister, A. K., Katz, L. C., & Lo, D. C. (1999). Neurotrophins and synaptic plasticity. *Proc Natl Acad Sci USA, 96*, 13600–13602.

McClure, E., Rogeness, G. A., & Thompson, N. M. (1997). Characteristics of adolescent girls with depressive symptoms in a so-called "normal" sample. *J Affect Disord, 42*(2–3), 187–197.

McGee, R., Anderson, J., Williams, S., & Silva, P. A. (1986). Cognitive correlates of depressive symptoms in 11-year-old children. *J Abnorm Child Psychol, 14*(4), 517–524.

Mervaala, E., Fohr, J., Kononen, M., Valkonen-Korhonen, M., Vainio, P., Partanen, K., Partanen, J., Tiihonen, J., Viinamaki, H., Karjalainen, A. K., & Lehtonen, J. (2000). Quantitative MRI of the hippocampus and amygdala in severe depression. *Psychol Med, 30*, 117–125.

Meyer, W. J. D., Richards, G. E., Cavallo, A., Holt, K. G., Hejazi, M. S., Wigg, C., & Rose, R. M. (1991). Depression and growth hormone [letter; comment]. *J Am Acad Child Adolesc Psychiatry, 30*(2), 335.

Patchev, V. K., & Almeida, O. F. (1998). Gender specificity in the neural regulation of the response to stress: new leads from classical paradigms. *Mol Neurobiol, 16*(1), 63–77.

Petty, F. (1995). GABA and mood disorders: a brief review and hypothesis. *J Affect Disord, 34*(4), 275–281.

Petty, F., McChesney, C., & Kramer, G. (1985). Intracortical glutamate injection produces helpless-like behavior in the rat. *Pharmacol Biochem Behav, 22*(4), 531–533.

Pierpaoli, C., Jezzard, P., Basser, P. J., Barnett, A., & Di Chiro, G. (1996). Diffusion tensor MR imaging of the human brain. *Radiology, 201*(3), 637–648.

Pine, D. S., Coplan, J. D., Wasserman, G. A., Miller, L. S., Fried, J. E., Davies, M., Cooper, T. B., Greenhill, L., Shaffer, D., & Parsons, B. (1997). Neuroendocrine response to fenfluramine challenge in boys. Associations with aggressive behavior and adverse rearing [see comments] [published erratum appears in Arch Gen Psychiatry 1998 Jul;55(7):625]. *Arch Gen Psychiatry, 54*(9), 839–846.

Plotsky, P. M., Owens, M. J., & Nemeroff, C. B. (1998). Psychoneuroendocrinology of depression. Hypothalamic-pituitary-adrenal axis. *Psychiatr Clin North Am, 21*(2), 293–307.

Post, R. M. (1992). Transduction of psychosocial stress into the neurobiology of recurrent affective disorder. *Am J Psychiatry, 149*(8), 999–1010.

Prosser, J., Hughes, C. W., Sheikha, S., Kowatch, R. A., Kramer, G. L., Rosenbarger, N., Trent, J., & Petty, F. (1997). Plasma GABA in children and adolescents with mood, behavior, and comorbid mood and behavior disorders: a preliminary study. *J Child Adolesc Psychopharmacol, 7*(3), 181–199.

Puig-Antich, J., Dahl, R., Ryan, N., Novacenko, H., Goetz, D., Goetz, R., Twomey, J., & Klepper, T. (1989a). Cortisol secretion in prepubertal children with major depressive disorder. Episode and recovery. *Arch Gen Psychiatry, 46*(9), 801–809.

Puig-Antich, J., & Gittleman, R. (1982). Depression in childhood and adolescence. In E. Paykel (Ed.), *Handbook of affective disorders*. New York: Guilford Press.

Puig-Antich, J., Goetz, D., Davies, M., Kaplan, T., Davies, S., Ostrow, L., Asnis, L., Twomey, J., Iyengar, S., & Ryan, N. D. (1989b). A controlled family history study of prepubertal major depressive disorder. *Arch Gen Psychiatry, 46*(5), 406–418.

Puig-Antich, J., Goetz, R., Hanlon, C., Davies, M., Thompson, J., Chambers, W. J., Tabrizi, M. A., & Weitzman, E. D. (1982). Sleep architecture and REM sleep measures in prepubertal children with major depression: a controlled study. *Arch Gen Psychiatry, 39*(8), 932–939.

Puig-Antich, J., Kaufman, J., Ryan, N. D., Williamson, D. E., Dahl, R. E., Lukens, E., Todak, G., Ambrosini, P., Rabinovich, H., & Nelson, B. (1993). The psychosocial functioning and family environment of depressed adolescents. *J Am Acad Child Adolesc Psychiatry, 32*(2), 244–253.

Puig-Antich, J., Novacenko, H., Davies, M., Chambers, W. J., Tabrizi, M. A., Krawiec, V., Ambrosini, P. J., & Sachar, E. J. (1984). Growth hormone secretion in prepubertal children with major depression. I. Final report on response to insulin-induced hypoglycemia during a depressive episode. *Arch Gen Psychiatry, 41*(5), 455–460.

Raja, S. N., Feehan, M., Stanton, W. R., & McGee, R. (1992). Prevalence and correlates of premenstrual syndrome in adolescence. *J Am Acad Child Adolesc Psychiatry, 31*, 783–789.

Rajkowska, G., Miguel-Hidalgo, J. J., Wei, J., Dilley, G., Pittman, S. D., Meltzer, H. Y., Overholser, J. C., Roth, B. L., & Stockmeier, C. A. (1999). Morphometric evidence for neuronal and glial prefrontal cell pathology in major depression [see comments]. *Biol Psychiatry, 45*(9), 1085–1098.

Rao, U., Dahl, R. E., Ryan, N. D., Birmaher, B., Williamson, D. E., Giles, D. E., Rao, R., Kaufman, J., & Nelson, B. (1996). The relationship between longitudinal clinical course and sleep and cortisol changes in adolescent depression. *Biol Psychiatry, 40*(6), 474–484.

Rao, U., Ryan, N. D., Birmaher, B., Dahl, R. E., Williamson, D. E., Kaufman, J., Rao, R., & Nelson, B. (1995). Unipolar depression in adolescents: clinical outcome in adulthood. *J Am Acad Child Adolesc Psychiatry, 34*(5), 566–578.

Rao, U., Weissman, M. M., Martin, J. A., & Hammond, R. W. (1993). Childhood depression and risk of suicide: a preliminary report of a longitudinal study. *J Am Acad Child Adolesc Psychiatry, 32*(1), 21–27.

Rende, R., Weissman, M., Rutter, M., Wickramaratne, P., Harrington, R., & Pickles, A. (1997). Psychiatric disorders in the relatives of depressed probands. II. Familial loading for comorbid non-depressive disorders based upon proband age of onset. *J Affect Disord, 42*(1), 23–28.

Reynolds, C., Gillen, J., & Kupfer, D. (1987). Sleep and affective disorders. In H. Meltzer (Ed.), *Psychopharmacology: The third generation*. New York: Raven Press.

Robbins, D. R., Alessi, N. E., Yanchyshyn, G. W., & Colfer, M. V. (1983). The dexamethasone suppression test in psychiatrically hospitalized adolescents. *J Am Acad Child Psychiatry, 22*(5), 467–469.

Rosenberg, D. R., & Lewis, D. A. (1995). Postnatal maturation of the dopaminergic innervation of monkey prefrontal and motor cortices: a tyrosine hydroxylase immunohistochemical analysis. *J Comp Neurol, 358*(3), 383–400.

Rosenberg, D. R., Sweeney, J. A., Gillen, J. S., Kim, J., Varanelli, M. J., O'Hearn, K. M., Erb, P. A., Davis, D., & Thulborn, K. R. (1997). Magnetic resonance imaging of children without sedation: preparation with simulation. *J Am Acad Child Adolesc Psychiatry, 36*(6), 853–859.

Rubinow, D. R., Schmidt, P. J., & Roca, C. A. (1998). Estrogen-serotonin interactions: implications for affective regulation. *Biol Psychiatry, 44*(9), 839–850.

Ryan, N., & Dahl, R. (1993). The biology of depression in children and adolescents. In J. Mann & D. Kupfer (Eds.), *The biology of depressive disorders*. New York: Plenum.

Ryan, N. D., Birmaher, B., Perel, J. M., Dahl, R. E., Meyer, V., al-Shabbout, M., Iyengar, S., & Puig-Antich, J. (1992). Neuroendocrine response to L-5-hydroxytryptophan challenge in prepubertal major depression. Depressed vs normal children. *Arch Gen Psychiatry, 49*(11), 843–851.

Ryan, N. D., Dahl, R. E., Birmaher, B., Williamson, D. E., Iyengar, S., Nelson, B., Puig-Antich, J., & Perel, J. M. (1994). Stimulatory tests of growth hormone secretion in prepubertal major depression: depressed versus normal children. *J Am Acad Child Adolesc Psychiatry, 33*(6), 824–833.

Ryan, N. D., Puig-Antich, J., Ambrosini, P., Rabinovich, H., Robinson, D., Nelson, B., Iyengar, S., & Twomey, J. (1987). The clinical picture of major depression in children and adolescents. *Arch Gen Psychiatry, 44*(10), 854–861.

Ryan, N. D., Puig-Antich, J., Rabinovich, H., Ambrosini, P., Robinson, D., Nelson, B., & Novacenko, H. (1988). Growth hormone response to desmethylimipramine in depressed and suicidal adolescents. *J Affect Disord, 15*(3), 323–337.

Sallee, F. R., Vrindavanam, N. S., Deas-Nesmith, D., Odom, A. M., Carson, S. W., & Sethuraman, G. (1998). Parenteral clomipramine challenge in depressed adolescents: mood and neuroendocrine response. *Biol Psychiatry, 44*(7), 562–567.

Sanacora, G., Mason, G. F., Rothman, D. L., Behar, K. L., Hyder, F., Petroff, O. A., Berman, R. M., Charney, D. S., & Krystal, J. H. (1999). Reduced cortical gamma-aminobutyric acid levels in depressed patients determined by proton magnetic resonance spectroscopy. *Arch Gen Psychiatry, 56*(11), 1043–1047.

Sanchez, M. M., Hearn, E. F., Do, D., Rilling, J. K., & Herndon, J. G. (1998). Differential rearing affects corpus callosum size and cognitive function of rhesus monkeys. *Brain Res, 812*(1–2), 38–49.

Schildkraut, J., Green, A., & Mooney, J. (1989). Mood disorders: Biochemical aspects. In H. Kaplan & B. Sadock (Eds.), *Comprehensive textbook of psychiatry* (Vol. I, pp. 868–879). Baltimore: Williams and Wilkins.

Seidman, S. N., & Rabkin, J. G. (1998). Testosterone replacement therapy for hypogonadal men with SSRI-refractory depression. *J Affect Disord, 48*(2–3), 157–161.

Serretti, A., Macciardi, F., Verga, M., Cusin, C., Pedrini, S., & Smeraldi, E. (1998). Tyrosine hydroxylase gene associated with depressive symptomatology in mood disorder. *Am J Med Genet, 81*(2), 127–130.

Shah, P. J., Ebmeier, K. P., Glabus, M. F., & Goodwin, G. M. (1998). Cortical grey matter reductions associated with treatment-resistant chronic unipolar depression. Controlled magnetic resonance imaging study. *Br J Psychiatry, 172,* 527–532.

Sheline, Y. I., Gado, M. H., & Price, J. L. (1998). Amygdala core nuclei volumes are decreased in recurrent major depression [published erratum appears in Neuroreport 1998 Jul 13;9(10):2436]. *Neuroreport, 9*(9), 2023–2028.

Sheline, Y. I., Wang, P. W., Gado, M. H., Csernansky, J. G., & Vannier, M. W. (1996). Hippocampal atrophy in recurrent major depression. *Proc Natl Acad Sci U S A, 93*(9), 3908–3913.

Silberg, J., Pickles, A., Rutter, M., Hewitt, J., Simonoff, E., Maes, H., Carbonneau, R., Murrelle, L., Foley, D., & Eaves, L. (1999). The influence of genetic factors and life stress on depression among adolescent girls. *Arch Gen Psychiatry, 56*(3), 225–232.

Simon, N. G., Cologer-Clifford, A., Lu, S. F., McKenna, S. E., & Hu, S. (1998). Testosterone and its metabolites modulate 5HT1A and 5HT1B agonist effects on intermale aggression. *Neurosci Biobehav Rev, 23*(2), 325–336.

Souery, D., Lipp, O., Mahieu, B., Mendelbaum, K., De Bruyn, A., De Maertelaer, V., Van Broeckhoven, C., & Mendlewicz, J. (1996). Excess tyrosine hydroxylase restriction fragment length polymorphism homozygosity in unipolar but not bipolar patients: a preliminary report. *Biol Psychiatry, 40*(4), 305–308.

Steingard, R. J., & Renshaw, P. F. (1996). MRS in depressed adolescents (abstract). *Biol Psychiatry, 34S,* 1042.

Steingard, R. J., Renshaw, P. F., Yurgelun-Todd, D., Appelmans, K. E., Lyoo, I. K., Shorrock, K. L., Bucci, J. P., Cesena, M., Abebe, D., Zurakowski, D., Poussaint, T. Y., & Barnes, P. (1996). Structural abnormalities in brain magnetic resonance images of depressed children. *J Am Acad Child Adolesc Psychiatry, 35*(3), 307–311.

Strober, M., Lampert, C., Schmidt, S., & Morrell, W. (1993). The course of major depressive disorder in adolescents: I. Recovery and risk of manic switching in a follow-up of psychotic and nonpsychotic subtypes. *J Am Acad Child Adolesc Psychiatry, 32*(1), 34–42.

Susman, E. J., Inoff-Germain, G., Nottelmann, E. D., Loriaux, D. L., Cutler, G. B., Jr., & Chrousos, G. P. (1987). Hormones, emotional dispositions, and aggressive attributes in young adolescents. *Child Dev, 58*(4), 1114–1134.

Sweeney, J. A., Strojwas, M. H., Mann, J. J., & Thase, M. E. (1998). Prefrontal and cerebellar abnormalities in major depression: evidence from oculomotor studies. *Biol Psychiatry, 43*(8), 584–594.

Thase, M. E., Kupfer, D. J., Buysse, D. J., Frank, E., Simons, A. D., McEachran, A. B., Rashid, K. F., & Grochocinski, V. J. (1995). Electroencephalographic sleep profiles in single-episode and recurrent unipolar forms of major depression: I. Comparison during acute depressive states. *Biol Psychiatry, 38*(8), 506–515.

Thomas, K. M., Drevets, W. C., Dahl, R. E., Ryan, N. D., Birmaher, B., Eccard, C. H., Axelson, D., Whalen, P. J., & Casey, B. J. (2001). Amygdala response to fearful faces in anxious and depressed children. *Arch Gen Psychiatry, 58,* 1057–1063.

Vakili, K., Pillay, S. S., Lafer, B., Fava, M., Renshaw, P. F., Bonello-Cintron, C. M., & Yurgelun-Todd, D. A. (2000). Hippocampal volume in primary unipolar major depression: a magnetic resonance imaging study. *Biol Psychiatry, 47,* 1087–1090.

Warren, M. P., & Brooks-Gunn, J. (1989). Mood and behavior at adolescence: evidence for hormonal factors. *J Clin Endocrinol Metab, 69*(1), 77–83.

Waterman, G. S., Ryan, N. D., Puig-Antich, J., Meyer, V., Ambrosini, P. J., Rabinovich, H., Stull, S., Novacenko, H., Williamson, D. E., & Nelson, B. (1991). Hormonal responses to dextroamphetamine in depressed and normal adolescents. *J Am Acad Child Adolesc Psychiatry, 30*(3), 415–422.

Watson, S. J., & Akil, H. (1999). Gene chips and arrays revealed: a primer on their power and their uses. *Biol Psychiatry, 45*(5), 533–543.

Weissman, M. M., Leckman, J. F., Merikangas, K. R., Gammon, G. D., & Prusoff, B. A. (1984). Depression and anxiety disorders in parents and children. Results from the Yale family study. *Arch Gen Psychiatry, 41*(9), 845–852.

Weissman, M. M., Warner, V., Wickramaratne, P., & Prusoff, B. A. (1988). Early-onset major depression in parents and their children. *J Affect Disord, 15*(3), 269–277.

Weissman, M. M., Wolk, S., Goldstein, R. B., Moreau, D., Adams, P., Greenwald, S., Klier, C. M., Ryan, N. D., Dahl, R. E., & Wickramaratne, P. (1999). Depressed adolescents grown up. *JAMA, 281*(18), 1707–1713.

Williamson, D. E., Birmaher, B., Frank, E., Anderson, B. P., Matty, M. K., & Kupfer, D. J. (1998). Nature of life events and difficulties in depressed adolescents. *J Am Acad Child Adolesc Psychiatry, 37*(10), 1049–1057.

Williamson, D. E., Ryan, N. D., Birmaher, B., Dahl, R. E., Kaufman, J., Rao, U., & Puig-Antich, J. (1995). A case-control family history study of depression in adolescents. *J Am Acad Child Adolesc Psychiatry, 34*(12), 1596–1607.

Winokur, G. (1982). The development and validity of familial subtypes in primary unipolar depression. *Pharmacopsychiatria, 15*(4), 142–146.

Young, W., Knowles, J. B., MacLean, A. W., Boag, L., & McConville, B. J. (1982). The sleep of childhood depressives: comparison with age-matched controls. *Biol Psychiatry, 17*(10), 1163–1168.

TWENTY

Psychosocial Stressors as Predisposing Factors to Affective Illness and PTSD

Potential Neurobiological Mechanisms and Theoretical Implications

Robert M. Post, Gabriele S. Leverich, Susan R. B. Weiss, Li-Xin Zhang, Guoqiang Xing, He Li, and Mark Smith

SENSITIZATION IN THE AFFECTIVE DISORDERS

Stressor and Episode Sensitization in the Unmedicated State

At the beginning of the twentieth century, Kraepelin (1921) laid out the fundamentals of the sensitization hypothesis of affective disorders:

> the attacks begin not infrequently after the illness or death of near relatives ... we must regard all alleged injuries as possibly sparks for the discharge of individual attacks, but the real cause of the malady must be sought in *permanent internal changes*, which at least very often, perhaps always, are innate ... in spite of the removal of the discharging cause, the attack follows its independent development. But, finally, the appearance of wholly similar attacks on wholly dissimilar occasions or quite without external occasion shows that even there where there has been external influence, it must not be regarded as a necessary presupposition for the appearance of the attack. (pp. 180–181)

In this terse and insightful paragraph, he outlines four different components of the sensitization hypothesis: (1) initial episodes of affective illness are often precipitated by psychosocial stressors; (2) as recurrences emerge, later episodes do not require the same psychosocial precipitation, but may occur more spontaneously; (3) episodes tend to occur with a characteristic similarity; and (4) innate neurobiological mechanisms mediate these vulnerabilities and recurrences, and presumably these could occur both on an inherited and an experiential basis.

Other aspects of this sensitization hypothesis are outlined in additional passages from his work. Although Kraepelin noted the "sheer immeasurable multiplicity of clinical pictures," (p. 114) and "the frequency, with which the different clinical forms of

The invaluable support of these projects and the salaries of Li-Xin Zhang, Guoqiang Xing, and He Li by the Theodore and Vada Stanley Foundation is gratefully acknowledged.

Editorial and manuscript assistance of Chris Gavin and Harriet Brightman is very much appreciated.

manic-depressive insanity here described occur in a fairly large series of observations, is naturally very various ..." (p. 133), "... for the most part the disease shows the tendency later on to run its course more quickly and to shorten the intervals, even to their complete cessation" (p. 137). "When the disease has lasted for some time and the attacks have been frequently repeated, the psychic changes usually become more distinct during the intervals also" (p. 149).

Thus, Kraepelin (1921) recognized both the inherent variability and unpredictability of bipolar episode presentation and course among and within individual patients; but within this seeming randomness, he noted a tendency for well intervals to decrease as a function of the successive number of episodes (i.e., sensitization) with a particularly striking effect after the first, second, and third episodes. Kraepelin recognized the poor prognostic implications of the occurrence of dysphoric mania and its high rate of hospitalization and chronicity, particularly in females. Herein he applied another postulate of the sensitization model, that with greater number of recurrences there may be a malignant progression and treatment resistance in the illness. We have summarized these essential elements of the sensitization hypothesis in Figure 20.1, with the more explicit hypothesis that greater numbers and/or faster cycling of episodes will be associated with greater treatment resistance, particularly to the classical modality of pharmacoprophylaxis – lithium carbonate.

Illness Progression During Tolerance Development

There is an additional component of the sensitization hypothesis in affective illness based on episodes breaking through previously effective pharmacoprophylaxis in a pattern that resembles tolerance. In these instances, patients who had previously been severely ill experience a good response to prophylactic monotherapy or combination therapy and remain well for a period of years, and then begin to experience breakthrough episodes of increasing severity or duration (Post et al., 1999; Post, Ketter, Denicoff, Leverich, & Mikalauskas, 1993; Post, Leverich, Rosoff, & Altshuler, 1990). These recurrences may progress to the point of complete loss of efficacy to what had previously been a highly effective treatment regimen.

A number of predictions in affective illness are based on a preclinical model of tolerance (Weiss, Clark, Rosen, Smith, & Post, 1995) to the anticonvulsant effects of mood stabilizing anticonvulsants on amygdala-kindled seizures (Table 20.1). These postulates, which remain to be further specifically examined for their clinical applicability, include:

1. A greater number of prior episodes (a marker of increased pathological illness drive) will be associated with a greater likelihood and more rapid onset of tolerance development;
2. Higher rather than minimally effective doses of a treatment will be more likely to prevent or delay tolerance development (for some, but not all drugs [e.g., with lamotrigine being a possible exception]);
3. Stable (or possibly descending) dose regimens will be preferable to minimally effective dosing followed by dose escalation in an attempt to treat breakthrough episodes;

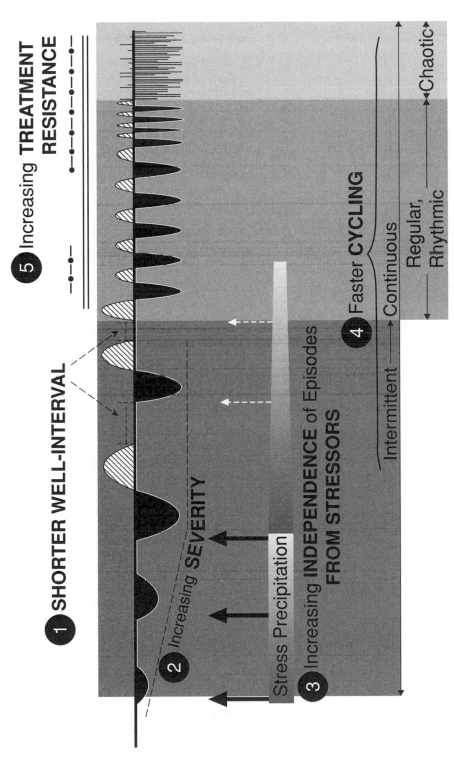

Figure 20.1. Sensitization in affective illness. Evidence of the tendency for the illness to progress is based on a variety of observations, including: (1) increases in episode frequency; (2) increases in episode severity, quality, or complexity; (3) early episodes precipitated by psychosocial stressors, but later ones occurring more spontaneously; (4) transition from intermittent to continuous to chaotic cycling patterns; and (5) possibly increasing treatment resistance, especially to lithium.

Table 20.1. Clinical Predictions[a] to Be Explored Based on Observations from a Preclinical Model of Amygdala-Kindled Seizures[b]

Tolerance to anticonvulsant effects slowed by:	Future studies; is there predictive validity for clinical tolerance in affective illness?
Higher doses (but lower doses w/LTG)	Maximum tolerated doses
Not escalating doses	Stable dosing
More efficacious drugs (VPA > CBZ)	Different rate of treatment resistance?
Treatments initiated early in illness	Sarantidis and Waters, 1981; Gelenberg et al., 1989; O'Connell et al., 1991; Denicoff et al., 1997; Swann et al., 1999
Combination treatment (CBZ plus VPA)	Combination > monotherapy?
Reducing illness drive	Treat comorbidities
Response restored by:	
Period of drug discontinuation then re-exposure	Randomized study of continuation treatment vs. discontinuation and re-exposure
Agents with different mechanisms of action (no cross-tolerance)	Cross tolerance from lamotrigine to CBZ, not VPA

[a] Right side of table.
[b] Left side of table.
VPA, valproic acid; CBZ, carbamazepine; LTG, lamotrigine.

4. Drugs with different mechanisms of action will have different potency in preventing tolerance development;

5. Combination treatments employing multiple and differential mechanisms of action will be more effective in delaying tolerance development than similar doses of several monotherapies;

6. When loss of efficacy via a tolerance mechanism has occurred, renewal of efficacy may be achieved by switching to or adding another drug with a different mechanism of action (i.e., one that does not show cross tolerance); and

7. In instances in which loss of efficacy has developed gradually via a purported tolerance mechanism, effectiveness of the initial drug may be re-achieved following a period of treatment with other agents and then reinstitution of the initial drug.

As noted below, some of these predictions based on the preclinical kindled seizure model have been preliminarily explored and partially validated, but a number remain to be directly tested in the clinic. Moreover, to the extent that these predictions of the model do prove valid, a third round of predictions could be derived based on presumed neurobiological and experiential effects on gene expression mechanisms involved. These also will be elaborated in a later section of the chapter.

Episode Sensitization

Kraepelin's empirical observations which form the basis of the sensitization model in affective illness have now been largely validated and confirmed by many investigators using a variety of study methodologies. Most studies support a greater role of psychosocial stressors in initial, compared with later, episodes, with few exceptions (Table 20.2). Studies that have found that stressors continued to be associated with later episodes of affective illness have misinterpreted these observations as a refutation of the model (Hammen & Gitlin, 1997; Swendsen, Hammen, Heller, & Gitlin, 1995). This refutation is not true because the sensitization model is based on the assumption that over the course of illness, patients become *increasingly* sensitive to the role of stressors in the precipitation of episodes. To the extent that stressors are involved and documented, it supports the model; to the extent that later episodes are associated with or precipitated by symbolic stressors, conditioned stressors, or occur in the relative absence of exogenous stressors, this finding would also be consistent with the model. The model only suggests that there is a reduced need for the involvement of and direct triggering by stressors in later episodes.

Numerous studies support the general provision of cycle acceleration with shorter well intervals between successive episodes (Table 20.3), although, again, as Kraepelin and others have pointed out, there would be many individual exceptions to this rule. For example, we have observed a subgroup of patients who begin their illness with rapid or continuous cycling from the outset (Roy-Byrne, Post, Uhde, Porcu, & Davis, 1985) and, therefore, we would not expect any notable further degree of cycle acceleration; in fact, it might not be possible to demonstrate such a phenomenon in patients with continuous cycling from the outset because of a ceiling effect.

Moreover, Kraepelin (1921) made his observations in an era before major psychopharmacological interventions were available. Thus, many investigators who fail to observe this pattern or report that there is a lack of progression in the illness, or a failure of rapid cycling patients to continue in this pattern, have often not taken treatment into account (Coryell, Endicott, & Keller, 1992). Whenever effective treatment interventions are employed, the natural course of the illness would be altered, which is the goal of modern pharmacotherapeutic interventions. For example, Angst and Sellaro (2000) report that duration of the well interval only decreases over the first two episodes and then stabilizes thereafter.

Failure of well-treated patients to demonstrate this pattern of cycle acceleration and malignant progression of the illness cannot be taken as a refutation of the sensitization hypothesis. The fact that we and others have continued to observe this pattern of sensitization in treatment-refractory patients is predicated on their lack of adequate response to pharmacotherapy, presumably yielding a course and pattern of illness not entirely dissimilar from what might have been expected if they were untreated (as in the Kraepelinian era). It is also possible, however, that some treatment such as antidepressants could modify the course in an adverse fashion similar to that observed with levodopa treatment in Parkinson's disease, generating an increased rapidity of cycling of the on-off phenomenon (Nissenbaum et al., 1987).

The prediction that greater number of episodes prior to institution of lithium pharmacoprophylaxis is a negative prognosticator for response has also been widely replicated in the literature in two different types of studies. In the first type, studies overwhelmingly indicate that rapid cycling patients are less responsive to lithium than those without a rapid cycling pattern (Post, Ketter, Speer, Leverich, & Weiss, 2000; Post, Kramlinger, Altshuler, Ketter, & Denicoff, 1990). In addition, there is a considerable literature indicating that the number of episodes prior to institution of lithium

Table 20.2. Greater Association Between Life Events and First versus Subsequent Episodes of Affective Disorder

Author	Disorder	Number of Episodes	N	% Patients for Whom Major Life Events Preceded Episode		p Value	Assessment
				First Episode	Later Episode		
Matussek et al. (1965)	Depression	1	242	44		—	Stressors (138 psychologic; 58 somatic) had to clearly precede onset of episode
		2	135		34	—	
		3	82		24	—	
		4	119		19	—	
Angst (1966)	Depression	1	103	60		—	No inventory
		≥4			38	—	
Okuma and Shimoyama (1972)	Manic Depression	1	134	45		—	Any event (3 months prior)
		2	134		26	—	
		3	134		13	—	
Glassner et al. (1979)	Manic Depression	1	25	75		—	Event rated stressful by patient and on Holmes and Rahe Scale (1 year prior; usually 2–24 days); role loss critical in patients and comparison subjects
		≥1[a]			56	—	
Ambelas (1979)[b]	Mania	1	14	50			Paykel Life Events Scale (4 weeks prior); one-third of cases followed bereavement
		≥2		67	28	< 0.01	
Ayuso et al. (1981)	Depression	1	43	55.8	40.0	< 0.05	Social and somatic stressors; patients with late onset had more events than did those with early onset
		2	35		38.8		
		3	18		29.7		
		≥4	47				
Perris (1984)	Depression	1	37	62	50[c]	< 0.02	Semistructured interview; 56 item inventory (3 months prior)
		≥2	112	43	19[d]	< 0.001	

Study	Diagnosis	Episodes	n	%	p	Instrument
Dolan et al. (1985)	Depression	1 / ≥2	21 / 57	62 / 29	<0.05	Bedford College-Life Events and Difficulties Schedule (6 months prior) (Brown, Harris, 1978)
Ezquiaga et al. (1987)	Depression	<3 / ≥3	52 / 45	50 / 16	<0.01	Semistructured interview (Brown, Harris); no effect on chronic stress
Ambelas (1987)	Mania	1 / ≥2	50 / 40	66 / 20	<0.001	Paykel Life Events Scale (4 weeks prior)
Ghaziuddin et al. (1990)	Depression	1 / ≥2	33 / 40	91 / 50	<0.05	Paykel Life Events Scale (6 months prior)
Cassano et al. (1989)	Depression	1 / ≥2	94 / 173	66.0 / 49.4	<0.05	Paykel Life Events Scale
Hammen & Gitlin (1997)	Bipolar	0–8 / ≥9	52	40	0.05	More episodes, more stressors and relapsed faster
Castine et al. (1998)	Schizophrenia	≤3	32	76 more recent life events	0.01	Paykel Life Events Scale
Nierenberg et al. (1998)	Depression	1st vs. >3 episodes	176	1st episode had more stressful negative life events compared with recurrent	0.037	Life Events Scale, Perceived Stress Scale

[a] For this group, the most recent hospitalization was preceded by a life event resulting in role loss.
[b] Of surgical comparison subjects, 6.6% had experienced recent major life events.
[c] Percentage for negative or undesirable events.
[d] Percentage for events involving psychological conflict.

Table 20.3. Early Studies of Life Course of Manic-Depressive Illness

Study	# of pts.	High UP/BP Pt. Ratio	Sex	Age of Onset (Peak or Mean Years)	Decreasing Well Interval	Observational Time (years) Retrospective (R) Prospective (P)	Late Age at Onset Predicts Increased Relapse	Comments
Swift (1907)	105	No	74 F 31 M		Yes	R	Yes	Study examined first episode in terms of prognosis. Prognosis is better if first episode is a depression than if it is mania.
Kraepelin (1921)	903	Yes	648 F 255 M	20–30	Yes	Variable up to a lifetime R,P	Yes	Study contained both a large number of patients and extended periods of observation. Few patients were observed for their complete life course.
Malzberg (1929)	11,393		6513 F 4880 M	mean = 40			Yes	Study examined only first admissions and reviewed relationship to duration of episode and recovery.
Paskind (1930)	633			21–30	Yes	R	Yes	Nonhospitalized patients studied – may be helpful as a comparison group to the hospitalized patients. *Late age of onset predicts increased duration of episodes.
Pollock (1931)	8438	No	519 F 3274 M	20–24		11 R	Yes	Study examined a large number of patients. Many unrecovered cases were discharged as improved. Age of onset between 20 and 40 years – better prognosis than patients younger or older.
Steen (1933)	493			20–40		8 R	Yes	Study confused other diagnostic groups (i.e., schizophrenia, schizoaffective) with BP patients. Twenty to 30-year age of onset predicts high rate of recovery.

Study	N		Sex	Age		R		Comments
Rennie (1942)	208	Yes	117 F 91 M	45–55		20 R		Seventy-nine percent of patients will have more than 1 episode during their lifetime; 50% will have less than 3 episodes; 93% (193) recovered from first episode; 21% (62) never had another recurrence.
Poort (1945)	141	No		20–30		10–15 R	No	Fifty percent (71) were recurrent UP or BP; 19% (27) went on to develop another type of psychosis such as schizophrenia, "hysteria," or sociopathy.
Lundqvist (1945)	319		196 F 123 M	<30/mania >50/depression	Yes	14–32 R	Yes	Patient population is difficult to assess because 28% (89) became chronic following their first episode and 7% (22) developed schizophrenia. First episode of mania predicts increased risk for relapse.
Stenstedt (1952)	216	Yes	126 F 90 M	mean = 38.7 F		29 R		Study does not detail polarity of episodes in UP and manics who relapse; 11.7% was the morbidity risk of the illness among siblings and children of probands; 83% (117) had first episode as a depression; 53% (114) had one episode.
Astrup et al. (1959)	270	Yes				5–19 R	No	Study separates schizoaffective from manic-depressive illness; emphasizes the need for long-term follow-up to make separation

(continued)

Table 20.3 *(continued)*

Study	# of pts.	High UP/BP Pt. Ratio	Sex	Age of Onset (Peak or Mean Years)	Decreasing Well Interval	Observational Time (years) Retrospective (R) Prospective (P)	Late Age at Onset Predicts Increased Relapse	Comments
Angst and Weiss (1967)	388	Yes		mean = 38.5 (BP)	Yes	7 R	Yes	Study clarifies set of definitions for episode, interval, cycle. Confirms by use of statistics the earlier observations of the relationship of age of onset and number of episodes with prognosis. Only 12% (45) of patients were BP type.
Bratfos and Haug (1968)	207	Yes	116 F 91 M	mean = 35	Yes	6 P	No	Patients had various types of somatic therapy (ECT, antidepressant, and neuroleptics). Study did not distinguish between the type of therapy received in terms of risk for relapse; 20% (41) remained chronically ill.
Perris (1968)	270	No	144 F 126 M	mean = 37.7		20 R		Eighty-four percent of UP patients will convert to BP illness before 3 episodes, i.e., 16% of BP patients will be misdiagnosed as UP with up to 3 observations of depressive episodes. BP patients are at higher risk for relapse than UP.
Grof et al. (1974)	987	Yes			Yes	Up to 45	Yes	Patients were treated only during the acute phases of their illness and not prophylactically. Each succeeding cycle length is shorter on the average than the preceding one.

Study	N		Sex				Description
Taschev (1974)	652	Yes	350 F 323 M	Yes	R	Yes	Retrospective evaluation of cyclothymic depression (122, 18.7%), recurrent depression (134, 20.5%), involutional depression (335, 51.3%), reactive depression (23, 3.5%), recurrent mania (38, 5.8%); 26.4% (172) of depressives committed suicide; 16% (104) became chronic; no mention if patients were treated.
Angst et al. (1978)	254	Yes		Yes	12–16 P		Study of the number of episodes before conversion of UP or BP. Conversion of UP to BP > 3 episodes = 70%; > 6 episodes = 83%. Conversion of BP to schizoaffective: 3 of 40 (7.5%).
Angst (1978)	95	No	58 F 37 M mean = 61	Yes	26 R, P		Statistical description of long-term observation of BP illness. Study examines the heterogeneity of BP illness. Females exhibit more depression than mania. Males exhibit a symmetrical distribution of mania/depression.
Zis et al. (1980)	334	Yes		Yes		Yes	Increased risk of relapse is a function of number of previous episodes.
Maj et al. (1992)	72	Yes	42 F 30 M mean = 32.6	Yes	P	No	Increasing severity from the index episode to the first, second, and third prospective episodes.
Angst and Sellaro (2000)	549	No		Yes	329 R 220 P	No	Increased rapidity of episode recurrence only after the first 2 episodes.

Key: UP = Unipolar; BP = Biploar; ECT = Electroconvulsive Therapy.

Table 20.4. More Episodes Prior to Starting Lithium Is Associated with Poor
Prophylactic Response

Investigator	Correlates of Poor Response to Lithium
Prien et al., 1974	High frequency of hospitalizations
Sarantidis and Waters, 1981	More episodes per year
Abou-Saleh and Coppen, 1986	Higher number of episodes (7.0 ± 1.3) in bipolar patients
Gelenberg et al., 1989	> 3 prior episodes
O'Connell et al., 1991	≥ 3.8 mean episodes
Goldberg et al., 1996	≥ 2 prior hospitalizations
Denicoff et al., 1997	• Older age at first treatment
	• Longer duration of illness
	• More than 1 hospitalization for mania
Maj et al., 1998	≥ 7.2 mean episodes
Swann et al., 1999	≥ 10 prior episodes

prophylaxis is a negative predictor of lithium response (Table 20.4). Of course, it is
also possible in these uncontrolled studies that a greater number of episodes is only a
marker for a subsequent adverse course that would have been manifest even if lithium
prophylaxis were instituted after the first or second episode.

Although the study of Kessing, Bolwig, and colleagues (1998) involving more than
20,000 patients in the Danish Case Registry did not initially control for treatment, it
is striking that they found a direct relationship between the number of prior episodes
and both the incidence of and latency to relapse into another episode in unipolar and
bipolar patients. These data from a country in which lithium is very widely used provide
some of the strongest evidence of an overall sensitization effect, that is, greater number
of prior episodes is associated with a greater risk of relapse in both of these affective
disorders. This trend apparently emerges irrespective of whether or not patients were
treated in the community with sustained prophylactic medication (although the direct
analysis of this inference remains to be reported).

Stressor and Episode Sensitization

In another seminal study, in more than 600 female identical twin pairs, Kendler et al.
(1993) showed that strong predictors of major depression included both stressors and
number of prior episodes. They also documented that a variety of early life stressors
such as lack of parental warmth and parental loss were associated with the onset of
initial or minor (neurotic) depressions and that more concurrent psychosocial stressors
were involved in the precipitation of recurrent episodes. Thus, these data appear to
support an early vulnerability factor of the environment, perhaps leaving the patient at
a higher risk for subsequent stressor-related induction of depression. Kendler et al. also
found that neurotic or minor depression predisposed to major depression and prior
major depressive episodes predisposed to further depressions. A genetic component
accounted for part of the variance in both the initial and recurrent episodes.

Thus, there is substantial evidence for two types of sensitization: (1) most promi-
nently, early childhood and subsequent adult life stressors can act as precipitants or
vulnerability factors (stressor sensitization), and (2) episode sensitization, in which the
number of prior episodes correlates with the likelihood of relapse and a shortening of

Table 20.5. Sensitization Phenomena in Affective Illness

Observation	Evidence	Investigators
↑ FREQUENCY OF RECURRENCE		
Well interval	+++	Kraepelin; Grof; Post
↑ SEVERITY		
As function of episode number	+	Maj
↑ CHRONICITY		
Each new episode carries added 10% risk of nonrecovery	++	Thase
↑ TREATMENT RESISTANCE		
First major depression more responsive than second	+	Angst
Greater number and frequency of prior episodes associated with lithium nonresponse	+	Gelenberg; O'Connell; Denicoff
↑ ABNORMAL NEUROBIOLOGY		
More Episodes:		
− More sleep abnormalities	++	Armitage; Thase
− Greater hypercortisolism	+	Ribeiro; Gurguis

the well interval. Preliminary data (Table 20.4) also suggest greater treatment refractoriness as a function of number of prior episodes.

Given these two major perspectives of the model (i.e., stressor and episode sensitization), it is then necessary to ascertain which underlying neurobiological mechanisms could mediate such long-term vulnerability from early stressors and episodes of affective illness themselves. Kraepelin (1921) wrote "... the real, the deeper cause of the malady is to be sought in a permanent morbid state which must also continue to exist in the intervals between the attacks" (p. 117). Although there are only a modicum of data available on the neurobiological correlates of episode sensitization in man, as outlined in Table 20.5, there is a very considerable preclinical literature that at least provides a basis for examining their potential relevance to the clinic.

There is considerable evidence for cross-sensitization between some types of stressors and cocaine administration, suggesting that elements of cocaine sensitization may parallel phenomena observed in stressor sensitization (Antelman, Eichler, Black, & Kocan, 1980; Kalivas & Duffy, 1989; Post, Ketter, Speer, Leverich, & Weiss, 2000). However, episodes of cocaine-induced hyperactivity and stereotypy can, in addition, serve as models of brief episodes of manic-like hyperactivity and frantic psychomotor drive that are not unlike those that occur in some patients with mania and dysphoric mania, respectively. As such, cocaine sensitization may be examined from the perspective that it could model aspects of both stressor sensitization and manic episode sensitization, and direct one toward the examination of whether some parallel neurobiological mechanisms are involved in all three types.

Sensitization and Kindling Phenomena Differences

We will only briefly allude to the neurobiology of another model of long-lasting neuronal learning and memory – amygdala kindling, which differs considerably (in behavior, biochemistry, neural pathways, and pharmacology involved) from sensitization

(Weiss & Post, 1994). The kindling model is an interesting model not only for examining the development of epileptogenesis, but also for observing lasting changes in neural and behavioral responsivity in response to very brief periods of brain stimulation. In amygdala kindling, repeated administration of subthreshold amygdala stimulation evokes afterdischarges of increasing frequency, duration, and complexity which then spread throughout the brain, involving other limbic and cortical structures in association with the development of increasingly robust and complex behavioral phenomena, culminating in a full-blown generalized seizure (Goddard, McIntyre, & Leech, 1969; Racine, 1972a, 1972b). Following sufficient numbers of amygdala stimulations associated with completed kindled seizures, a phase of spontaneity may emerge in which animals exhibit true epilepsy and have spontaneous seizures in the absence of exogenous physiological stimulation.

Thus, the kindling model provides a readily identifiable set of physiological and behavioral concomitants of neuronal learning and memory, each of which demonstrates an obvious augmented response to repeated brain stimulation and then culminates in a further progression to spontaneous episodes. At the level of both physiology (amygdala excitability thresholds and afterdischarges as well as their spread to other brain areas) and behavior (seizure stage evolution from partial to full-blown and then to spontaneous), increases in responsivity occur.

Although these electrophysiological and behavioral progressions present clear evidence for neuronal learning and memory phenomena, it is equally clear that they do not represent endpoints directly parallel to those that occur in bipolar illness (Weiss & Post, 1994). Complex partial seizures of the temporal lobe are often associated with prominent affective symptoms, but, conversely, primary affective illness is rarely associated with seizure-like manifestations. Moreover, the induced seizures of electroconvulsive therapy are used as a prominent treatment for severe manic and depressive episodes. Thus, kindling to a seizure endpoint must be considered a nonhomologous model for the affective disorders, since neither the inducing phenomena, nor the behaviors or their temporal domains, nor the pharmacological interventions between the two are identical or even highly similar.

However, kindling may be useful in understanding how a complex behavioral phenomenon such as a major motor seizure comes to be evoked by previously subthreshold stimuli upon repetition and, as well, how such precipitated episodes may proceed to the spontaneous variety. In addition, the kindled seizure model is particularly appropriate for examining tolerance development to the anticonvulsant effects of a variety of effective antiepileptic agents (Weiss, Clark, Rosen, Smith, & Post, 1995) many of which are now also used for the treatment of affective disorders (Dunn et al., 1998; Post et al., 1996, 1998a, 1998b). One can examine the principles and underlying neural mechanisms of tolerance development to these agents in the seizure realm and ask whether or not similar phenomena exist for tolerance development in other models or clinical situations, such as the tolerance that can occur in the prevention of paroxysmal pain syndromes (Pazzaglia & Post, 1992), migraine headaches (Post & Silberstein, 1994), breakthrough panic attacks, and most pertinent to the current discussion, episodes of recurrent affective disorder (Post, Ketter, Denicoff, Leverich, & Mikalauskas, 1993; Post & Weiss, 1996).

Thus, the stressor and cocaine sensitization models have direct parallels and homologies to phenomena that occur in the clinical realm in the course of unipolar and bipolar affective disorders, whereas kindling must be considered only as an analogy and used for its indirect parallels. The kindling model's degree of predictive validity in this indirect realm remains to be determined, but will in turn reveal its ultimate utility.

NEUROBIOLOGICAL MECHANISMS FOR LONG-LASTING BEHAVIORAL AND BIOCHEMICAL VULNERABILITIES FOLLOWING EARLY LIFE STRESSORS

Levine et al. (1991) have used a paradigm of a single 24-hour period of maternal deprivation in rat pups as an inducer of long-lasting altered behavior and biochemical responsivity. These animals, like those of Plotsky and colleagues (Francis, Caldji, Champagne, Plotsky, & Meaney, 1999; Ladd et al., 2000; Plotsky, 1997) which are subjected to repeated episodes of three hours of maternal deprivation in the first weeks of life, show long-lasting hypercortisolism and increased anxiety-like behaviors.

Neurobiology of Repeated Maternal Separation: Parallels to the GR Knock-out Mouse

The studies of Plotsky and Meaney are particularly interesting from the perspective of adaptive and homeostatic mechanisms, because animals subjected to only fifteen minutes of daily maternal separation are protected against age-related loss of hippocampal anatomy and associated decline in learning and memory skills (Anisman, Zaharia, Meaney, & Merali, 1998; Liu et al., 1997; Meaney, Aitken, Van Berkel, Bhatnagar, & Sapolsky, 1988). Meaney has demonstrated that the mechanism of this effect is an increase in maternal licking behavior that occurs following the fifteen-minute separation, but not after a three-hour separation. After three hours, the previously separated pups are apparently not well identified and maternal behavior is degraded, with increased agitation in the mother and, in some instances, apparent frantic trampling of her offspring. It appears that this element of maternal behavior and neglect is a crucial element in producing the long-lasting hypercortisolism and anxiety-like behaviors in the separated offspring. This behavior can be remedied or prevented if the mother is given substitute rat pups during the three-hour period of separation from her own pups. In this case, when the separated pups are returned, the mother's behavior is normal and no lasting behavioral or biochemical alterations in the offspring are produced (Meaney, 1999).

In the three-hour separated pup that receives the full separation/maternal malbehavior, it is remarkable that these animals as adults show an increased proclivity to self-administer alcohol and cocaine compared with litter mates without such early stressors (Meaney, Brake, & Gratton, 2002; Huot, Thrivikraman, Meaney, & Plotsky, 2000). The entire biobehavioral syndrome, including hypercortisolism, is reversed by serotonin-selective antidepressants. However, if the antidepressant drug treatment is discontinued, animals revert to their prior anxious and hypercortisolemic state.

This model thus provides a dramatic illustration of how experiences in the environment can induce lasting behavioral and neurobiological changes at the level of gene expression. Increases in corticotropin-releasing factor (CRF) mRNA, for example, have recently been demonstrated in the hypothalamus of these animals (Francis, Caldji, Champagne, Plotsky, & Meaney, 1999). Moreover, the ability of these early stressors to alter the expression of these behavioral and biochemical changes in a life-long fashion parallels a related syndrome that can be induced genetically using transgenic animals.

For example, Barden and colleagues (Pepin, Pothier, & Barden, 1992) have developed a strain of animals with deficient glucocorticoid receptor number that also have resultant hypercortisolemia and increases in anxiety and depressive-like behaviors. These behaviors can also be reversed by treatment with antidepressant medications (Beaulieu, Rousse, Gratton, Barden, & Rochford, 1994; see also Figure 20.2). Thus, these two different animal models of life-long hypercortisolemia and lasting behavioral aberrations illustrate that hereditary genetic as well as experiential alterations in gene expression based on environmental insults, can each be sufficient to induce fairly similar phenotypic syndromes.

Neurobiology of One-Day Maternal Separation in the One-Day-Old Rat Pup

Further insight into the way isolated stressful life events occurring early in an animal's development could produce temporary to long-lasting neurobiological alterations is revealed by studies with the single-day separation model (Levine, Huchton, Wiener, & Rosenfeld, 1991). Zhang et al. (2002) have demonstrated a doubling of apoptosis (preprogrammed cell death) in widely distributed cells in the brain of separated rat pups after maternal deprivation. Double staining techniques show that this involves both neurons and glia.

In white matter areas of brain, the degree of induction of nerve growth factor (NGF) as measured by *in situ* hybridization of mRNA is directly proportional to the degree of apoptosis (Zhang, Xing, Levine, Post, & Smith, 1998). This apparently paradoxical finding of increased neurotrophic factor gene induction associated with greater degrees of apoptosis is understandable from the perspective that the NGF receptor trk A is not fully developed at this time and NGF potently binds instead to the lower affinity p75 receptor component, which is an executor of a death program rather than a neurotrophic one typical of the trk A receptor (Barrett, 2000). These data are thus of considerable interest in suggesting that mal-timed induction of neurotrophic substances may be as harmful as their deficiency of expression in other instances.

The one-day separation stress is also associated with increased expression of the proto-oncogene c-fos mRNA and the cell death factor Bax mRNA. In addition, in the hippocampus, there is decreased gene expression of calcium calmodulin kinase-II (CaMKII), the growth factor brain-derived neurotrophic factor (BDNF), and the inducible form of nitric oxide synthase (iNOS) (Xing et al., 1998, and unpublished data, 2000). These substances are of potentially great interest in relation to their important roles in long-term potentiation and other models of learning and memory. In this regard, the decrease in neurotrophic factors and increase in cell death factors following the one-day separation stress could be pertinent to findings that some individuals with posttraumatic stress disorder (PTSD) may have decreased volume of their hippocampus assessed by magnetic resonance imaging (MRI) (Bremner et al., 1995, 1997; Gurvits et al., 1996) and an associated impairment in learning and memory. However, the cause and effect relationships in these instances remain to be elucidated (Bremner, 2001).

Although there has been no direct pathophysiological link between decrements in BDNF (or any other neurotrophic factor) and the size of the hippocampal alterations in learning and memory in this paradigm, the ability of stressors to decrease BDNF at least provides a potential explanatory mechanism that can be further examined for

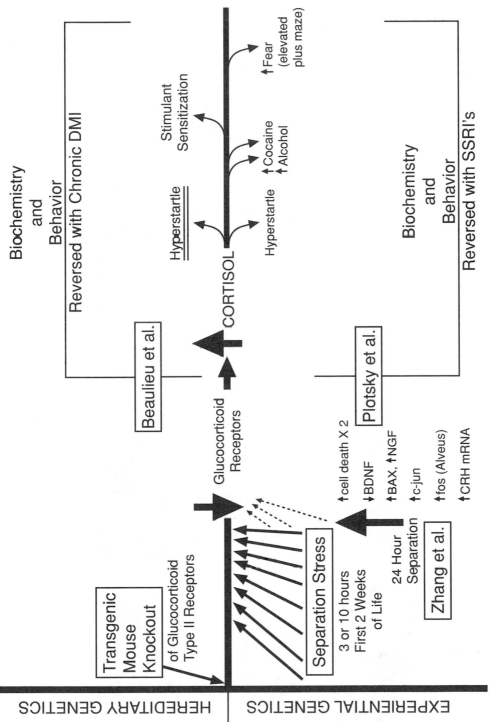

Figure 20.2. Convergent genetic and environmental models of depression. Either heredity or experiential genetics may lead to compounding behavioral and biochemical end points similar to those seen in depression and reversible by antidepressants. DMI, desipramine; BDNF, brain-derived neurotrophic factor; NGF, nerve growth factor; CRH, corticotropin-releasing hormone; SSRIs, serotonin selective reuptake inhibitors.

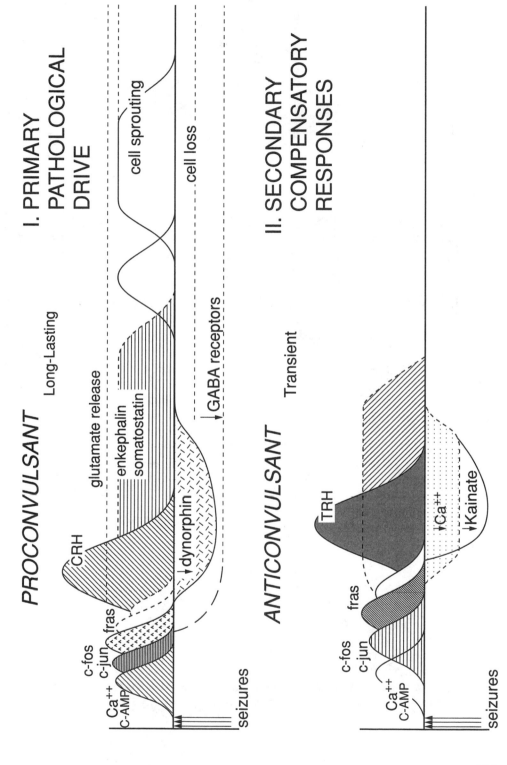

its putative role in such a relationship. Supporting the possibility that BDNF could be a crucial factor in learning and memory defects are the observations of Korte et al. (1998) indicating that transgenic animals with an absence of BDNF have both deficient long-term potentiation (LTP), and an inability to navigate accurately in the Morris maze test, indicating a deficit in the ability to perform normal tasks that are ordinarily well within the animal's normal repertoire.

One is now in a position to ask questions such as what are the crucial degrees of BDNF, CaMKII, or iNOS decrement that might be etiopathological to the observed behavioral and biochemical alterations. We would imagine that there is a considerable range of different parameters that may influence the ultimate impact and outcome of a stressor, including severity, duration, quality, and timing, as well as the number of repetitions and recurrences later in development. The degree of both genetic vulnerability and stressor resistance or resilience (Luthar, Cicchetti, & Becker, 2000) in conjunction with the potential for adaptation to the stressor and the support provided by others (Breier et al., 1988) may all be crucial variables in whether long-term pathological neurochemical and behavioral alterations become manifest.

Pathological versus Adaptive Alterations in Gene Expression in Kindled Seizures

It is perhaps useful to discriminate between changes in gene expression that are related to the primary pathology of sensitization versus those that are compensatory and adaptive. A similar distinction is more readily identifiable for amygdala-kindled seizures. Here we have provisionally divided the many changes in gene expression into these two components (Figure 20.3). One is based on whether they are primary and important to the maintenance of the kindled "memory" trace, or whether they reflect endogenous anticonvulsant adaptations that attempt to return the animal to homeostasis (Post & Weiss, 1992, 1996).

This separation has potential clinical importance from a number of perspectives, perhaps the most significant of which is that it provides new, dual, and differential targets of therapeutics. One can attempt to both block the primary pathological changes of kindling progression and, conversely, enhance the endogenous anticonvulsant or adaptive processes.

We have preliminarily identified thyrotropin-releasing hormone (TRH) as an endogenous anticonvulsant substance because it transiently increases in the hippocampus after seizures and has been reported to be anticonvulsant (Kubek, Liang, Byrd, & Domb, 1998). We have extended these observations with the finding that intra-hippocampal injection of TRH suppresses amygdala-kindled seizures (Wan, Noguera, & Weiss, 1998).

Figure 20.3. Schematic illustration of potential genomic, neurotransmitter, and peptidergic alterations that follow repeated kindled seizures. Putative mechanisms related to the primary pathological drive (i.e., kindled seizure evolution) are illustrated on top and those thought to be related to the secondary compensatory responses (i.e., anticonvulsant effects) are shown on the bottom. The horizontal line represents time. Sequential transient increases in second messengers and immediate early genes (IEGs) are followed by longer lasting alterations in peptides, neurotransmitters, and receptors or their mRNAs, as illustrated above the line, whereas decreases are shown below the line. Given the potential unfolding of these competing mechanisms in the evolution of seizure disorders, the question arises regarding whether parallel opposing processes also occur in the course of affective illness of other psychiatric disorders. Endogenous adaptive changes (bottom) may be exploited in the design of the new treatment strategies.

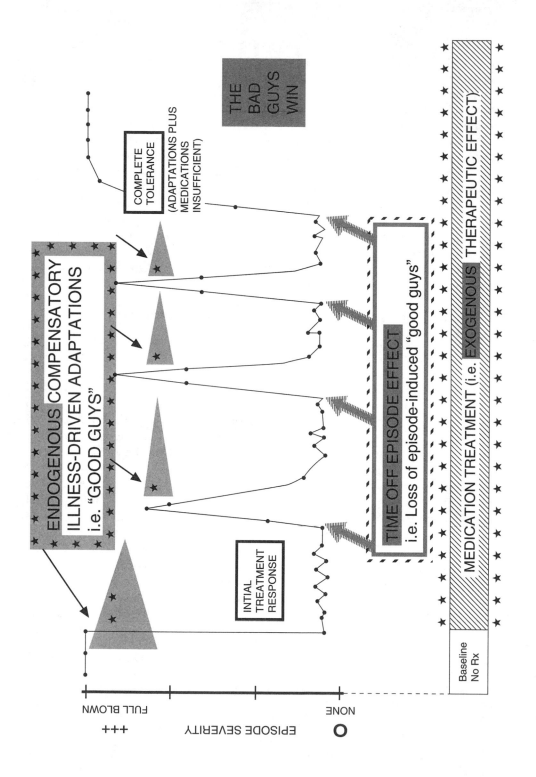

This is of additional interest because, in animals that have become tolerant to the anti-convulsant effects of either carbamazepine or diazepam, seizures that normally increase TRH mRNA no longer do so (Weiss, Clark, Rosen, Smith, & Post, 1995). It is postulated that the failure to induce some compensatory adaptive changes in gene expression (such as TRH, GABA$_A$ receptors, etc.) may be intimately involved with the tolerance process. This would also provide a conceptual mechanism for how the therapeutic efficacy of a drug may be revived after tolerance has developed following a period of time off the drug (which would theoretically allow seizures to again induce the TRH mRNA and other adaptive changes in gene expression) and thus facilitate carbamazepine's effectiveness.

Pathological versus Adaptive Changes in Gene Expression in Affective Disorders?

Not only have we postulated that the relative balance and predominance of primary pathological compared with the secondary and adaptive alterations in gene expression are associated with the development of loss of efficacy to some classes of anticonvulsants in the tolerance model, but this ratio might also be relevant in determining, in the medication-free state as well, whether seizures are manifest or not during kindling development and expression. Do parallels exist in the progressive evolution of illness in other syndromes? In this regard, we would surmise that the increases in CRF (in turn driving increases in cortisol) may be representative of one of the primary pathological processes of depression evolution and progression, particularly since hypercortisolemia has been associated with depression and cognitive impairment in other syndromes, such as Cushing's disease (Starkman, 1993).

Conversely, the increases in TRH directly reported in cerebrospinal fluid (CSF; Banki, Bissette, Arato, & Nemeroff, 1988) or inferred from the associated blunting of TSH response to TRH (suggestive of subclinical hyperthyroidism; Loosen, 1985), may be part of an endogenous set of antidepressant mechanisms that help to naturally terminate a depressive episode. Thus, as schematized in Figure 20.3, we again hypothesize that it is the ratio of the primary pathological versus secondary adaptive changes in gene expression that determine whether an individual remains in a relatively euthymic state or proceeds toward the recurrence of further episodes of affective disorder (Figure 20.4).

Figure 20.4. Hypothetical schema of the role of endogenous regulatory factors in the generation and progression of illness cyclicity. After an illness episode, adaptive compensatory mechanisms are induced (i.e., "good guys"; shaded triangle with two stars), which together with drug treatment suppress the illness (initial treatment response; box). The "good guys" dissipate with time (i.e., the time-off seizure effect), and episodes of illness re-emerge. Although this re-elicits illness-related compensatory mechanisms, the concurrent drug treatment prevents some of the illness-induced adaptive responses from occurring (smaller triangles with one star). As tolerance proceeds (associated with the loss of adaptive mechanisms), faster illness re-emergence occurs. Thus, the drug is becoming less effective in the face of less robust compensatory mechanisms. The primary pathology is progressively re-emerging, driven both by additional stimulations and episodes (i.e., the kindled memory trace, or the "bad guys") along with a loss of illness-induced adaptations. Because this cyclic process is presumably driven by the ratio of the "bad vs. good guys" at the level of changes in gene expression, we postulate that such fluctuations in the "battle of the oncogenes" arising out of illness and treatment-related variables could account for individual patterns in illness cyclicity.

Table 20.6. Incidence of Traumatic Stressors in Bipolar
Patients in the Stanley Foundation Bipolar Network

	Child N (%)	Adolescent N (%)	Adult N (%)
Physical Abuse			
Not Abused	228 (76)	242 (80)	246 (88)
Abused	71 (24)	59 (20)	37 (12)
Sexual Abuse			
Not Abused	241 (76)	247 (83)	242 (82)
Abused	59 (20)	51 (17)	55 (18)

IMPACT OF EARLY STRESSFUL EXPERIENCES IN BIPOLAR AFFECTIVE DISORDER

Although a number of studies outlined in Table 20.2 have examined the relative role of stressors in initial versus later episodes of both unipolar and bipolar depression, there has been less examination of the impact of early stressful life events on the subsequent course of bipolar illness. In the Stanley Foundation Bipolar Treatment Outcome Network, which now follows more than 500 patients on a detailed daily basis with the NIMH-LCMp (prospective version of the life chart method) (Leverich et al., 2001), we had the opportunity to address this question in 631 consecutive outpatients who completed a detailed questionnaire which included items related to whether or not they were exposed to physical or sexual abuse in childhood or adolescence (Leverich et al., 2002).

The incidence rate of these types of extraordinary psychosocial stressors listed in Table 20.6 is parenthetically and disappointingly not that different from the rate observed in many unselected nonclinical populations. However, in the context of patients with bipolar illness, the reported occurrence of either early physical or sexual abuse in childhood or adolescence was highly associated with an earlier onset of affective illness and more rapid, ultrarapid, and ultradian cycling patterns (Table 20.7). In the univariate analyses subjected to Bonferroni correction and in the logistic regression analysis, other

Table 20.7. Type of Early Abuse (Childhood or Adolescence) and Characteristics of Early Abuse

	Physical Abuse N (%)	Sexual Abuse N (%)
Early Onset	92 (50)***	96 (50)***
Ultradian Cycling	52 (41)**	43 (34)
Increased Severity of Mania	116 (63)***	106 (56)**
Increased Severity of Depression	119 (64)	123 (64)**
Attempted Suicide	90 (49)***	90 (48)***

*** $p < .001$
** $p < .01$
* $p < .05$

variables remain significant as well. Physical abuse included self-reports of a pattern of increasing severity of mania and a family history of bipolar disorder, alcoholism, drug abuse, or other psychiatric illnesses. Sexual abuse included self-reports of an increased incidence of attempted suicide (45%) and a family history of drug abuse and other psychiatric illnesses.

There was also an increase in the number of clinician-rated Axis I lifetime comorbidities (2.0) in those experiencing these early traumatic life experiences versus those without these early stressors (1.3, $p < 0.002$). Physical abuse was associated with a significant increase in anxiety disorder, drug abuse, alcoholism, and a diagnosis of PTSD. Sexual abuse was selectively associated with a lifetime history of drug abuse. Those with early stressor history also had greater numbers of Axis II comorbidities. Physical abuse had a strong association with increased presence of cluster A disorders (i.e., the odd, eccentric) including paranoid, schizoid, and schizotypical disorders. Sexual abuse was most strongly associated with the presence of cluster B disorders (i.e., dramatic, emotional, including histrionic, narcissistic, borderline, and antisocial disorders).

Moreover, in addition to the retrospective self-reported illness variables related to earlier onset and greater severity in the unfolding of bipolar illness (mania and suicidality), in the prospective year of clinician ratings we observed that those with a history of physical and/or sexual abuse in childhood and adolescence were more ill than those without such a history (Leverich et al., 2002). This was revealed in both an increased percentage of time well measured on the LCM as well as on the increased levels of depression severity measured on the Inventory of Depressive Symptomatology (IDS) (Rush et al., 1986, 1996).

CLINICAL APPROACHES TO BIPOLAR ILLNESS AND ITS PREVENTION

Caveats

The causal relationships in the data described above are not easily discerned or readily disentangled. Although it is highly plausible to first think that these early life experiences could lead to altered neurochemistry through some of the mechanisms described in the previous preclinical sections, and thus change the likelihood and severity of bipolar symptom development and evolution, it is also possible that traits associated with increased severity of later illness could evoke increased physical or sexual abuse. Lastly, it is possible that another or third variable, such as genetic loading, could determine both the more severe pattern of illness and the tendency for increased physical or sexual abuse (either evoked or directly related to parental illness), rather than any direct causal relationship between early abuse and more severe course of illness characteristics.

Notwithstanding these causal ambiguities, the strong relationships suggest the importance of attempts at earlier intervention. Those who were physically or sexually abused had a longer period of time from first affective symptoms to first treatment (13 ± 11 years) than those who were not abused (8 ± 9 years; $p = .0003$). Even eight years in the nonabused group is far too long; the average treatment delay in many populations is about ten years, including the Stanley Network (Suppes et al., 2001), the surveyed members of the National DMDA (Lish, Dime-Meenan, Whybrow, Price, & Hirschfeld, 1994), or other clinical research cohorts (Egeland, Hostetter, Pauls, & Sussex, 2000).

Early Intervention

Thus, there is a great need for earlier recognition and initiation of treatment in patients with bipolar illness in general. It would appear even more critical for those at high risk for more severe illness progression and negative prospective outcomes based on high genetic loading or the occurrence of early stressors. Yet it is just these adolescents and adults who are likely to have the longest delays in beginning treatment.

In addition to helping prevent serious affective dysfunction, earlier intervention may help a child avoid the variety of Axis I (McElroy et al., 2001), Axis II (Leverich et al., 2000), and medical comorbidities that are associated with these early stressful life experiences. In particular, the increased rate of substance abuse is already a problem in general in bipolar illness (Regier et al., 1990), and now we have found there is an additional greater risk for those with these earlier adverse life experiences. Forty-eight percent of those with a history of sexual abuse versus 19 percent without ($p = 0.00025$) have a lifetime diagnosis of drug abuse in the Stanley Foundation Bipolar Network; 40 percent of those with a history of physical abuse compared with 22 percent without have a history of drug abuse, and 52 percent versus 31 percent have a history of alcohol abuse ($p = 0.025$) (Leverich et al., 2000).

Thus, it would appear prudent to recommend primary substance abuse prevention techniques in the child and adolescent with bipolar illness, particularly in the presence of a history of physical and/or sexual abuse in childhood and/or adolescence. One can only wonder about the potential parallels of these vulnerabilities to the findings of increased alcohol and cocaine self-administration in the adult rodents that had previously experienced repeated maternal separation as pups (Meaney et al., 2002; Huot et al., 2002).

The association between stressful episodes and precipitation of the first episode of illness, as well as the current episode of illness in those with a history of early physical or sexual abuse compared with those without, also provides an important area for pharmacotherapeutic and psychotherapeutic intervention. To the extent that these individuals are particularly vulnerable to stressor precipitation of episodes and/or at increased risk of exposure to more stressors in general (Table 20.8), as our data would suggest ($p < 0.0001$ for physical abuse and $p < 0.001$ for first sexual abuse [Leverich et al., 2002]), dealing with this likelihood on a direct basis with appropriate cognitive, behavioral, interpersonal, or other focused psychotherapeutic techniques, as well as pharmacotherapeutics, may be of great assistance in raising the threshold for episode precipitation. Putting coping strategies and alternative perspectives into place that would enable the individual to be more comfortable in the face of stressor occurrence may be particularly valuable. The great potential for therapeutic benefit of these types of interventions are delineated in Cicchetti, Rogosch, and Toth (2000) and Luthar, Cicchetti, and Becker (2000).

Opposite Effects of Stress and Psychotrophic Drugs on Gene Expression and Neurogenesis

New data suggest additional theoretical rationales for psychotherapy besides providing additional psychosocial support based on the general therapeutic relationship and specialized techniques employed. To the extent that therapy and the development of

Table 20.8. Incidence of Stressful Life Events prior to First Episode and Most Recent Episode in Patients with or without a History of Early Abuse (Data from Leverich et al., 2002)

	Prior to First Episode	Prior to Most Recent Episode
History of Early Physical Abuse		
Absent	2.5	2.8
	]***	]***
Present	4.2	4.8
History of Early Sexual Abuse		
Absent	2.5	2.8
	]***	]***
Present	3.9	4.4

*** $= p < 0.001$

coping strategies can lessen the impact of stressors, they could ultimately lessen the effects of stressors on gene expression. Although this remains only a theoretical possibility, it has been demonstrated that antidepressant compounds have a variety of effects on neurotrophic factor gene expression that are opposite to those of stress (Duman, 1998; Smith et al., 1995). For example, stress depletes BDNF in the hippocampus while chronic antidepressant treatment increases BDNF in this area. Moreover, both Smith and colleagues in our laboratory (Smith et al., 1995) and Duman (1998) have demonstrated that pretreatment with antidepressants may block some or all of the associated effects of stress on neurotrophic factor gene expression. Most recently, this paradigm has been extended by Gould and Tanapat (1999) and others, indicating that the antidepressants (and lithium) increase neurogenesis even in the adult animal, whereas stressors produce the opposite effect (Table 20.9).

Table 20.9. Impact of Stress and Psychotropic Drugs on Gene Expression and Brain Structure

	STRESS	Gluco-corticoids	LITHIUM	VPA	TCAs
Transcription Factor CREB	↓	↓	↑		↑
Neurotrophic Factor BDNF	↓	↓	↑		↑
Neuroprotective Factor BCL-2 (Anti-Apoptotic)			↑↑	↑	
Neurite Sprouting (in vitro)		↓	↑		
Neurogenesis (in vivo)	↓	↓	↑		↑
Neuronal Viability (NAA by MRS in humans)			↑		
Increased Grey Matter (in humans)			↑		

Based on studies of Smith et al., 1995; Duman, 1998; Chen and Chuang, 1999; Gould and Tanapat, 1999; Moore et al., 2000a,b; Chuang et al., 2002

Lithium as a Neuroprotectant

Significant effects are not unique to the antidepressant substances because some mood stabilizers also appear to have neurotrophic and neuroprotective properties. Chuang and his collaborators reported neuroprotective effects of lithium in a variety of cell culture systems (Nonaka, Katsube, & Chuang, 1998) and then went on to demonstrate that this occurred *in vivo* as well. Chronic treatment with lithium in rats subjected to ligation of the middle cerebral artery (Nonaka & Chuang, 1998) reduced the size of ischemic infarct by approximately 50 percent. In addition, they observed marked neuroprotective effects of lithium in an animal model of Huntington's disease involving the intrastriatal administration of the neurotoxic compound quinolinic acid (Wei et al., 2001). For example, lithium increases the expression of BDNF and Bcl2 mRNA (two neuroprotective factors), whereas it decreases the mRNA levels of Bax and p53 (two proteins that promote cell death or apoptosis) (Chen & Chuang, 1999; Chen et al., 1999). Lithium increases neurite sprouting in culture and in humans also increases a marker of neural integrity in levels of N-acetyl aspartate (NAA) measured by MRS (Moore et al., 2000b). Taken together, these converging *in vitro* and *in vivo* data in animals and humans suggest the possibility that lithium's neuroprotective properties could be important to its therapeutic effects, although this remains to be more directly demonstrated.

Potential Liabilities of Lithium Discontinuation

These preclinical data are of great interest in relation to the clinical findings that lithium not only helps to bring the markedly elevated suicide rate in the unipolar and bipolar affective disorders back toward normal (Baldessarini, Tondo, & Hennen, 1999; Tondo et al., 1998), but also normalizes the mortality rate from associated medical conditions in patients with primary affective disorders (Ahrens et al., 1995; Coppen et al., 1991). These data raise the possibility that the antistroke and neuroprotective effects of lithium observed in animal models could play a role in the normalization of medical mortality in patients who remain on long-term lithium prophylaxis. These observations provide other secondary reasons for continuing lithium pharmacotherapy, even in the absence of a complete clinical response. New meta-analytic data from Baldessarini, Tondo, and Hennen (1999) have indicated that there is a twenty-fold increased risk of suicide in those individuals who discontinue lithium in the first year, compared with those who remain on lithium treatment.

Thus, there would appear to be a variety of potential liabilities of lithium discontinuation, including: (1) increasing the likelihood of a new episode of mania and depression and its associated morbidity; (2) provoking a serious episode requiring rehospitalization; (3) destabilizing the illness for the long term; and (4) contributing to the lethality of the illness from death by suicide. As to point 3, there are increasing data suggesting that a small percentage of patients who are doing well on lithium, but decide to discontinue their medicine and experience a relapse, will not have as robust a response when they resume treatment as they previously had (Post, Ketter, Speer, Leverich, & Weiss, 2000; Post, Leverich, Altshuler, & Mikalauskas, 1992; Post, Leverich, Pazzaglia, Mikalauskas, & Denicoff, 1993). Even in the study of Tondo et al. (1997), reporting no difference in episodes on lithium prior to and after the lithium discontinuation, a significantly higher dose of neuroleptics was required after the period off lithium.

Table 20.10. Prevalence of Lithium Discontinuation-Induced Refractoriness

Study	Length of Lithium Trial (years)	Induced Refractoriness		Patients	Notes
Post et al., 1992, 1993	6–15	9/66	13.6%	All Refractory	Depression or mania
Bauer, 1994	12	1/1	–	–	Single case
Koukopoulos et al., 1995	8.8	13/145	9%	All	Depression or mania
Maj et al., 1995	5.9	10/54	18.5%	Responders	Depression or mania; D/C refractory patients had longer lithium trials
Berghofer and Muller-Oerlinghausen, 1996	5	1/24	4.2%	All	2 initial nonresponders responded in second trial
		1/10	10.0%	Responders	Depression or mania
Tondo et al., 1997	4.6	16/86	18.6%	All	11 initial nonresponders responded in second trial; depression or mania
Coryell et al., 1998	?	1/28	3.6%	Responders	Mania
Overall incidence		39/321	12.1%	All Patients	
		12/92	13.0%	Responders Only	

In our studies and those of a variety of others, 5–15 percent of patients appeared to experience lithium discontinuation-induced refractoriness, in which even the reinstitution of lithium at higher doses than previously needed was without adequate effect (Table 20.10). Coryell et al (1998) reported little evidence for this phenomenon in their report. However, because their study: (a) was under-powered to observe this effect on a statistically reliable basis; (b) used episode criteria that were not optimal; and (c) chose subjects who were not necessarily well-established, long-term lithium responders, one wonders about the strength of the conclusions that can be drawn from that study. Moreover, (d) one of the patients reported in their study failed to re-respond, yielding a refractoriness rate of 3.6 percent even in this negative study (see Table 20.10).

Such a phenomenon of lithium discontinuation-induced refractoriness, when it does occur in an individual, can be particularly devastating, as it was for the patient illustrated in our report (Post, Leverich, Altshuler, & Mikalauskas, 1992). This patient had been completely asymptomatic for eight years during lithium monotherapy treatment, after it was initiated for a series of incapacitating depressions of 2–3 months duration as well as interposed hypomanic episodes. Ten years after restarting her lithium and subsequently adding or substituting a vast array of other treatments, she still continues to be highly symptomatic from her bipolar II illness.

Thus, in addition to the four clinical reasons enumerated above, there is a potential fifth reason for not stopping lithium prophylaxis – to the extent that lithium's neuroprotective effects are related to its mechanisms of action in the affective disorders, one could be losing such a potential long-term protective effect. Could lithium be preventing not only episodes, but also the neural and glial loss associated with the illness, as described below? Even if lithium's neuroprotective effects were mediated separately from its therapeutic actions in bipolar affective disorders, such discontinuation of lithium might also put the patient at greater medical risk from stroke (separate from the risk of relapse, rehospitalization, refractoriness, or suicide).

Affective Illness and Brain Structure

Alterations in neurochemical content (Knable, Torrey, Webster, & Bartko, 2001; Xing et al., 2002) and in the structure of the brain (Ketter, George, Kimbrell, Benson, & Post, 1997; Soares & Mann, 1997) are increasingly being documented in the affective disorders, and therefore the potential effects of antidepressants and mood stabilizers on neurotrophic factors, neurogenesis, glial survival, and neuronal structure take on added interest. A series of studies have suggested deficient size, area, and number of glia or neurons in areas of the brain including ventral (Drevets, Ongur, & Price, 1998) and dorsal aspects of the anterior cingulate gyrus (Rajkowska et al., 1999) and mixed reports on the size of the hippocampus. Two studies (but not Pearlson et al., 1997) report increased size of the amygdala (Altshuler et al., 2000; Strakowski et al., 1999), one in proportion to the number of hospitalizations for mania (Altshuler et al., 2000).

   Thus, we return to the preclinical data reviewed above indicating that experiential effects on gene expression could induce long-lasting changes in behavioral and neurochemical set points, as well as in synaptic and neuroanatomical structure and altered numbers of neuronal and glial cells. The impact of life events on brain biochemistry and microstructure could likewise be of either pathological or adaptive importance for the clinical course of the affective disorders as well. The plasticity of the brain is extraordinary and ongoing throughout one's life. With better understanding of not only the genetic underpinning of vulnerability to affective disorders, but also their interaction with crucial life events and recurrent episodes of illness, we should ultimately be able to design more rational approaches to psychological and pharmacological interventions at the appropriate opportunities.

The Possibility of Primary Prevention

As clinical and genetic markers of high vulnerability become better recognized, perhaps a role for primary prevention in those at highest risk (even before full expression of the illness) should begin to be considered. To the extent that early intervention (such as at first symptoms yielding dysfunction) helps prevent the development of more full-blown recurrent affective disorders and their progression toward treatment-refractoriness even in only a subgroup of patients, an important impact on many lives would be achieved.

   Although most of the links between preclinical models and pathophysiological mechanisms in the affective disorders discussed here remain at the level of hypothesis generation and require more direct examination and testing, their ability to engender appropriate clinical questions and conceptualize the longer time domains of vulnerability (including over the entire lifetime of an individual) gives them value, even beyond their direct predictive validity. We hope that this speculative discussion will foster a wide range of questions and concepts that ultimately will lead to earlier, more focused, and rational interventions in the recurrent affective disorders. Perhaps with such early intervention, the magnitude of the problem affective disorders pose for individuals and society – at both the level of immense suffering and in the billions of dollars they cost each year – can be very substantially lessened.

REFERENCES

Abou-Saleh, M. T. & Coppen, A. (1986). Who responds to prophylactic lithium? *Journal of Affective Disorders 10,* 115–125.

Ahrens, B., Muller-Oerlinghausen, B., Schou, M., Wolf, T., Alda, M., Grof, E., Grof, P., Lenz, G., Simhandl, C., & Thau, K. (1995). Excess cardiovascular and suicide mortality of affective disorders may be reduced by lithium prophylaxis. *Journal of Affective Disorders, 33,* 67–75.

Altshuler, L. L., Bartzokis, G., Grieder, T., Curran, J., Jimenez, T., Leight, K., Wilkins, J., Gerner, R., & Mintz, J. (2000). An MRI study of temporal lobe structures in men with bipolar disorder or schizophrenia. *Biological Psychiatry, 48,* 147–162.

Ambelas, A. (1979). Psychologically stressful events in the precipitation of manic episodes. *British Journal of Psychiatry, 135,* 15–21.

Ambelas, A. (1987). Life events and mania. A special relationship? *British Journal of Psychiatry, 150,* 235–240.

Angst, J. (1966). *Atiologie und Nosologie endogener depressiver Psychosen.* Berlin: Springer Verlag.

Angst, J. (1978). The course of affective disorders. II. Typology of bipolar manic-depressive illness. *Archiv Fur Psychiatrie und Nervenkrankheiten, 226,* 65–74.

Angst, J. & Sellaro, R. (2000). Historical perspectives and natural history of bipolar disorder. *Biological Psychiatry, 48,* 445–457.

Angst, J., Felder, W., Frey, R., & Stassen, H. H. (1978). The course of affective disorders. I. Change of diagnosis of monopolar, unipolar, and bipolar illness. *Archiv Fur Psychiatrie und Nervenkrankheiten, 226,* 57–64.

Angst, J. & Weiss, P. (1967). Periodicity of depressive psychoses. In H. Brill, J. O. Cole, P. Deniker, et al. (Eds.), *Proceedings of the Fifth International Medical Foundation; International Congress Series* (pp. 702–710). Amsterdam: Excerpta Medica.

Anisman, H., Zaharia, M. D., Meaney, M. J., & Merali, Z. (1998). Do early-life events permanently alter behavioral and hormonal responses to stressors? *International Journal of Developmental Neuroscience, 16,* 149–164.

Antelman, S. M., Eichler, A. J., Black, C. A., & Kocan, D. (1980) Interchangeability of stress and amphetamine in sensitization. *Science, 207,* 329–331.

Astrup, C., Fossum, A., & Holmboe, R. (1959). A follow-up study of 270 patients with acute affective psychoses. *Acta Psychiatrica Scandinavica, 34,* 7–62.

Ayuso, G. J., Fuentenebro, D. D., Mendez, B. R., & Marteo, M. I. (1981). [Analysis of precipitating factors in a sample of patients hospitalized for endogenous depression] Analyse des Facteurs declencheurs sur un echantillon de patients hospitalises pour depression endogene. *Annales Medico-Psychologiques, 139,* 759–769.

Baldessarini, R. J., Tondo, L., & Hennen, J. (1999). Effects of lithium treatment and its discontinuation on suicidal behavior in bipolar manic-depressive disorders. *Journal of Clinical Psychiatry, 60 Supplement 2,* 77–84.

Banki, C. M., Bissette, G., Arato, M., & Nemeroff, C. B. (1988). Elevation of immunoreactive CSF TRH in depressed patients. *American Journal of Psychiatry, 145,* 1526–1531.

Barrett, G. L. (2000). The p75 neurotrophin receptor and neuronal apoptosis. *Progress in Neurobiology, 61,* 205–229.

Bauer, M. (1994). Refractoriness induced by lithium discontinuation despite adequate serum lithium levels [letter]. *American Journal of Psychiatry, 151,* 1522.

Beaulieu, S., Rousse, I., Gratton, A., Barden, N., & Rochford, J. (1994). Behavioral and endocrine impact of impaired type II glucocorticoid receptor function in a transgenic mouse model. *Annals of the New York Academy of Sciences, 746,* 388–391.

Berghofer, A. & Muller-Oerlinghausen, B. (1996). No loss of efficacy after discontinuation and reinstitution of long-term lithium treatment? In V. S. Gallicchio & N. J. Birch (Eds.), *Lithium: biochemical and clinical advances* (pp. 39–46). Cheshire: Weidner Publishing.

Bratfos, O. & Haug, J. O. (1968). The course of manic-depressive psychosis: Follow-up investigation of 215 patients. *Acta Psychiatrica Scandinavica, 44*, 89–112.

Breier, A., Kelsoe, J. R., Jr., Kirwin, P. D., Beller, S. A., Wolkowitz, O. M., & Pickar, D. (1988) Early parental loss and development of adult psychopathology. *Archives of General Psychiatry, 45*, 987–993.

Bremner, J. D. (2001). Hypotheses and controversies related to effects of stress on the hippocampus: an argument for stress-induced damage to the hippocampus in patients with posttraumatic stress disorder. *Hippocampus, 11*, 75–81.

Bremner, J. D., Randall, P., Scott, T. M., Bronen, R. A., Seibyl, J. P., Southwick, S. M., Delaney, R. C., McCarthy, G., Charney, D. S., & Innis, R. B. (1995). MRI-based measurement of hippocampal volume in patients with combat-related posttraumatic stress disorder. *American Journal of Psychiatry, 152*, 973–981.

Bremner, J. D., Randall, P., Vermetten, E., Staib, L., Bronen, R. A., Mazure, C., Capelli, S., McCarthy, G., Innis, R. B., & Charney, D. S. (1997). Magnetic resonance imaging-based measurement of hippocampal volume in posttraumatic stress disorder related to childhood physical and sexual abuse – a preliminary report. *Biological Psychiatry, 41*, 23–32.

Brown, G. W. & Harris, T. O. *Social origins of depression.* London: Tavistock Press, 1978.

Cassano, G. B., Akiskal, H. S., Musetti, L., Perugi, G., Soriani, A., & Mignani, V. (1989). Psychopathology, temperament, and past course in primary major depressions. 2. Toward a re-definition of bipolarity with a new semistructured interview for depression. *Psychopathology, 22*, 278–288.

Castine, M. R., Meador-Woodruff, J. H., & Dalack, G. W. (1998). The role of life events in onset and recurrent episodes of schizophrenia and schizoaffective disorder. *Journal of Psychiatric Research, 32*, 283–288.

Chen, R. W. & Chuang, D. M. (1999). Long term lithium treatment suppresses p53 and Bax expression but increases Bcl-2 expression. A prominent role in neuroprotection against excitotoxicity. *Journal of Biological Chemistry, 274*, 6039–6042.

Chen, G., Zeng, W. Z., Yuan, P. X., Huang, L. D., Jiang, Y. M., Zhao, Z. H., & Manji, H. K. (1999). The mood-stabilizing agents lithium and valproate robustly increase the levels of the neuroprotective protein bcl-2 in the CNS. *Journal of Neurochemistry, 72*, 879–882.

Chuang, D. M., Chen, R. W., Chalecka-Franaszek, E., Ren, M., Hashimoto, R., Senatorov, V., Kanai, H., Hough, C., Hiroi, T., & Leeds, P. (2002). Neuroprotective effects of lithium in cultured cells and animal models of diseases. *Bipolar Disorders, 4*, 129–136.

Cicchetti, D., Rogosch, F. A., & Toth, S. L. (2000). The efficacy of toddler-parent psychotherapy for fostering cognitive development in offspring of depressed mothers. *Journal of Abnormal Child Psychopathology, 28*, 135–148.

Coppen, A., Standish-Barry, H., Bailey, J., Houston, G., Silcocks, P., & Hermon, C. (1991). Does lithium reduce the mortality of recurrent mood disorders? *Journal of Affective Disorders, 23*, 1–7.

Coryell, W., Endicott, J., & Keller, M. (1992). Rapidly cycling affective disorder. Demographics, diagnosis, family history, and course. *Archives of General Psychiatry, 49*, 126–131.

Coryell, W., Solomon, D., Leon, A. C., Akiskal, H. S., Keller, M. B., Scheftner, W. A., & Mueller, T. (1998). Lithium discontinuation and subsequent effectiveness. *American Journal of Psychiatry, 155*, 895–898.

Denicoff, K. D., Smith-Jackson, E. E., Disney, E. R., Ali, S. O., Leverich, G. S., & Post, R. M. (1997). Comparative prophylactic efficacy of lithium, carbamazepine, and the combination in bipolar disorder. *Journal of Clinical Psychiatry, 58*, 470–478.

Dolan, R. J., Calloway, S. P., Fonagy, P., De Souza, F. V., & Wakeling, A. (1985). Life events, depression and hypothalamic-pituitary-adrenal axis function. *British Journal of Psychiatry, 147*, 429–433.

Drevets, W. C., Ongur, D., & Price, J. L. (1998). Neuroimaging abnormalities in the subgenual prefrontal cortex: implications for the pathophysiology of familial mood disorders. *Molecular Psychiatry, 3*, 220–221.

Duman, R. S. (1998). Novel therapeutic approaches beyond the serotonin receptor. *Biological Psychiatry, 44*, 324–335.

Dunn, R. T., Frye, M. S., Kimbrell, T. A., Denicoff, K. D., Leverich, G. S., & Post, R. M. (1998). The efficacy and use of anticonvulsants in mood disorders. *Clinical Neuropharmacology, 21*, 215–235.

Egeland, J. A., Hostetter, A. M., Pauls, D. L., & Sussex, J. N. (2000). Prodromal symptoms before onset of manic-depressive disorder suggested by first hospital admission histories. *Journal of the American Academy of Child and Adolescent Psychiatry, 39,* 1245–1252.

Ezquiaga, E., Ayuso, G. J., & Garcia, L. A. (1987). Psychosocial factors and episode number in depression. *Journal of Affective Disorders, 12,* 135–138.

Francis, D. D., Caldji, C., Champagne, F., Plotsky, P. M., & Meaney, M. J. (1999). The role of corticotropin-releasing factor – norepinephrine systems in mediating the effects of early experience on the development of behavioral and endocrine responses to stress. *Biological Psychiatry, 46,* 1153–1166.

Gelenberg, A. J., Kane, J. M., Keller, M. B., Lavori, P., Rosenbaum, J. F., Cole, K., & Lavelle, J. (1989). Comparison of standard and low serum levels of lithium for maintenance treatment of bipolar disorder. *New England Journal of Medicine, 321,* 1489–1493.

Ghaziuddin, M., Ghaziuddin, N., & Stein, G. S. (1990). Life events and the recurrence of depression. *Canadian Journal of Psychiatry, 35,* 239–242.

Glassner, B., Haldipur, C. V., & Dessauersmith, J. (1979). Role loss and working-class manic depression. *Journal of Nervous and Mental Disease, 167,* 530–541.

Goddard, G. V., McIntyre, D. C., & Leech, C. K. (1969). A permanent change in brain function resulting from daily electrical stimulation. *Experimental Neurology, 25,* 295–330.

Goldberg, J. F., Harrow, M., & Leon, A. C. (1996). Lithium treatment of bipolar affective disorders under naturalistic followup conditions. *Psychopharmacology Bulletin, 32,* 47–54.

Gould, E. & Tanapat, P. (1999). Stress and hippocampal neurogenesis. *Biological Psychiatry, 46,* 1472–1479.

Grof, P., Angst, J., & Haines, T. (1974). The clinical course of depression: Practical issues. In J. Angst (Ed.), *Classification and prediction of outcome of depression/Symposium Schloss Reinhartshausen/Rhein, September 23–26, 1973* (pp. 141–148). Stuttgart: F.K. Schattauer Verlag.

Gurvits, T. V., Shenton, M. E., Hokama, H., Ohta, H., Lasko, N. B., Gilbertson, M. W., Orr, S. P., Kikinis, R., Jolesz, F. A., McCarley, R. W., & Pitman, R. K. (1996). Magnetic resonance imaging study of hippocampal volume in chronic, combat-related posttraumatic stress disorder. *Biological Psychiatry, 40,* 1091–1099.

Hammen, C. & Gitlin, M. (1997). Stress reactivity in bipolar patients and its relation to prior history of disorder. *American Journal of Psychiatry, 154,* 856–857.

Huot, R. L., Thrivikraman, K. V., Meaney, M. J., & Plotsky, P. M. (2001). Development of adult ethanol preference and anxiety as a consequence of neonatal maternal separation in Long Evans rats and reversal with antidepressant treatment. *Psychopharmacology (Berl), 158,* 366–373.

Kalivas, P. W. & Duffy, P. (1989). Similar effects of daily cocaine and stress on mesocorticolimbic dopamine neurotransmission in the rat. *Biological Psychiatry, 25,* 913–928.

Kendler, K. S., Kessler, R. C., Neale, M. C., Heath, A. C., & Eaves, L. J. (1993). The prediction of major depression in women: toward an integrated etiologic model. *American Journal of Psychiatry, 150,* 1139–1148.

Kessing, L. V., Andersen, P. K., Mortensen, P. B., & Bolwig, T. G. (1998). Recurrence in affective disorder. I. Case register study. *British Journal of Psychiatry, 172,* 23–28.

Ketter, T. A., George, M. S., Kimbrell, T. A., Benson, B. E., & Post, R. M. (1997). Functional brain imaging in mood and anxiety disorders. *Current Review of Mood and Anxiety Disorders, 1,* 95–112.

Knable, M. B., Torrey, E. F., Webster, M. J., & Bartko, J. O. (2001). Multivariate analysis of prefrontal cortical data from the Stanley Foundation Neuropathology Consortium. *Brain Research Bulletin, 55,* 651–659.

Korte, M., Kang, H., Bonhoeffer, T., & Schuman, E. (1998). A role for BDNF in the late-phase of hippocampal long-term potentiation. *Neuropharmacology, 37,* 553–559.

Koukopoulos, A., Reginaldi, D., Minnai, G., Serra, G., Pani, L., & Johnson, F. N. (1995). The long term prophylaxis of affective disorders. *Advances in Biochemical Psychopharmacology, 49,* 127–147.

Kraepelin, E. (1921). *Manic-depressive insanity and paranoia.* Edinburgh: E.S. Livingstone.

Kubek, M. J., Liang, D., Byrd, K. E., & Domb, A. J. (1998). Prolonged seizure suppression by a single implantable polymeric-TRH microdisk preparation. *Brain Research, 809,* 189–197.

Ladd, C. O., Huot, R. L., Thrivikraman, K. V., Nemeroff, C. B., Meaney, M. J., & Plotsky, P. M. (2000). Long-term behavioral and neuroendocrine adaptations to adverse early experience. *Progress in Brain Research, 122,* 81–103.

Leverich, G. S., Altshuler, L. L., McElroy, S. L., Keck, P. E., Jr., Suppes, T., Denicoff, K. D., Nolen, W. A., Rush, A. J., Kupka, R., Frye, M. A., Autio, K. A., & Post, R. M. (2000). Prevalence of Axis II comorbidity in bipolar disorder: relationship to mood state and course of illness. Presented at the Second European Stanley Foundation Conference on Bipolar Disorder, Amsterdam, The Netherlands, September 21–22.

Leverich, G. S., McElroy, S. L., Suppes, T., Keck, P. E., Jr., Denicoff, K. D., Nolen, W. A., Altshuler, L. L., Rush, A. J., Kupka, R., Frye, M., Autio, K., & Post, R. M. (2002). Early physical and sexual abuse associated with an adverse course of bipolar illness. *Biological Psychiatry, 51,* 288–297.

Leverich, G. S., Nolen, W. A., Rush, A. J., McElroy, S. L., Keck, P. E., Denicoff, K. D., Suppes, T., Altshuler, L. L., Kupka, R., Kramlinger, K. G., & Post, R. M. (2001). The Stanley Foundation Bipolar Treatment Outcome Network. I. Longitudinal methodology. *Journal of Affective Disorders, 67,* 33–44.

Levine, S., Huchton, D. M., Wiener, S. G., & Rosenfeld, P. (1991). Time course of the effect of maternal deprivation on the hypothalamic-pituitary-adrenal axis in the infant rat. *Developmental Psychobiology, 24,* 547–558.

Lish, J. D., Dime-Meenan, S., Whybrow, P. C., Price, R. A., & Hirschfeld, R. M. (1994). The National Depressive and Manic-depressive Association (DMDA) survey of bipolar members. *Journal of Affective Disorders, 31,* 281–294.

Liu, D., Diorio, J., Tannenbaum, B., Caldji, C., Francis, D., Freedman, A., Sharma, S., Pearson, D., Plotsky, P. M., & Meaney, M. J. (1997). Maternal care, hippocampal glucocorticoid receptors, and hypothalamic-pituitary-adrenal responses to stress. *Science, 277,* 1659–1662.

Loosen, P. T. (1985). The TRH-induced TSH response in psychiatric patients: a possible neuroendocrine marker. *Psychoneuroendocrinology, 10,* 237–260.

Lundqvist, G. (1945). Prognosis and course in manic-depressive psychosis. *Acta Psychiatrica Neurologica, 35,* 1–96.

Luthar, S. S., Cicchetti, D., & Becker, B. (2000). The construct of resilience: a critical evaluation and guidelines for future work. *Child Development, 71,* 543–562.

Maj, M., Pirozzi, R., & Magliano, L. (1995). Nonresponse to reinstituted lithium prophylaxis in previously responsive bipolar patients: prevalence and predictors. *American Journal of Psychiatry, 152,* 1810–1811.

Maj, M., Pirozzi, R., Magliano, L., & Bartoli, L. (1998). Long-term outcome of lithium prophylaxis in bipolar disorder: a 5-year prospective study of 402 patients at a lithium clinic. *American Journal of Psychiatry, 155,* 30–35.

Maj, M., Veltro, F., Pirozzi, R., Lobrace, S., & Magliano, L. (1992). Pattern of recurrence of illness after recovery from an episode of major depression: a prospective study. *American Journal of Psychiatry, 149,* 785–800.

Malzberg, B. (1929). A statistical study of the factor of age in manic-depressive psychoses. *Psychiatric Quarterly, 3,* 590–604.

Matussek, P., Halbach, A., & Troger, U. (1965). *Endogene depression.* Munchen: Urban and Schwarzenberg.

McElroy, S. L., Altshuler, L., Suppes, T., Keck, P. E., Frye, M. A., Denicoff, K. D., Nolen, W. A., Kupka, R., Leverich, G. S., Rochussen, J., Rush, A. J., & Post, R. M. (2001). Axis I psychiatric comorbidity and its relationship to historical illness variables in 288 patients with bipolar disorder. *American Journal of Psychiatry, 158,* 420–426.

Meaney, M. J. (1999). Early environmental experience and lifelong changes in behavior and in gene expression (abstract). Presented at the 38th Annual American College of Neuropsychopharmacology Meeting, Acapulco, Mexico, December 12–16.

Meaney, M. J., Aitken, D. H., Van Berkel, C., Bhatnagar, S., & Sapolsky, R. M. (1988). Effect of neonatal handling on age-related impairments associated with the hippocampus. *Science, 239,* 766–768.

Meaney, M. J., Brake, W., & Gratton, A. (2002). Environmental regulation of the development of mesolimbic dopamine systems: a neurobiological mechanism for vulnerability to drug abuse? *Psychoneuroendocrinology, 27,* 127–138.

Moore, G. J., Bebchuk, J. M., Wilds, I. B., Chen, G., & Manji, H. K. (2000a). Lithium-induced increase in human brain grey matter. *Lancet, 356,* 1241–1242.

Moore, G. J., Bebchuk, J. M., Hasanat, K., Chen, G., Seraji-Bozorgzad, N., Wilds, I. B., Faulk, M. W., Koch, S., Glitz, D. A., Jolkovsky, L., & Manji, H. K. (2000b). Lithium increases N-acetyl-aspartate in the human brain: in vivo evidence in support of bcl-2's neurotrophic effects? *Biological Psychiatry, 48*, 1–8.

Nierenberg, A. A., Pingol, M. G., Baer, H. J., Alpert, J. E., Pava, J., Tedlow, J. R., & Fava, M. (1998). Negative life events initiate first but not recurrent depressive episodes. *APA New Research Program and Abstracts, Abstract NR236*, 132.

Nissenbaum, H., Quinn, N. P., Brown, R. G., Toone, B., Gotham, A. M., & Marsden, C. D. (1987). Mood swings associated with the "on-off" phenomenon in Parkinson's disease. *Psychological Medicine, 17*, 899–904.

Nonaka, S. & Chuang, D. M. (1998). Neuroprotective effects of chronic lithium on focal cerebral ischemia in rats. *Neuroreport, 9*, 2081–2084.

Nonaka, S., Katsube, N., & Chuang, D. M. (1998). Lithium protects rat cerebellar granule cells against apoptosis induced by anticonvulsants, phenytoin and carbamazepine. *Journal of Pharmacology and Experimental Therapeutics, 286*, 539–547.

O'Connell, R. A., Mayo, J. A., Flatow, L., Cuthbertson, B., & O'Brien, B. E. (1991). Outcome of bipolar disorder on long-term treatment with lithium. *British Journal of Psychiatry, 159*, 123–129.

Okuma, T. & Shimoyama, N. (1972). Course of endogenous manic-depressive psychosis, precipitating factors and premorbid personality – a statistical study. *Folia Psychiatrica et Neurologica Japonica, 26*, 19–33.

Paskind, H. A. (1930). Manic-depressive psychosis in a private practice. *Archives of Neurological Psychiatry, 23*, 699–794.

Pazzaglia, P. J. & Post, R. M. (1992). Contingent tolerance and reresponse to carbamazepine: a case study in a patient with trigeminal neuralgia and bipolar disorder. *Journal of Neuropsychiatry and Clinical Neurosciences, 4*, 76–81.

Pearlson, G. D., Barta, P. E., Powers, R. E., Menon, R. R., Richards, S. S., Aylward, E. H., Federman, E. B., Chase, G. A., Petty, R. G., & Tien, A. Y. (1997). [Ziskind-Somerfeld Research Award 1996]. Medial and superior temporal gyral volumes and cerebral asymmetry in schizophrenia versus bipolar disorder. *Biological Psychiatry, 41*, 1–14.

Pepin, M. C., Pothier, F., & Barden, N. (1992). Impaired type II glucocorticoid-receptor function in mice bearing antisense RNA transgene. *Nature, 355*, 725–728.

Perris, C. (1968). The course of depressive psychoses. *Acta Psychiatrica Scandinavica, 44*, 238–248.

Perris, H. (1984). Life events and depression. Part 2. Results in diagnostic subgroups, and in relation to the recurrence of depression. *Journal of Affective Disorders, 7*, 25–36.

Plotsky, P. M. (1997). Long-term consequences of adverse early experience: A rodent model (abstract). *Biological Psychiatry, 41*, 77S.

Pollock, H. M. (1931). Recurrence of attacks in manic-depressive psychoses. *American Journal of Psychiatry, 11*, 567–573.

Poort, R. (1945). Catamnestic investigations on manic-depressive psychoses with special reference to the prognosis. *Acta Psychiatrica et Neurologica Scandinavica, 20*, 59–74.

Post, R. M., Denicoff, K. D., Frye, M. A., Dunn, R. T., Leverich, G. S., Osuch, E., & Speer, A. (1998a). A history of the use of anticonvulsants as mood stabilizers in the last two decades of the 20th century. *Neuropsychobiology, 38*, 152–166.

Post, R. M., Frye, M. A., Denicoff, K. D., Leverich, G. S., Kimbrell, T. A., & Dunn, R. T. (1998b). Beyond lithium in the treatment of bipolar illness. *Neuropsychopharmacology, 19*, 206–219.

Post, R. M., Denicoff, K., Frye, M., Leverich, G. S., Cora-Locatelli, G., & Kimbrell, T. A. (1999). Long-term outcome of anticonvulsants in affective disorders. In J. F. Goldberg & M. Harrow (Eds.), *Bipolar disorders: clinical course and outcome* (pp. 85–114). Washington, D.C.: American Psychiatric Press.

Post, R. M., Ketter, T. A., Denicoff, K., Leverich, G. S., & Mikalauskas, K. (1993). Assessment of anticonvulsant drugs in patients with bipolar affective illness. In I. Hindmarch & P. D. Stonier (Eds.), *Human psychopharmacology: methods and measures* (pp. 211–245). Chichester: Wiley.

Post, R. M., Ketter, T. A., Denicoff, K., Pazzaglia, P. J., Leverich, G. S., Marangell, L. B., Callahan, A. M., George, M. S., & Frye, M. A. (1996). The place of anticonvulsant therapy in bipolar illness. *Psychopharmacology (Berl.), 128*, 115–129.

Post, R. M., Ketter, T. A., Speer, A. M., Leverich, G. S., & Weiss, S. R. (2000). Predictive validity of the sensitization and kindling hypotheses. In J. C. Soares & S. Gershon (Eds.), *Bipolar disorders: basic mechanisms and therapeutic implications* (pp. 387–432). New York: Marcel Dekker.

Post, R. M., Kramlinger, K. G., Altshuler, L. L., Ketter, T., & Denicoff, K. (1990). Treatment of rapid cycling bipolar illness. *Psychopharmacology Bulletin, 26,* 37–47.

Post, R. M., Leverich, G. S., Altshuler, L., & Mikalauskas, K. (1992). Lithium-discontinuation-induced refractoriness: preliminary observations. *American Journal of Psychiatry, 149,* 1727–1729.

Post, R. M., Leverich, G. S., Pazzaglia, P. J., Mikalauskas, K., & Denicoff, K. (1993). Lithium tolerance and discontinuation as pathways to refractoriness. In N. J. Birch, C. Padgham, & M. S. Hughes (Eds.), *Lithium in medicine and biology* (1st ed., pp. 71–84). Lancashire, UK: Marius Press.

Post, R. M., Leverich, G. S., Rosoff, A. S., & Altshuler, L. L. (1990). Carbamazepine prophylaxis in refractory affective disorders: a focus on long-term follow-up. *Journal of Clinical Psychopharmacology, 10,* 318–327.

Post, R. M. & Silberstein, S. D. (1994). Shared mechanisms in affective illness, epilepsy, and migraine. *Neurology, 44,* S37–S47.

Post, R. M. & Weiss, S. R. (1992). Ziskind-Somerfeld Research Award 1992. Endogenous biochemical abnormalities in affective illness: therapeutic versus pathogenic. *Biological Psychiatry, 32,* 469–484.

Post, R. M. & Weiss, S. R. B. (1996). A speculative model of affective illness cyclicity based on patterns of drug tolerance observed in amygdala-kindled seizures. *Molecular Neurobiology, 13,* 33–60.

Prien, R. F., Caffey, E. M. J., & Klett, C. J. (1974). Factors associated with treatment success in lithium carbonate prophylaxis. Report of the Veterans Administration and National Institute of Mental Health collaborative study group. *Archives of General Psychiatry, 31,* 189–192.

Racine, R. J. (1972a). Modification of seizure activity by electrical stimulation. I. After-discharge threshold. *Electroencephalography and Clinical Neurophysiology, 32,* 269–279.

Racine, R. J. (1972b). Modification of seizure activity by electrical stimulation. II. Motor seizure. *Electroencephalography and Clinical Neurophysiology, 32,* 281–294.

Rajkowska, G., Miguel-Hidalgo, J. J., Wei, J., Dilley, G., Pittman, S. D., Meltzer, H. Y., Overholser, J. C., Roth, B. L., & Stockmeier, C. A. (1999). Morphometric evidence for neuronal and glial prefrontal cell pathology in major depression. *Biological Psychiatry, 45,* 1085–1098.

Regier, D. A., Farmer, M. E., Rae, D. S., Locke, B. Z., Keith, S. J., Judd, L. L., & Goodwin, F. K. (1990). Comorbidity of mental disorders with alcohol and other drug abuse. Results from the Epidemiologic Catchment Area (ECA) Study. *Journal of the American Medical Association, 264,* 2511–2518.

Rennie, T. (1942). Prognosis in manic-depressive psychoses. *American Journal of Psychiatry, 98,* 801–814.

Roy-Byrne, P., Post, R. M., Uhde, T. W., Porcu, T., & Davis, D. (1985). The longitudinal course of recurrent affective illness: life chart data from research patients at the NIMH. *Acta Psychiatrica Scandinavica, Suppl, 71,* 1–34.

Rush, A. J., Giles, D. E., Schlesser, M. A., Fulton, C. L., Weissenburger, J., & Burns, C. A. (1986). The inventory for depressive symptomatology (IDS): Preliminary findings. *Psychiatry Research, 18,* 65–87.

Rush, A. J., Gullion, C. M., Basco, M. R., Jarrett, R. B., & Trivedi, M. H. (1996). The Inventory of Depressive Symptomatology (IDS): psychometric properties. *Psychological Medicine, 26,* 477–486.

Sarantidis, D. & Waters, B. (1981). Predictors of lithium prophylaxis effectiveness. *Progress in Neuropsychopharmacology, 5,* 507–510.

Smith, M. A., Makino, S., Altemus, M., Michelson, D., Hong, S. K., Kvetnansky, R., & Post, R. M. (1995). Stress and antidepressants differentially regulate neurotrophin 3 mRNA expression in the locus coeruleus. *Proceedings of the National Academy of Sciences of the United States of America, 92,* 8788–8792.

Soares, J. C. & Mann, J. J. (1997). The anatomy of mood disorders – review of structural neuroimaging studies. *Biological Psychiatry, 41,* 86–106.

Starkman, M. N. (1993). The HPA axis and psychopathology: Cushing's syndrome. *Psychiatric Annals, 23,* 691–701.

Steen, R. B. (1933). Prognosis in manic-depressive psychoses. *Psychiatric Quarterly, 7,* 419–429.

Stenstedt, A. (1952). A study in manic-depressive psychosis. *Acta Psychiatrica et Neurologica Scandinavica, Supp, 79,* 1–111.

Strakowski, S. M., DelBello, M. P., Sax, K. W., Zimmerman, M. E., Shear, P. K., Hawkins, J. M., & Larson, E. R. (1999). Brain magnetic resonance imaging of structural abnormalities in bipolar disorder. *Archives of General Psychiatry, 56,* 254–260.

Suppes, T., Leverich, G. S., Keck, P. E., Jr., Nolen, W., Denicoff, K. D., Altshuler, L. L., McElroy, S. L., Rush, A. J., Kupka, R., Frye, M. A., Bickel, M., & Post, R. M. (2001). The Stanley Foundation Bipolar Treatment Outcome Network: II. Demographics and illness characteristics of the first 261 patients. *Journal of Affective Disorders, 67,* 45–59.

Swann, A. C., Bowden, C. L., Calabrese, J. R., Dilsaver, S. C., & Morris, D. D. (1999). Differential effect of number of previous episodes of affective disorder on response to lithium or divalproex in acute mania. *American Journal of Psychiatry, 156,* 1264–1266.

Swendsen, J., Hammen, C., Heller, T., & Gitlin, M. (1995). Correlates of stress reactivity in patients with bipolar disorder. *American Journal of Psychiatry, 152,* 795–797.

Swift, J. M. (1907). The prognosis of recurrent insanity of the manic-depressive type. *American Journal of Insanity, 64,* 311–326.

Taschev, T. (1974). The course and prognosis of depression on the basis of 652 patients decreased. In F. K. Schattauer (Ed.), *Symposia Medica Hoest: Classification and prediction of outcome of depression* (8th ed., pp. 156–172). New York: Schattauer.

Tondo, L., Baldessarini, R. J., Floris, G., & Rudas, N. (1997). Effectiveness of restarting lithium treatment after its discontinuation in bipolar I and bipolar II disorders. *American Journal of Psychiatry, 154,* 548–550.

Tondo, L., Baldessarini, R. J., Hennen, J., Floris, G., Silvetti, F., & Tohen, M. (1998). Lithium treatment and risk of suicidal behavior in bipolar disorder patients. *Journal of Clinical Psychiatry, 59,* 405–414.

Wan, R. Q., Noguera, E. C., & Weiss, S. R. (1998). Anticonvulsant effects of intra-hippocampal injection of TRH in amygdala kindled rats. *Neuroreport, 9,* 677–682.

Wei, H., Qin, Z., Senatorov, V. V., Wei, W., Wang, Y., Qian, Y., & Chuang, D. (2001). Lithium suppresses excitotoxicity-induced striatal lesions in a rat model of Huntington's disease. *Neuroscience, 106,* 603–612.

Weiss, S. R., Clark, M., Rosen, J. B., Smith, M. A., & Post, R. M. (1995). Contingent tolerance to the anticonvulsant effects of carbamazepine: relationship to loss of endogenous adaptive mechanisms. *Brain Research, Brain Research Reviews, 20,* 305–325.

Weiss, S. R. & Post, R. M. (1994). Caveats in the use of the kindling model of affective disorders. *Toxicology and Industrial Health, 10,* 421–447.

Xing, G. Q., Russell, S., Hough, C., O'Grady, J., Zhang, L., Yang, S., Zhang, L. X., & Post, R. M. (2002). Decreased prefrontal CaMKII α mRNA in bipolar illness. *NeuroReport, 13,* 501–505.

Xing, G. Q., Smith, M. A., Levine, S., Yang, S. T., Post, R. M., & Zhang, L. X. (1998). Suppression of CaMKII and nitric oxide synthase by maternal deprivation in the brain of rat pups (abstract). *Society for Neuroscience Abstracts, 24* [176.9], 452.

Zhang, L. X., Levine, S., Dent, G., Zhan, Y., Xing, G., Okimoto, D., Kathleen, G. M., Post, R. M., & Smith, M. A. (2002). Maternal deprivation increases cell death in the infant rat brain. *Developmental Brain Research, 133,* 1–11.

Zhang, L. X., Xing, G. Q., Levine, S., Post, R. M., & Smith, M. A. (1998). Effects of maternal deprivation on neurotrophic factors and apoptosis-related genes in rat pups (abstract). *Society for Neuroscience Abstracts, 24* [176.8], 451.

Zis, A. P., Grof, P., & Webster, M. (1980). Prediction of relapse in recurrent affective disorder. *Psychopharmacology Bulletin, 16,* 47–49.

TWENTY-ONE

Neurohormonal Aspects of the Development of Psychotic Disorders

Elaine F. Walker and Deborah Walder

The major mental illnesses, most notably schizophrenia and other psychotic disorders, typically have their onset in young adulthood, and often lead to a lifetime of chronic disability. The possibility of preventing these illnesses has received increasing attention in the past few years (McGorry & Edwards, 1998; Wyatt, Apud, & Potkin 1996). This trend has been fueled by evidence that the longer the duration of the initial untreated episodes of psychosis, the worse the long-term prognosis (Wyatt, 1995). Also, the availability of atypical antipsychotic medications that have fewer immediate side effects has contributed to interest in psychosis prevention.

The first step in the prevention process is the identification of vulnerable individuals. It is well established that the clinical onset of schizophrenia is preceded by behavioral dysfunction. In some cases, preschizophrenic individuals manifest consistent dysfunction that is apparent within the first few years of life, extends throughout childhood, and becomes more pronounced in adolescence (Larsen, McGlashan, Johannessen, & Vibe-Hansen, 1996; Walker, Baum, & Diforio, 1998). Others show relatively normal childhood development, then a precipitous decline that begins in adolescence. Based on the best available evidence, about 70 percent of adult-onset patients manifested behavioral dysfunction in adolescence (Larsen et al., 1996; Neumann, Grimes, Walker, & Baum, 1995; Yung & McGorry, 1996). Thus, many view adolescence/early adulthood as the most plausible developmental stage for initiating prevention.

In parallel with the increasing emphasis on prevention, there has been a resurgence of interest in the neurodevelopmental changes that accompany pubertal maturation. There is mounting evidence that adolescence is a critical developmental period for onset of adjustment problems because it is associated with significant normative changes in brain function (Spear, 2000a,b; Walker, in press). Neuroimaging studies have revealed changes in the volume and neuronal organization of various brain regions, as well as changes in neurotransmitter systems. The post-pubertal rise in gonadal hormones is well documented, and recent findings indicate that the release of cortisol, an adrenal hormone, also increases at this time (Walker, 2002). Cross-sectional and longitudinal studies of normal children reveal a gradual rise in salivary and urinary cortisol during middle childhood, then a marked increase in adolescence (Kenny, Gancayo, Heald & Hung, 1966; Kenny, Preeyasombat, & Migeon, 1966; Kiess, Meidert, Dressendorfer,

Scheiver, Kessler, & Konig, 1995; Lupien, King, Meaney, & McEwen, 2001; Wajs-Kuto, De Beeck, Rooman, & Caju, 1999; Walker, 2002). Those that have examined pubertal stage find a positive correlation between pubertal stage and cortisol level (Kenny, et al., 1966; Kiess, et al., 1995). These findings suggest that the hypothalamic–pituitary–adrenal (HPA) axis, which governs the release of cortisol, is showing heightened activity following the onset of puberty.

It has been suggested that neuromaturational processes contribute to the marked escalation in risk for psychotic and affective disorders through adolescence (Walker, in press). Specifically, it is possible that the neurodevelopmental changes that accompany the post-pubertal period are triggering the expression of latent vulnerabilities. Biological indicators, in conjunction with behavioral markers, may prove useful in the identification of at-risk groups. In this chapter, we review some key trends in the literature on early stages of psychotic disorder, with an emphasis on neurohormonal processes in vulnerable individuals. We also present recent results from our longitudinal study of youth presumed to be at behavioral risk for schizophrenia. This study is aimed at determining whether biological measures can enhance the prediction of Axis I disorder in adolescents with schizotypal personality disorder (SPD).

BEHAVIORAL INDICATORS OF RISK

The chief question that has challenged prevention researchers in the field of psychopathology is how to identify persons at imminent risk. The nature of the prodrome for psychotic disorders is variable, but retrospective research has shown that a substantial proportion of preschizophrenic youth show a behavioral syndrome that is comparable to SPD as defined by the *Diagnostic and Statistical Manual of Mental Disorders*, revised, 4th edition (*DSM-IV*; Davidson, et al., 1999; Neumann et al., 1995; Tyrka, Cannon, Haslam, & Mednick, 1995; Walker, Baum, & Diforio, 1998; Wolfradt & Straub, 1998). This syndrome includes interpersonal deficits and social withdrawal, as well as perceptual and ideational abnormalities.

Given the possibility that individuals at risk for psychotic disorders could be identified on the basis of subclinical behavioral characteristics, investigators have launched longitudinal studies of adolescents/young adults who show a prodromal syndrome (Miller & McGlashan, 2000; Yung & McGorry, 1996). Yung and colleagues identified individuals, ranging in age from 15 to 26 years (mean age 18 years), who showed one or more attenuated psychotic symptoms as defined by the *DSM III-R* for prodromal signs of schizophrenia (Yung & McGorry, 1996). These signs included magical thinking, perceptual disturbance, social isolation, or impaired role function. A follow-up assessment conducted 20 months later revealed that 21 percent (7 out of 33) showed at least one frank psychotic symptom (hallucinations, delusions, or significant abnormality of thought content as defined by *DSM-IV*).

In a subsequent study, the researchers recruited individuals at risk through general community announcements, primary care practitioners, and school counselors (Yung et al., 1998). The *DSM-IV* criteria for SPD were used to select a risk sample with attenuated psychotic symptoms (e. g., ideas of reference, odd beliefs or magical thinking, perceptual disturbances, odd thinking and speech, paranoid ideation, and odd behavior or appearance). Although the inclusion criteria were less stringent than those for a *DSM-IV* diagnosis of SPD, the participants were significantly impaired. Twelve-month follow-up data indicated that 48 percent met criteria for an Axis I psychotic disorder; schizophreniform ($n = 6$), brief psychosis ($n = 1$), schizophrenia ($n = 1$), schizoaffective disorder ($n = 1$), bipolar disorder ($n = 1$), and major depression with psychotic features ($n = 1$). Analysis of the intake data revealed that those who became psychotic did not differ on initial levels of pre-psychotic, affective, or negative symptoms. Thus, there was little evidence that further refinement of the behavioral criteria would yield better prediction. Consistent with these findings, a subsequent report on a community sample indicated that 45 percent of adolescents (mean age 13.8) who met *DSM-IV* diagnostic criteria for a cluster A personality disorder met criteria for an Axis I disorder 8–10 years later (Johnson et al., 1999). However, in this study the investigators did not explore the relation between specific Axis II categories and subsequent psychiatric status.

Biological Risk Indicators. The results of the above studies indicate that the use of behavioral criteria for identifying at-risk youth holds promise, but that further refinement of vulnerability criteria is needed. In the "Emory Study of Adolescent Development," an ongoing longitudinal study of youth at risk, we measured several physical indicators of vulnerability to schizophrenia in adolescents with SPD (Weinstein et al., 1999). One objective was to determine whether the SPD youth, like schizophrenia patients, showed more dysmorphic features; namely, minor physical anomalies (MPAs) and dermatoglyphic abnormalities. Dysmorphic features are of interest to psychopathologists because they have their origins in prenatal neurodevelopment, and thus suggest the presence of a congenital vulnerability. At the same time that the fetal central nervous system (CNS) is undergoing genesis from cells in the ectoderm, various external morphological features are forming from the same cell mass (Nowakowski & Hayes, 1999). MPAs are irregularities in the structure of the face, head, hands, and feet. These external features of the head and extremities undergo rapid development during the first and second trimesters – the same periods when the CNS undergoes significant development (Moore, 1982). The most widely used measure of MPAs, the Waldrop scale (Waldrop & Halverson, 1971), indexes anomalies such as steepled palate, asymmetric ears, and wide-spaced eyes. Research has provided evidence that MPAs are a consequence of fetal exposure to prenatal insult, as well as genetic factors (Smith, 1982). MPAs occur at an elevated rate in individuals with a variety of disorders, including autism (Gualtieri et al., 1982), attention deficit disorder (Deutsch et al., 1990), childhood adjustment disorder (Fogel, Mednick, & Michelsen, 1985; Halverson & Victor, 1976; Pomeroy et al., 1988), aggressive behavior (Kandel et al., 1989), schizophrenia and other psychotic disorders (Griffiths et al., 1998), and SPD (Weinstein et al., 1999). Taken together, the research findings suggest that MPAs are nonspecific indicators of abnormal fetal CNS development that can compromise postnatal CNS function, thereby conferring an increased risk for behavioral dysfunction.

Irregularities in palm and fingerprints are additional dysmorphic signs associated with mental illness (Schaumann & Alter, 1976). Among the most commonly measured aspects of dermal patterns are differences in finger ridge counts between corresponding digits on the right and left hands (fluctuating asymmetries – FAs), total finger ridge counts, and palmar a-b ridge count. Like MPAs, these irregularities have their origins in prenatal development (primarily the first part of the second trimester), and appear to be a consequence of both genetic factors and prenatal insult (Cummins & Midlow, 1961; Mellor, 1968). In addition, a causal effect of prenatal stress is indicated by findings that exposure of pregnant monkeys to stress results in an increase in dermatoglyphic abnormalities in offspring (Newell-Morris et al., 1989).

In our study of SPD adolescents, the SPD group was compared with age-matched normals, in addition to adolescents with other disorders (Weinstein et al., 1999). Diagnostic group comparisons revealed that the SPD group showed a higher rate of both MPAs and FAs. The group suffering from other disorders fell midway between the SPD and control groups. These findings are generally consistent with those obtained from studies of adult schizophrenia patients, and provide support for the assumption that the vulnerability to SPD is, in part, congenital.

Several lines of evidence point to the presence of HPA axis dysfunction in schizophrenia. Adult patients with the illness manifest elevated baseline and post-dexamethasone cortisol levels (Walker & Diforio, 1997). We therefore sought to determine whether cortisol hypersecretion was present in youth with SPD. Consistent with predictions, when compared to normal participants, the SPD group showed higher salivary cortisol levels, and this was most pronounced for the first sample obtained. The latter finding suggests that the SPD participants were more responsive to the novelty of the testing situation.

It is noteworthy that several investigators have reported that higher rates of dysmorphic features in children and adolescents are linked with greater vulnerability to stress. In a longitudinal study by Pine et al. (1997), MPAs were measured when participants were seven years of age, and psychiatric status was measured when they were seventeen years. The relation between environmental risk factors (e.g., familial discord and stressors) and psychiatric disorder was stronger in participants with high MPA scores. Significant interactive effects of MPAs and environmental stress on behavior problems are also reported by Brennan et al. (1997), Mednick and Kandel (1988), and Sandberg et al. (1980). It thus appears that MPAs are associated with more pronounced behavioral sequelae of stress exposure. As with MPAs, there is evidence that the presence of dermatoglyphic abnormalities in children is associated with heightened sensitivity to stressful experiences (Alexander et al., 1997). Taken together, these research findings raise the possibility that the presence of dysmorphic features might be linked with a more pronounced cortisol response to stressful events. Thus, dysmorphic features may reflect the presence of the "diathesis" which, in interaction with elevated cortisol, can lead to the expression of behavioral dysfunction. We therefore sought to test the interactive relation of cortisol levels and dysmorphic features with Axis I outcomes in at-risk youth.

In conceptualizing the role of stress and stress hormones in psychiatric disorder, it is important to emphasize that elevated cortisol secretion is not specific to schizophrenia or spectrum disorders. Several lines of evidence suggest that activation of biological stress systems can serve to trigger symptom expression in youth at risk for a variety of mental disorders. Longitudinal studies have shown that elevated cortisol levels are linked with later onset or exacerbation of depressive symptoms (Goodyer, Herbert, Tamplin, & Altham, 2000; Susman et al., 1997), panic disorder (Abelson & Curtis, 1996), anorexia (Steiner & Levine, 1988), mixed childhood adjustment disorders (Granger et al., 1996), and psychotic symptoms (Franzen, 1971; Sachar et al., 1970). Taken together, these results suggest that the HPA axis acts as a generalized moderating system that has the potential to augment the expression of vulnerability to multiple forms of psychopathology (Stansbury & Gunnar, 1994; Walker & Diforio, 1997). Further, the normative postpubescent increase in HPA activity may be one of the maturational factors contributing to the rise in prodromal features of mental illness during adolescence (Kenny, Gancayo, Heald, & Hung, 1966; Kenny, Preeyasombat, & Migeon, 1966; Kiess et al., 1995; Lupien et al., 2001; Walker et al., 2001; Weinstein et al., 1999).

The Emory Study of Adolescent Development: Interim Diagnostic Follow-Up. We recently conducted a diagnostic follow-up of the adolescent participants in our study of youth at risk for psychosis. The primary goals were (1) to determine the rate of Axis I diagnoses in this sample during the late adolescence/early adult period, and (2) to test the hypothesis that elevated cortisol levels and dysmorphic signs would be associated with progression to Axis I disorder. Detailed descriptions of the study participants are provided in earlier reports on the study (e.g., Diforio, Kestler, & Walker, 2000; Weinstein et al., 1999), so only general information will be presented here.

The sample was recruited from the local community in 1995 and 1996, primarily through announcements directed at clinicians and at parents who had concerns about their child's adjustment. Following procedures used in previous studies, the announcement described signs of schizotypal personality disorder in lay terms (i.e., "problems in social relationships," "unusual ideas," "suspiciousness"). A screening interview was administered to parents over the phone, and appropriate participants were scheduled for assessment. The goal was to obtain a sample of participants with SPD, as well as a sample with other personality disorders. A comparison group of adolescents with no Axis I or II disorder was recruited through a register maintained by the Department of Psychology for studies of normal child development. For all subjects, including normal controls, diagnostic status was determined with administration of the Structured Clinical Interview for *DSM III-R* Personality Disorders (SCID-II) questionnaire (Spitzer, Williams, Gibbon, & First, 1990), the SCID-II interview, and the SCID Psychotic Screen.

The resultant samples were composed of 20 participants (12 males) who met *DSM-IV* diagnostic criteria for SPD, 20 (13 males) who met criteria for one or more other Axis II disorder (Other disorder – OD group), and 26 (17 males) who did not meet criteria for any Axis II disorder (Normal control – NC group). The diagnoses of the OD group were: Paranoid, $n = 3$; Schizoid, $n = 3$; Borderline, $n = 1$; Antisocial/Conduct disorder, $n = 6$; Dependent, $n = 1$; Passive-Aggressive, $n = 5$; Obsessive-Compulsive, $n = 4$; NOS, $n = 2$. As expected, there was a high rate of comorbidity, so the sum of these numbers exceeds the number of OD participants. Similarly, consistent with evidence of comorbidity in personality disorders, some of the participants in the SPD group also met criteria for other Axis II disorders. However, none of the participants met criteria for an Axis I disorder at the first assessment.

Mean ages for the SPD, OD, and NC groups were 14.2 (SD = 1.2), 14.7 (SD = 2.2), and 13.9 (SD = 1.6), respectively. Of the 20 SPD participants, 10 had previous outpatient contact (pediatrician, psychiatrist, or psychologist) because of parental concerns about the child's adjustment. There were no significant differences among the diagnostic groups in IQ scores, or the occupational status of the parents.

INITIAL ASSESSMENT PROCEDURES

Dysmorphic Features. The techniques used to index MPAs and FAs are described in detail in Wienstein et al. (1999). Briefly, the measurement of MPAs was based on standard procedures. Following Green et al. (1994), the modified Waldrop Scale was administered (Waldrop et al., 1968). It assesses six body regions, including the head, eyes, mouth, ears, hands, and feet.

Dermatoglyphics. To assess dermatoglyphic abnormalities, prints of each palm and each finger were obtained from participants using an inkless method (Cummins & Midlow, 1961). An amplification screen was used to enhance the prints, and inter-rater reliability was almost 100 percent. The index of primary interest derived from the prints was fluctuating asymmetry (FAs), the sum of the absolute differences in ridge counts between the corresponding left and right fingers.

Saliva Sampling. In order to control for normal diurnal variation in cortisol, all assessments were scheduled to begin at the same time of day. Participants were instructed to abstain from caffeinated beverages and all medication the day of the assessment. Saliva samples were obtained in specimen tubes at predetermined points throughout the assessment (one each hour). At least four samples were obtained from each subject. The assay used to measure cortisol levels is described in detail in earlier publications (Weinstein et al., 1999).

   It should be noted that plasma, urinary, and salivary cortisol measures are highly interrelated (Shipley et al., 1992), suggesting that all are indexing activity of the HPA axis. However, salivary cortisol appears to be a more sensitive measure of stress reactivity than either urinary (Bassett et al., 1987) or plasma cortisol (Rahe et al., 1990). Also, saliva cortisol shows a higher correlation with ratings of psychiatric symptoms (Rahe et al., 1990). This may indicate that the more invasive nature of obtaining plasma and urine samples results in increased measurement error.

1997 Follow-up Assessment. Between February and August 1997, follow-up assessments were conducted in the research center, 1 1/2 to 2 years after the first assessment. As in the initial assessment, saliva cortisol was measured four times, at hourly intervals.

   Of the total sample of 66 participants, 44 were able to return to our laboratory for assessment. The breakdown of followed participants by initial diagnostic group was 12 SPD, 11 OD, and 21 from the NC group. Information on current status for an additional 19 participants was obtained in telephone interviews with the parent and child. Of these 19 participants, 5 did not undergo follow-up evaluation in the clinic because they were either hospitalized ($n = 3$) or in a detention facility ($n = 2$) at the time. The other 14 youths were characterized by oppositional and withdrawn tendencies and resisted scheduling a follow-up assessment, despite the encouragement of research personnel and their parents. Three participants could not be reached by telephone or mail at the time.

1999 Diagnostic Follow-up. In 1999, telephone interviews were conducted with the parents of 37 of the original 40 participants in the SPD and OD groups. The mean age of the participants in 1999 was 18.5 years (SD = 1.8), with a range of 16 to 24.

   Systematic data on diagnostic outcome were obtained in telephone interviews, rather than at the research center, in order to maximize the number of participants for whom information was obtained. The mode of follow-up ascertainment has special relevance for longitudinal studies of psychiatric disorder, because the psychiatric

Table 21.1. Axis I Diagnostic Outcome by Group

Axis II Diagnostic Group	Axis I Diagnostic Outcome
SPD ($n = 19$)	No Axis I disorder or Mental Health Treatment $n = 7$ Outpatient psychotherapy, but no diagnosis, $n = 4$ Schizophrenia, $n = 3$ Schizophreniform psychosis, $n = 2$ Bipolar disorder, $n = 1$ Psychotic disorder NOS, $n = 1$ Major depression, $n = 1$
OD ($n = 18$)	No Axis I disorder or Mental Health Treatment, $n = 10$ Inpatient treatment, but no Axis I diagnosis, $n = 1$ Outpatient psychotherapy, but no diagnosis, $n = 3$ Major depression, $n = 2$ Psychosis (NOS), $n = 1$ Schizophrenia, $n = 1$

outcomes of participants are often associated with their willingness/ability to participate in a follow-up interview. In the present sample, some of the most severely disturbed participants were in hospitals or detention facilities, and thus unavailable. In all cases, however, the parent-informant had regular contact with the participant.

Previous research has compared medical history and diagnostic interviews conducted over the telephone with those conducted in person, and the results indicate that the reliability of diagnostic information obtained over the phone is very good (Fenig, Levav, Kohn, & Yelin, 1993; King, Hovey, Brand, & Ghaziuddin, 1997; Potts, Daniels, Burnam, & Wells, 1990; Revicki, Tohen, Gyulai, & Thompson, 1997; Sobin, Weissman, Goldstein, & Adams, 1993). This includes interviews with parents about their adolescent's psychiatric symptoms and history (Fendrich, Johnson, Wislar, & Nageotte, 1999).

A semistructured interview was administered to obtain information on the subject's medical history, behavior, and psychiatric symptoms. The following information was collected: current school/occupational performance, inpatient and outpatient mental health treatment history, current and past psychiatric diagnoses, type and dosage of medication.

The Transition from Axis II to Axis I Disorder. Although most of the study participants have not yet entered their early twenties, the peak risk period for onset of psychotic symptoms, we found that a substantial number had received an Axis I diagnosis. Of the SPD participants for whom follow-up data were obtained in 1999 ($n = 19$), eight (42 percent) had received an Axis I diagnosis since the initial assessment. Six of the eight had received treatment at an inpatient psychiatric facility, one was treated at a juvenile detention facility, and another in a state prison. The diagnoses are listed in Table 21.1. Seven of the eight SPD adolescents with Axis I disorders (i.e., 36% of the total) were reported to have psychotic symptoms. The eighth participant with an Axis I diagnosis (major depression) was described as having highly debilitating symptoms.

Five (28%) of the eighteen OD adolescents had been hospitalized, and four (22%) received an Axis I diagnosis. (For diagnoses, see Table 21.1.) According to parental reports, the hospitalized adolescent who did not receive an Axis I diagnosis has been

Table 21.2. Mean Cortisol Levels, MPA Scores, and Dermatoglyphic Scores by Axis II Group and Axis I Diagnostic Outcome

| | MPA Score | | Fluctuating Asymmetry | | Mean Cortisol Assessment | | | |
| | | | | | 1 | | 2 | |
	M	(SD)	M	(SD)	M	(SD)	M	(SD)
Combined SPD and OD groups								
No Axis I disorder	2.2	(1.76)	16.86	(7.7)	.25	(.08)	.29	(.15)
Axis I disorder	2.2	(1.87)	16.25	(9.37)	.35	(.09)	.44	(.20)
SPD group								
No Axis I disorder	2.66	(2.27)	16.75	(7.32)	.25	(.10)	.33	(.12)
Axis I disorder	2.85	(1.86)	19.60	(9.31)	.36	(.07)	.42	(.17)
OD group								
No Axis I disorder	1.88	(1.27)	16.94	(8.25)	.25	(.09)	.26	(.16)
Axis I disorder	.68	(.57)	10.67	(6.66)	.33	(.04)	.47	(.39)

diagnosed as having a conduct disorder. Psychotic symptoms were reported in two of the four hospitalized participants. (It is noteworthy that four other OD participants had been in juvenile detention facilities for short periods of time. Based on parental descriptions, two of these may have manifested significant psychiatric symptoms, but because no diagnosis was made they are classified as having no Axis I diagnosis.)

Group Differences Based on Axis I Outcomes. Group comparisons were conducted in order to determine whether cortisol levels and/or dysmorphic features were linked with Axis I outcome based on the 1999 follow-up interviews. Because of the small number of subjects in any single *DSM* category, all of those with an Axis I diagnosis were combined for purposes of data analysis. Mean values for cortisol (averaged across four saliva samples), MPAs, and FAs, by diagnostic outcome, are presented in Table 21.2.

T tests were first conducted with the SPD and OD groups combined. Comparisons of those with and without Axis I diagnoses showed that the participants *with* Axis I diagnosis had significantly higher cortisol values at the first, $t(36) = 4.44$, $p < .01$, and second, $t(22) = 1.86$, $p < .05$, assessments. However, the two outcome groups did not differ in MPA or FAs.

Comparing the outcome groups from the SPD sample only, those with an Axis I diagnosis showed a trend toward higher cortisol at the second assessment, $t(10) = 1.04$, $p = .15$, and significantly higher cortisol at the first assessment, $t(18) = 4.16$, $p < .01$. There were no differences in MPAs or FAs. It is important to note that substantially fewer participants were assessed at the second laboratory follow-up. Thus, statistical power for detecting group differences in cortisol at the second assessment was low. Also, when the analyses were conducted excluding the one participant with an Axis I diagnosis but no reported psychotic symptoms, the statistical results were the same.

A similar pattern of diagnostic group differences was observed in the OD group; those with Axis I diagnosis had higher cortisol levels at the first, $t(17) = 2.68$, $p < .05$,

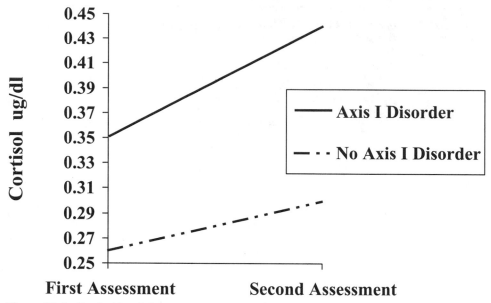

Figure 21.1. Cortisol levels by outcome group and assessment time

but not the second assessment, $t(10) = .73$, $p = .25$. Again, there was no significant difference in MPAs or FAs.

Developmental Changes in Cortisol and Outcome. It is of interest to know whether the developmental change in cortisol over time is linked with Axis I outcome. Because not all of the participants received the second assessment, mean cortisol scores were computed separately for those who participated in *both* assessments. This allowed us to examine developmental changes over time. The mean values are presented in Figure 21.1 for the combined SPD and OD participants. A repeated measures ANOVA revealed a significant main effects for diagnostic outcome, $F(1, 22) = 5.46$, $p < .05$, with Axis I outcome participants showing higher levels. Although the interaction did not reach statistical significance, $F(1, 22) = .86$, $p = .25$, it is clear that there was a more marked increase in cortisol values for the subjects who progressed to Axis I diagnoses.

As mentioned, there is evidence from previous research that higher levels of dysmorphic features are linked with a greater susceptibility to stress. It was therefore of interest to test the interaction between dysmorphic signs and cortisol in predicting Axis I diagnostic outcomes. Regression analyses were conducted to test for an interaction effect, with mean cortisol, MPA, and FA scores from the initial assessment as the predictors, and Axis I classification as the dependent variable. These analyses did not reveal any significant interactions.

A SYNTHESIS: THE EARLY DEVELOPMENTAL COURSE OF PSYCHOSIS

The Transition from Axis II to Axis I. A central question in longitudinal studies of samples at risk for psychosis concerns the eventual rate of Axis I outcomes. A variety of methodologic factors pose challenges in our attempts to obtain accurate estimates. Two of these factors are the duration of the follow-up period and subject ascertainment for diagnosis. Because our study participants were relatively young at the most recent telephone follow-up, we must assume that diagnostic status will undergo substantial change in the future. Thus, their 1999 diagnostic status must be considered to be a measure of interim outcome. Furthermore, in order to obtain information on a larger proportion of the sample, the Axis I diagnostic data are based on parental reports, and these may not correspond to what would be obtained with direct diagnostic interviews. Nonetheless, our findings are consistent with previous reports of a high rate of Axis I diagnostic outcomes in youth with Axis II disorder. For example, the proportion with Axis I outcomes among the SPD adolescents was similar to that reported by McGorry and colleagues in their follow-up of an older group (mean age of 18 years at study inception; McGorry & Edwards, 1998). Although the younger age of the participants in our investigation (14 years at study inception) would lead to the expectation of fewer Axis I outcomes, our more stringent inclusion criteria for the SPD group may have yielded a more severely disturbed sample. (Our inclusion criteria were those for *DSM-IV* SPD, whereas participants in the McGorry study were not required to meet the full SPD criteria.)

It has been shown that patients with a younger age-at-onset of schizophrenia have poorer premorbid function (Gupta et al., 1995). Given that our sample is young, with a relatively severe level of disturbance, we expect that their mean age-at-onset of clinical disorder will be below the average age-at-onset for Axis I psychotic disorder. The eventual rate of disorder may also be higher. In sum, it should be assumed that these participants will undergo further change in psychiatric status, such that additional Axis I diagnoses will emerge, and some current diagnoses will change. Assuming a population base-rate of 1–2 percent for psychotic disorders (with late adolescent/young adult onset), our findings of a 36 percent rate of psychotic disorders in the SPD sample represents a major increase. Thus, the presence of SPD alone contributes significantly to the prediction of Axis I outcomes, especially psychotic disorders.

At the same time, we must acknowledge that the rates of Axis I outcome from studies of at-risk populations are all under 50 percent. In our study sample, some youth who met criteria for SPD in the initial assessment were functioning at above-average levels at the 1999 follow-up. This is consistent with the assumption that many adolescents manifest transient adjustment problems. Beyond this, we addressed the question of whether physical risk indicators, cortisol, and dysmorphic features, enhanced the prediction of Axis I outcomes.

Cortisol and Axis I Outcome. Group comparisons revealed differences in cortisol levels between those with and without Axis I disorders. As predicted, the PD adolescents who later developed Axis I disorders showed a higher mean cortisol level up to four years prior to receiving an Axis I diagnosis. This held for both the combined groups, and the SPD and OD groups examined separately. These findings are consistent with previous reports that elevated cortisol predicts worse outcomes for youth with a variety of psychiatric syndromes that involve internalized symptoms.

As shown by this and previous studies, there is an association between cortisol secretion and the expression of a broad spectrum of psychopathologies. This suggests that the HPA axis is a nonspecific moderating system. Although the neural mechanisms mediating the relations between cortisol secretion and symptom expression are unknown, it is likely that they involve the effects of glucocorticoids on various neurotransmitter systems. A discussion of the empirical literature in this area is beyond the scope of this chapter; however, it should be mentioned that plausible neural mechanisms have been hypothesized for both depression (Post et al., 1994) and psychotic disorders (Benes, 1994; Walker & Diforio, 1997).

In the case of schizophrenia, over-activity of the dopamine (DA) system has been implicated in the neuropathophysiology (Davis et al., 1991; Den Boer, 1995). As described by Walker and Diforio (1997), cortisol augments DA activity (Mittleman et al., 1992; Rothschild et al., 1985; Schatzberg et al., 1985; Wolkowitz, 1994), so that DA is enhanced by stress exposure (Antelman & Chiodo, 1984; Grossman, 1993; McMurray et al., 1991; Sorg & Kalivas, 1995). Several lines of animal research suggest that activation of the HPA axis can also alter DA receptors in some strains, indicating a role for individual differences in the neural consequences of stress exposure (Biron et al., 1992; Cabib, Oliverio, Ventura, Lucchese, & Puglisi-Allegra, 1997; Cabib & Puglisi-Allegra, 1991). For example, Cabib & Puglisi-Allegra (1991) have shown that repeated stressful experiences lead to a hyposensitivity of brain DA receptors in one mouse strain (DBA), while they produced a hypersensitivity of DA receptors in another strain (C57). This group of investigators have thus concluded that genotype influences the interaction between the organism and the environment by modulating individual differences in responsiveness to stressors and by determining the neurochemical consequences of stressful experiences. These and other findings support the notion that activation of the HPA axis can contribute to the expression of psychotic symptoms when there is a pre-existing vulnerability to abnormalities in the DA system (Walker & Diforio, 1997).

Dysmorphic Features. Contrary to prediction, those with Axis I diagnosis were not characterized by higher rates of dysmorphic features. MPAs and FAs failed to distinguish the two outcome groups, either independently or in interaction with cortisol. Thus, although these dysmorphic features were previously found to be elevated in the SPD youth (Weinstein et al., 1999), they are not linked with progression to more severe psychopathology in this sample. Analyses also failed to reveal an interaction between dysmorphic signs and cortisol in predicting outcome.

Coupled with the past findings, the present results suggest that dysmorphic signs are indicators of vulnerability, but that later developmental processes independently determine the course of the psychopathological process. As noted, dysmorphic features arise during prenatal development and are thus assumed to reflect congenital vulnerability. They are static indicators of risk. In contrast, cortisol levels undergo developmental change that is partially driven by post-pubertal maturation. Thus, the ultimate psychiatric outcome may be the cumulative result of events that occur during periods when neurodevelopmental change is most pronounced, namely the fetal period and the adolescent period. Abnormalities in fetal neurodevelopment may set the stage for vulnerability, but the onset of more serious psychopathology might depend upon environmental factors and maturational processes that arise much later. Of course, this interpretation must be considered tentative, given that we do not know the long-term clinical outcome for this sample.

CONCLUSIONS AND DIRECTIONS FOR FUTURE RESEARCH

The results of the research described in this chapter add to the rapidly accumulating literature on the role of neurohormones in the genesis of psychopathology. It appears that the incorporation of the HPA system into diathesis-stress models of developmental psychopathology has the potential to explain several key findings. First, it suggests a biological mechanism for explaining the relation between stress and psychopathology. Second, the demonstrated effects of persistent HPA over-activation on hippocampal morphology and on subsequent stress-sensitivity provide an explanation for the apparent worsening of the prognosis for depression and schizophrenia when episodes recur or go untreated (Post et al., 1994; Wyatt, 1995). Finally, neuromaturational changes in HPA function may be implicated in the gradually escalating behavior problems observed in adolescents who subsequently show serious psychopathology (Neumann et al., 1995).

As noted, there is a growing body of research which indicates that the adolescent period is associated with an increase in biological sensitivity to stress (Spear, 2000a,b, in press; Walker, in press). This has been attributed to maturational changes in the frontal and limbic regions of the brain, as well as to changes in neurotransmitter systems. These maturational changes are influenced by the effects of hormones on the expression of genes.

It has been shown that the behavioral influences exerted by gonadal and adrenal hormones are partially mediated by their effects on the expression of genes that control brain function (McEwen, 1994; Watson & Gametchu, 1999). There are hormone receptors on the surface of neurons as well as in the nucleus. In general, it appears that the surface receptors mediate short-term effects on behavior. These are referred to as *nongenomic* effects. The hormone receptors that reside in the cell's nucleus are responsible for their *genomic* effects. These receptors are transcription factors that influence the expression of genes. When hormones bind to them, they can increase gene expression. The genomic effects of hormones involve changes in the expression of messenger RNA that codes for specific proteins. These proteins, in turn, influence neuronal structure and function, including neuron growth, neurotransmitter synthesis, receptor density and sensitivity, and neurotransmitter reuptake. Thus, some of the normative brain changes observed in human adolescents are assumed to result from the effects of hormones on the expression of genes that govern maturational processes, such as the proliferation and elimination of neuronal processes.

One of the most fascinating findings from behavioral genetic studies is that the heritability of some behavioral propensities and mental disorders increases with age. In other words, the proportion of the variance accounted for by genetic factors rises, particularly during adolescence. This holds for cognitive and personality traits, as well as for clinical depression (Silberg et al., 1999). This raises the possibility that the hormonal changes occurring during adolescence may also be capable of triggering genes that contribute to vulnerability for mental disorders. The post-pubescent increase in heritability for behavioral traits and disorders suggests that hormonal maturation results in the expression of genes that were previously silent. If the individual possesses genes that code for aberrant brain function, and gonadal or adrenal hormones trigger the expression of these "vulnerability" genes, then signs of behavioral disorder may first become apparent in adolescence. For example, the rise in hormones during puberty may result in the expression of a gene that codes for abnormal dopamine neurotransmission. This, in turn, may give rise to the brain abnormality that confers susceptibility to schizophrenia. Via the same mechanism, vulnerability to mood disorder might result if hormone surges trigger the expression of a gene that leads to a defect in the serotonin system.

Hormonal deficiency may also be involved in neurodevelopmental abnormality. It is plausible that psychopathology results from insufficient levels of gonadal or adrenal hormones that lead to the failure of expression of genes that are critical for adolescent brain maturation. In this connection, it has been suggested that schizophrenia involves a deficit in neuronal "pruning" that is normally triggered by puberty, thus resulting in faulty neuronal interconnections because there is deficient elimination of neuronal processes (Feinberg, 1990; Keshavan & Hogarty, 1999).

Clearly, further research on the link between adjustment and hormonal changes during adolescence is needed. Our longitudinal study of at-risk youth focused on a relatively small sample, and the participants have not yet passed through the major risk period for the onset of major mental illness. Thus, any conclusions drawn from the results must be considered tentative. Nonetheless, the findings point to some promising leads in the search for the epigenesis of psychopathology. The combination of behavioral and biological risk indicators may prove to be the most productive approach for charting the prodromal course of major mental disorders. Furthermore, if risk for mental disorders is indeed influenced by maturational or environmentally induced changes in neurohormone systems, then new models for research and preventive intervention are likely to emerge.

Leaders in the field of developmental psychopathology have pointed to the critical interface among social, psychological, and biological factors in determining human development (Cicchetti & Sroufe, 2000). The rapid advances that have been made in the study of gene expression provide new frontiers for research on the epigenesis of psychopathology. Molecular genetic techniques now allow researchers to examine the expression of specific genes or large numbers of genes ("gene profiles") through the use of DNA microarrays (Mirnics, Middleton, Lewis, & Levitt, 2001; Raychaudhuri, Sutphin, Chang, & Altman, 2001). DNA microarrays are produced with the use of markers that label mRNA in cell nuclei, thus revealing which genes are "turned on." The procedure permits the examination of the expression of target genes or the individual's full complement of genes from a tissue or fluid sample. Microarrays can be compared from different tissue samples from the same individual, or from different individuals.

As an example, Kwak, Koo, Choi, and Sunwoo (2001) compared the expression of dopamine receptor genes on lymphocytes from normals and schizophrenia patients before and after antipsychotic medication. After medication, mRNA expression for certain dopamine receptor genes increased in lymphocytes, whereas for normal controls the expression of these genes remained stable. The researchers also found that patients with increased dopamine receptor expression had more severe psychiatric symptoms. These findings are very important, because they suggest that lymphocytes obtained with blood sampling can be used to index changes in the expression of genes that are critical for brain function.

It is also possible to examine developmental changes with microarray techniques. Recently, developmental processes in the expression of genes in the mouse hippocampus have been studied with microarrays, and the investigators found that 1,926 genes showed changes during hippocampal development (Mody et al., 2001). Cluster analysis was used to group these genes into distinct groups that were linked with major developmental events such as neuronal proliferation, differentiation, and synapse formation.

Given that hormones alter the expression of genes, microarray technology may yield important new information about gene expression in adolescence. It will allow investigators to examine changes in the expression of genes during this critical developmental period. By tracking behavioral, hormonal, and gene expression changes in at-risk populations, we may be able to elucidate the unfolding of aberrant biodevelopmental processes – both vulnerability genes and their neurohormonal triggers. Extending the paradigm further, environmental factors can be simultaneously measured to determine how biodevelopmental processes are altered by context, especially stressful events.

There is little doubt that progress in molecular genetics has set the stage for behavioral scientists to apply their skills in research on complex interactional processes. As investigators begin to integrate multiple levels of analysis – social, behavioral, macrobiological, and microbiological – we may be on the threshold of important new discoveries about the developmental origins of psychopathology.

REFERENCES

Abelson, J. L., & Curtis, G. C. (1996). Hypothalamic-pituitary-adrenal axis activity in panic disorder: Predication of long-term outcome by pretreatment cortisol levels. *American Journal of Psychiatry, 153,* 69–73.

Alexander, D. B., Viken, R. E., & Bates, J. E. (April, 1997). Children's dermatoglyphic asymmetry interacts with family stress in predicting school adjustment. Paper presented at the Society for Research in Child Development. Washington, DC.

Angold, A., Costello, E. J., Erkanli, A., & Worthman, C. M. (1999). Pubertal changes in hormone levels and depression in girls. *Psychological Medicine, 29,* 1043–1053.

Antelman, S. M., & Chiodo, L. A. (1984). Stress: Its effects on interactions among biogenic amines and role in the induction and treatment of disease. In S. I. Iverson, L. L. Iverson, & S. H. Snyder (Eds.) *Handbook of psychopharmacology* (pp. 279–334). New York: Plenum.

Bassett, J. R., Marshall, P. M., & Spillane, R. (1987). The physiological measurement of acute stress in bank employees. *International Journal of Psychophysiology, 5,* 265–273.

Benes, F. M. (1994). Developmental changes in stress adaptation in relation to psychopathology. *Development and Psychopathology, 6,* 723–739.

Biron, D., Dauphin, C., & Di Paolo, T. (1992). Effects of adrenalectomy and glucocorticoids on rat brain dopamine receptors. *Neuroendocrinology, 55:* 468–476.

Brennan, P. A., Mednick, S. A., & Raine, A. (1997). Biosocial interactions and violence: A focus on perinatal factors. In A. Raine. (Ed.) *Biosocial bases of violence* (pp. 163–174). New York: Plenum.

Cabib, S., Oliverio, A., Ventura, R., Lucchese, F., & Puglisi-Allegra, S. (1997). Brain dopamine receptor plasticity: Testing a diathesis-stress hypothesis in an animal model. *Psychopharmacology, 132,* 153–160.

Cabib, S., & Puglisi-Allegra, S. (1991). Genotype-dependent effects of chronic stress on apomorphine-induced alterations of striatal and mesolimbic dopamine metabolism. *Brain Research, 542,* 91–96.

Cicchetti, D., & Sroufe, L. A. (2000). The past as prologue to the future: The times, they've been a-changin'. *Development and Psychopathology, 12,* 255–264.

Cummins, H., & Midlow, C. (1961). *Fingerprints, palms and soles: An introduction to dermatoglyphics.* New York: Dover.

Davidson, M., Reichenberg, A., Rabinowitz, J., Weiser, M., Kaplan, Z., & Mordehai, M. (1999). Behavioral and intellectual markers for schizophrenia in apparently healthy male adolescents. *American Journal of Psychiatry, 156,* 1328–1335.

Davis, K. L., Khan, R. S., Ko, G., & Davidson, M. (1991). Dopamine in schizophrenia: A review and reconceptualization. *American Journal of Psychiatry, 148,* 1474–1486.

Den-Boer, J. A. (1995). *Advances in the neurobiology of schizophrenia.* Chichester: Wiley.

Deutsch, C. K., Matthysse, S., Swanson, J. M., & Farkas, L. G. (1990). Genetic latent structure analysis of dysmorphology in attention deficit disorder. *Journal of the American Academy of Child and Adolescent Psychiatry, 29,* 189–194.

Diforio, D., Kestler, L., & Walker, E. (2000). Executive functions in adolescents with schizotypal personality disorder. *Schizophrenia Research, 42,* 125–134.

Feinberg, I. (1990). Cortical pruning and the development of schizophrenia. *Schizophrenia Bulletin, 16,* 567–568.

Fendrich, M., Johnson, T., Wislar, J., & Nageotte, C. (1999). Accuracy of parent mental health service reporting: Results from a reverse record-check study. *Journal of the American Academy of Child and Adolescent Psychiatry, 38,* 147–155.

Fenig, S., Levav, I., Kohn, R., & Yelin, N. (1993). Telephone versus face-to-face interviewing in a community psychiatric survey. *American Journal of Public Health, 83,* 896–898.

Fogel, C. A., Mednick, S. A., & Michelsen, N. (1985). Hyperactive behavior and minor physical anomalies. *Acta Psychiatrica Scandinavica, 72,* 551–556.

Franzen, G. (1971). Serum cortisol in chronic schizophrenia: Changes in the diurnal rhythm and psychiatric mental status on withdrawal of drugs. *Psychiatrica Clinica, 4,* 237–246.

Goodyer, I. M., Herbert, J., Tamplin, A., & Altham, P. M. E. (2000). Recent life events, cortisol, dehydroepiandrosterone and the onset of major depression in high-risk adolescents. *British Journal of Psychiatry, 177,* 499–504.

Granger, P. A., Weis, J. R., McCracken, J. T., & Ikeda, S. C. (1996). Reciprocal influences among adrenocortical activation, psychosocial processes, and the behavioral adjustment of clinic-referred children. *Child Development, 67,* 3250–3262.

Green, M. F., Satz, P., & Christenson, C. (1994). Minor physical anomalies in schizophrenia patients, bipolar patients, and their siblings. *Schizophrenia Bulletin, 20,* 433–440.

Griffiths, T. D., Sigmundsson, T., Takei, N., Frangou, S., Birkett, P. B., Sharma, T., Reveley, A. M., & Murray, R. M. (1998). Minor physical anomalies in familial and sporadic schizophrenia: The Maudsley family study. *Journal of Neurology, Neurosurgery, and Psychiatry, 65,* 56–60.

Grossman, R. (1993). The relationship between hormonal mediators and systemic hypermetabolism after severe head injury. *Journal of Trauma, 34,* 806–816.

Gualtieri, C. T., Adams, A., Chen, C. D., & Loiselle, D. (1982). Minor physical anomalies in alcoholic and schizophrenic adults and hyperactive and autistic children. *American Journal of Psychiatry, 139,* 640–643.

Gupta, S., Rajaprabhakaran, R., Arndt, S., & Flaum, M. (1995). Premorbid adjustment as a predictor of phenomenological and neurobiological indices in schizophrenia. *Schizophrenia Research, 16,* 189–197.

Halverson, C., & Victor, J. B. (1976). Minor physical anomalies and problem behavior in elementary school children. *Child Development, 47,* 281–285.

Johnson, J. G., Cohen, P., Skodol, A. E., Oldham, J. M., Kasen, S., & Brook, J. S. (1999). Personality disorders in adolescence and risk of major mental disorders and suicidality during adulthood. *Archives of General Psychiatry, 56,* 805–811.

Kandel, E., Brennan, P. A., Mednick, S. A., & Michelson, N. M. (1989). Minor physical anomalies and recidivistic adult violent criminal behavior. *Acta Psychiatrica Scandinavica, 79,* 103–107.

Kenny, F. M., Gancayo, G., Heald, F. P., & Hung, W. (1966). Cortisol production rate in adolescent males in different stages of sexual maturation. *Journal of Clinical Endocrinology, 26,* 1232–1236.

Kenny, F. M., Preeyasambat, C., & Migeon, C. J. (1966). Cortisol production rate: II. Normal infants, children and adults. *Pediatrics, 37,* 34–42.

Keshavan M. S., & Hogarty G. E. (1999). Brain maturational processes and delayed onset in schizophrenia. *Development and Psychopathology, 11,* 525–543.

Kiess, W., Meidert, A., Dressendorfer, R. A., Scheiver, K., Kessler, U., & Konig, A. (1995). Salivary cortisol levels throughout childhood and adolescence: Relation with age, pubertal stage and weight. *Pediatric Research, 37,* 502–506.

King, C. A., Hovey, J. D., Brand, E., & Ghaziuddin, N. (1997). Prediction of positive outcomes for adolescent psychiatric inpatients. *Journal of the American Academy of Child and Adolescent Psychiatry, 36,* 1434–1442.

Kwak, Y. T., Koo, M. S., Choi, C. H., & Sunwoo, I. (2001). Change of dopamine receptor mRNA expression in lymphocyte of schizophrenic patients. *BMC Medical Genetics, 2,* 3.

Larsen, T. K., McGlashan T. H., Johannessen J. O., & Vibe-Hansen, L. (1996). First-Episode Schizophrenia: II. Premorbid patterns by gender. *Schizophrenia Bulletin, 22,* 257–269.

Lupien, S. J., King, S., Meaney, M., & McEwen, B. S. (2001). Can poverty get under your skin?: Basal cortisol levels and cognitive function in children from low and high socioeconomic status. *Development and Psychopathology, 13*, 653–676.

McEwen, B. (1994). Steroid hormone actions on the brain: when is the genome involved? *Hormones and Behavior, 28*, 396–405.

McGorry, P. D., & Edwards, J. (1998). The feasibility and effectiveness of early intervention in psychotic disorders: the Australian experience. *International Clinical Psychopharmacology, 13 (suppl.1)*, S47–S52.

McMurray, R. G., Newbould, E., & Bouloux, G. M. (1991). High-dose naloxone modifies cardiovascular and neuroendocrine function in ambulant subjects. *Psychoneuroendocrinology, 16*, 447–455.

Mednick, S. A. & Kandel, E. S. (1988). Congenital determinants of violence. *Bulletin of the American Academy of Psychiatry and the Law, 16*, 101–109.

Mellor, C. S. (1968). Dermatoglyphics in schizophrenia: I. Qualitative aspects. *British Journal of Psychiatry, 14*, 1387–1397.

Miller, T. J., & McGlashan, T. H. (2000). Early identification and intervention in psychotic illness. *Connecticut Medicine, 64* (6), 339–341.

Mirnics, K., Middleton, F. A., Lewis, D. A., & Levitt, P. (2001). Analysis of complex brain disorders with gene expression microarrays: schizophrenia as a disease of the synapse. *Trends in Neurosciences, 24*, 479–486.

Mittleman, G., Blaha, C., & Phillips, A. (1992). Pituitary-adrenal and dopaminergic modulation of schedule-induced polydipsia: Behavioral and neurochemical evidence. *Behavioral Neuroscience, 106*, 408–420.

Mody, M., Cao, Y., Cui, Z., Tay, K. Y., Shyong, A., Shimizu, E., Pham, K., Schultz, P., Welsh, D., & Tsien, J. Z. (2001). Genome-wide gene expression profiles of the developing mouse hippocampus. *Proceedings of the National Academy of Sciences of the United States of America, 98*, 8862–8867.

Moore K. L. (1982). *The developing human: clinically oriented embryology.* Philadelphia: WB Saunders.

Neumann, C. S., Grimes, K., Walker, E. F., & Baum, K. (1995). Developmental pathways to schizophrenia: Behavioral subtypes. *Journal of Abnormal Psychology, 104*, 1–9.

Newell-Morris, L. L., Fahrenbruch, C. E., & Sackett, G. P. (1989). Prenatal psychological stress, dermatoglyphic asymmetry and pregnancy outcome in the pigtailed macaque. *Biology of the Neonate, 56*, 61–75.

Nowakowski R. S., & Hayes N. L. (1999). CNS development: an overview. *Development and Psychopathology. 11*, 395–417.

Pine, D. S., Shaffer, D., Schonfeld, I. S., & Davies, M. (1997). Minor physical anomalies: Modifiers of environmental risks for psychiatric impairment? *Journal of the American Academy of Child and Adolescent Psychiatry, 36*, 395–403.

Pomeroy, J. C., Sprafkin, J., & Gadow, K. D. (1988). Minor physical anomalies as a biological marker for behavior disorders. *Journal of the American Academy of Child and Adolescent Psychiatry, 27*, 466–473.

Post, R. M., Weiss, S. R., & Leverich, G. S. (1994). Recurrent affective disorder: roots in developmental neurobiology and illness progression based on changes in gene expression. Special issue: Neural plasticity, sensitive periods, and psychopathology. *Development and Psychopathology, 6*, 781–813.

Potts, M., Daniels, M., Burnam, M., & Wells, K. (1990). A structured interview version of the Hamilton Depression Rating Scale: Evidence of reliability and versatility of administration. *Journal of Psychiatric Research, 24*, 335–350.

Rahe, R. H., Karson, S., Howard, N. S., Rubin, R. T., & Poland, R. E. (1990). Psychological and physiological assessments on American hostages freed from captivity in Iran. *Psychosomatic Medicine, 52*, 1–16.

Raychaudhuri, S., Sutphin, P. D., Chang, J. T., & Altman, R. B. (2001). Basic microarray analysis: grouping and feature reduction. *Trends in Biotechnology, 19*, 189–193.

Revicki, D. A., Tohen, T. M., Gyulai L., & Thompson, C. (1997). Telephone versus in-person clinical and health status assessment interviews in patients with bipolar disorder. *Harvard Review of Psychiatry, 5* (2), 75–81.

Rothschild, A. J., Langlais, P., Schatzberg, A. F., Miller, M., Salomon, M. S., Lerbinger, J. E., Cole, J. O., & Bird, E. D. (1985). The effects of a single dose of dexamethasone on monoamine and metabolite levels in rat brain. *Life Sciences, 36,* 2491.

Sachar, E. J., Kanter, S. S., Buie, D., Engle, R., & Mehlman, R. (1970). Psychoendocrinology of ego disintegration. *American Journal of Psychiatry, 126,* 1067–1078.

Sandberg, S. T., Wieselberg, M., & Shaffer, D. (1980). Hyperkinetic and conduct problem children in a primary school population: Some epidemiological considerations. *Journal of Child Psychology and Psychiatry and Allied Disciplines, 21,* 293–311.

Schatzberg, A. F., Rothschild, A., Langlais, P. J., Bird, E. D., & Cole, J. O. (1985). A corticosteroid/dopamine hypothesis for psychotic depression and related states. *Journal of Psychiatric Research, 19*: 57–64.

Schaumann, B., & Alter, M. (1976). *Dermatoglyphics in medical disorders.* New York: Springer-Verlag.

Shipley, J. E., Alessi, N., Wade, S. E., Haegle, A. D., & Helmbold, B. (1992). Utility of an oral diffusion sink (ODS) device for quantification of saliva corticosteroids in human subjects. *Journal of Clinical Endocrinology and Metabolism, 74,* 698–700.

Silberg, J., Pickles, A., Rutter, M., Hewitt, J., Simonoff, E., Maes, H., Carbonneau, R., Murrelle, L., Foley, D., & Eaves, L. (1999). The influence of genetic factors and life stress on depression among adolescent girls. *Archives of General Psychiatry, 56,* 225–232.

Smith, D. (1982). *Recognizable patterns of human malformation.* London: WB Saunders.

Sobin, C., Weissman, M. M., Goldstein, R. B., & Adams, P. (1993). Diagnostic interviewing for family studies: Comparing telephone and face-to-face methods for the diagnosis of lifetime psychiatric disorders. *Psychiatric Genetics, 3,* 227–233.

Sorg, B. A., & Kalivas, P. W. (1995). Stress and neuronal sensitization. In M. J. Friedman, D. S. Charney, & A. Y. Deutch (Eds.), *Neurobiological and clinical consequences of stress* (pp. 83–102). Philadelphia: Lippincott-Raven.

Spear, L. P. (2000a). The adolescent brain and age-related behavioral manifestations. *Neuroscience and Biobehavioral Reviews, 24,* 417–463.

Spear, L. P. (2000b). Neurobehavioral changes in adolescence. *Current Directions in Psychological Science, 9,* 111–114.

Spitzer, R. L., Williams, J. B., Gibbon, M., & First, M. B. (1990). *Structured Clinical Interview for DSM-III-R Personality Disorders Questionnaire.* Washington, D.C.: American Psychiatric Press.

Stansbury, K., & Gunnar, M. R. (1994). Adrenocortical activity and emotion regulation. *Monographs of the Society for Research in Child Development, 59,* 108–134.

Steiner, H., & Levine, S. (1988). Acute stress response in anorexia nervosa: A pilot study. *Child Psychiatry and Human Development, 18,* 208–218.

Susman, E. J., Dorn, L. D., Inoff-Germain, G., Nottelmann, E. D., & Chrousos, G. P. (1997). Cortisol reactivity, distress behavior, and behavioral and psychological problems in young adolescents: A longitudinal perspective. *Journal of Research on Adolescence, 7,* 81–105.

Tyrka, A. R., Cannon, T. D., Haslam, N., & Mednick, S. A. (1995). The latent structure of schizotypy: I: Premorbid indicators of a taxon of individuals at risk for schizophrenia-spectrum disorders. *Journal of Abnormal Psychology, 104,* 173–183.

Wajs-Kuto, E., De Beeck, L. O., Rooman, R. P. & Caju, M. V. (1999). Hormonal changes during the first year of oestrogen treatment in constitutionally tall girls. *European Journal of Endocrinology, 141* (6), 579–584.

Waldrop, M. F., & Halverson, C. F. (1971). Minor physical anomalies and hyperactive behavior in young children. In J. Helmuth (Ed.), *Exceptional infant: Studies in abnormalities.* New York: Brunner/Mazel.

Waldrop, M. P., Pederson, F. A., & Bell, R. Q. (1968). Minor physical anomalies and behavior in preschool children. *Child Development, 39,* 391–400.

Walker, E. (2002). Adolescent neurodevelopment and psychopathology. *Current Directions in Psychological Science, 11,* 24–28.

Walker, E., Baum, K., & Diforio, D. (1998). Developmental changes in the behavioral expression of vulnerability for schizophrenia. In M. Lenzenweger and B. Dworkin (Eds.), *Origins and development of schizophrenia: Advances in experimental psychopathology* (pp. 469–491). Washington, D.C.: American Psychological Association Press.

Walker, E., & Diforio, D. (1997). Schizophrenia: A neural diathesis-stress model. *Psychological Review 104*, 1–19.

Walker, E., Walder, D. & Reynolds, F. (2001). Adolescent changes in stress sensitivity and the expression of vulnerability to psychopathology. *Development and Psychopathology, 13*, 721–732.

Watson, C., & Gametchu, B. (1999). Membrane-initiated steroid actions and the proteins that mediate them. *Proceedings of the Society for Experimental Biology & Medicine, 220*, 9–19.

Weinstein, D., Diforio, D., Schiffman, J., Walker, E., & Bonsall, B. (1999). Minor physical anomalies, dermatoglyphic abnormalities and cortisol levels in adolescents with schizotypal personality disorder. *American Journal of Psychiatry 156*, 617–623.

Wolfradt, U., & Straube, E. (1998). Factor structure of schizotypal traits among adolescents. *Personality and Individual Differences, 24*, 201–206.

Wolkowitz, O. (1994). Prospective controlled studies of the behavioral and biological effects of exogenous corticosteroids: Review. *Psychoneuroendocrinology, 19*, 233–255.

Wyatt, R. (1995). Antipsychotic medication and the long-term course of schizophrenia. In C. L. Shriqui & H. A. Nasrallah (Eds.), *Contemporary issues in the treatment of schizophrenia* (pp. 385–410). Washington, D.C.: American Psychiatric Association Press.

Wyatt, R. J., Apud, J. A., & Potkin, S. (1996). New directions in the prevention and treatment of schizophrenia: A biological perspective. *Psychiatry, 59*, 357–370.

Yung, A. R., & McGorry, P. D. (1996). The initial prodrome in psychosis: descriptive and qualitative aspects. *Australian and New Zealand Journal of Psychiatry, 30*, 587–599.

Yung, A. R., Phillips, L. J., McGorry, P. D., Hallgren, M. A., McFarlane, C. A., Jackson, H. J., Francey, S., & Patton, G. C. (1998). Can we predict the onset of first-episode psychosis in a high-risk group? *International Clinical Psychopharmacology, 13(suppl 1)*, S23–S30.

Index

Abernethy, L. J., 40
acetazolamide, 11
acquired (specific) immunity, 297
addiction, 18–19, 336–7
adolescence: behavioral changes in, 63,
    64, 67, 68–71; defining of, 62–3;
    hormonal changes with, 63–4,
    537–8
adolescent neurodevelopment: amygdala
    and, 66, 70–1; cannabinoid receptor
    systems and, 70; cerebellar cognitive
    affective syndrome and, 73; DA/GABA
    systems interactions and, 390; DA
    systems, 67–70, 73, 75; disease
    prevention and, 526–7; drug sensitivity
    and, 71–2; efficiency changes in, 65–6;
    future research directions in, 75–6;
    metabolic decline during, 65–6;
    overview, 64–5; prefrontal cortex
    changes with, 66–7; schizophrenia and,
    72, 125–7, 384–5, 526; stress sensitivity
    and, 64, 69, 70–1, 73, 74–5, 76;
    symptomatology and, 72–4; synapse
    elimination during, 65–6, 125–6, 128,
    377f, 538
adoption studies, 247, 261, 408
adrenal androgens, 64
adrenocorticotropic hormone (ACTH): in
    child maltreatment, 205; cytokines
    and, 302; social deprivation effects on,
    193; stress and, 158, 171, 172
affective disorders: adaptive/pathological
    alterations with, 510f, 511;
    amygdala-kindled seizure model and,

494t, 503–5; causes of, 86–7, 101;
    cocaine sensitization and, 503, 504–5;
    Dutch famine and, 87, 90, 91; early
    bipolar studies, 498–501t; episode
    sensitization in, 494–5, 496–7t, 502–3,
    503t; future research directions in,
    103–4; genetics and, 101; sensitization
    in, 491–2, 493f, 494; stress effects on,
    491, 493f, 502, 503; stress mechanism
    and, 505–6, 507–8f, 509, 510f, 511;
    timing of teratogen, 104, 140. *See also*
    bipolar disorders
aggressive behavior: in BPD, 414, 415–16;
    cortisol link to, 333–5, 336;
    neurotransmitter systems and, 415–16;
    variants of, 327
Akbarian, S., 139
alcohol exposure (prenatal): effects of, 22,
    177, 178, 179; measuring exposure,
    14–15; mechanism of, 10
alcoholism: depression and, 476–7;
    genetic susceptibility of, 18; physical
    abuse association, 513, 514
Allebeck, P., 36
allelic heterogeneity, 242
Alzheimer's disease, 395
amphetamines, 98, 411
amygdala: adolescent neurodevelopment
    and, 66, 70–1; autism and, 224;
    depression and, 473, 474;
    GABA/DA/serotonin systems
    interactions and, 385; social
    cognition/behavior and, 217, 218t,
    219, 221